The Receptors

Series Editor: *David B. Bylund,* University of Missouri,
Columbia, Missouri

Board of Editors

S. J. Enna, Nova Pharmaceuticals, Baltimore, Maryland
Morley D. Hollenberg, University of Calgary, Calgary,
Alberta Canada
Bruce S. McEwen, Rockefeller University, New York, New York
Solomon H. Snyder, Johns Hopkins University,
Baltimore, Maryland

The alpha-2 Adrenergic Receptors, edited by **Lee Limbird,
1988**
The Opiate Receptors, edited by *Gavril W. Pasternak,* **1988**
The alpha-1 Adrenergic Receptors, edited by
Robert R. Ruffolo, Jr., 1987
The GABA Receptors, edited by *S. J. Enna,* 1983

The Opiate Receptors

Edited by

Gavril W. Pasternak

Memorial Sloan-Kettering Cancer Center and
Cornell University Medical College,
New York, New York

THE HUMANA PRESS • CLIFTON, NEW JERSEY

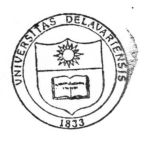

Library of Congress Cataloging in Publication Data
Main entry under title:

The Opiate receptors.

 (The Receptors)
 Includes bibliographies and index.
  1. Endorphins—Receptors.   2. Opioids—Receptors.
I. Pasternak, Gavril W.   II. Series.
QP552.E53064 1988   615'.7822   87-3095
ISBN 0-89603-120-9

© 1988 The Humana Press Inc.
Crescent Manor
PO Box 2148
Clifton, NJ 07015

Printed in the United States of America

Preface

The growth of the opiate field over the past decade has been enormous. Initial interest focused upon the strategic clinical importance of morphine and its analogs, but the discovery of the enkephalins and the other endogenous opioid peptides with their widespread actions within brain has expanded the field to investigators in almost all areas of neuroscience as well as pharmacology. Unfortunately, this field of research with its vast literature has become progressively more complex. The receptors are no longer limited to opiates, but include many subtypes selective for the opioid peptides. Indeed, they might be better termed opioid, rather than opiate, receptors. Many controversies have emerged and been settled; others remain. Early studies must now be interpreted on the basis of current information. Thousands of papers examining various aspects of opiates and the endogenous opioids present separate pieces of a large puzzle. The goal of this volume is to put the pieces together to give a coherent overview of opiate receptor pharmacology and to provide insights into both the molecular and classical pharmacology of opiates and the opioid peptides.

The issue of multiple classes of opiate and opioid peptide receptors and their importance in understanding mechanisms of action provides the major focus of the book. The study of opiates and opioid peptides provides a unique research opportunity in the neuropharmacology of drug receptors. The availability of a wide variety of agonist and antagonist ligands has permitted studies not possible in other systems. Second, the close association of opiate drugs with easily measurable pharmacological bioassays and behavioral responses permits the correlation of binding studies with pharmacological actions and helps to bridge the gap between molecular and classical pharmacology. In this regard, the opiate system is relatively unique. Sections of the book cover historical perspectives in the concept of multiple opiate receptors along with a general overview of the opioid peptides, biochemical characterization of the binding sites and their regional distribution, biochemical and electrophysiological mechanisms of action, and correlations of binding sites with function. Throughout the entire volume, we have attempted to provide an integrated approach that pulls together the biochemical, physiological, and pharmacological studies of opiate action. We feel that this volume will be a valuable resource for scientists actively working in the opiate field, as well as others interested in neuroscience and pharmacology in general.

Gavril W. Pasternak

Contents

Preface v

List of Contributors. xvii

Section 1: Historical Perspectives

Chapter 1
The Evolution of Concepts of Opioid Receptors
W. R. Martin

1. Introduction 3
2. Reflections 17
   2.1. Pharmacologic Implications. 17
   References 19

Chapter 2
The Opioid Peptides
**Christopher J. Evans, Donna L. Hammond, and
Robert C. A. Frederickson**

1. Introduction 23
2. History of Opioid Peptides 23
3. Peptides Derived from Proopiomelanocortin 26
4. Processing Products Derived from Proenkephalin 34
5. Processing Products Derived from Prodynorphin 41
6. Receptor Interactions and Further Considerations 45
7. Pharmacological and Physiological Effects of the
   Endogenous Opioid Peptides 47
   7.1. Effects of Naloxone 48
   7.2. Effects of Inhibitors of Opioid Degradation 49

    7.3. Effects of the Endogenous Opioid Peptides and
           Structural Analogs.............................50
    References 57

Section 2: Characterization of Opioid Receptor Binding Sites

Chapter 3
Early Studies of Opioid Binding
Gavril W. Pasternak

  1. Introduction......................................75
  2. Early Attempts To Demonstrate Opiate
      Binding Sites 75
  3. Identification and Characterization of Opiate
      Binding Sites 76
  4. Correlating Opiate Binding Sites with Opiate
      Actions 82
  5. Discrimination of Agonist and Antagonist
      Binding 82
  6. Membrane Lipids and Opiate Binding 86
  7. Binding Heterogeneity 88
  8. Conclusion.......................................89
    References 89

Chapter 4
Multiple Opioid Binding Sites
Yossef Itzhak

  1. Introduction......................................95
  2. Ligand–Receptor Binding Assays......................97
  3. Multiple Opioid Binding Sites........................99
      3.1. Mu and Delta Binding Sites 99
      3.2. Multiple Mu Receptors: Mu_1 and Mu_2 Sites 107
      3.3. Kappa Binding Sites 112
      3.4. Sigma [(+)-*N*-Allylnormetazocine]-Specific
           Binding Sites.................................116
      3.5. β-Endorphin Binding Sites 119
  4. Regional Distribution of Opioid Binding Sites
      Within the Brain....................................119
  5. Biochemical Properties of Opioid Binding Sites 124
      5.1. Physical and Chemical Properties 124
      5.2. Effect of Ions and Nucleotides 124
      5.3. Effect of Alcohols and Detergents...............127

6. Developmental Appearance of Opioid Binding
   Sites 128
7. Opiate Binding in Pathological States 130
8. Concluding Remarks 131
   References 131

Chapter 5
The σ Receptor
R. Suzanne Zukin and Stephen R. Zukin

1. Introduction 143
2. The PCP/σ Receptor 145
   2.1. PCP/σ Receptors Labeled with [³H]PCP 145
   2.2. Receptors Labeled with (−)-[³H]SKF 10,047 147
3. The Haloperidol-Sensitive non-PCP σ Site 151
   3.1. Sites Labeled with (+)-[³H]SKF 10,047 151
   3.2. Sites Labeled with (+)-[³H]3-(3-hydroxyphenyl)-
        N-(l-propyl)piperidine [(+)-[³H]3PPP] 153
4. A Biological Function of σ Receptors 154
5. The Question of Endogenous Ligands 155
6. Nomenclature 158
   References 158

Chapter 6
Solubilization and Purification of Opioid Binding Sites
Eric J. Simon and Jacob M. Hiller

1. Introduction 165
2. Solubilization 166
   2.1. Prebound Opioid Binding Sites 166
   2.2. Active Opioid Binding Sites in Solution 167
   2.3. Characteristics of Solubilized Opioid
        Receptors 170
   2.4. Separation of Opioid Receptor Types 171
3. Covalent Labeling 172
   3.1. Affinity Labeling 173
   3.2. Photoaffinity Labeling 177
   3.3. Affinity Crosslinking 180
4. Purification 182
   4.1. Partial Purification 182
   4.2. Purification to Homogeneity 185
5. Conclusions 187
   References 189

Section 3: Location of Opioid Receptors

Chapter 7
Regional Distribution of Opioid Receptors
**Robert R. Goodman, Benjamin A. Adler,
and Gavril W. Pasternak**

1. Introduction..197
2. Early Autoradiographic Studies 199
   2.1. In Vivo Autoradiography........................199
   2.2. In Vitro Autoradiography 201
3. Ontogeny of Opioid Receptors.......................202
4. Presynaptic and Postsynaptic Localization of
   Opioid Binding Sites 203
   4.1. Striatum and Limbic System....................203
   4.2. Spinal Cord...................................205
   4.3. Other Studies 205
5. Localization of Multiple Opioid Receptor
   Subtypes..206
   5.1. Mu and Delta Receptors 206
   5.2. Mu$_1$ Receptors 207
   5.3. Kappa Receptor Autoradiography................211
   5.4. Epsilon Receptors 215
6. Opioid Receptors and Opioid Peptides...............218
7. Conclusion...222
   References 223

Section 4: Mechanisms of Receptor Action

Chapter 8
Opioid-Coupled Second Messenger Systems
Steven R. Childers

1. Introduction.......................................231
2. Receptor-Coupled Adenylate Cyclase: The Ternary
   Complex Models....................................232
3. Actions of N-Proteins on Opioid Receptor Binding
   Sites 240
   3.1. Effects of Guanine Nucleotides 240
   3.2. Sodium Regulation of Opioid Binding 243
4. Opioid-Inhibited Adenylate Cyclase 246
   4.1. Studies in Cell Culture.......................246
   4.2. Studies in Brain Membranes....................250
   4.3. Opioid-Stimulated GTPase 256

5. Other Opioid Receptor-Coupled Second Messenger
   Systems..258
   5.1. Cyclic GMP 258
   5.2. Protein Phosphorylation 259
   5.3. Effects of Opioids on Calcium Uptake 260
   5.4. Opioid-Mediated Changes in Membrane
        Lipids 261
6. Conclusions 262
   References 263

Chapter 9
Electrophysiology of Opiates and Opioid Peptides
Charles Chavkin

1. Overview 273
2. Receptor Identification 274
3. Opioid Actions on Cells in Enteric Ganglia..........278
4. Opioid Actions in Locus Ceruleus....................280
5. Opioid Actions in Dorsal Root Ganglia and Spinal
   Cultures 282
6. Opioid Actions in the CA1 Region of the
   Hippocampus 284
7. Opioid Actions in the CA3 Region of the
   Hippocampus 287
8. Opioid Actions in Dentate Region of the
   Hippocampus 290
9. Role of Adenylate Cyclase in the Electrophysiological
   Actions of Opioids..................................291
10. Summary 294
    References 295

Section 5: Pharmacological Correlation
of Binding Sites with Function

Chapter 10
Central Actions of Opiates and Opioid Peptides: In Vivo
Evidence for Opioid Receptor Multiplicity
Paul L. Wood and Smriti Iyengar

1. Introduction...307
2. Analgesia...308
   2.1. Mu and Delta Agonists 308
   2.2. Kappa Agonists 310

2.3. Agonist/Antagonist Analgesics.................311
3. Behavioral/Autonomic Actions 312
   3.1. Respiratory Depression 312
   3.2. Catalepsy......................................314
   3.3. Substance P-Induced Scratching 315
   3.4. Feeding..316
4. Neuroendocrinology 316
   4.1. Corticosterone-ACTH...........................317
   4.2. Thyroid-Stimulating Hormone (TSH)............321
   4.3. Prolactin......................................323
   4.4. Growth Hormone (GH) 326
   4.5. Luteinizing Hormone (LH) 329
5. Neurochemistry....................................330
   5.1. Acetylcholine (ACh) 330
   5.2. Dopamine (DA) 332
   5.3. Serotonin.....................................337
6. Overview 338
   References 338

Chapter 11
Peripheral Actions Mediated by Opioid Receptors
Brian M. Cox

1. Introduction.......................................357
2. Opioid Actions Related to the Enteric Nervous
   System...361
   2.1. Endogenous Opioids in the Gastrointestinal
        Tract 361
   2.2. Effects of Opioids on Gastrointestinal
        Motility...................................... 362
   2.3. Effects of Opioids on Gastrointestinal
        Secretion..................................... 373
   2.4. Actions of Antidiarrheal Agents............... 375
3. Opioid Actions Related to the Sympathetic Nervous
   System...377
   3.1. Endogenous Opioids and the Sympathetic
        Nervous System...............................377
   3.2. Actions of Opioids on Transmission at
        Sympathetic Ganglia..........................378
   3.3. Actions of Opioids in Adrenal Gland..........379
   3.4. Actions of Opioids on Blood Vessels 381
   3.5. Actions of Opioids on Cat Nictitating
        Membrane 383
4. Actions of Opioids on the Heart 383

4.1. Endogenous Opioids and Opioid Binding in the
      Heart. 383
4.2. Actions of Opioids on the Vagal Innervation
      of the Heart. 384
4.3. Actions of Opioids on the Sympathetic
      Innervation of the Heart 386
4.4. Reflex Regulation of Heart Rate by Opioids 386
4.5. Effects of Opioids on Blood Pressure 387
5. Actions of Opioids on Sensory Nerves. 388
   5.1. Endogenous Opioids in Sensory Nerves 388
   5.2. Opioid Receptors on Sensory Neurons 388
   5.3. Peripheral Antinociception by Opioids 390
   5.4. Antagonism of Neurogenic Edema 392
6. Opioid Receptors in Pars Nervosa of Pituitary 393
   6.1. Endogenous Opioids in Pars Nervosa 393
   6.2. Regulation by Opioids of AVP and OXY
        Secretion 393
7. Actions of Opioids on Reproductive Tract
   Tissues 396
   7.1. Endogenous Opioids in Reproductive Tract
        Tissues 396
   7.2. Opioid Actions on Vas Deferens 397
   7.3. Receptors in Other Reproductive Tract
        Tissues 404
8. Interactions of Opioids with Blood Cells and the
   Immune System 405
9. Summary 406
   References 407

Section 6: Regulation of Opioid Receptors

Chapter 12
Regulation of Opioid Receptors
Steven G. Blanchard and Kwen-Jen Chang

1. Introduction. 425
2. Modulation of Receptor–Ligand Interactions. 425
   2.1. Effects of Cations on Opioid Binding. 426
   2.2. Regulation of Opioid Binding by Guanyl
        Nucleotides 427
   2.3. Relationship of Opioid Binding to N_1. 427
3. Ligand-Induced Down-Regulation 429
   3.1. Opioid Peptides and Neuroblastoma Cells 429
   3.2. Mechanism of Down-Regulation 430

     3.3. Down-Regulation in Other Tissues 431
     3.4. Possible Significance of Down-Regulation 432
  4. Receptor Up-Regulation 432
      References 434

Chapter 13
Role of Opioid Receptors in Narcotic Tolerance/ Dependence
Andrew P. Smith, Ping-Yee Law, and Horace H. Loh

  1. Introduction 441
  2. Chronic Opioid Effects in Clonal Neuroblastoma-
      Glioma Cell Lines 442
     2.1. Desensitization 444
     2.2. Down-Regulation 445
     2.3. Increase of Adenylate Cyclase Activity 447
     2.4. Summary and Conclusions 450
  3. Chronic Opioid Effects in Isolated Tissue
      Systems 452
     3.1. Guinea Pig Ileum and Mouse Vas Deferens 453
     3.2. Central Nervous System Tissue 459
     3.3. Summary and Conclusions 461
  4. Chronic Opioid Effects in Whole Animals 462
     4.1. Down-Regulation of Opioid Receptors in the
         Brain 464
     4.2. Up-Regulation of Opioid Receptors in the
         Brain 465
  5. Toward a Theory of Opioid Tolerance/
      Dependence 467
     5.1. Receptor Models 469
     5.2. Homeostatic Models 472
     5.3. Combined Models 474
      References 476

Section 7: Future Vistas

Chapter 14
Opiate and Opioid Peptide Receptors: The Past, the Present, and the Future
Gavril W. Pasternak

  1. The Classical Era 489
  2. The Molecular Era 491

3. The Future 492
  3.1. Receptor Heterogeneity 492
  3.2. Receptor Function 492
  3.3. Tolerance and Dependence 493
  3.4. Clinical Perspectives 493
  References 493
Index 497

Contributors

BENJAMIN A. ADLER • *The Cotzias Laboratory of Neuro-Oncology, Memorial Sloan-Kettering Cancer Center, New York, New York*

STEVEN G. BLANCHARD • *Department of Molecular Biology, Burroughs Wellcome Company, Research Triangle Park, North Carolina*

DAVID B. BYLUND • *Department of Pharmacology, School of Medicine, University of Missouri, Columbia, Missouri*

KWEN-JEN CHANG • *Department of Molecular Biology, Burroughs Wellcome Company, Research Triangle Park, North Carolina*

CHARLES CHAVKIN • *Department of Pharmacology, University of Washington, Seattle, Washington*

STEVEN R. CHILDERS • *Department of Pharmacology and Therapeutics, University of Florida College of Medicine, Gainesville, Florida*

BRIAN M. COX • *Department of Pharmacology, Uniformed Services University, Bethesda, Maryland*

CHRISTOPHER J. EVANS • *Department of Psychiatry and Behavioral Science, Stanford University, Stanford, California*

ROBERT C. A. FREDERICKSON • *Searle Research and Development, G. D. Searle & Company, Skokie, Illinois*

ROBERT R. GOODMAN • *Department of Neurosurgery, College of Physicians and Surgeons, Columbia University, New York, New York*

DONNA L. HAMMOND • *Searle Research and Development, G. D. Searle & Company, Skokie, Illinois*

JACOB M. HILLER • *Department of Psychiatry, New York University Medical Center, New York, New York*

YOSSEF ITZHAK • *Department of Pharmacology, Hadassah School of Medicine, The Hebrew University, Jerusalem, Israel*

SMRITI IYENGAR • *Neuroscience Research Department, Pharmaceuticals Division, Ciba Geigy, Summit, New Jersey*

PING-YEE LAW • *Department of Pharmacology, University of California, San Francisco, California*

HORACE H. LOH • *Department of Pharmacology, University of California, San Francisco, California*

W. R. MARTIN • *Department of Pharmacology, University of Kentucky College of Medicine, Lexington, Kentucky*

GAVRIL W. PASTERNAK • *The Cotzias Laboratory of Neuro-Oncology, Memorial Sloan-Kettering Cancer Center and Departments of Neurology and Pharmacology, Cornell University Medical College, New York, New York*

ERIC J. SIMON • *Departments of Psychiatry and Pharmacology, New York University Medical Center, New York, New York*

ANDREW P. SMITH • *Department of Pharmacology, University of California, San Francisco, California*

PAUL L. WOOD • *Neuroscience Research Department, Pharmaceuticals Division, Ciba Geigy, Summit, New Jersey*

STEPHEN R. ZUKIN • *Departments of Neuroscience and Psychiatry, Albert Einstein College of Medicine/Montefiore Medical Center and Bronx Psychiatric Center, Bronx, New York*

R. SUZANNE ZUKIN • *Department of Neuroscience, Albert Einstein College of Medicine, Bronx, New York*

SECTION 1
HISTORICAL
PERSPECTIVES

Chapter 1

The Evolution of Concepts of Opioid Receptors

W. R. Martin

1. Introduction

The early evolution of concepts of endogenous opioids and multiple opioid receptors had its inception in a concerted program to develop safe, nonaddicting substitutes for opiates (*see* Eddy, 1973). This endeavor was initiated by the Bureau of Social Hygiene and subsequently supported by the United States Public Health Service under the auspices of the National Research Council. An empiric approach was taken in which a large number of chemicals, synthesized by University-based chemists and the pharmaceutical industry, were examined for their pharmacologic effects, particularly their analgesic activity and their abuse potential. Although heroin and morphine addiction were the initial driving force of this endeavor, the economic gains associated with the marketing of a less-addicting analgesic became the most important factor of the pharmaceutical industries large synthetic effort. From a societal perspective, however, the economics of drug abuse is by far the most important economic factor, since drug abuse costs the United States well over $100 billion dollars a year. The search for safer and less-abusable analgesics has not been entirely successful. The evolution of ideas concerning multiple opioid receptors and endogenous opioid transmitters is still active.

3

The critical opioids in the pharmacologic dissection of multiple opioid receptors were N-allylnorcodeine, N-allylnormorphine, naloxone, cyclazocine, ethylketazocine, N-allylnormetazocine, and buprenorphine. Proceeding on the concept that allyl substitutions functioned as respiratory stimulants, von Braun (1916) synthesized N-allylnorcodeine, and Pohl (1915) studied the interactions between N-allylnorcodeine and morphine and first demonstrated that N-allylnorcodeine was capable of antagonizing the respiratory depressant effects of morphine. Although Pohl's important observations were published in 1915 and were confirmed by Meissner (1923), these findings lay dormant until they were resurrected again by Chauncy Leake. Doctor Leake, then of the University of California in San Francisco, stimulated efforts to synthesize N-allylnorcodeine and N-allylnormorphine. These endeavors have been briefly recounted (Leake, 1967) and, like Pohl's concept, were based on the hypothesis that allyl groups are respiratory stimulants. The initial synthesis of N-allylnormorphine was controversial. As a consequence of resolving the synthetic issues, N-allylnormorphine (nalorphine) was independently synthesized by Weijlard and Erickson (1942) of Merck Laboratories and by Hart (1941) and Hart and McCauley (1944) of the University of California. Both Unna (1943) and Hart and McCauley (1944) also studied the pharmacology of this interesting compound and extended the observations of Pohl by showing that nalorphine antagonized other actions of morphine. The issue of the respiratory stimulant action of allyl substitutions is still not entirely resolved and will be subsequently discussed. Nalorphine's respiratory stimulant action can be clearly differentiated from its morphine antagonistic effects and from the respiratory stimulant actions of dinitrophenol. The observations of nalorphine's antagonistic effects were reluctantly accepted, as were speculations concerning its mechanism of action (Unna, personal communication). The clinical use of nalorphine for the treatment of acute morphinism was not pursued despite Unna's urging and was not demonstrated until Eckenhoff et al. (1952) conducted the critical experiments in man.

To further elaborate on the importance of opiate addiction in stimulating research on opioid drugs, a committee on Drug Addiction was formed by the Committee on Social Hygiene in 1920 to increase the understanding of addiction processes. Following the passage of the Harrison Narcotic Act and on the recommendations of the American Medical Association, clinics that provided narcotics to addicts were closed, leaving most addicts without a legitimate source for their narcotics. As part of this Committee's activities, they proposed a strategy for identifying new analgesics that would be devoid of the toxic and dependence-producing actions of the opium analgesics. Subsequently the Federal government assumed the responsibility of continuing the activities of this committee. Among the important activities of the committee were the initiation and continuation of a synthetic program, the development of an animal screening program, and finally the assessment of new analgesics in humans for their ability to produce or sustain physical dependence. Many compounds were synthesized and evaluated by Dr. Eddy's laboratory at the National Institutes of Health, by Dr. Seevers laboratory at the University of Michigan, and by investigators at the Addiction Research Center in humans. Most of the drugs that were studied were sufficiently like morphine that they were judged not to have any marked advantage. In retrospect, there may have been significant differences between the drugs; these were either not detected using the methods at hand, however, or differences were not pursued. Two examples of compounds that had unique pharmacological properties in humans were meperidine and normorphine. It was much more difficult to produce physical dependence on these drugs than it was to produce physical dependence on morphine.

Doctor Harris Isbell had developed an interest in the use of N-allylnormorphine as an analgesic. He obtained the drug, however, at a time when he was very much involved in conducting his studies on alcohol and barbiturate dependence. Lasagna and Beecher (1954) did study the analgesic actions of nalorphine and found it to be nearly as potent as morphine. Doctor Abraham Wikler attempted to substitute nalorphine for morphine in a dependent subject and observed that it precipitated a violent abstinence syndrome that could not be antidoted by morphine. He (Wikler et al., 1953; Wikler and Carter, 1953) subsequently characterized precipitated abstinence in humans and the spinal dog. These observations provided an important clue in the development of nonaddicting, safer analgesics and were pursued by several pharmaceutical firms that synthesized a number of compounds with antagonistic effects.

Thus the driving force for the enormous commitment for development of opioid antagonists as analgesics was that they had analgesic activity and did not appear to substitute for morphine in morphine-dependent subjects. It is important to recognize the importance of the substitution technique for identifying morphine-like drugs devised by C. K. Himmelsbach (1939). Although Himmelsbach did not couch his concepts in receptor theory, his work was one of the first critical pieces of evidence that strongly indicated that opioids were exerting their effects by acting through a common mechanism. Himmelsbach (1978) attributes the development of this technique to the observations of Downs and Eddy (1928), who demonstrated cross-tolerance between morphine, codeine, and heroin in the dog. Himmelsbach reasoned that cross-dependence could also exist, and that dependence was a major determinant of the addictiveness of analgesics. He demonstrated that a number of morphine congeners substituted for morphine in morphine-dependent subjects. These studies had several major implications. One of the drugs studied by Dr. Himmelsbach was desomorphine. Desomorphine did not produce dependence in the monkey; it substituted for morphine in morphine-dependent subjects, however. This was to be only the first of several drugs whose ability to sustain dependence was much greater in humans than in the monkey. These observations, and others, led to the suggestion that opioid receptors differed in the intimate details of their configuration from one species to another (Martin and Jasinski, 1977; Martin, 1983).

Another important innovation was the application of bio-assay statistical techniques to not only suppression and precipitation data, but to subjective effects data as assessed by questionnaires. Harris Isbell introduced this technique to help strengthen the conclusions that had been reached concerning the abuse potentiality of phenazocine, the first of a series of benzomorphans that had a critical role in the formulation of concepts concerning multiple opioid receptors. Phenazocine was much less potent than morphine in suppressing abstinence in the monkey and more potent than morphine as an analgesic in humans. In humans, however, phenazocine was three to four times more potent than morphine in constricting pupils and producing subjective effects and was eight times more potent in suppressing abstinence (Fraser and Isbell, 1960). In addition to emphasizing the large differences in response to opioids among species, several other important lessons were learned through this quantitative comparison between drug measure and species. (1) Different experimental variables (e.g., pupillary diameter vs. subjective effects) that were measured using different scales (e.g., ordinal, nominal, or ratio) yield potency estimates that were not only equivalent, but had similar confidence limits. (2) The use of dose–response relationships became an important criterion for identifying changes in subjective states that were relevant to the drugs effect. (3) The concomitant use of both a physiologic and behavioral measure provided an internal validation of the behavioral measures (Martin and Fraser, 1961). The effects of opioids on subjective states became an important criterion for differentiating the receptor subtypes.

Isbell's (Fraser and Isbell, 1960) use of bioassay statistics and techniques to compare the relative potencies of opioids to suppress abstinence, to alter subjective states, and to induce physiologic changes provided a powerful tool for quantitatively characterizing the pharmacologic profiles of drugs. The use of crossover designs allowed for the simultaneous and efficient assessment of relative potencies on several experimental parameters. Thus, valid assays could be obtained on studies employing four to six subjects using a four-point assay (Bliss, 1952; Finney, 1964). This design allowed for the partitioning out of the between-subjects variance, and the error term for calculating the confidence limits of the potency estimate was the residual part of the between-doses variance.

This seminal approach, however, had a major statistical problem in that different pharmacologic effects were measured with different types of scales. For example, pupils were photographed and measured with a ruler (ratio scale). Some subjective states were measured using a nominal scale; others using an ordinal scale. Isbell's first effort (Table 1) revealed that the confidence

TABLE 1
The Relative Potency of Phenazocine and Levophenacylmorphan
in Comparison to Morphine in Constricting Pupils (Interval Scale),
Altering Signs and Symptoms (Nominal Scale),
and Suppressing Abstinence (Mixed Scale)[a]

	Pupils (miosis)	Questions	Suppression
Phenazocine (NIH-75/4)	3.8 (1.3–5.6)	3.2 (2.3–5.0)	8.2 (4.2–17.2)
Levophenacylmorphan (NIH-7525)	5.2 (2.7–8.0)	6.11 (5.0–7.5)	9.1 (4.8–20.0)

[a]From Fraser and Isbell, 1960.

limits of the potency estimates for the different types of measurement scales were similar despite differences in the inherent properties of the scales.

From a practical and empirical perspective, potency estimates obtained from dose–response relationships employing data bearing on the frequency of occurrence of signs and symptoms using nominal scales, data bearing on the subjectively estimated intensity of feeling states using ordinal scales, and the measurement of pupillary diameter from polaroid photographs were in close agreement and had similar confidence limits (Martin and Fraser, 1961). These potency estimates further agreed with estimates of analgesic potency obtained in patients suffering from both acute and chronic pain. These observations were taken to mean that (1) the miotic phenomenon and changes in subjective states were probably the consequence of the drugs acting through a similar mechanism and that measures of subjective states were valid measures of drug effect; (2) any lack of additivity among signs and symptoms, and deviations from linearity for nominal and ordinal scales, was probably small compared to between-subjects and across-times variance. These later issues were pursued experimentally. Thus the frequency of occurrence of various signs or the intensity of symptoms and the degree of miosis produced by both morphine and heroin were found to be linearly related to the logarithm of dose. Hence, we knew that the principle additivity was applicable to data obtained using nominal and ordinal ratio scales. We began to apply the criterion of dose responsiveness for the selection of questionnaire items (Martin and Fraser, 1961; Martin et al., 1971), yet another approach that enhanced the rigor of additivity for our behavioral scales. Different signs were weighted such that the signs that exhibited lesser sensitivity were given greater weight. Thus, by weighting, different responses could be equated (e.g., pupils and liking).

The Himmelsbach method for scoring the intensity of opioid abstinence is composed of data derived from nominal, interval, and ratio scales that have different weighting values that are related to the severity of abstinence. A similar system for assessing abstinence was developed for precipitation and suppression studies in the dog (Martin et al., 1974; Martin et al., 1976; Gilbert and Martin, 1976) that was composed of changes that were suppressed or precipitated in a dose-related way by agonists and antagonists and that were measured using nominal, ordinal, interval, and ratio scales. Those signs of abstinence, whose frequency or intensity were related to the dose of the agonists in suppression studies and the dose of antagonists in precipitation studies, were selected for measuring the intensity of abstinence, and each sign was weighted such that all signs made an approximately equal contribution to the abstinence syndrome score. Thus, the criterion of additivity and linearity were fulfilled. By establishing linearity and additivity for items of subjective effects questionnaires, through weighting and dose relationship, a report of itchy skin can be equated to a feeling of drive, and reports of the two effects can be added. In a similar manner, the abstinence signs yawning, pilorection, and temperature can be added. Through the technique of mapping, we have shown that there is a linear relationship between dose-related changes in scores on the nominal, ordinal, interval, and ratio scales. This relationship is implicit when valid parallel line assays are obtained for different measures and effects. This is illustrated in Table 1. These issues of measures and statistics have been discussed by Stevens (1968). Two important principles emerged. (1) Deviations from additivity and linearity for nominal and ordinal data are small compared to the unaccounted-for variance and (2) the frequency of occurrence or intensity of report are linearly related to the dose (logarithm) of the drug.

The use of pharmacologic syndromes has played a critical role in identifying receptor subtypes and in identifying specific drugs. In detailed studies of cyclazocine in humans, it was apparent that cyclazocine produced effects that were not produced by morphine (Martin et al., 1965). Although cyclazocine was a potent miotic (10–15 times more potent than morphine and nalorphine), valid potency assays of this activity were not obtained. Further, cyclazocine in higher doses produced overt ataxia, and subjects reported that they were sleepy and felt drunk. These signs and symptoms were not commonly observed in, or reported by, postaddicts who had been administered morphine or heroin. Cyclazocine and nalorphine produced feelings of well-being in some subjects, but not in others. They also produced feelings of dysphoria in most subjects when the dose was sufficient. The dysphoric effects of cyclazocine and nalorphine are complex. The most commonly reported symptom, with minimally dysphoric doses, is recall of disturbing memories. The patient can be distracted, but has difficulty suppressing these thoughts. With larger doses, delusions, hallucinations, sleep with disturbing dreams, and anxiety states may be reported. Cyclazocine was found to be

10–20 times more potent than morphine in equivalent measures. An attempt was made to make patients dependent on an equivalent dose of cyclazocine based on single-dose relative potency. A daily dose of 13.2 mg/70 kg was attained in six subjects. Some subjects found the dysphoric effects of cyclazocine especially disturbing, and the dose of cyclazocine was incremented slowly. At the time these studies were initiated, we did not realize that cyclazocine had much longer duration of action than morphine, and hence our estimates of the equipotent dose of cyclazocine may have been high. Regardless, when the administration of cyclazocine was terminated, we were presented with several surprises. The first was a long latency to onset of signs of abstinence. In fact, signs were not perceptible until the third day of withdrawal and were not maximal until the seventh day of withdrawal. Second, the abstinence syndrome was not associated with drug need. Most subjects were glad the study was over and none sought medication for relief of their symptoms. The third issue was the nature of the abstinence syndrome.

Doctors Eddy and Isbell took the position that the cyclazocine abstinence syndrome was just mild abstinence. To help resolve this issue, Dr. Isbell provided me with unpublished data of E. G. Williams (cf., Martin, 1966), who had studied the abstinence syndrome of subjects dependent on different stabilization doses of morphine in an attempt to determine the smallest dose of morphine that produced a clinically significant degree of physical dependence. A sign analysis of Williams' data and the cyclazocine abstinence data was done. This analysis indicated that the relative magnitude of the signs of cyclazocine abstinence was different from that of morphine abstinence, regardless of the level of dependence (Martin et al., 1965; Martin, 1966).

The effects of cyclazocine shared certain characteristics with those of nalorphine (Martin and Gorodetzky, 1965), except that nalorphine was less potent and the maximum degree of ataxia was less. Whereas cyclazocine could produce overt drunkenness, nalorphine produced liminal ataxia that was only demonstrable with tandem gate walking. This latter difference was subsequently explained when studies were conducted in the chronic spinal dog, in which it was shown that nalorphine showed partial agonistic activity (McClane and Martin, 1967b; Gilbert and Martin, 1976a). When nalorphine was administered chronically in doses of 240 mg/kg/day and then withdrawn, an abstinence syndrome emerged within 24 h and was qualitatively different from the morphine abstinence syndrome and similar to the cyclazocine abstinence syndrome.

Several investigators studied mixtures of morphine and nalorphine in human subjects and in animals, administered acutely and chronically (cf., Martin, 1967). Of particular importance were the observations of Houde and Wallenstein (1956), who found that low doses of nalorphine antagonized the effects of 10 mg of morphine, whereas higher doses produced a lesser antagonism. The nalorphine biphasic dose–response antagonism of morphine's analgesic action could not be explained by assuming that nalorphine was a competitive antagonist or a partial agonist of morphine. Houde and Wallenstein's (1956) observation stimulated a mathematical formulation of receptor dualism (Martin, 1967; Martin et al., 1972).

Naloxone antagonized the actions of cyclazocine in the chronic spinal dog (McClane and Martin, 1967) and in human subjects (Jasinski et al., 1968). Naloxone in a high dose (15 mg/70 kg) antagonized the miotic, respiratory depressant and subjective effects produced by 1 mg/70 kg of cyclazocine in human subjects. Naloxone (0.2 mg/kg) partially antagonized the depressant effects of cyclazocine (0.063 mg/kg) on the flexor reflex of the chronic spinal dog. The same dose of naloxone completely antagonized the effects of 1.0 mg/kg of morphine. Blumberg et al. (1965) showed that naloxone antagonized the analgesic effects of cyclazocine, nalorphine, and pentazocine in mice.

Thus, four lines of evidence suggested that nalorphine and cyclazocine differed from morphine in their actions. (1) The nature of the subjective effects that they produced were different; (2) they produced different types of dependence; (3) interaction studies between morphine and nalorphine yielded biphasic dose response curves; and (4) the effects of several agonist–antagonists could be antagonized by large doses of naloxone. These observations lead to the suggestions that there were two opioid receptors, an M (morphine) and N (nalorphine). Further, the M and N receptors operated in concert in some, but not all, physiologic systems. The process of a concerted action was called "pharmacologic dualism." It was suggested that morphine acted as an agonist and nalorphine as a competitive antagonist at the M receptor. Further, nalorphine acted as a partial agonist at the N receptor (Martin, 1967). This concept (pharmacologic dualism) was an elaboration on my concept of pharmacologic redundancy, which postulated parallel neuronal pathways employing different transmitters, as well as cotransmitter and coreceptors, as alternative mechanisms for the conduct of function (Martin, 1970).

The hypothesis that there are two opioid receptors that exhibit the principle of receptor dualism reconciled many observations. It was soon apparent, however, that it left other observations unexplained in terms of receptor theory.

The first analgesic with predominantly N agonistic activity to be marketed was pentazocine. It was not scheduled as a narcotic because studies at the Addiction Research Center indicated that it did not produce as much euphoria as morphine, did not substitute for morphine in morphine-dependent subjects, did not appear to produce physical dependence, and was not liked by postaddict subjects when administered chronically (Fraser and Rosenberg, 1964). There were sporadic case reports of the abuse of pentazocine. For this reason, and because we had new techniques for measuring subjective effects and had developed new concepts, we decided to reinvestigate the abuse potentiality of pentazocine. One of the important developments in opioid pharmacology was the synthesis of naloxone and the elucidation of its pharmacology. Blumberg (cf., Blumberg and Dayton, 1974) had encouraged the synthesis of naloxone with the end of obtaining a more potent antagonist with fewer side effects (e.g., respiratory depression and psychotomimetic effects). Foldes et al. (1963) conducted extensive studies with naloxone showing that it antagonized the respiratory depressant actions of opiate analgesics. Lasagna (1965) found that naloxone produced a modest degree of both analgesia and hyperalgesia in patients with pain. Our task was to assess the abuse potentiality of naloxone. We found that it did not induce subjective changes, did not produce miosis when administered chronically, did not produce physical dependence, and, when administered to morphine-dependent subjects, was seven times more potent than nalorphine in precipitating abstinence (Jasinski et al., 1967). We concluded that naloxone was an opioid antagonist that was devoid of agonistic activity. Naloxone was of great importance in further clarifying the mechanism of action of pentazocine and provided critical proof that morphine was acting as an agonist.

In our reinvestigations of pentazocine, we confirmed several of the observations of Fraser and Rosenberg (1964). Low doses of pentazocine produced a subjective state similar to that produced by low doses of morphine characterized by elevations of MBG scale scores, which measure feelings of well being. In this regard pentazocine was about one fourth as potent as morphine (Jasinski et al., 1970). Further, doses above 40 mg produced dose-related elevation on the LSD and PCAG scale scores, which measure, respectively, hallucinations, delusions, and anxiety (LSD) and apathetic sedation (PCAG), and a decrease in the MBG scale scores. The fact that lower doses of pentazocine produced elevations of MBG scale scores raised the question of whether pentazocine could be a weak partial agonist at the M receptor and a less potent, but strong agonist, at the N receptor. To test this hypothesis, subjects were made dependent on decreasingly lower doses of morphine and the ability of pentazocine to suppress the morphine abstinence syndrome was assessed. In short, pentazocine did not clearly suppress abstinence in subjects dependent on morphine in doses as low as 30 mg/d and as high as 240 mg/d. When subjects who were dependent and stabilized on 240 mg/d of morphine were administered pentazocine, it precipitated an abstinence syndrome and in this regard was 1/50 as potent as nalorphine. Thus the doses of pentazocine that were necessary to precipitate abstinence were greater than those necessary to cause miosis, analgesia, and subjective effects. When subjects were administered pentazocine in doses of 522–684 mg/d and then abruptly withdrawn, a mild abstinence syndrome emerged that was qualitatively similar to that seen in cyclazocine- and nalorphine-dependent subjects. Further, an abstinence syndrome could be precipitated in pentazocine-dependent subjects with naloxone in doses approximately 10 times larger than necessary to precipitate an abstinence syndrome in morphine-dependent subjects. At this juncture our operating hypothesis was that pentazocine, like nalorphine and cyclazocine, was a competitive antagonist at the M receptor and either a partial or a strong agonist at the N receptor.

We had been aware that cyclazocine and nalorphine produced a subjective syndrome consisting of a dysphoria and an apathetic sedation. The fact that pentazocine produced more feeling of well being than did nalorphine and cyclazocine, and yet resembled them in many other ways, was a problem—"the pentazocine problem." To determine if this problem had a receptor-based explanation, an extensive group of studies was initiated in the chronic spinal dog (Martin et al., 1974, 1976, 1978, 1980; Gilbert and Martin, 1976a,b). These studies developed methods that yielded data in the dog that provided potency estimates on a variety of physiologic parameters (pupillary diameter, pulse rate, respiratory rate, body temperature, amplitude of the flexor reflex, and the latency of the skin twitch reflex). In addition, procedures were developed for conducting valid assays of the potency of drugs in suppressing signs of abstinence in the maximally abstinent chronic spinal dog and in precipitating abstinence in the stabilized chronic spinal dog. A large group of dogs was made dependent on morphine; a prototypic "M" agonist: another group was made dependent on cyclazocine; a prototypic "N" agonist. Over 20 prototypic drugs were studied. Morphine-like drugs (see Table 2) by and large produced a similar pattern of effects suppressing the flexor and skin twitch reflexes constricting pupils, lowering body temperature, and slowing pulse rate. Further these agents as well as others that resemble morphine suppressed the morphine abstinence syndrome in a dose-related way. Of some importance were the observations that neither meperidine nor normorphine produced morphine-like effects or suppressed the morphine abstinence syndrome. Hence, although they are morphine-like drugs in other species, they do not appear to be morphine-like in the dog.

Buprenorphine in single doses also produced a morphine-like pattern of effects, but differed from morphine in that it produced a lesser maximal effect. Further it suppressed abstinence signs; the slope of its suppression dose–response line was less than that of morphine, however. Buprenorphine also precipitated abstinence in stabilized morphine-dependent dogs; the slope of the precipitation dose–response line, however, was less than that of naloxone and naltrexone. These data were consistent with the hypothesis that buprenorphine was a partial agonist of the morphine-type.

In contrast to morphine-like drugs, cyclazocine, nalorphine, and pentazocine were relatively ineffective in suppressing the thermally evoked skin twitch reflex, but produced a profound depression of the pressure-evoked flexor reflex. They also, especially in larger doses, dilated pupils and increased heart and respiratory rate, but did not depress body temperature to the degree morphine did.

Keats and Telford (1964) in their study of the analgesic properties of a series of N-substituted benzomorphans had observed that N-allylnormetazocine (NANM; SKF 10,047) produced severe dysphoria and little analgesia. NANM was selected as a proto-

TABLE 2

Relative Potency of μ and κ Agonists in Suppressing and Precipitating Abstinence in Morphine (A)- and Cyclazocine (B)-Dependent Dogs and in Producing Changes in the Nondependent Dog (C)[a]

| Drug | Morphine-dependent dogs (A) | | Cyclazocine-dependent dogs (B) | | (C) |
	Suppression potency	Precipitation potency	Suppression potency	Precipitation potency	Single dose
D-Propoxyphene	0.2				0.12
Propiram					0.14
Codeine					0.06–0.1
Morphine	1.0		1		1
Oxycodone	1.2				
Methadone	4.9				
Ketobemidone	5.1				
Phenazocine	8.1				
Levorphanol	9.0				
Dilaudid	15.4				
Fentanyl	70.5				
Etorphine	200.3				
Buprenorphine					257
Pentazocine		0.002	0.19		0.3
Nalorphine		0.08	0.24 (PA)	0.009	0.5
NANM		0.13			
Cyclazocine		0.47	1.0		3.3
Naloxone		1			
Naltrexone		3.4		1	0
Ethylketazocine			4.4		9
Ketazocine			0.2		1

[a]Potency estimates for suppression studies are expressed as milligrams of morphine or cyclazocine that are necessary to produce the same degree of suppression as the experimental drug. Naloxone is used as the standard drug in precipitation studies in morphine-dependent dogs and naltrexone in cyclazocine-dependent dogs. PA indicates nalorphine is a partial agonist.

typic and relatively selective dysphoriant and was studied in the chronic spinal dog. It produced less depression of the flexor reflex than morphine or ethylketazocine, did not depress the skin twitch reflex, increased pupillary diameter, pulse rate, and respiratory rate, and produced a canine delirium. NANM's respiratory stimulant action probably has a different mechanism of action than morphine's in the dog. Morphine causes panting by resetting the hypothalamic thermoregulatory center that downregulates the set point and thus body temperatures. In contrast, NANM stimulates respiration, while producing a modest hyperthermic reaction. In all probability the respiratory stimulant actions of nalorphine, which are seen in relatively high doses, are a consequence of nalorphine's σ activity (Gilbert and Martin, 1976a,b).

Other prototypic drugs studied were ketazocine and ethylketazocine, which depressed the flexor reflex, had little effect on the latency of the skin twitch reflex, produced sedation, and were potent miotics.

Studies in the morphine- and cyclazocine-dependent dog are summarized in Table 2. Several points are of importance. Nalorphine precipitated abstinence in both the morphine- and cyclazocine-dependent dog. In the cyclazocine-dependent spinal dog, however, it exhibited a ceiling effect. These observations were in keeping with the observations in the nondependent dog, namely that nalorphine's agonistic effects exhibited a ceiling and that it was probably a partial agonist of the κ type (see below). Of great importance were the observations that three groups of drugs suppressed the cyclazocine abstinence; (1) morphine, (2) cyclazocine, nalorphine, and pentazocine, which exhibited excitatory effects such as mydriasis and tachycardia, and (3) ethylketazocine and ketazocine, which constricted pupils, but did not suppress the morphine abstinence syndrome. The excitatory effects of cyclazocine, nalorphine, and to some extent pentazocine resembled the effects of NANM.

To further compare the pharmacologic properties of NANM with those of the prototypic drugs, morphine and cyclazocine, dogs were made dependent on 10 mg/kg/day of NANM administered in equally divided iv doses six times a day (Martin et al., 1980). This proved to be a difficult experiment to execute. As the dose levels were increased, dogs exhibited canine delirium and loss of appetite and weight. By slowly escalating the dose, a stabilization dose of 10 mg/kg was eventually obtained and precipitation and withdrawal studies were conducted. This study showed that chronic administration of NANM induced tolerance to its ability to produce canine delirium, tachypnea, and anorexia. The withdrawal abstinence was mild, consisting of a decrease in body temperature, miosis, bradycardia, tachypnea, and an increase in the amplitude of the flexor reflex. This syndrome was unlike that seen in either morphine- or cyclazocine-dependent animals. The naltrexone-precipitated abstinence syndrome was yet different, consisting of hyperthermia, tachycardia, tachypnea, and an increase in the amplitude of the flexor reflex. These data further showed that some of the effects of chronically administered NANM could be antagonized by naltrexone, whereas others could not. These observations led to the suggestion that NANM might have multiple modes of action.

These and other observations could be reconciled by the hypothesis that (1) there were three opioid-related receptors: μ, κ, and σ (Martin et al., 1976; Gilbert and Martin, 1976a), (2) these receptors could exert their effects on several physiologic systems through different but converging pathways (receptor dualism and pharmacologic redundancy) (Martin, 1967), and (3) drugs that interacted with opioid receptors could act as competitive antagonists, partial agonists, and strong agonists.

2. Reflections

In the relatively brief time, two decades, since these hypotheses were proposed, an enormous body of data has been generated that supports them. Further, they have been extended in two major directions; additional types of opioid or opioid-related receptors have been identified, and endogenous opioid transmitter substances have been discovered. These observations have had, and will continue to have, an enormous impact on neurochemistry, physiology, neuropsychopharmacology, and psychology, as well as mental health.

2.1. Pharmacologic Implications

The first clues concerning the existence of multiple opioids came from studies in humans that were subsequently elaborated on using the chronic spinal dog. The conclusions were drawn from analyses of the patterns of pharmacologic effects using agonists and antagonists of differing specificities and differed from other classic analyses of receptor subtypes only in that these comparisons used signs derived from changes in central nervous function for the comparisons. For these pattern comparisons to become meaningful, valid bioassay techniques had to be developed for the various central nervous system functions under study such as subjective effects, pupillary diameter, function of homeostats, and reflex activity. The second element was the use of receptor theory in the design of experiments and conceptualization of hypotheses. The third major ingredient in this endeavor was the very large synthetic effort that yielded a rich diversity of structural modification of important drugs. In this regard the synthetic efforts of Sidney Archer, William Michne, Jack Fishman, John Lewis, and Everett May were particularly important. In a relatively short time it was demonstrated that relatively minor structural modifications of opioid drugs could change the specificities for μ, κ, δ, and σ receptors and could alter their activity yielding agonists, partial agonists, and competitive antagonists. It was also apparent that opioid ligands had a number of reactive sites that could interact with a variety of moieties on opioid receptors. These general observations lead to the formulation of the steric theory of multiple opioid receptors, which offers a theoretical basis for explaining not only the multiplicity of opioid receptors, but differences in their efficacy and activity (Martin, 1983). The steric theory has several components. (1) It assumes that the opioid receptor has nuclear sites that are responsible for initiating the pharmacologic action of the drug or transmitter, as well as satellite sites that play two roles: (a) determination of the affinity of the drug for the receptor and (b) the orientation of the drug on the receptors. (2) Changes in the configuration of these two components of the receptors may have several effects on drug receptor interactions. The following terms are coined to designate the possible types of changes. *Allomorphism* is a change in the position of the active moieties of the nuclear part of the receptor. Such changes will result in a change in the specificity of drugs for the receptor. *Allosterism* is a change in the positions of moieties of the satellite sites. These result in changes of affinity of the drug for the receptor and in the orienting properties of the receptor toward the drug. *Allotaxia* is the property whereby the drug can occupy the receptor in several positions.

These types of changes in the receptor can hypothetically be interactive. Clearly, changes in the relative positions of satellite moieties could alter both the affinity and the allotaxic properties of a family of drugs and hence alter both the K_d values and the activity of the drug. On the other hand, allomorphic changes will result in a change in the number of receptors of different specificities. These types of changes may result in complicated dose–response curves.

Depending on one's perspective, the concept of opioid antagonists had a slow acceptance by the medical and pharmacologic community. The concept of multiple opioid receptors and the application of receptor theory to opioids had a somewhat more rapid acceptance. The delineation of each receptor subtype has extended our basic understanding of general receptor theory, as well as the complexity of body function and evolution. In turn, the complexities of microstructure and function have provided those who have a bent for using pharmacologic approaches to function and evolution a wonderful opportunity for identifying drugs with unique specificities. I believe that a strong case can be made for the proposition that the discovery of most multiple receptor types has been a consequence of pattern identification using tissues of diverse origins and responses to drugs.

I have tried in this account to remember most of the critical events that either directly or indirectly influenced my thinking and conclusions about multiple opioid receptors and receptor dualism. It was my very good fortune to have had Dr. Klaus Unna, Harris Isbell, and Abraham Wikler as my teachers, collaborators, and friends. They played critical roles and had seminal influences in the development of opioid antagonists and agonist–antagonists as therapeutic agents and pharmacologic tools. They also recognized the importance of systematic, quantitative, and reliable observations in drug comparison, both in humans and animals, a perspective that was essential in the analysis of the mechanisms of action of opioid receptors.

References

Bliss, C. I. (1952) *The Statistics of Bioassay: With Special Reference to the Vitamins* Academic Press, New York.

Blumberg, H. and Dayton, H. B. (1974) Naloxone, Naltrexone and Related Noroxymorphones, in *Narcotic Antagonists* (Braude, M. C., Harris, L. S., May, E. L., Smith, J. P., and Villarreal, J. E., eds.) *Advances in Biomedical Psychopharmacology* vol. 8, Raven, New York.

Blumberg, H., Wolfe, P. S., and Dayton, H. B. (1965) Use of writhing test for evaluating analgesic activity of narcotic antagonists. *Proc. Soc. Exp. Biol. Med.* **118,** 763–766.

Downs, A. W. and Eddy, N. B. (1928) Morphine tolerance. II. The susceptibility of morphine-tolerant dogs to codeine, heroin and scopolamine. *J. Lab. Clin. Med.* **13,** 745.

Eckenhoff, J. E., Elder, J. D., and King, B. D. (1952) N-Allylnormorphine in treatment of morphine or demerol narcosis. *Am. J. Med. Sci.* **223,** 191–197.

Eddy, N. B. (1973) The National Research Council Involvement in the Opiate Problem, 1928–1971. The National Academy of Sciences, Washington.

Finney, D. J. (1964) *Statistical Methods of Biological Assay* 2nd Ed., Hafner, New York.

Foldes, F. F., Lunn, J. N., Moore, J., and Brown, I. M. (1963) N-Allylnoroxymorphone: A new potent narcotic antagonist. *Am. J. Med. Sci.* **245,** 23–30.

Fraser, H. F. and Isbell, H. (1960) Human pharmacology and addiction liabilities of phenazocine and levophenacylmorphan. *Bull. Narcot.* **12,** 15–23.

Fraser, H. F. and Rosenberg, D. E. (1964) Studies on the human addiction liability of 2-hydroxy-5,9-dimethyl-2-(3,3 dimethylallyl)-6,7-benzomorphan (Win 20 228). *J. Pharmacol. Exp. Ther.* **143,** 149–156.

Gilbert, P. E. and Martin, W. R. (1976a) The effects of morphine- and nalorphine-like drugs in the nondependent, morphine-dependent and cyclazocine-dependent chronic spinal dog. *J. Pharmacol. Exp. Ther.* **198,** 66–82.

Gilbert, P. E. and Martin, W. R. (1976b) Sigma effects of nalorphine in the chronic spinal dog. *Drug Alc. Depend.* **1,** 373–376.

Hart, E. R. (1941) N-Allylnorcodeine and N-allylnormorphine, two antagonists to morphine. *J. Pharmacol. Exp. Ther.* **72,** 19.

Hart, E. R. and McCauley, E. L. (1944) The pharmacology of N-allylnormorphine as compared with morphine. *J. Pharmacol. Exp. Ther.* **82,** 339–348.

Himmelsbach, C. K. (1939) Studies of certain addiction characteristics of: (a) dihydromorphine ("paramorphan"), (b) dihydrodesoxymorphine-*d* ("desomorphine"), (c) dihydrodesoxycodeine-*d* ("desocodeine"), (d) methyldihydromorphinone ("metopon"). *J. Pharmacol. Exp. Ther.* **67,** 239–249.

Himmelsbach, C. K. (1978) Summary of Chemical, Pharmacological and Clinical Research, in *Drug Addiction and the U. S. Public Health Service* (W. R. Martin and H. Isbell, eds.) National Institute on Drug Abuse, Washington.

Houde, R. W. and Wallenstein, S. L. (1956) Clinical studies of morphine-nalorphine combinations. *Fed. Proc.* **15,** 440–441.

Jasinski, D. R., Martin, W. R., and Haertzen, C. A. (1967) The human pharmacology and abuse potential of N-allylnoroxymorphone (naloxone). *J. Pharamcol. Exp. Ther.* **157,** 420–426.

Jasinski, D. R., Martin, W. R., and Hoeldtke, R. D. (1970) Effects of short- and long-term administration of pentazocine in man. *Clin. Pharmacol. Ther.* **11**, 385–403.

Jasinski, D. R., Martin, W. R., and Sapira, J. D. (1968) Antagonism of the subjective, behavioral, pupillary and respiratory depressant effects of cyclazocine by naloxone. *Clin. Pharmacol. Ther.* **9**, 215–222.

Keats, A. S. and Telford, J. (1964) Narcotic Antagonists as Analgesics, in *Molecular Modification in Drug Design,* Advances in Chemistry Series no. 45, (Gould, R. F., ed.) American Chemical Society.

Lasagna, L. (1965) Drug interaction in the field of analgesic drugs. *Proc. Roy. Soc. Med.* **58**, 978–983.

Lasagna, L. and Beecher, H. K. (1954) Analgesic effectiveness of nalorphine and nalorphine-morphine combinations in man. *J. Pharmacol. Exp. Ther.* **112**, 356–363.

Leake, C. D. (1967) Introduction, in *New Concepts in Pain and Its Clinical Management* (Way, E. L., ed.) F. A. Davie Co., Philadelphia.

McClane, T. K. and Martin, W. R. (1967a) Antagonism of the spinal cord effects of morphine and cyclazocine by naloxone and thebaine. *Int. J. Neuropharmacol.* **6**, 325–327.

McClane, T. K. and Martin, W. R. (1967b) Effects of morphine, nalorphine, cyclazocine and naloxone on the flexor reflex. *Int. J. Neuropharmacol.* **6**, 89–98.

Martin, W. R. (1966) Assessment of the Dependence Producing Potentiality of Narcotic Analgesics, in *International Encyclopedia of Pharmacology and Therapeutics* (Radouco-Thomas, C. and Lasagna, L., eds.) Pergamonn, Glasgow.

Martin, W. R. (1967) Opioid antagonists. *Pharmacol. Rev.* **19**, 463–521.

Martin, W. R. (1970) Pharmacological redundancy as an adaptive mechanism in the central nervous system. *Fed. Proc.* **29**, 13–18.

Martin, W. R. (1983) Pharmacology of opioids. *Pharmacol. Rev.* **35**(4), 283–323.

Martin, W. R. and Fraser, H. F. (1961) A comparative study of physiological and subjective effects of heroin and morphine administered intravenously in postaddicts. *J. Pharmacol. Exp. Ther.* **133**, 388–399.

Martin, W. R. and Gorodetzky, C. W. (1965) Demonstration of tolerance to and physical dependence on N-allylnormorphine (nalorphine). *J. Pharmacol. Exp. Ther.* **150**, 437–442.

Martin, W. R. and Jasinski, D. R. (1977) Assessment of the Abuse Potential of Narcotic Analgesics in Animals, in *Drug Addiction I* sect. II (Martin, W. R., ed.) Springer Verlag, Berlin.

Martin, W. R., Eades, C. G., Gilbert, P. E., and Thompson, J. A. (1980) Tolerance to and physical dependence on N-allylnormetazocine (NANM) in chronic spinal dogs. *Subst. Alcohol Actions Misuse* **1**, 269–279.

Martin, W. R., Eades, C. G., Thompson, W. O., Thompson, J. A., and Flanary, H. G. (1974) Morphine physical dependence in the dog. *J. Pharmacol. Exp. Ther.* **189**, 759–771.

Martin, W. R., Eades, C. G., Thompson, J. A., Huppler, R. E., and Gilbert, P. E. (1976) The effects of morphine- and nalorphine-like drugs in the nondependent and morphine-dependent chronic spinal dog. *J. Pharmacol. Exp. Ther.* **197**, 517–532.

Martin, W. R., Fraser, H. F., Gorodetzky, C. W., and Rosenberg, D. E. (1965) Studies of the dependence producing potential of the narcotic antagonist 2-cyclopropylmethyl-2'-hydroxy-5, 9-dimethyl-6,7-benzomorphan (cyclazocine, WIN 20, 740; ARC II-C-3). *J. Pharmacol. Exp. Ther.* **150**, 426–436.

Martin, W. R., Gilbert, P. E., Thompson, J. A., and Jessee, C. A. (1978) Use of the chronic spinal dog for the assessment of the abuse potentiality and utility of narcotic analgesics and narcotic antagonists. *Drug Alcohol Depend.* **3**, 23–35.

Martin, W. R., Gorodetzky, C. W., and Thompson, W. O. (1972) Receptor Dualism: Some Kinetic Implications, in *Agonist and Antagonist Actions of Narcotic Analgesic Drugs:* Proceedings of the Symposium of the British Pharmacological Society, (Kosterlitz, H. W., Collier, H. O. J., and Villarreal, J. E., eds.) Aberdeen, July 1971, Macmillan, London.

Martin, W. R., Sloan, J. W., Sapira, J. D., and Jasinski, D. R. (1971) Physiologic, subjective and behavioral effects of amphetamine, methamphetamine, ephedrine, phenmetrazine and methylphenidate in man. *Clin. Pharmacol. Ther.* **12**, 245–258.

Meissner, R. (1923) Ueber atmungserregende heilmettel. *J. Gesamte Exp. Med.* **31**, 159–214.

Pohl, J. (1915) Ueber das N-allylnorcodeine, einin antagonisten des morphins. *Z. Exp. Pathol. Ther.* **17**, 370–382.

Stevens, S. S. (1968) Measurement, statistics and the schemapiric view. *Science* **161**, (3844), 849–856.

Unna, K. (1943) Antagonistic effect of N-allylnormorphine upon morphine. *J. Pharmacol. Exp. Ther.* **79**, 27–31.

von Braun, J. (1916) Unter suchungen uber morphium-alkalvide. III. Mitteilung. *Berlin Deut. Chem. Ges.* **49**, 977–989.

Wikler, A. and Carter, R. L. (1953) Effects of single doses of N-allylnormorphine on hindlimb reflexes of chronic spinal dogs during cycles of morphine addiction. *J. Pharmacol. Exp. Ther.* **109**, 92–101.

Wikler, A., Fraser, H. F., and Isbell, H. (1953) N-Allylnormorphine: Effects of single doses and precipitation of acute "abstinence syndromes" during addiction to morphine, methadone or heroin in man (post-addicts). *J. Pharmacol. Exp. Ther.* **109**(1), 8–20.

Weijlard, J. and Erickson, A. E. (1942) N-Allylnormorphine. *J. Am. Chem. Soc.* **64**, 869–870.

Chapter 2

The Opioid Peptides

Christopher J. Evans, Donna L. Hammond, and Robert C. A. Frederickson

1. Introduction

The discovery of endogenous opioids has begun an intricate saga involving multiple ligands and multiple receptors that form an extensive neuronal network in both the central and peripheral nervous systems. This intricacy is reflected in the complex pharmacology and diverse physiological effects of opioids in mammals. The aim of this chapter is to consolidate the immense literature on endogenous opioid ligands and attempt to rationalize the multiple forms of these bioactive substances. A number of recent reviews on endogenous opioids reflect different perspectives to this extensive field (Weber et al., 1983b; Frederickson, 1984; Akil et al., 1984; Offermeier and Van Rooyen, 1984; Imura et al., 1985; Herbert et al., 1985; Barchas et al., 1986).

2. History of Opioid Peptides

Morphine (named after Morpheus, the Greek god of dreams), was the first natural opioid to be identified and characterized. This alkaloid was isolated as one of the analgesic components of opium, the infamous product of the poppy, *Papaver somniferum.*

The question of why a plant alkaloid should bind to stereospecific receptors on neuronal membranes and display such dramatic effects on the mammalian nervous system, was answered by an extensive search for an opioid ligand endogenous to the mammalian system. Initial studies were understandably aimed at the isolation of alkaloids, but it soon became apparent from many experiments, including enzyme degradation studies, that peptides may be endogenous ligands for the opiate receptor.

Indeed, in the early 1970s, two pentapeptides with opiate-like activity were extracted from porcine brain and characterized (Hughes et al., 1975). These peptides differed only in the C-terminal amino acid and were named methionine enkephalin (Tyr-Gly-Gly-Phe-Met) and leucine enkephalin (Tyr-Gly-Gly-Phe-Leu). Numerous analogs were synthesized in order to determine the structural requirements of these peptide opioids. Among the general conclusions from these studies was that activity remained following modification of the C-terminus of enkephalin via amidation or addition of amino acids. The N-terminal tyrosine residue, however, appeared to be an absolute requirement, in that removal of the N-terminal positive charge either by acetylation or other means completely obliterated opioid bioactivity. These two simple conclusions from the structure–activity relationships of enkephalin are useful to remember when viewing the activity of various products of the opioid peptide precursors.

Following the discovery of the enkephalins, multiple opioid receptors, originally demonstrated by Martin et al. (1976), using the alkaloid opiates, were established as a focus in opioid biochemistry. Based on bioassay and binding assays, several opioid receptors were postulated. Characterization and identity of these opioid receptors are the subjects of other chapters in this book. Suffice to say there is still much discussion on the nature of opioid binding sites that will undoubtedly be resolved by chemical characterization of the receptor proteins and genes.

The observation that a fragment of β-lipotropin (β-LPH) shared the same N-terminal structure with enkephalin initiated considerable interest (Bradbury et al., 1975). As one might expect from the structure–activity relationships deduced from enkephalin analogs, this 31-amino acid peptide named β-endorphin (β-end) bound to opioid receptors and, in addition, proved to be a potent, long-lasting analgesic, an opiate property not shared with the unmodified enkephalins. Analgesic activity could also be demonstrated after high doses of the enkephalins given directly into the brain, but the activity was fleeting because of rapid degradation. Initially, it was considered that β-end may be a precursor of methionine enkephalin in brain, but this seemed improbable from several standpoints. Foremost, the distribution of enkephalin immunoreactive material was distinctly different from that of β-end (Watson et al., 1978). A second consideration was that the processing to form enkephalin from β-end would be highly unusual, requiring demanding cleavage at a methionyl/serine linkage. Processing of neuropeptide precursors accrues almost exclusively at basic residues. The general belief that enkephalin was the product of a different precursor than β-end was subsequently shown to be correct. The convincing evidence stemmed from a series of studies initiated by an observation that [Met]enkephalin could be immunologically detected in adrenal glands (Schultzberg et al., 1978). This observation focused on adrenals as a good tissue for the isolation of enkephalin-like peptides and resulted in the characterization of a whole tribe of peptides containing the enkephalin nucleus, either embedded within the structure or at the N-terminus (Stern et al., 1981, 1979; Lewis et al., 1980; Kimura et al., 1980; Jones et al., 1982). The enkephalin nuclei embedded within many of the characterized adrenal peptides were flanked at both the N- and C-termini by paired basic residues, making these peptides strong candidates for precursors of the enkephalins.

The isolation of a third class of opioid peptides, the dynorphins, was initiated prior to the complete characterization of enkephalin, with the identification of a pituitary peptide with intriguing opiate-like activity on the guinea pig ileum (Cox et al., 1975). Nearly a decade later, dynorphin A, a sticky peptide with properties very different from any of the other opioid peptides was isolated and characterized (Goldstein et al., 1981). Dynorphin A was shown to be a potent ligand for the kappa class of receptors. Using antisera raised to dynorphin A, a C-terminally extended peptide was sequenced that contained a second [Leu]enkephalin opioid nucleus, separated from dynorphin A by a pair of basic residues (Fischli et al., 1982a). This second [Leu]enkephalin-containing opioid, dynorphin-B (rimorphin), was isolated as a discrete peptide by Kilpatrick et al. (1982). Preceding the purification and complete structural analysis of the dynorphins, two peptides with a [Leu]enkephalin sequence at the N-terminus had been isolated and characterized from hypothalamus. These peptides were named α- and β-neoendorphin and differed only in the additional lysine residue present on the C-terminus of α-neoendorphin (Kangawa et al., 1979, 1981; Minamino et al., 1981). The colocalization of α-neoendorphin with dynorphin immunoreactivity suggested that these peptides may be derived from a common precursor (Weber et al., 1982d).

The differentiation of the three opioid families was finalized by the cloning of the representative opioid precursors. Proopiomelanocortin (Nakanishi et al., 1979) possessed β-end at the C-terminus of a 31-kdalton protein, also containing the sequence of ACTH. Technical problems conquered, the other two opioid precursors were quickly sequenced, proenkephalin by Noda et al. (1982) and prodynorphin by Kakidani et al. (1982). Proenkephalin contained all the enkephalin-containing sequences isolated from the bovine adrenal gland, and, as expected, the prodynorphin precursor contained the sequences of α-neoendorphin, dynorphin A, and dynorphin B. The precise sequences of the three opioid precursors laid sound foundation for both immunological and processing studies.

This introduction would be incomplete if we omitted to mention that morphine and perhaps other similar alkaloids can be found in various mammalian and amphibian tissues (Oka et al., 1985; Gintzler et al., 1976; Goldstein et al., 1985). Although it remains unclear whether these alkaloids are produced endogenously or exogenously, they can certainly be detected in vertebrate tissues. Very recently, Donnerer et al. (1986) demonstrated a marked increase in the levels of codeine and morphine in rat tissues after administration of salutaridine and thebaine, suggesting that there is a biosynthetic pathway to morphine in mammals. Perhaps morphine, the plant alkaloid responsible for the birth of opioid research, retains some influence on the highly diversified and specialized opioid system that has developed in vertebrates.

3. Peptides Derived from Proopiomelanocortin

Proopiomelanocortin, or POMC, is a glycoprotein of 31 kdalton that has been identified as the precursor of adrenocorticotrophic hormone (ACTH), β-lipotropin (β-LPH), β-endorphin (β-end), γ-melanocyte-stimulating hormone (γ-MSH), α-MSH, γ-LPH, and corticotropin-like intermediate lobe peptide (CLIP) (Fig. 1). The precursor–product relationships were first identified through radiolabeling studies of mouse pituitary ACTH-producing tumor cells (AtT-20) and through cell-free biosynthesis directed by messenger RNA from bovine pituitary or AtT-20 cells (for review of these studies, *see* Eipper and Mains, 1980). The structural assumptions from these data were completely corroborated by the nucleotide sequence representing either mRNA or DNA encoding the precursor. The nucleotide sequence now has been determined for the bovine, human, rat, and mouse precursors (*see* Eberwine and Roberts, 1983, for review). It appears that there is only one gene encoding the POMC sequence, and alternative splicing probably accounts for different messenger sizes found in certain tissues (Jingami et al., 1984).

Unlike proenkephalin and prodynorphin, which have gene-duplicated the enkephalin nucleus, the duplication in POMC is for the MSH portion of the molecule. It therefore seems an appropriate question to ask whether the precursor has had evolutionary pressure to be an opioid precursor, or an MSH precursor. One could postulate that both activities are used by animals, albeit on different neurons. Alternatively, both bioactive molecules may function in the same areas and interact synergistically, as suggested by some experiments demonstrating analgesia by α-MSH (Walker et al., 1980). In any event, it seems appropriate when discussing the forms of endorphins to include some information on MSH.

With the exception of γ- and α-endorphin, the known bioactive fragments generated from POMC are flanked at both the C-terminal and N-terminal by pairs of basic residues (*see* Fig. 1). Furthermore, ACTH and β-end, both potent biologically active molecules, contain pairs of basic residues within their structures. This would suggest that not all pairs of basic residues are equally susceptible to enzymic cleavage by the processing enzymes, an important issue that will recur when analyzing the products of the other opioid precursors. Pulse-chase labeling studies in primary pituitary cell cultures have outlined a processing pathway in this tissue. Initial cleavage occurs at the C-terminus of ACTH, leaving β-LPH, the C-terminal non-opioid fragment containing the sequence of the opioid β-end at the C-terminus. Subsequent cleavages of the resulting fragments give rise to ACTH and β-end (1-31), and in turn these can be processed down to α-MSH and smaller endorphins (*see* Eipper and Mains, 1980, for review). It is

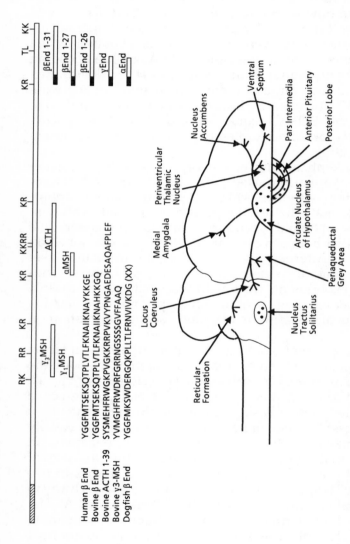

Human β End YGGFMTSEKSQTPLVTLFKNAIIKNAYKGE
Bovine β End YGGFMTSEKSQTPLVTLFKNAIIKNAHKKGQ
Bovine ACTH 1-39 SYSMEHFRWGKPVGKKRRPVKVYPNGAEDESAQAFPLEF
Bovine γ3-MSH YVMGHFRWDRFGRRNGSSSSGVFFAAQ
Dogfish β End YGGFMKSWDERGQKPLLTLFRNVIVKDG (XX)

Fig. 1. Diagram representing the structure of bovine POMC and distribution of POMC-containing cell bodies (stippled area) and projections (tridents) in rat brain and pituitary. The primary amino acid sequence of the bioactive molecules are represented by the single-letter code such that the sequence of all bioactive processing products can be deduced. Also included for comparison are sequences of β-end found in a selection of other species. Symbols: cross-hatched bars, signal peptide; solid black bars, opiate-active enkephalin nucleus; A, alanine; D, aspartic acid; E, glutamic acid; F, phenylalanine; G, glycine; H, histidine; I, isoleucine; K, lysine; L, leucine; S, methionine; N, asparagine; P, proline; Q, glutamine; R, arginine; S, serine; T, threonine; V, valine; W, tryptophan; Y, tyrosine; X, unknown.

by no means clear, however, whether this processing pathway is used by every POMC-producing cell.

The majority of experiments on POMC have been conducted on rodents. Considerable variability in opiate receptor distribution, precursor expression, and posttranslational processing has been observed in the same tissues of different species. It therefore may be inappropriate to assign activities to a particular endorphin source between species. Several examples of these processing differences will be given throughout the chapter, especially when they may have direct relevance to possible in vivo functions.

Peptides derived from POMC have a comparatively narrow distribution. In all the mammals that have been investigated, the highest concentration of POMC products has been found in the pituitary. Both the anterior and intermediate lobe of the pituitary synthesize POMC, albeit the final precursor products are considerably different in each tissue. In the anterior lobe of the pituitary, the production of ACTH is considered to be the physiologically important synthesis to control circulating steroids released from the adrenal cortex. The cells in the anterior lobe accordingly process POMC to ACTH via two cleavages at lysyl-arginine residues (see Fig. 1). In the intermediate lobe, however, ACTH is further cleaved at a Lys-Lys-Arg-Arg sequence to form α-MSH. This 13-residue peptide is amidated at the C-terminus, and, in the rat intermediate lobe, acetylated at the N-terminus—a modification that considerably increases its melanocyte-stimulating activity in vivo (Guttman and Boissonnas, 1961).

The endorphin-containing region of POMC follows a somewhat parallel processing pattern to the ACTH region. In the anterior lobe, β-LPH [an opiate-inactive precursor of β-end (1-31)] predominates (for synopsis, see Smyth, 1983). In the intermediate lobe, more extensive processing occurs to form β-end (1-27), via a cleavage at a Lys-Lys bond, and in some species, β-end (1-26) (Smyth, 1983; Evans et al., 1981). The formation of β-end (1-26) probably results from exopeptidase attack on the C-terminal histidine residue of β-end (1-27) by a carboxy peptidase E-like enzyme (Fricker et al., 1982). Like α-MSH, the endorphins are also found to be acetylated at the N-terminal residue (Smyth et al., 1979). This is an extremely critical posttranslational modification of endorphin, since it prevents the N-terminal amino group from ionizing. As reviewed in the introduction, the positive charge at the N-terminus of enkephalins and endorphins is an absolute requirement for opioid activity, and, consequently, acetylation completely inactivates the endorphins as opioid peptides.

The analysis of α-N-acetylated endorphins has been greatly facilitated by a specific radioimmunoassay that does not cross-react with opioid active (nonacetylated) endorphins. The assay used in conjunction with a middle region or C-terminally directed β-end radioimmunoassay that detects both forms allows the ratio of acetylated to nonacetylated endorphins to be measured in various tissues (Weber et al., 1982c). Studies using this antisera confirm that it is predominantly the intermediate lobe of the pituitary that is responsible for the high concentrations of acetyl endorphins in this tissue (*see* Table 1). The human pituitary is at variance from many other mammalian species in that it has no classical neurointermediate lobe. It is important to note that in the adult human pituitary, no acetylated endorphin or acetylated α-MSH can be detected (Weber et al., 1982c; Evans et al., 1982). The question of an activity for acetylated endorphins other than as opiates has been raised many times, but at present no satisfactory role for these peptides has been discovered.

Aside from the pituitary gland, POMC products have been detected immunologically in other peripheral tissues, including the pancreas, gastric antrum, placenta, testes, and adrenal medulla. In pancreas, multiple forms of β-end immunoreactive peptides have been observed, the principal products in rat pancreas assigned as derivatives of β-end (1-27) and β-end (1-26) (Smyth, 1983). There appears to be very little β-LPH in this tissue. In gastric antrum, there are conflicting data as to whether the β-end immunoreactive material is β-LPH- or β-end-sized, and there have been suggestions of O-sulfation of β-end tyrosyl residues in this tissue (for overview, *see* Smyth, 1983).

Considerably more studies have been directed at the POMC products in placental tissue. The presence of ACTH in the placenta was first observed in the early 1970s, and placenta was postulated as the primary source for increased circulating ACTH during pregnancy (Rees et al., 1975). Later studies revealed that immunoreactive peptides corresponding to β-end and β-LPH were present in placental extracts (Nakai et al., 1978). Placental cells kept in primary culture synthesize glycosylated POMC and appear to process the precursor to form peptides with immunological and gel filtration chromatographic properties identical to β-LPH, β-end, ACTH (1-39), and α-MSH (Liotta and Krieger, 1980). It appears from further analysis of this immunoreactivity that α-N-acetylation does not occur in these cells. The processing in placenta is apparently more extensive than in anterior pituitary

TABLE 1
Distribution of α-N-Acetylation of β-Endorphin in Areas of Pituitary
in the Pituitary Adrenal Axis in Different Species[a]

Tissue	Immunoreactivity, nmol/g tissue		Relative degree of acetylation, %
	Middle region β-endorphin RIA	α-N-Acetyl β-endorphin RIA	
Rat pituitary			
Posterior lobe			
Intermediate lobe	1100.0 ± 121.5	1011.0 ± 106.51	92
Anterior lobe	39.2 ± 4.6	4.1 ± 0.35	10
Bovine pituitary			
Posterior lobe	2.18 ± 0.4	1.16 ± 0.5	53
Intermediate lobe	664.8 ± 58.4	323.9 ± 42.3	49
Anterior lobe	56.0 ± 8.4	1.78 ± 0.3	3
Human pituitary			
Posterior lobe	31.0 ± 7.3	ND	0
Anterior lobe	112.0 ± 16.8	ND	0
Rat adrenal	ND	ND	
Human adrenal medulla	0.14 ± 0.014	ND	0
Bovine adrenal	ND	ND	

[a]For references regarding these values, see Evans et al. (1985b).

cells, both as determined by primary cell culture labeling studies and analysis of tissue extracts.

The Leydig cells of the rat testis have been shown by immunocytochemistry and *in situ* hybridization to express both POMC protein and POMC RNA (Pintar et al., 1984; Tsong et al., 1982). Although the message is slightly shorter than the POMC and mRNA found in rat pituitary and hypothalamus, there apparently is still expression of this message form (Chen et al., 1984). It is interesting that the concentrations of POMC peptides in this tissue are 2–3 orders of magnitude lower than in the hypothalamus, although the message levels are approximately equivalent in the two tissues. The major forms of POMC in rat testis extract are β-end and α-MSH, both found in the nonacetylated forms (Margioris et al., 1983).

In the adrenal medulla, the expression of POMC-derived peptides appears to be very species-specific and has been observed only in human and monkey adrenal extracts (Evans et al., 1983, 1985b). It should be noted, however, that bovine adrenals contain a short form of POMC message that appears not to be expressed (Jingami et al., 1984). The major forms of stored bioactive peptides in human adrenal appear to be β-end (1-31) and desacetyl α-MSH. There is no evidence for significant amounts of β-LPH or shorter forms of β-end in this tissue, and authentic ACTH (1-39) is present in very low concentrations (Evans et al., 1983). Immunocytochemistry indicates that cells staining for α-MSH and β-end are not the same population as those staining for proenkephalin (unpublished observation).

Production of POMC in such close proximity to the adrenal cortex, the target organ for ACTH, raises questions as to the possible role of POMC in this tissue. This role may be in the adult or perhaps the developing fetus when α-MSH is a potent secretagogue of corticosteriods (Glickman et al., 1979).

The major sites of cell bodies synthesizing POMC peptides in brain are located in the arcuate nucleus of the hypothalamus. An extensive fiber system originating from these cell bodies terminates in many areas of the brain (*see* Fig. 1). A more minor group of cell bodies is located in the nucleus tractus solitarius of the brain stem. The arcuate POMC-producing cells have recently been nicely visualized by *in situ* hybridization and immunocytochemistry demonstrating colocalization of cDNA to POMC message and POMC peptides (Gee et al., 1983). Figure 1 shows a cartoon of the areas of brain containing POMC products, but detailed anatomical and RIA data can be obtained from the following references: Frederickson (1984); Akil et al. (1984); O'Donohue and Dorsa (1982); Bloom et al. (1978a,b).

Although β-end and α-MSH have been known to be present in the brain for nearly a decade, there is still much controversy as to the molecular variants in different brain regions. This may be because of very low concentrations of POMC products in this tissue; consequently, differences in extraction techniques and RIA protocols become important factors in the analysis of the peptides. The major controversy is whether or not α-N-acetylation is a major modification of endorphins and α-MSH in brain. The α-MSH immunoreactive material was originally analyzed by Loh et al. (1980) and O'Donohue et al. (1982). Both groups found substantial quantities of a α-N-acetylated α-MSH in brain. Using acid acetone extracts of both hypothalamus and midbrain, we have been unable to repeat these results and find only one form of α-MSH material that possesses identical chromatographic properties to desacetyl α-MSH (Evans et al., 1982). The absence of acetylated α-MSH in rat brain has now been reported by another group (Geis et al., 1984).

A more relevant issue to this chapter is whether β-end is α-N-acetylated in brain. Initial analyses were performed by Zakarian and Smyth (1979) using cation-exchange chromatography and analyzing the β-end immunoreactive profiles. The conclusions from these studies were that acetylation occurs in terminal areas where β-end may be released. Using the acetyl-specific antisera in an RIA, we found less than 2% acetylation of β-end immunoreactive material in brain, and this disappeared following hypophysectomy of the animals, indicating a pituitary origin (Weber et al., 1981). In immunohistochemical studies, the acetyl antisera showed no staining in either cell body or terminal POMC areas unless the sections had been chemically acetylated with acetic anhydride prior to staining (Weber et al., 1981). Other groups have indicated variable degrees of acetylation in brain areas (Akil et al., 1983, 1984; O'Donohue et al., 1982, for reviews). The acetylation of β-end would have very interesting implications if this were indeed a mechanism for controlling activity, especially when viewed together with the possible enhancement of biological activity by the same modification of α-MSH.

The issue of posttranslation processing of β-end at the C-terminus has received some attention (Zakarian and Smyth, 1982). The majority of studies agree that β-end immunoreactive material is processed down from β-LPH to β-endorphin-sized peptides. In hypothalamus, the major form of β-end appears to be β-end (1-31), which is the most potent analgesic of the endogenous endorphins (Geisow et al., 1977). In more terminal regions, such as the limbic system and brain stem, C-terminal processing to form β-end (1-27) has been reported (Zakarian and Smyth, 1979). In any event, the processing in brain seems to be very different from that found either in the intermediate lobe of the pituitary or the anterior lobe of the pituitary.

The interest in β-end has resulted in the sequencing of this opioid peptide from several species, including salmon, ostrich, dogfish, human, camel, bovine, ovine, porcine, and equine sources (*see* Kawauchi, 1983, for overview). In all species the [Met]enkephalin sequence is present at the N-terminus. There are important species differences, however, with regard to α-N-acetylation. For example, salmon β-end found in the pituitary is almost invariably α-N-acetylated (Kawauchi, 1983). This contrasts with the absence of α-N-acetylated β-endorphins in the dogfish pituitary (Lorenz et al., 1986). Both the salmon and the dogfish β-end sequence have a basic residue (a lysine) following the N-terminal [Met]enkephalin sequence. Analysis of the processing products of POMC in the shark pituitary show there is a product representing cleavage at a single lysine residue at the C-terminus (Lorenz et al., 1986). If the single lysine at position 6 in shark β-end were cleaved, this would result in the pentapeptide [Met]-enkephalin, an opioid peptide with very different characteristics from β-end (*see* Fig. 1). With this in mind, it is conceivable that β-end may have played a crucial role during the evolution of the vertebrate enkephalinergic opioid system.

4. Processing Products Derived from Proenkephalin

Proenkephalin is an opioid peptide precursor of very similar molecular weight to POMC, but with multiple copies of the enkephalin nucleus. In mammals, proenkephalin has six copies of Tyr-Gly-Gly-Phe-Met and one copy of Tyr-Gly-Gly-Phe-Leu. Interestingly, in frog all seven of the enkephalin nuclei correspond to Tyr-Gly-Gly-Phe-Met (*see* Herbert et al., 1985, for review on genetic structure). There is some structural similarity with POMC at the N-terminus of the precursor relating to the pattern of cysteine residues. Proenkephalin gives rise to a large spectrum of opioid peptides, including [Met]enkephalin, peptide F, amidorphin, [Met]enkephalin-Arg-Gly-Leu, peptide E, BAM 22, BAM 18, BAM 12, metorphamide, [Leu]enkephalin, and [Met]enkephalin-Arg-Phe (*see* Fig. 2). The processing varies considerably between tissues and often results in the formation of nonopioid fragments with enkephalin nuclei embedded within the body of the sequence.

Proenkephalin products have a wide distribution throughout the central and peripheral nervous system (for review, *see* Frederickson et al., 1981; Herbert et al., 1985; Akil et al., 1984; Hokfelt et al., 1977). High concentrations of proenkephalin-derived peptides and mRNA are found in the adrenals of many mammals, although extremely variable processing and different absolute concentrations exist between species (Evans et al., 1985b). In some tissues, such as rat heart, there are very high concentrations of mRNA-encoding proenkephalin, but only very low peptide concentrations, underlining an emerging recognition that mRNA levels are not necessarily good indicators of stored peptide levels.

Probably the most systematic and useful method of dissecting the processing of proenkephalin is to start at the N-terminus and gradually work to the C-terminus (*see* Fig. 2). Some important studies have been undertaken with antisera generated to a N-terminal fragment (NTF) of proenkephalin, originally isolated from bovine adrenal by virtue of a single enkephalin nucleus embedded within the sequence (Liston et al., 1983). In extracts of bovine striatum, antisera directed to NTF detect a peptide of molecular weight similar to that isolated from adrenal glands. The brain immunoreactive fragment lacks the enkephalin nucleus, however, and was therefore named syn-enkephalin. Results obtained using this antisera provided early evidence that the adrenal proenkephalin was structurally similar to the brain precursor, although the processing was somewhat different.

The enkephalin nucleus situated closest to the N-terminal in proenkephalin (residues 100–104 of the human precursor and residues 97–101 of the bovine precursor) has not been a focus of interest. This enkephalin nucleus is flanked at the C-terminus by Lys-Arg and at the N-terminus by Lys-Arg in the human sequence and Lys-Lys in the bovine sequence. In bovine adrenal this enkephalin nucleus likely constitutes the C-terminus of NTF because Lys-Lys is not a favored cleavage site. It should be noted

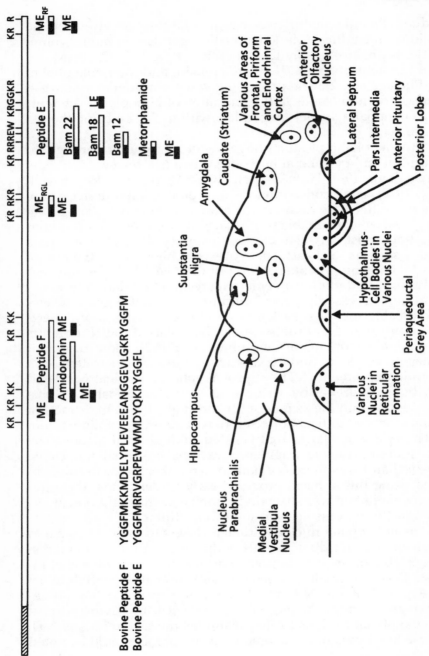

Fig. 2. Structure of bovine proenkephalin and distribution of proenkephalin in the rat brain (*see* Fig. 1 for symbols).

that in bovine caudate, however, this pair of lysine residues does represent a processing site, as evidenced by the characterization of syn-enkephalin.

The second enkephalin nucleus in proenkephalin separated only by a Lys-Arg from the first enkephalin nucleus is followed by an Arg-Arg sequence. Analysis of the peptides generated from the processing of prodynorphin and other neuroactive peptide precursors suggests that Arg-Arg is not a favored precusor processing site. It is, therefore, not surprising that C-terminally extended forms of this enkephalin nucleus have been shown to be present in various tissues. One such opiate, peptide F, a 3.8-kdalton peptide isolated from bovine adrenal, is interesting in that it has enkephalin nuclei from both the C- and N-terminus (Kilpatrick et al., 1981). Although peptide F can be detected in relatively high concentrations in bovine adrenal extracts, this processing product exists only in negligible concentrations in brain extracts (Hollt et al., 1982b).

Studies on an N-terminal fragment of peptide F, namely amidorphin, have shed more light on the processing of this area of proenkephalin. The structure of amidorphin was predicted from the cDNA sequence of proenkephalin using the following rationale. Just prior to the C-terminal enkephalin nucleus of peptide F (the third enkephalin nucleus in proenkephalin) is the sequence X_1-Gly-Lys-Arg-X_2. This sequence is a consensus sequence found in many precursors for C-terminal amidation. The series of events thought to occur are cleavage at the carboxyl site of lysine or arginine followed by carboxy peptidase B-like activity exposing the free C-terminal glycine. The glycine residue is then enzymatically decarboxylated to X_1-amide (Bradbury et al., 1981). In order to demonstrate the existence of this processing product, amidorphin was synthesized, antisera generated, and an RIA developed that was utilized to isolate immunoreactive material from various bovine tissues (Seizinger et al., 1985). The immunoreactivity was characterized by sequencing and shown to correspond to intact amidorphin in bovine adrenal. When amidorphin immunoreactivity material was analyzed in bovine brain, the major product proved not to be amidorphin, but the C-terminal 19 amino acids lacking the N-terminal enkephalin sequence (Liebisch et al., 1986). In this case, the immunoreactive material in brain is not opiate-active and provides an example of an amidated peptide that may not be biologically active. In the human precursor, the C-terminus of amidorphin is preceded by alanine, not glycine, and this exchange probably renders the peptide unable to be amidated. Whether the C-terminal amidaton of amidorphin affects the stability and/or receptor interaction of this fragment has not yet been investigated.

For the following reasons, it would be reasonable to assume that in striatum, and probably many other areas of brain, the major brain processing product of the N-terminal three enkephalin nuclei is the pentapeptide [Met]enkephalin itself.

1. The high concentration of amidorphin (7-26) in brain.
2. The absence of enkephalin on the N-terminus of proenkephalin in striatum (syn-enkephalin).
3. The absence of peptide F in brain.
4. The very high concentrations of [Met]enkephalin in many brain areas.

The fourth [Met]enkephalin nucleus (proenkephalin residues 182–186 of the bovine sequence) is one of two enkephalin nuclei that have no pairs of basic residues immediately following the enkephalin sequence. A pair of arginine residues occur three residues downstream, however, following an arginine, glycine, and leucine residue. The octapeptide, [Met]enkepahlin-Arg-Gly-Leu, is found in high concentrations in many brain areas (Lindberg and Yang, 1984). The original identification of this sequence was from extracts of bovine adrenal. In this tissue, the sequence is found at the C-terminus of a nonopioid 3.6-kdalton peptide (Stern et al., 1981). In brain, multiple forms of [Met]enkephalin-Arg-Gly-Leu immunoreactive material exist (Lindberg and Yang, 1984). In striatum and hypothalamic extracts, the octapeptide appears to be the major stored processing product. In pons medulla, however, a large proportion of the immunoreactivity is, according to gel filtration analysis of higher molecular weight (>2 kdalton), possibly identical to peptide B described by Stern et al., 1981.

In guinea pig adrenal, the high molecular weight species is the predominant form of [Met]enkephalin-Arg-Gly-Leu immunoreactivity. In this tissue, the [Met]enkephalin-Arg-Gly-Leu immunoreactive material, when acetylated with acetic anhydride, does not react with antisera recognizing α-N-acetyl Tyr-Gly-Gly-Phe-X (unpublished results). This observation suggests there is no enkephalin nucleus at the N-terminus, and consequently this processing product as stored in the adrenal is not opiate-active. In brain, there are no conclusive experiments to determine if this high molecular weight species is opiate-active or not.

The region between the [Met]enkephalin nucleus residues 296–300 and the only [Leu]enkephalin nucleus residue in bovine proenkephalin has been a major focus of study. Peptide E isolated from bovine adrenal is analogous to peptide F in that there is an enkephalin nucleus at each end of the molecule, a [Met]enkephalin sequence at the N-terminus and a [Leu]enkephalin at the C-terminus (Kilpatrick et al., 1981). This peptide produces analgesia, but like peptide F, is not found in high concentrations in brain (Hollt et al., 1982a). There is a series of opioid-active fragments of this region of proenkephalin that are endogenous to both brain and adrenals of many species. These include [Leu]enkephalin, BAM 22, BAM 12, metorphamide (BAM 1-8 Amide or adrenophin), and [Met]enkephalin.

The opioid peptides BAM 12 and BAM 22 are found in only very low concentrations in brain compared to other proenkephalin processing products (Hollt et al., 1982b; Baird et al., 1982). It should be recognized that if the processing in any tissue goes entirely via BAM 22 (Mizumo et al., 1980), no [Leu]enkephalin would be formed from proenkephalin.

Recently we have isolated and characterized BAM 18 from bovine adrenal glands. Specific antisera were generated to BAM 18, and this peptide was found as a major product in bovine adrenal and rat brain tissues. Table 2 shows the ratio of metorphamide to BAM 18 in various rat brain regions. Preliminary studies show the receptor profile of BAM 18 to be very similar to that of

TABLE 2

Concentration of Immunoreactive BAM 18 and Metorphamide in Rat Brain Regions

Brain region	Immunoreactivity, pmol per g tissue	
	BAM 18	Metorphamide
Spinal cord	86.6 ± 7.84	8.7 ± 0.4
Midbrain	63.3 ± 6.80	5.2 ± 0.4
Cerebellum	18.6 ± 2.40	Undetectable
Hippocampus	16.9 ± 2.66	Undetectable
Pons/medulla	122.0 ± 4.50	5.4 ± 0.9
Hypothalamus	156.7 ± 18.50	5.7 ± 1.3
Striatum	165.7 ± 13.40	7.0 ± 0.6
Cortex	10.0 ± 1.63	Undetectable
Pituitary	6.7 ± 2.50	Undetectable
Adrenal	Undetectable	Undetectable

metorphamide (Hurlbut et al., submitted). It is unclear, however, whether the in vivo stability of these two peptides could influence their biological activity. To determine if this portion of proen-kephalin is converted to metorphamide or [Met]enkephalin, we raised antisera to the C-terminus of BAM 18, residues 10–18. The material in brain recognized by this antisera was isolated, charac-terized, and found to correspond entirely to BAM 8-18, sug-gesting cleavage at the pair of arginine residues to release the C-terminus of [Met]enkephalin and not metorphamide.

Somewhat surprising was the lack of BAM 10-18 or BAM 11-18 in the bovine caudate extracts. If processing proceeded via BAM 18, one of these peptides would be expected to be present as a result of production of metorphamide, originally isolated from the same tissue (Weber et al., 1983a). An explanation of this may be that the processing of metorphamide occurs via a different route, since the techniques employed should have detected BAM 10-18 or 11-18 if they were present in concentrations equivalent to those of metorphamide. It is important to note that metorph-amide is a result of cleavage at a single arginine residue that is preceded in the sequence by a glycine residue. Cleavage of single arginines appears to be common in many neuroactive precursors; the amidation process has been discussed earlier in this section in connection with amidorphin.

[Met]Enkephalin-Arg-Phe represents the C-terminus of pro-enkephalin. This enkephalin nucleus was originally identified from bovine adrenal as part of a 3.6-kdalton nonopioid-active peptide corresponding to cleavage at the C-terminus of [Leu]en-kephalin sequence residues 231–232 of bovine proenkephalin (Jones et al., 1982). Immunoreactive material with chromato-graphic properties similar to the 3.6-kdalton peptide has been identified in guinea pig adrenal (Evans et al., 1985c). In rat, the ratio of authentic heptapeptide to a larger molecular weight mate-rial varies throughout the brain in a similar manner to that found for [Met]enkephalin-Arg-Gly-Leu immunoreactivity. In hypothal-amus and striatum, the immunoreactivity is predominantly the heptapeptide size. In other regions, multiple forms of [Met]en-kephalin-Arg-Phe are present that are of considerably greater mo-lecular weight. The exact nature of these forms remains to be investigated (Yang et al., 1983). Conceivably, both the octapep-tide [Met]enkephalin-Arg-Gly-Leu and the heptapeptide [Met]-enkephalin-Arg-Phe may be further processed at the single argi-nine residue to form enkephalin. This processing step has not been demonstrated, however.

In summary, the processing of proenkephalin in brain seems to give rise to mostly smaller opioid products representing cleavages at all pairs of basic residues and some single arginine residues. BAM 18 and higher molecular weight peptides containing octapeptide and heptapeptide immunoreactivity also appear to be present in brain. In bovine adrenal, processing appears to be much less complete, resulting in high molecular weight species containing opioid nuclei. In the adrenals of other species such as humans, however, more extensive processing does seem to occur (*see* Imura et al., 1985, for overview).

5. Processing Products Derived from Prodynorphin

Prodynorphin is a precursor with characteristics very similar to both proenkephalin and POMC, both with regard to size and message construction (*see* Herbert el al., 1985, for a recent review). The active peptides are clustered at the C-terminus of the precursor, and the pattern of cysteine residues at the N-terminus is very reminiscent of those found in POMC and proenkephalin. Two species of prodynorphin mRNA have been reported. In the rat brain, a mRNA of ~2.8 kbases predominates (Jingami et al., 1984). In the rat adrenal, a smaller message is present in high concentrations (Jim Douglas, personal communication), although there are no prodynorphin products detectable in this tissue (Evans et al., 1985b). In guinea pig adrenal that does express prodynorphin, the larger message and the smaller message are present (Eberwine, unpublished observation). The data available indicate that the smaller message may not be translated. If this is true, only probes differentiating the two messages should be used for localization of the biologically relevant message. Immunoreactive material corresponding to the neoendorphins and dynorphins is widely distributed throughout the brain and spinal cord, the highest concentrations being in the anterior hypothalamic nuclei, in which axons project to the posterior pituitary (*see* Akil et al., 1984; Khachaturian et al., 1982). Dynorphin-derived peptides can also be observed in the anterior pituitary, reticular formation, caudate, hippocampus, and many regions of cortex (*see* Fig. 3).

The processing of prodynorphin is relatively simple compared with that of POMC or proenkephalin. There is no evidence for α-N-acetylation of any prodynorphin fragments. In parallel with many of the enkephalin nuclei in proenkephalin, all three of the opioid core sequences in prodynorphin are followed by pairs

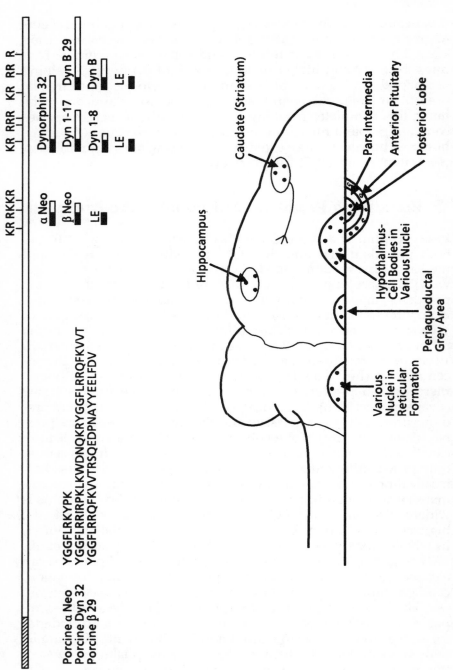

Fig. 3. Structure of porcine prodynorphin and distribution in rat brain (*see* Fig. 1 for symbols).

of basic residues. The question of [Leu]enkephalin being a product of this precursor is important given the very different receptor selectivity and in vivo activity of [Leu]enkephalin compared to the C-terminally extended neoendorphins and dynorphins. Evidence that prodynorphin does indeed give rise to [Leu]enkephalin has been obtained by lesioning the nigrostriatal pathway and demonstrating parallel changes in [Leu]enkephalin and other prodynorphin products in the caudate (Zamir et al., 1984). Dehydration experiments also show that [Leu]enkephalin in posterior pituitary is probably derived from prodynorphin (Lorenz et al., 1985). The production of [Leu]enkephalin from prodynorphin does not appear to be a major pathway, however.

The first peptide fragment of prodynorphin isolated was α-neoendorphin. This 10-residue peptide has a C-terminal lysine residue preceded in sequence by a proline residue (*see* Fig. 3). The sister peptide β-neoendorphin lacks the basic residue. The proline immediately preceding the lysine in α-neoendorphin probably renders this site unattractive to enzymic cleavage. The ratio between α-neoendorphin and β-neoendorphin differs widely throughout the brain (Weber et al., 1982b). This may be attributed either to different concentrations or ratios of available enzyme(s) performing this cleavage, differences in rates of turnover of the precursor peptide, or other factors regulating the processing.

Dehydration, a physiological stimulus inducing vasopressin release from the posterior pituitary, results in co-secretion of the co-stored prodynorphin products from the posterior pituitary. This provides an excellent model for studying the dynamics of the prodynorphin system. Dehydration has recently been shown to change the ratio of α-neoendorphin and β-neoendorphin stored in the posterior pituitary lobe. Although the issue is complex, it is conceivable that the ratio of these products may be useful as some measure of turnover of the precursor in certain tissues, a physiologically relevant measurement at present unavailable (Lorenz et al., 1985).

Dynorphin A [dynorphin (1-17)], from which the precursor has been named, was the second opioid-active peptide from prodynorphin to be characterized. Most studies have been aimed at this peptide. The single arginine residue at position 9 appears particularly susceptible to processing enzymes such that dynorphin (1-8) is the major product in rat brain and pituitary. Table 3 shows the ratio of dynorphin (1-8) to dynorphin (1-17) in various areas of rat brain (Weber et al., 1982a). In posterior pituitary, the

TABLE 3
Concentration of Immunoreactive Dynorphin (1-17)
and Dynorphin (1-8) in Rat Brain Regions

Brain region	Immunoreactivity, pmol per g tissue	
	Dynorphin (1-17)	Dynorphin (1-8)
Spinal cord	12.1 ± 2.3	22.7 ± 1.6
Midbrain	6.2 ± 1.0	59.6 ± 3.7
Cerebellum	<0.2	<1.2
Hippocampus	3.4 ± 0.7	26.5 ± 2.2
Pons/medulla	3.9 ± 0.4	22.5 ± 0.6
Hypothalamus	10.3 ± 1.1	65.5 ± 1.8
Striatum	7.3 ± 0.7	64.1 ± 4.1
Cortex	2.6 ± 0.6	21.0 ± 1.9
Posterior pituitary	503.6 ± 32.9	1384.0 ± 84.4

ratio of dynorphin (1-8) to dynorphin (1-17) is 3:1. But this ratio is not consistent throughout the brain. In midbrain, for example, the ratio is 9:1.

A third product from this portion of the precursor is an extended form of dynorphin (1-17), dynorphin (1-32), which has been isolated from hypothalamic extracts (Fischli et al., 1982a). This product (*see* Fig. 3) has a lysyl-arginine residue following the dynorphin (1-17) portion, in turn followed by the dynorphin B sequence. Dynorphin (1-32) appears to be in higher concentrations in whole rat brain than is authentic dynorphin (1-17) (Cone et al., 1983). The existence of dynorphin (1-32) argues that the single arginine cleavage site at position 14 in dynorphin B (*see* Fig. 3) is a very susceptible cleavage in some areas of brain and proceeds in favor to the lysyl-arginine cleavage at the C-terminus of dynorphin A. This processing step has been the subject of intense studies by Devi and Goldstein, 1984.

Yet a fourth species of approximately 7 kdaltons, containing both dynorphin (1-17) and dynorphin B immunoreactive material, is present in rat brain (Fischli et al., 1982b). In guinea pig adrenal glands, this species may be the sole processing product of this area of prodynorphin (Evans et al., 1985c). It is questionable whether this species is opiate-active or has α-neoendorphin at the N-terminus.

Dynorphin B itself is a 13-amino acid peptide generated by a single arginine cleavage of prodynorphin. This opioid is found in high concentrations in many brain areas (Cone et al., 1983). Some studies indicate that an extended form of dynorphin B, leumorphin, is a major product in brain and, because of its highly acidic nature, requires neutral extraction prior to RIA (Nakao et al., 1983). In acid extracts of rat brain, leumorphin is reported to be a very minor processing product (Cone et al., 1983). Employing an antisera to the C-terminus of prodynorphin (residues 242–256 of the porcine sequence), a single product was detected in acid acetone extracts of bovine caudate. This peptide has been isolated and characterized, and shown to correspond to the 15 C-terminal residues of leumorphin, the expected product from cleavage at the single arginine required for release of dynorphin B from the precursor (Evans et al., 1985a). It appears that in parallel with cleavages at paired basic residues, the arginine cannot be found on either prodynorphin C fragment or dynorphin B, suggesting that either the enzyme cleaves on both sides of the arginine residue (suggested by studies by Devi and Goldstein, 1984) or, alternatively, that a carboxy-peptidase B or amino-peptidase B cleaves at the arginine residue following a trypsin-like clip.

Although proenkephalin and prodynorphin have many structural similarities, and the precursors are often colocalized (Basbaum and Fields, 1984; Evans et al., 1985c), the processing patterns are distinctly different. The major products of proenkephalin in brain are the enkephalins [Met]enkephalin-Arg-Gly-Leu and [Met]enkephalin-Arg-Phe, representing cleavages at all paired basic residues. The processing of prodynorphin appears to be considerably less complete, with the major opioid products retaining paired basic residues linking C-terminal extensions to the enkephalin nuclei. These C-terminal extensions have endowed many of the prodynorphin-derived opioid peptides with high affinity for kappa receptors (James et al., 1984).

6. Receptor Interactions and Further Considerations

In this chapter, we have concentrated on the three characterized precursors of opioid peptides. Although, increasing evidence suggests the presence of other endogenous opioids. Immunoreactive dermorphin—an opioid peptide isolated from frog skin—has been detected in vertebrate tissue (Buffa et al., 1982; Negri et al., 1981). Antibodies are notoriously promiscuous, however, and this immunoreactivity requires further characterization. With regard to morphine and associated alkaloids in vertebrates, experiments are in progress to determine if these opiates are stored and made in secretory vesicles or are merely drifting around under no effective biological control.

From the preceding information in this chapter, it is clear that the processing of the three opioid precursors is not homogeneous, giving rise to different tribes of peptides in different tissues. Some products appear to be stored in an inactive form because of either incomplete processing or deactivation by posttranslational modifications. The question of whether activation can occur extracellularly following release of these peptides has been considered. To date, however, there has not been convincing evidence to demonstrate postrelease activation. A related issue is whether there is a discrete subset of granules released, or if this is a random event. The studies cited here have focused on stored peptide pools, and the issue of the actual peptides released is crucial. Several reviews have dealt with this issue and with opioids in CSF and blood (Frederickson and Geary, 1982; Akil et al., 1984). Following release, the opioid peptides are subjected to a battery of extracellular enzymes. In brain, the attack seems to be most virulent by exopeptidases. Small unblocked peptides have proved to be very susceptible to attack by brain aminopeptidase and carboxypeptidases (*see* Frederickson and Geary, 1982, for review). Consequently, endogenous opioids such as enkephalin would not be expected to have effects at sites distant from their release because of rapid degradation by peptidases such as metalloendopeptidase ("enkephalinase") or aminopeptidase. Larger peptides, such as β-end appear to be relatively stable and, consequently, may function in a more neurohormonal-type role.

The question of whether a particular precursor is tailor-made for a particular receptor type is often raised. The evidence would indicate that endogenous opioids are pure agonists at all receptor types, albeit very different concentrations are required for activation of the different receptor types. The concept of receptor selectivity for each opioid peptide is only relevant if the opioid peptide has a choice. The issue then becomes one of localization of receptors with regard to the site of release and of stability of the ligands in the extracellular matrix. The techniques of immunocytochemistry and receptor autoradiography are helping us understand the microdistribution of receptor types and the opioid ligands in closest proximity.

The processing of opioid peptides can drastically influence their receptor affinity and selectivity. This has been the subject of a previous review (Weber et al., 1983b). Pharmacologically, the endogenous opioid peptides have very different actions. Analgesia, perhaps the best studied pharmacological action of opioids, is discussed later in this chapter. In the pharmacological testing of analgesia, multiple receptor sites are available for interaction with the exogenous peptides, and consequently, receptor selectivity, as well as stability and site of injection, are crucial factors that may not be significant for endogenous peptides confined to the microenvironment of the synapse. The issue of receptor–ligand interactions in vivo is presently very complex and is addressed in a separate chapter.

7. Pharmacological and Physiological Effects of the Endogenous Opioid Peptides

Elucidation of the pharmacological and physiological actions of the dynorphins, enkephalins, and endorphins was hampered initially by their metabolic instability and relatively low potency. The introduction of more stable and potent structural analogs of the endogenous opioid peptides has revealed more fully the diversity of their actions. In addition, studies of the effects of opioid antagonists and inhibitors of opioid peptide degradation have provided insight into the tonic nature of their involvement. Studies using these experimental approaches have implicated endogenous opioid peptides in the regulation of seizure threshold (Frenk, 1983; Tortella et al., 1981, 1985; Olson et al., 1985), motor behavior (Sandyk, 1985; Olson et al., 1985), feeding and drinking (Olson et al., 1985; Baile et al., 1986), mental disorders (Frederickson and Geary, 1982; Olson et al., 1985; Schmauss and Emrich, 1985), and immune responses (Plotnikoff et al., 1985; Wybran, 1985). The endogenous opioid peptides have also been implicated in the regulation of gastrointestinal (Porreca and Burks, 1983; Olson et al., 1985; Schick and Schusdziarra, 1985), cardiovascular (Holaday, 1983; Bernton et al., 1985; Johnson et al., 1985), neuroendocrine (Grossman and Rees, 1983; Bicknell, 1985; Millan and Herz, 1985; Yen et al., 1985), and cognitive (Olson et al., 1985; Izquierdo and Netto, 1985) functions.

A comprehensive discourse on the pharmacological and physiological actions of the endogenous opioid peptides is beyond the scope of this chapter. The succeeding discussion will therefore focus only on the involvement of enkephalins, dynorphins, and endorphins in analgesia, perhaps the best-recognized effect of the endogenous opioid peptides. The experimental approaches used in these studies are representative of those used to elucidate the involvement of the endogenous opioid peptides in other functions.

7.1. Effects of Naloxone

Some of the earliest evidence for an involvement of the endogenous opioid peptides in the regulation of nociceptive threshold was obtained from studies of the effects of naloxone on preclinical and clinical measures of pain and analgesia. This evidence, which has been reviewed extensively by Frederickson and Geary (1982), is briefly summarized here. In the rodent, administration of naloxone produces hyperalgesia (Jacob et al., 1974; Berntson and Walker, 1977; Frederickson et al., 1977; Grevert and Goldstein, 1977a; Kokka and Fairhurst, 1977; Woolf, 1980a). This effect, however, is dependent on the measure of nociception (Jacob et al., 1974; Goldstein et al., 1976; Frederickson et al., 1977). In clinical studies of *experimental pain threshold,* naloxone does not produce hyperalgesia (El-Sobky et al., 1976; Grevert and Goldstein, 1977b, 1978). In studies of *clinical* pain resulting from oral surgery, however, naloxone produces hyperalgesia, suggesting that an endogenous opioid system is activated by postoperative pain (Levine et al., 1978b, Levine, 1979; Gracely et al., 1983). This observation is supported by findings that stimulation of peripheral nerves at intensities that are noxious evokes the release of opioid peptides and opioid-like material from the CNS (Yaksh and Elde, 1981; Yaksh et al., 1983; Cesselin et al., 1982, 1985). Although activation of an endogenous opioid system is suggested to mediate placebo-induced analgesia (Levine et al., 1978a), this interpretation has been challenged by observations that naloxone can produce hyperalgesia independent of the placebo effect, and that a placebo effect can occur in the presence of hidden infusions of naloxone (Gracely et al., 1983).

In retrospect, it is not surprising that the results of many of these studies were often at variance. More recent studies have illustrated the influence on nociceptive threshold and opioid-induced analgesia of age (Kavaliers and Hirst, 1983, Hamm and Knisley, 1985), diurnal rhythm (Frederickson et al., 1977; Procacci et al., 1972; Kavaliers and Hirst, 1983), the measure of nociception (Frederickson et al., 1977), the type of pain (Tyers, 1980; Ward and Takemori, 1983; Yaksh and Noueihed, 1985), the dose and receptor selectivity of the antagonist employed (Paterson et al.,

1984), the route of administration of the antagonist (Woolf, 1980a,b), and environmental factors (Watkins and Mayer, 1982). Furthermore, many of these studies were based on the assumption that the endogenous opioid system was not only tonically active in the quiescent state, but that its activation contributed significantly to the production of analgesia. It is now recognized that bulbospinal serotonergic and noradrenergic systems also exert a powerful influence on nociceptive threshold and are involved in the production of analgesia (Hammond, 1986). Thus, it is not surprising that it is difficult to demonstrate alterations in nociceptive threshold following administration of one class of pharmacological antagonist.

7.2. Effects of Inhibitors of Opioid Degradation

The hyperalgesic effect of naloxone suggests that, under certain conditions, an endogenous opioid system is tonically active. Given this assumption, one might conversely expect that administration of agents that inhibit the degradation of the endogenous opioid peptides would produce analgesia. Several hydrolytic enzymes have been identified that degrade the endogenous opioid peptides and for which specific inhibitors have been synthesized. These enzymes include, but are not limited to, neutral metalloendopeptidase ("enkephalinase," EC 3.4.24.11), which hydrolyzes the Gly^3-Phe^4 bond of the enkephalins, and an aminopeptidase, which hydrolyzes the Tyr^1-Gly^2 bond of the opioid peptides (Frederickson and Geary, 1982; De La Baume et al., 1983; Schwartz et al., 1985; Turner et al., 1985). Intracerebroventricular (icv) or intrathecal (it) administration of inhibitors of aminopeptidase (e.g., bestatin, amastatin) or of metalloendopeptidase (e.g., thiorphan, retro-thiorphan, kelatorphan, phosphoramidon) produces analgesia in the rodent, as measured by several different tests, including writhing, tail-flick, paw-pressure, and hot-plate (Roques et al., 1980, 1983; Yaksh and Harty, 1982; Ruprecht et al., 1983; Chaillet et al., 1983; Fournie-Zaluski et al., 1983, 1984, 1985; Mendelsohn et al., 1985; Scott et al., 1985). Intrathecal administration of thiorphan also diminishes the intensity and occurrence of headache and nausea that accompany myelography in humans (Floras et al., 1983). The analgesic activity of these agents is attributed to their ability to inhibit the degradation of the endogenous opioid peptides. This hypothesis is supported by observations that these inhibitors potentiate the actions of exogenously administered enkephalins. For example, thiorphan, phosphoramidon, kelatorphan, retro-thiorphan, and bestatin potentiate the analgesia produced by icv or it injection of enkephalins (Roques et al., 1980; Chipkin et al., 1982; Yaksh and Harty, 1982; Chaillet et al., 1983; Fournie-Zaluski et al., 1983, 1984, 1985; Mendelsohn et al., 1985). Moreover, these effects are naloxone-reversible, further supporting the hypothesis that they enhance the activity of an endogenous opioid system. These studies support an involvement of endogenous opioid peptides in analgesia and suggest that the system may be tonically active.

7.3. Effects of the Endogenous Opioid Peptides and Structural Analogs

The results of studies of the effects on nociceptive threshold of opioid antagonists and of inhibitors of opioid degradation suggest that endogenous opioid peptides modulate pain sensitivity. These studies do not provide insight into the relative contributions of the different families of endogenous opioid peptides, however, nor do they provide insight into the involvement of different opioid receptor subtypes in the production of analgesia. Rather, such information is provided by studies in which the endogenous opioid peptides themselves, or their structural analogs, are administered. In the majority of these studies, the opioid peptides have been administered centrally to minimize (but not eliminate) the problems of degradation and distribution encountered with systemic administration (Frederickson, 1984).

Numerous structural analogs of the endogenous opioid peptides exist for which analgesic activity has been demonstrated, particularly after central administration. Rather than document this voluminous literature, it is of greater interest to examine how these peptides have been used to define the opioid receptor subtypes involved in the production of analgesia. Therefore, this section will deal with studies of the peptides that offer insight into the relative contribution of mu, delta, and kappa opioid receptors to the production of analgesia. Recently, several laboratories have provided evidence that different opioid receptors may be involved in the suppression of different types of pain (Tyers, 1980; Ward and Takemori, 1983; VonVoigtlander et al., 1983; Yaksh and Noueihed, 1985). Kappa agonists appear more effective in suppressing visceral, chemically induced pain of prolonged duration (e.g., writhing test), than in suppressing cutaneous, thermally induced pain of transient duration (tail-flick test, hot-plate test). Thus, conclusions concerning the involvement of different opioid receptors must be tempered by a recognition of the influence of the measure of nociception.

7.3.1. Endorphins

β-Endorphin is restricted largely to neurons of the arcuate nucleus (Bloom et al., 1978a). Consequently, significant reductions in the levels of β-endorphin in the CNS can be produced by lesions of this one nucleus. This restricted localization of β-endorphin contrasts with the widespread distribution of enkephalinergic and dynorphinergic neurons in the CNS (Watson et al., 1982) and has facilitated studies of its involvement in the regulation of nociceptive threshold and the production of analgesia to an extent that has not been feasible with either the enkephalins or the dynorphins. Employing lesions of the arcuate nucleus, Millan et al. (1980) demonstrated that the lesion-induced reduction in β-endorphin levels is accompanied by an enhanced sensitivity to pain (hyperalgesia), as measured by a decrease in the threshold for vocalization to noxious tail shock. Microinjection of anti-β-endorphin antiserum into the periaqueductal gray, a nucleus to which arcuate neurons project and one that has been previously implicated in the production of analgesia, antagonizes electroacupuncture analgesia in the rabbit (Xie et al., 1983). This observation provides additional evidence for the involvement of β-endorphin in the regulation of nociceptive threshold.

β-Endorphin has preferential affinity for the mu and delta opioid receptors (Paterson et al., 1983) and has been proposed to be the prototypic ligand for the epsilon receptor identified in rat vas deferens (Wuster et al., 1979). When administered icv, β-endorphin produces analgesia and is the most potent of the endogenous opioid peptides in this respect (Feldberg and Smyth, 1976; Loh et al., 1976; Jacquet, 1978; Kuraishi et al., 1980; Tseng et al., 1980; Hollt et al., 1985). Recently, Hollt et al. (1985) demonstrated an excellent correlation between the analgesic activity of icv administered β-endorphin and other opioid peptides and their inhibitory potency on the rat vas deferens, but not the mouse vas deferns or the guinea pig ileum. On the basis of this correlation, these authors postulate that the analgesic action of icv administered endogenous opioid peptides is mediated by opioid receptors resembling those in the rat vas deferens, i.e., the epsilon receptor. Recently, Tseng and Fujimoto (1985) reported that the analgesia produced by icv administration of morphine and β-endorphin is differentially sensitive to antagonism by intrathecally administered naloxone. This finding suggests that opioid receptors and neuronal circuitry that mediate the analgesic activity of β-endorphin and morphine differ.

β-Endorphin also produces analgesia when administered intrathecally, despite the absence of β-endorphinergic neurons or terminals in the spinal cord (Bloom et al., 1978b). This effect has been documented in rat (Yaksh and Henry, 1978; Kuraishi et al., 1980; Tseng, 1981; Belcher et al., 1982), cat (Yaksh and Henry, 1978), monkey (Yaksh et al., 1982; Yaksh, 1983), and human (Oyama et al., 1980; Wen et al., 1985). Interestingly, the apparent pA_2 value for naloxone vs β-endorphin is the same as that for morphine, a mu-selective ligand (Yaksh and Henry, 1978; Yaksh et al., 1982). This finding suggests that the analgesic effect of intrathecally administered β-endorphin is mediated by a mu opioid receptor, in contrast to the epsilon receptor that is postulated to mediate its supraspinal effects.

7.3.2. Enkephalins

Several products of the posttranslational processing of proenkephalin A produce analgesia when administered icv or it. These products include [Met[5]]enkephalin and [Leu[5]]enkephalin (Malick and Goldstein, 1977; Yaksh et al., 1977; Takagi et al., 1978; Hylden and Wilcox, 1983; Kuraishi et al., 1985), as well as [Met[5]]enkephalyl-Arg[6]-Phe[7], [Met[5]]enkephalyl-Arg[6]-Gly[7]-Leu[8], BAM 12P, BAM-22P, peptide E, and peptide F (Hollt et al., 1985). Metorphamide, a novel amidated octapeptide fragment of proenkephalin A, has also produced analgesia when administered icv or it (Xu et al., 1985; Porreca, personal communication). The enkephalins are largely inactive as analgesics following systemic administration. The fact is attributed to their metabolic instability (Morley, 1980), although factors such as poor blood–brain barrier permeability are cited as contributing causes (Zlokovic et al., 1985).

Structural modifications have been made to the enkephalins in attempts to bestow metabolic stability. These attempts have been fairly successful, and a wide variety of enkephalin analogs are now available with which to probe the CNS. Among the best known of these analogs are [Met[5]]enkephalinamide, [D-Ala[2]-D-Leu[5]]enkephalin and [D-Ala[2]-Met[5]]enkephalinamide. Perhaps the most notable results of synthetic efforts to endow [Met[5]]-

enalin with metabolic stability are the two enkephalin analogs FK 33-824 [Tyr-D-Ala-Gly-N(Me)Phe-Met(S-O)carbinol: Sandoz] (Roemer et al., 1977) and metkephamid (Tyr-D-Ala-Gly-Phe-N(Me)Met-amide, LY 127623) (Frederickson et al., 1981). Both of these analogs are systemically active analgesics in laboratory animals and have been demonstrated to be clinically effective analgesics. The preclinical and clinical pharmacology of these drugs has been reviewed by Frederickson (1984).

Structural modifications have also been made to the enkephalins to yield opioid peptides having very high selectivity for the mu and delta opioid receptors (Paterson et al., 1984). The opioid peptide currently thought to be the most selective for the mu opioid receptor is DAGO or DAMPGO [Tyr-D-Ala-Gl y-MePhe-NH(CH$_2$)$_2$OH] (Handa et al., 1981). Several opioid peptides with high selectivity for the delta opioid receptor have also been synthesized. These peptides include DSLET (Tyr-D-Ser-Gly-Phe-Leu-Thr) (Fournie-Zaluski et al., 1981) and DTLET (Tyr-D-Thr-Gly-Phe-Leu-Thr) (Zajac et al., 1983), the dimeric pentapeptide DPE$_2$ [Tyr-D-Ala-Gly-Phe-LeuNH]$_2$·(CH$_2$)$_2$] (Rodbard et al., 1983), and the dimeric tetrapeptide DTE$_{12}$ [Tyr-D-Ala-Gly-PheNH]$_2$·(CH$_2$)$_{12}$] (Shimohigashi et al., 1982). Using penicillamine residues, conformationally constrained analogs of enkephalin have been synthesized. Two *bis*-penicillamine analogs that are highly selective for the delta opioid receptor are [D-Pen^2, L-Pen^5]- and [D-Pen^2, D-Pen^5]-enkephalin (Mosberg et al., 1983).

Numerous investigators have administered receptor selective peptides either icv or it in order to examine further the role of mu and delta opioid receptors in the production of analgesia. As noted by Yaksh (1984), differences in technique (e.g., strain of animal, type of test, volume of injection, and so on) hamper comparison of results among these laboratories. This problem is particularly acute for studies in which only one or two peptides were administered and, for this reason, these studies will not be extensively reviewed. The studies of greatest importance are those in which extensive structure–activity relationships have been generated by the same laboratory using the very highly selective opioid peptides and in which apparent pA_2 values have been calculated. (Even these studies, however, cannot control the fact that the different peptides have different physicochemical properties that will affect important variables such as distribution and susceptibility to degradation, and hence the results.) Recently, Chaillet and coworkers (1984) examined the opioid receptor subtype that mediates the increase in hot-plate latency produced by icv injection of DAGO, DADLE, DSLET, and DTLET in mice. Intracerebroventricular administration of the delta opioid antagonist ICI 154129 does not antagonize the analgesia produced by DTLET. More importantly, the apparent pA_2 value of naloxone is similar for both DAGO and for DTLET. Finally, no correlation exists between the analgesic effects of these opioid peptides and either their relative potency on mouse vas deferens or their affinity for delta opioid receptors. In an interesting addition to the study, these authors also computed the apparent pA_2 value of naloxone for the analgesia produced by concomitant administration of bestatin and thiorphan, a treatment that would be expected to augment the levels of endogenous opioid peptides. The apparent pA_2 value is similar to that computed for DAGO and DSLET. In addition, the analgesia is not antagonized by ICI 154129. Chaillet and colleagues therefore conclude that the analgesic effects of the icv-administered opioid peptides and of the endogenous opioid peptides are mediated by the mu rather than the delta opioid receptors. Schuman et al. (1987) have similarly observed that the pA_2 values for icv-administered DSLET, morphine, and fentanyl are the same in the tail-flick test in the rat. They further observed that DPDPE was inactive in this test. These results also support the conclusion that the analgesic effects of opioid peptides in this test are mediated predominantly by mu receptors.*

However, it must be noted that this conclusion is valid only for thermal pain in the rodent, and that different measures of antinociception may yield different conclusions (*see* Hollt et al., 1985). Indeed, although Ward and Takemori (1983) conclude that the analgesic action of icv-administered DADLE is mediated by mu receptors, they observe test-dependent differences in the apparent pA_2 values of naloxone for morphine as compared to DADLE.

The pharmacology of spinally administered opioids has been examined also. Yaksh and colleagues have conducted extensive studies of the structure–activity relationships of it-administered opioids in the rodent and primate, the results of which have re-

---

*Porreca has argued for an additional involvement of delta receptors in the suppression of both thermal and chemical pain in the rodent (Porreca et al., 1984, 1987a). Most recently, he has demonstrated that the analgesia produced by icv administration of DPDPE is antagonized by ICI 174864 and not by pretreatment with β-FNA (Porreca et al. 1986b). pA_2 values would be a valuable adjunct to these data.

cently been summarized (Yaksh and Noueihed, 1985). Briefly, intrathecal administration of opioids having affinity for the mu or delta opioid receptor produces a monotonic, dose-dependent suppression of noxious cutaneous thermally induced pain (rodent tail-flick and hot-plate tests) or noxious cutaneous electrically induced pain (primate shock titration paradigm). Compounds having significant affinity for both the mu and delta receptors are frequently among the most efficacious in these tests, an observation that may have its basis in earlier observations of the synergistic interaction of mu- and delta-selective ligands (Larson et al., 1980; Vaught et al., 1982; Vaught and Barrett, 1986; Porrecca and Vaught, personal communication). In contrast, although mu- and mixed mu/delta-selective opioids produce a monotonic, dose-dependent suppression of noxious, visceral chemically induced pain, delta-selelctive opioids do not suppress this pain in doses that are without motor effect.

The computed apparent pA_2 values of naloxone for intrathecally administered DADL in the rodent tail-flick and hot-plate tests and in the primate shock titration test are nearly an order of magnitude less than the corresponding values for mu-selective ligands such as morphine (Tung and Yaksh, 1982; Yaksh, 1983). This observation suggests that activation of both mu and delta opioid receptors mediates the analgesic action of intrathecally administered opioids in these tests. Hylden and Wilcox (1983) reached a similar conclusion after observing that the highly selective mu receptor antagonist β-funaltrexamine does not antagonize the analgesia produced by intrathecal administration of DADL in mice. Finally, Yaksh and colleagues have reported that the dose–response function for it-administered DADL in morphine-tolerant animals is not significantly different from that in morphine-naive animals (Tung and Yaksh, 1982; Yaksh, 1983; Schmauss et al., 1985). Considered together, these studies indicate that there are *at least* two populations of spinal opioid receptors that mediate the production of analgesia, most likely mu and delta. This conclusion would be strengthened by additional studies conducted using the more highly selective delta agonists now available.

7.3.3. Dynorphins

When administered icv, the posttranslational products of prodynorphin such as dynorphin (1-17), dynorphin (1-13), dynorphin (1-9), dynorphin (1-8), α-neoendorphin, and β-neoendorphin are essentially inactive in measures of cutaneous thermally induced pain, such as the tail-flick and the hot-plate test, and shock-induced vocalization (Wuster et al., 1980; Friedman et al., 1981; Walker et al., 1982; Hayes et al., 1983; Nakazawa et al., 1985; Hollt et al., 1985). These products are effective in suppressing visceral chemically induced pain, however, as measured by the writhing test, and in suppressing noxious mechanical pain, as measured by the paw-pinch test (Hayes et al., 1983; Kaneko et al., 1983; Nakazawa et al., 1985) when administered icv.

Numerous laboratories have investigated the effects of it-administered dynorphin. In the rodent, it administration of dynorphin (1-17) and dynorphin (1-13) prolongs tail-flick latencies and latency to bite of a tail clip (Han and Xie, 1982; Piercey et al., 1982; Kaneko et al., 1983; Han et al., 1984; Przewlocki et al., 1983b; Herman and Goldstein, 1985; Spampinato and Candeletti, 1985), inhibits the writhing response to ip injection of an irritant (Przewlocki et al., 1983b), and increases the vocalization threshold to noxious tail shock (Spampinato and Candeletti, 1985) or noxious pinch (Herman and Goldstein, 1985). The analgesic effect is resistant to antagonism by low doses of naloxone, but can be antagonized by administration of the kappa antagonists Mr 2266 and Mr 1452, as would be expected of kappa-selective ligands (Han and Xie, 1982; Piercey et al., 1982; Przewlocki et al., 1983a,b; Han et al., 1984; Herman and Goldstein, 1985; Spampinato and Candeletti, 1985). It should be noted, however, that the majority of these studies also report that the analgesia produced by it administration of dynorphin is accompanied by a long-lasting paralysis or flaccidity of the hind limbs and tail. Several studies indicate that the analgesic effect is not dissociable from the motor dysfunction (Przewlocki et al., 1983a; Kaneko et al., 1983). Finally, similar effects are observed after administration of the non-opioid fragments des-Tyr[1]-dynorphin (1-13) (Przewlocki et al., 1983a) and des-Tyr[1]-dynorphin (1-17) (Faden and Jacobs, 1984), suggesting that these effects are not opioid-mediated. Such motor dysfunction clearly confounds measurements of analgesia, particularly those that rely on a reflexive action as the assay endpoint, and renders suspect conclusions of analgesia based on alterations in tail-flick latency, bite latency, or frequency of writhing. At least two investigators, however, report that it administration of dynorphin increases latency to vocalization, suggesting that analgesia may have been present. In addition, Wen et al. (1985) report that it-administered dynorphin (1-13) relieves intractable pain in humans. In contrast to the tridecapeptide and heptadecapeptide, it administration of dynorphin (1-8) produces a naloxone-reversible analgesia in the absence of motor deficits (Przewlocki et al., 1983a; Faden and Jacobs, 1984). The occurrence of motor dysfunction after it administration of the dynorphins appears unique to the peptide family, since it has not been observed after it administration of other kappa-selective ligands or of enkephalins (Faden and Jacobs, 1984).

Wood and colleagues (Wood et al., 1981) and Yaksh and coworkers have postulated an involvement of kappa opioid receptors in the spinal cord in the production of analgesia. Kappa agonists, when administered it, are more efficacious in suppressing visceral, chemically induced pain than cutaneous, thermally induced pain (Schmauss and Yaksh, 1984). The dose–response curves for it-administered dynorphin are not shifted in animals made tolerant to morphine (Han et al., 1984; Spampinato and Candeletti, 1985), suggesting that a third population of opioid receptors, the kappa receptor, is involved in the production of analgesia. In view of the uncertainty about the analgesic activity of dynorphin relative to its effects on motor dysfunction, it is important that these studies be replicated using highly selective kappa ligands such as dynorphin (1-8), U50488H, and U69593.

Acknowledgments

Many of the studies cited in this chapter were conducted in the Nancy Pritzker Laboratory, supported by NIDA 01207. We would like to thank Dr. Jack D. Barchas for continuing support, and Drs. James H. Eberwine, Karen L. Valentino, Mark Schaefer, and Elizabeth Erdelyi for critical reading of the manuscript.

We thank Grace Koek and Alicia Fritchle for assistance in preparation of the manuscript and graphic illustrations.

References

Akil, H., Lin, H. L., Veda, Y., Knoblock, M., Watson, S. J., and Coy, D. (1983) Some of the alpha-NH^2-acetylated beta-endorphin-like material in rat and monkey pituitary and brain is acetylated alpha- and beta-endorphin. *Life Sci.* **33** (suppl.), 9–12.

Akil, H., Watson, S. J., Young, E., Lewis, M. E., Khachaturian, H., and Walker, J. M. (1984) Endogenous opioids: Biology and function. *Ann. Rev. Neurosci.* **7**, 223–255.

Baile, C. A., McLaughlin, C. L., and Della-Fera, M. A. (1986) Role of cholecystokinin and opioid peptides in control of food intake. *Physiol. Rev.* **66**, 172–234.

Baird, A., Ling, N., Bohlen, P., Benoit, R., Klepper, R., and Guillemin, R. (1982) Molecular forms of the putative enkephalin precursor BAM-12P in bovine adrenal, pituitary, and hypothalamus. *Proc. Natl. Acad. Sci. USA* **79**, 2023–2025.

Barchas, J. D., Evans, C. J., Elliott, G. R., and Berger, P. A. (1986) Peptide neuroregulators: The opioid system as a model. *Yale J. Bio. Med.* **58**, 579–596.

Basbaum, A. I. and Fields, H. L. (1984) Endogenous pain control systems. *Ann Rev. Neurosci.* **7**, 309–338.

Belcher, G., Smock, T., and Fields, H. L. (1982) Effects of intrathecal ACTH on opiate analgesia in the rat. *Brain Res.* **247**, 373–377.

Bernton, E. W., Long, J. B., and Holaday, J. W. (1985) Opioids and neuropeptides: Mechanisms in circulatory shock. *Fed. Proc.* **44**, 290–299.

Berntson, G. G. and Walker, J. M. (1977) Effect of opiate receptor blockade on pain sensitivity in the rat. *Brain Res. Bull.* **2**, 157–159.

Bicknell, R. J. (1985) Endogenous opioid peptides and hypothalamic neuroendocrine neurones. *J. Endocrinol.* **107**, 437–446.

Bloom, F. E., Battenberg, E., Rossier, J., Ling, N., and Guillemin, R. (1978a) Neurons containing β-endorphin in rat brain exist separately from those containing enkephalin: Immunocytochemical studies. *Proc. Natl. Acad. Sci. USA* **75**, 1591–1595.

Bloom, F. E., Rossier, J., Battenberg, E., Bayon, A., French, E., Henricksen, S. J., Siggins, G. R., Segal, D., Browne, R., Ling, N., and Guillemin, R. (1978b) Beta-endorphin: Cellular localization, electrophysiological and behavioral effects. *Adv. Biochem. Psychopharmacol. Endorphins* **18**, 89–109.

Bradbury, A. F., Smyth, D. G., and Snell, C. R. (1975) *Peptides: Chemistry, Structure, and Biology* Proceedings of the Fourth American Peptide Symposium (Walter, R. and Meienhofer, J., eds.) Ann Arbor Science, Ann Arbor, Michigan.

Bradbury, A. F., Finnie, M. D. A., and Smyth, D. G. (1981) Mechanism of C-terminal amide formation by pituitary enzymes. *Nature* **298**, 686-688.

Buffa, R., Solcia, E., Magnoni, E., Rindi, G., Negri, L., and Melchiorri, P. (1982) Immunohistochemical demonstration of a dermorphin-like peptide in the rat brain. *Histochemistry* **76**, 273–276.

Cesselin, F., Oliveras, J. L., Bourgoin, S., Sierralta, F., Michelot, R., Besson, J. M., and Hamon, M. (1982) Increased levels of met-enkephalin-like material in the CSF of anesthetized cats after tooth pulp stimulation. *Brain Res.* **237**, 325–338.

Cesselin, F., LeBars, D., Bourgoin, S., Artaud, F., Gozlan, H., Clot, A. M., Besson, J. M., and Hamon, M. (1985) Spontaneous and evoked release of methionine-enkephalin-like material from the rat spinal cord in vivo. *Brain Res.* **339**, 305–313.

Chaillet P., Marcais-Collado, H., Costentin, J., Yi, C-C., de la Baume, S., and Schwartz, J.-C. (1983) Inhibition of enkephalin metabolism by, and antinociceptive activity of, bestatin, an aminopeptidase inhibitor. *Eur. J. Pharmacol.* **86**, 329–336.

Chaillet, P., Coulaud, A., Zajac, J-M., Fournie-Zaluski, M.-C., Costentin, J., and Roques, B. (1984) The μ rather than the δ subtype of opioid receptors appears to be involved in enkephalin-induced analgesia. *Eur. J. Pharmacol.* **101,** 83–90.

Chen, C.-L. C., Mather, J. P., Morris, P. L., and Bradin, C. W. (1984) Expression of pro-opiomelanocortin-like gene in the testis and epididymis. *Proc. Natl. Acad. Sci. USA* **81** (18), 5672–5675.

Chipkin, R. E., Latranyl, M. Z., Iorio, L. C., and Barnett, A. (1982) Potentiation of [D-Ala2]enkephalinamide analgesia in rats by thiorphan. *Eur. J. Pharmacol.* **83,** 283–288.

Cone, R. I., Weber, E., Barchas, J. D., and Goldstein, A. (1983) Regional distribution of dynorphin and neo-endorphin peptides in rat brain, spinal cord, and pituitary. *J. Neurosci.* **3,** 2146–2152.

Cox, B. M., Opheim, K. E., Teschemacher, H., and Goldstein, A. (1975) A peptide like substance from pituitary that acts like morphine; Purification and properties. *Life Sci.* **16,** 1777–1782.

De La Baume, S., Yi, C. C., Schwartz, J. C., Chaillet, P., Marcais-Collado, H., and Costentin, J. (1983) Participation of both enkephalinase and aminopeptidase activities in the metabolism of endogenous enkephalins. *Neuroscience* **8,** 143–151.

Devi, L. and Goldstein, A. (1984) Dynorphin-converting enzyme with unusual specificity from rat brain. *Proc. Natl. Acad. Sci. USA* **81,** 192–196.

Donnerer, J., Oka, K., Brossi, A., Rice, K. C., and Spector, S. (1986) Presence and formation of codeine and morphine in the rat. *J. Med. Chem.* **83,** 4556–4567.

Eberwine, J. H. and Roberts, J. L. (1983) Analysis of pro-opiomelanocortin gene structure and function. *dna* **2,** 1–8.

Eipper, B. A. and Mains, R. E. (1980) Structure and function of preadrenocorticotropin/endorphin and related peptides. *Endocr. Rev.* **1,** 247–262.

El-Sobky, A., Dostrovsky, J. O., and Wall, P. D. (1976) Lack of effect of naloxone on pain perception in humans. *Nature* **263,** 783–784.

Evans, C. J., Weber, E., and Barchas, J. D. (1981) Isolation and characterization of α-N-acetyl β-endorphin (1-26) from the rat posterior/intermediate pituitary lobe. *Biophys. Res. Commun.* **102,** 897–904.

Evans, C. J., Lorenz, R., Weber, E., and Barchas, J. D. (1982) Variants of alpha melanocyte stimulating hormone in rat brain and pituitary: Evidence that acetylated alpha MSH exists only in the intermediate lobe of the pituitary. *Biochem. Biophys. Res. Commun.* **106,** 910–919.

Evans, C. J., Erdelyi, E., Weber, E., and Barchas, J. D. (1983) Identification of pro-opiomelanocortin-derived peptides in the human adrenal medulla. *Science* **221,** 957–960.

Evans, C. J., Barchas, J. D., Esch, F. S., Bohlen, P., and Weber, E. (1985a) Isolation and characterization of an endogenous C-terminal fragment of the α-neo-endorphin/dynorphin precursor from bovine caudate nucleus. *J. Neurosci.* **5,** 1803–1807.

Evans, C. J., Erdelyi, E., and Barchas, J. D. (1985b) Opioid peptides in the adrenal pituitary axis. *Psychopharm. Bull.* **21**(3), 466–471.

Evans, C. J., Erdelyi, E., Hunter, J., and Barchas, J. D. (1985c) Co-localization and characterization of immunoreactive peptides derived from two opioid precursors in guinea pig adrenal glands. *J. Neurosci.* **5,** 3423–3427.

Faden, A. I. and Jacobs, T. P. (1984) Dynorphin related peptides cause motor dysfunction in the rat through a non-opiate action. *Br. J. Pharmac.* **81,** 271–276.

Feldberg, W. and Smyth, D. G. (1976) The C-fragment of lipotropin—a potent analgesic. *J. Physiol.* (Lond.) **260,** 30p–31p.

Fischli, W., Goldstein, A., Hunkapiller, M. W., and Hood, L. E. (1982a) Isolation and amino acid sequence analysis of a 4000 dalton dynorphin from porcine pituitary. *Proc. Natl. Acad. Sci. USA* **79,** 5435–5437.

Fischli, W., Goldstein, A., Hunkapiller, M. W., and Hood, L. E. (1982b) Two "big" dynorphins from porcine pituitary. *Life Sci.* **31,** 1769–1772.

Floras, P., Bidabe, A.-M., Caille, J.-M., Simonnet, G., Lecomte, J.-M., and Sabathie, M. (1983) Double-blind study of effects of enkephalinase inhibitor on adverse reactions to myelography. *Am. J. Neuroradiol.* **4,** 653–655.

Fournie-Zaluski, M.-C., Gacel, G., Maigret, B., Premilat, S., and Roques, B. P. (1981) Structural requirements for specific recognition of μ or δ opiate receptors. *Mol. Pharmacol.* **20,** 484–491.

Fournie-Zaluski, M.-C., Chaillet, P., Soroca-Lucas, E., Marcais-Callado, H., Costentin, J., and Roques, B. P. (1983) New carboxyalkyl inhibitors of brain enkephalinase: Synthesis, biological activity, and analgesic properties. *J. Med. Chem.* **26,** 60–65.

Fournie-Zaluski, M.-C., Chaillet, P., Bouboutou, R., Coulaud, A., Cherot, P., Waksman, G., Costentin, J., and Roques, B. P. (1984) Analgesic effects of kelatorphan, a new highly potent inhibitor of multiple enkephalin degrading enzymes. *Eur. J. Pharmacol.* **102,** 525–528.

Fournie-Zaluski, M.-C., Coulaud, A., Bouboutou, R., Chaillet, P., Devin, J., Waksman, G., Costentin, J., and Roques, B. P. (1985) New bidentates as full inhibitors of enkephalin-degrading enzymes: Synthesis and analgesic properties. *J. Med. Chem.* **28,** 1158–1169.

Frederickson, R. C. A. (1984) Endogenous Opioids and Related Derivatives, in *Analgesics: Neurochemical, Behavioral and Clinical Perspectives* (Kuhar, M. and Pasternak, G., eds.) Raven, New York.

Frederickson, R. C. A. and Geary, L. E. (1982) Endogenous opioid peptides: Review of physiological, pharmacological and clinical aspects. *Prog. Neurobiol.* **19,** 19–69.

Frederickson, R. C. A., Burgis, V., and Edwards, J. D. (1977) Hyperalgesia induced by naloxone follows diurnal rhythm in responsivity to painful stimuli. *Science* **198,** 756–758.

Frederickson, R. C. A., Smithwick, E. L., Shuman, R., and Bemis, K. G. (1981) Metkephamid, a systemically active analog of methionine enkephalin with potent δ receptor activity. *Science* **211,** 603–605.

Frenk, H. (1983) Pro- and anticonvulsant actions of morphine and the endogenous opioids: Involvement and interactions of multiple opiate and non-opiate systems. *Brain Res. Rev.* **6,** 197–210.

Fricker, L. D., Supattapore, S., and Snyder, S. H. (1982) Enkephalin convertase; a specific carboxypeptidase in adrenal chromaffin granules, brain and pituitary gland. *Life Sci* **31,** 1841–1844.

Friedman, H. J., Jen, M.-F., Chang, J.-K., Lee, N. M., and Loh, H. H. (1981) Dynorphin: A possible modulatory peptide on morphine or β-endorphin analgesia in mouse. *Eur. J. Pharmacol.* **69,** 357–360.

Gee, C. E., Chen, C.-L. C., Roberts, J. L., Thompson, R., and Watson, S. J. (1983) Identification of proopiomelanocortin neurones in rat hypothalamus by *in situ* cDNA-mRNA hybridization. *Nature* **306,** 374–376.

Geis, R., Martin, R., and Voigt, K. H. (1984) α-MSH-like peptides from the rat hypothalamus and pituitary: Differences in the degree of N-acetylation. *Horm. Metab. Res.* **16,** 266–267.

Geisow, M. J., Deakin, J. F. W., Dostrovsky, J. O., and Smyth, D. G. (1977) Analgesic activity of lipotropin C fragment depends on carboxyl terminal tetrapeptide. *Nature* **269,** 167–168.

Gintzler, A. R., Levy, A., and Spector, S. (1976) Antibodies as a means of isolating and characterizing biologically active substances: Presence of a non-peptide, morphine-like compound in the central nervous system. *Proc. Natl. Acad. Sci. USA* **73,** 2132–2136.

Glickman, J. A., Carson, G. D., and Challis, J. R. (1979) Differential effects of synthetic adrenocorticotropin 1-24 and alpha-melancyte-stimulating hormone on adrenal function in human and sheep fetuses. *Endocrinology* **104,** 34–39.

Goldstein, A., Barrett, R. W., James, I. F., Lowney, L. I., Weitz, C. J., Knipmeyer, L. L., and Rapoport, H. (1985) Morphine and other opiates from beef brain and adrenal. *Proc. Natl. Acad. Sci. USA* **82,** 5203–5207.

Goldstein, A., Fischli, W., Lowney, L. I., Hunkapiller, M., and Hood, L. (1981) Porcine pituitary dynorphin: Complete amino acid sequence of the biologically active heptadecapeptide. *Proc. Natl. Acad. Sci. USA* **78,** 7219–7223.

Goldstein, A., Pryor, G. T., Otis, L. S., and Larsen, F. (1976) On the role of endogenous opioid peptides: Failure of naloxone to influence shock escape threshold in the rat. *Life Sci.* **18,** 599–604.

Gracely, R. H., Dubner, R., Wolskee, P. J., and Deeter, W. R. (1983) Placebo and naloxone can alter postsurgical pain by separate mechanisms. *Nature* **306,** 264–265.

Grevert, P. and Goldstein, A. (1977a) Some effects of naloxone on behavior in the mouse. *Psychopharmacology* **53,** 111–113.

Grevert, P. and Goldstein, A. (1977b) Effects of naloxone on experimentally induced ischemic pain and on mood in human subjects. *Proc. Natl. Acad. Sci. USA* **74,** 1291–1294.

Grevert, P. and Goldstein, A. (1978) Endorphins: Naloxone fails to alter experimental pain or mood in humans. *Science* **199,** 1093–1095.

Grossman, A. and Rees, L. H. (1983) The neuroendocrinology of opioid peptides. *Br. Med. Bull.* **39,** 83–88.

Guttman, S. T. and Boissonnas, R. A. (1961) Influence of the structure of the N-terminal extremity of α-MSH on the melanophore-stimulating activity of this hormone. *Experientia* **17,** 265–267.

Hamm, R. J. and Knisely, J. S. (1985) Environmentally induced analgesia: An age-related decline in an endogenous opioid system. *J. Gerontol.* **40,** 268–274.

Hammond, D. L. (1986) Control Systems for Nociceptive Afferent Processing. The Descending Inhibitory Pathways, in *Spinal Afferent Processing* (Yaksh, T. L., ed.) Plenum, New York.

Han, J.-S. and Xie, C.-W. (1982) Dynorphin: Potent analgesic effect in spinal cord of the rat. *Life Sci.* **31**, 1781–1784.

Han, J.-S., Xie, G.-X., and Goldstein, A. (1984) Analgesia induced by intrathecal injection of dynorphin B in the rat. *Life Sci.* **34**, 1573–1579.

Handa, B. K., Lane, A. C., Lord, J. A. H., Morgan, B. A., Rance, M. J., and Smith, C. F. C. (1981) Analogues of β-LPH $_{61-64}$ possessing selective agonist activity at μ opiate receptors. *Eur. J. Pharmacol.* **70**, 531–540.

Hayes, A. G., Skingle, M., and Tyers, M. B. (1983) Antinociceptive profile of dynorphin in the rat. *Life Sci.* **33** (Suppl), 657–660.

Herbert, E., Civelli, O., Douglas, J., Martens, G., and Rosen, H. (1985) Generation of diversity of opioid peptides. *Biochemica Actions Horm.* **12**, 1–36.

Herman, B. H. and Goldstein, A. (1985) Antinociception and paralysis induced by intrathecal dynorphin A. *J. Pharmacol. Exp. Ther.* **232**, 27–32.

Hokfelt, T., Elde, R., Johansson, O., Terenius, L., and Stein, L. (1977) The distribution of enkephalin-immunoreactive cell bodies in the rat central nervous system. *Neurosci. Lett.* **5**, 25–31.

Holaday, J. W. (1983) Cardiovascular effects of endogenous opiate systems. *Annu. Rev. Pharmacol. Toxicol.* **23**, 541–594.

Hollt, V., Sanchez-Blazquez, P., and Garzon, J. (1985) Multiple opioid ligands and receptors in the control of nociception. *Phil. Trans. R. Soc. Lond. (Biol.)* **308**, 299–310.

Hollt, V., Tulunay, F. C., Woo, S. K., Loh, H. H., and Herz, A. (1982a) Opioid peptides derived from pro-enkephalin A but not that from pro-enkephalin B are substantial analgesics after administration into the brain of mice. *Eur. J. Pharmacol.* **85**, 355–356.

Hollt, V., Haarman, I., Grimm, C., Herz, A., Tulunay, F. C., and Loh, H. H. (1982b) Pro-enkephalin intermediates in bovine brain and adrenal medulla: Characterization of immunoreactive peptides related to BAM-22P and peptide F. *Life Sci.* **31**, 1883–1886.

Hughes, J., Smith, T. H., Kosterlitz, J. W., Fothergill, L. A., Morgan, B. A., and Morris, H. R. (1975) Identification of two related pentapeptides from the brain with potent opiate agonist activity. *Nature* **258**, 577–579.

Hylden, J. K. and Wilcox, G. L. (1983) Intrathecal opioids block a spinal action of substance P in mice: Functional importance of both μ and δ receptors. *Eur. J. Pharmacol.* **86**, 95–98.

Imura, H., Kato, Y., Nakai, Y., Kakao, K., Tanaka, I., Jingami, H., Koh, T., Yoshimasa, T., Suda, M., Sakamoto, M., Morii, N., Takahashi, H., Togo, K., and Sugawara, A. (1985) Endogenous opioids and related peptides: From molecular biology to clinical medicine. *J. Endocrinol.* **107**, 147–157.

Izquierdo, I. and Netto, C. A. (1985) Roles of β-endorphin in behavioral regulation. *Ann. NY Acad. Sci.* **444**, 162–177.

Jacob, J. J., Tremblay, E. C., and Colombel, M. C. (1974) Facilitation de reactions nociceptives par la naloxone chez la souris et chez le rat. *Psychopharmacologica* **37**, 217–223.

Jacquet, Y. F. (1978) Opiate effects after adrenocorticotropin or β-endorphin injection in the periaqueductal gray matter of rats. *Science* **201,** 1032–1034.

James, I. F., Fischli, W., and Goldstein, A. (1984) Opioid receptor selectivity of dynorphin gene products. *J. Pharmacol. Exp. Ther.* **228,** 88–93.

Jingami, H., Nakanishi, S., Imura, H., and Numa, S. (1984) Tissue distribution of messenger RNAs coding for opioid peptide precursors and related RNA. *Eur. J. Biochem.* **142,** 441–447.

Johnson, M. W., Mitch, W. E., and Wilcox, C. S. (1985) The cardiovascular actions of morphine and the endogenous opioid peptides. *Prog. Cardiovasc. Dis.* **27,** 435–450.

Jones, B. N., Shively, J. E., Kilpatrick, D. L., Kojima, K., and Udenfriend, S. (1982) Enkephalin biosynthetic pathway: A 5300-dalton adrenal polypeptide that terminates at its COOH end with the sequence [Met]enkephalin-Arg-Gly-Leu-COOH. *Proc. Natl. Acad. Sci. USA* **79,** 1313–1315.

Kakidani, H., Furutani, Y., Takahashi, H., Noda, M., Morimoto, Y., Horose, T., Asai, M., Inayama, S., Nakanishi, S., and Numa, S. (1982) Cloning and sequence analysis of cDNA for porcine β-neo-endorphin/dynorphin precursor. *Nature* **298,** 245–249.

Kaneko, T., Nakazawa, T., Ikeda, M., Yamatsu, K., Iwama, T., Wada, T., Satoh, M., and Takagi, H. (1983) Sites of analgesic action of dynorphin. *Life Sci.* **33** (suppl.), 661–664.

Kangawa, K., Matsuo, H., and Igarashi, M. (1979) α-Neo-endorphin: A "big" leu-enkephalin with potent opiate activity from porcine hypothalami. *Biochem. Biophys. Res. Comm.* **86,** 153–160.

Kangawa, K., Minamino, N., Chino, N., Sakakibara, S., and Matsuo, H. (1981) The complete amino acid sequence of α-neo-endorphin. *Biochem. Biophys. Res. Commun.* **99,** 871–888.

Kavaliers, M. and Hirst, M. (1983) Daily rhythms of analgesia in mice: Effects of age and photoperiod. *Brain Res.* **279,** 387–393.

Kawauchi, H. (1983) Chemistry of proopiocortin-related peptides in the salmon pituitary. *Arch. Biochem. Biophy.* **227,** 343–350.

Khachaturian, H., Watson, S. J., Lewis, M. E., Coy, D., Goldstein, A., and Akil, H. (1982) Dynorphin immunocytochemistry in the rat central nervous system. *Peptides* **3,** 941–954.

Kilpatrick, D. L., Taniguchi, T., Jones, B. N., Stein, A. S., Shirely, J. E., Hullihan, J., Kimura, S., Stein, S., and Udenfriend, S. (1981) A highly potent 3200-dalton adrenal opioid peptide that contains both a [Met]- and [Leu]enkephalin sequence. *Proc. Natl. Acad. Sci. USA* **78,** 3265–3268.

Kilpatrick, D. L., Wahlstrom, A., Lahm, H. W., Blacher, R. W., Ezra, E., Fleminger, G., and Udenfriend, S. (1982) Characterization of rimorphin, a new (leu)enkephalin-containing peptide from bovine posterior pituitary glands. *Life Sci.* **31,** 1849–1852.

Kimura, S., Lewis, R. V., Stern, A. S., Rossier, J., Stein, S., and Udenfriend, S. (1980) Probable precursors of [Leu]enkephalin and [Met]enkephalin in adrenal medulla: Peptides of 3-5 kilodaltons. *Proc. Natl. Acad. Sci. USA* **77,** 1681–1685.

Kokka, N. and Fairhurst, A. S. (1977) Naloxone enhancement of acetic acid-induced writhing in rats. *Life Sci.* **21,** 975–980.

Kuraishi, Y., Satoh, M., Harada, Y., Akaike, A., Shibata, T., and Takagi, H. (1980) Analgesic action of intrathecal and intracerebral β-endorphin in rats: Comparison with morphine. *Eur. J. Pharmacol.* **67,** 143–146.

Kuraishi, Y., Hirota, N., Satoh, M., and Takagi, H. (1985) Antinociceptive effects of intrathecal opioids, noradrenaline and serotonin in rats: Mechanical and thermal algesic tests. *Brain Res.* **326,** 168–171.

Larson, A. A., Vaught, J. L., and Takemori, A. E. (1980) The potentiation of spinal analgesia by leucine enkephalin. *Eur. J. Pharmacol.* **61,** 381–383.

Levine, J. D., Gordon, N. C., and Fields, H. L. (1978a) The mechanism of placebo analgesia. *Lancet* **ii,** 654–657.

Levine, J. D., Gordon, N. C., Jones, R. T., and Fields, H. L. (1978b) The narcotic antagonist naloxone enhances clinical pain. *Nature* **272,** 826–827.

Levine, J. D., Gordon, N. C., and Fields, H. L. (1979) Naloxone dose dependently produces analgesia and hyperalgesia in post operative pain. *Nature* **278,** 740–741.

Lewis, R. V., Stern, A. S., Kimura, S., Rossier, J., Stein, S., and Undenfriend, S. (1980) An about 50,000-dalton protein in adrenal medulla: A common precursor of [Met]- and [Leu]enkephalin. *Science* **208,** 1459–1460.

Liebisch, D. C., Weber, E., Kosica, B., Gramsh, C., Hertz, A., and Seizinger, B. R. (1986) Isolation and structure of a C-terminally amidated non-opioid peptide, amidorphin-(8-26), from bovine striatum: A major product of proenkephalin in brain but not adrenal medulla. *Proc. Natl. Acad. Sci. USA.* **83,** 1936–1940.

Lindberg, I. and Yang, H.-Y. T. (1984) Distribution of met^5-enkephalin-arg^6-gly^7-leu^8-immunoreactive peptides in rat brain: Presence of multiple molecular forms. *Brain Res.* **299,** 73–78.

Liotta, A. S. and Krieger, D. T. (1980) *In vitro* biosynthesis and comparative posttranslational processing of immunoreactive precursor corticotropin/β-endorphin by human placental and pituitary cells. *Endocrinology* **106,** 1504–1511.

Liston, D. R., Vanderhaeghen, J.-J., and Rossier, J. (1983) Presence in brain of synenkephalin, a proenkephalin-immunoreactive protein which does not contain enkephalin. *Nature* **302,** 62–65.

Loh, H. H., Tseng, L. F., Wei, W., and Li, C. H. (1976) β-Endorphin is a potent analgesic agent. *Proc. Natl. Acad. Sci. USA* **73,** 2895–2898.

Loh, Y.-P., Eskay, R. L., and Brownstein, M. (1980) A MSH-like peptides in rat brain: Identification and changes in level during development. *Science* **215,** 1125–1127.

Lorenz, R. G., Evans, C. J., and Barchas, J. D. (1985) Effects of dehydration on pro-dynorphin derived peptides in the neuro-intermediate lobe of the rat pituitary. *Life Sci.* **37,** 1523–1528.

Lorenz, R. G., Tyler, A. N., Faull, K. F., Makk, G., Barchas, J. D., and Evans, C. J. (1986) Characterization of endorphins from the pituitary of the spiny dogfish *Squalus acanthias. Peptides* **7,** 119–126.

Malick, J. B. and Goldstein, J. M. (1977) Analgesic activity of enkephalins following intracerebral administration in the rat. *Life Sci.* **20,** 827–832.

Margioris, A. N., Liotta, A. S., Vaudry, H., Bardin, C. W., and Krieger, D. T. (1983) Characterization of immunoreactive proopiomelanocortin-related peptides in rat testes. *Endocrinology* **113**, 663–671.

Martin, W. R., Eades, C. G., Thompson, J. A., Huppler, R. E., and Gilbert, P. E. (1976) The effects of morphine- and nalorphine-like drugs in the nondependent and morphine-dependent chronic spinal dog. *J. Pharmacol. Exp. Ther.* **197**, 517–532.

Mendelsohn, L. G., Johnson, B. G., Scott, W. L., and Frederickson, R. C. A. (1985) Thiorphan and analogs: Lack of correlation between potency to inhibit "enkephalinase A" in vitro and analgesic potency in vivo. *J. Pharmacol. Exp. Ther.* **234**, 386–390.

Millan, M. J. and Herz, A. (1985) The endocrinology of the opioids. *Int. Rev. Neurobiol.* **26**, 1–83.

Millan, M. J., Gramsch, C., Przewlocki, R., Hollt, V., and Herz, A. (1980) Lesions of the hypothalamic arcuate nucleus produce a temporary hyperalgesia and attenuate stress-evoked analgesia. *Life Sci.* **27**, 1513–1523.

Minamino, N., Kangawa, K., Chino, N., Sakakibara, S., and Matsuo, H. (1981) β-Neo-endorphin, a new hypothalamic "big" leu-enkephalin of porcine origin: Its purification and the complete amino acid sequence. *Biochem. Biophys. Res. Commun.* **99**, 864–870.

Mizumo, K., Minamino, N., Kangawa, K., and Matzuo, H. (1980) A new family of endogenous "big" met-enkephalins from bovine adrenal medulla: Purification and structure of Docosa (BAM-22P) and eicosapeptide (BAM-20P) with very potent opiate activity. *Biochem. Biophys. Res. Commun.* **97**, 1123–1290.

Morley, J. S. (1980) Structure–activity relationships of enkephalin-like peptides. *Ann. Rev. Pharmacol. Toxicol.* **20**, 81–110.

Mosberg, H. I., Hurst, R., Hruby, V. J., Gee, K., Akiyama, K., Yamamura, H. I., Galligan, J. J., and Burks, T. F. (1983) Bis-penicillamine enkephalins possess highly improved specificity toward δ receptors. *Proc. Natl. Acad. Sci. USA* **80**, 5871–5874.

Nakai, Y., Nakao, K., Oki, S., and Imura, H. (1978) Presence of immunoreactive lipotropin and endorphin in human placenta. *Life Sci.* **23**, 2013–2018.

Nakanishi, S., Inoue, A., Kita, T., Nakamura, M., Chang, A. C. Y., Cohen, S. W., and Numa, S. (1979) Nucleotide sequence of cloned cDNA for bovine corticotrophin-β-lipotropin precursor. *Nature* **278**, 423–427.

Nakao, K., Sudz, M., Sakamoto, M., Yoshimasi, T., Morii, N., Ikeda, Y., Yanaihara, C., Yanaihara, N., Numa, S., and Imura, H. (1983) Leumorphin is a novel endogenous opioid peptide derived from preproenkephalin B. *Biochem. Biophys. Res. Commun.* **117**, 695–701.

Nakazawa, T., Ikeda, M., Kaneko, T., and Yamatsu, K. (1985) Analgesic effects of dynorphin-A and morphine in mice. *Peptides* **6**, 75–78.

Negri, L., Melchiorri, F., Erspamer, G., and Erspamer, V. (1981) Radioimmunoassay of dermorphin-like peptides in mammalian and non-mammalian tissues. *Peptides* **2** (suppl.), 45–49.

Noda, M., Furatani, Y., Takahashi, H., Toyosato, M., Hirose, T., Inayama, S., Nakawishi, S., and Numa, S. (1982) Cloning and sequence analysis of cDNA for bovine adrenal preproenkephalin. *Nature* **295**, 202–206.

O'Donohue, T. L. and Dorsa, D. M. (1982) The opiomelanotropinergic neuronal and endocrine systems. *Peptides* **3,** 353–395.

O'Donohue, T. L., Handelmann, G. E., Miller, R. L., and Jacobowitz, D. M. (1982) N-Acetylation regulates the behavioral activity of α-melanotrophin in a multineurotransmitter neuron. *Science* **215,** 1125–1127.

Offermeier, J. and Van Rooyen, J. M. (1984) Opioid drugs and their receptors: A summary of the present state of knowledge. *South African Med. J.* **66,** 299–305.

Oka, K., Kandrowitz, J. D., and Spector, S. (1985) Isolation of morphine from toad skin. *Proc. Natl. Acad. Sci. USA* **82,** 1852–1854.

Olson, G. A., Olson, R. D., and Kastin, A. J. (1985) Endogenous opiates 1984. *Peptides* **6,** 769–791.

Oyama, T., Jin, T., Yamaya, R., Ling, N., and Guillemin, R. (1980) Profound analgesic effects of β-endorphin in man. *Lancet* **i,** 122–124.

Paterson, S. J., Robson, L. E., and Kosterlitz, H. W. (1983) Classification of opioid receptors. *Br. Med. Bull.* **39,** 31–36.

Paterson, S. J., Corbett, A. D., Gillan, M. G. C., Kosterlitz, H. W., McKnight, A. T., and Robson, L. E. (1984) Radioligands for probing opioid receptors. *J. Recept. Res.* **4,** 143–154.

Piercey, M. F., Varner, K., and Schroeder, L. A. (1982) Analgesic activity of intraspinally administered dynorphin and ethylketocyclozocine. *Eur J. Pharmacol.* **80,** 283–284.

Pintar, J. E., Schachter, B. S., Herman, A. B., Durgerian, S., and Krieger, D. T. (1984) Characterization and localization of proopiomelanocortin messenger RNA in the adult rat testis. *Science* **225,** 632–634.

Plotnikoff, N. P., Murgo, A. J., Miller, G. C., Cordes, C. N., and Faith, R. E. (1985) Enkephalins: Immunomodulators. *Fed. Proc.* **44,** 118–122.

Porreca, F. and Burks, T. F. (1983) The spinal cord as a site of opioid effects on gastrointestinal transit in the mouse. *J. Pharmacol. Exp. Ther.* **227,** 22–27.

Porreca, F., Mosberg, H. I., Hurst, R., Hruby, V. J., and Burks, T. F. (1984) Roles of mu, delta and kappa opioid receptors in spinal and supraspinal mediation of gastrointestinal transit effects and hot-plate analgesia in the mouse. *J. Pharmacol. Exp. Ther.* **230,** 341–348.

Porreca, F., Mosberg, H. I., Omnaas, J. R., Burks, T. F., and Cowan, A. (1987a) Supraspinal and spinal potency of selective opioid agonists in the mouse writhing test. *J. Pharmacol. Exp. Ther.* **240,** 890–894.

Porreca, F., Heyman, J. S., Mosberg, H. I., Omnaas, J. R., and Vaught, J. L. (1987b) Role of mu and delta receptors in the supraspinal and spinal analgesic effects of [D-Pen^2, D-Pen^5]enkephalin in the mouse. *J. Pharmacol. Exp. Ther.* **241,** 393–400.

Procacci, P., Della Corte, M., Zappi, M., Romano, S., Maresca, M., and Voegelin, M. R. (1972) Pain Threshold Measurements in Man, in *Recent Advances on Pain (Pathophysiology and Clinical Aspects)* (Bonica, J. T., Procacci, P., and Pagni, C. A., eds.) C. C. Thomas, Springfield, Illinois.

Przewlocki, R., Shearman, G. T., and Herz, A. (1983a) Mixed opioid/nonopioid effects of dynorphin and dynorphin related peptides after their intrathecal injection in rats. *Neuropeptides* **3,** 233–240.

Przewlocki, R., Stala, L., Greczek, M., Shearman, G. T., Przewlocka, B., and Herz, A. (1983b) Analgesic effects of μ, δ and κ-opiate agonists and, in particular, dynorphin at the spinal level. *Life Sci.* **33** (suppl.), 649–652.

Rees, L. H., Burke, C. W., Chard, T., Evans, S. W., and Letchworth, A. T. (1975) Possible placental origin of ACTH in normal human pregnancy. *Nature* **254**, 620.

Rodbard, D., Costa, T., Shimohigashi, Y., and Krumins, S. (1983) Dimeric pentapeptide and tetrapeptide enkephalins: New tools for the study of δ opioid receptors. *J. Recept. Res.* **3**, 21–33.

Roemer, D., Buscher, H. H., Hill, R. C., Pless, J., Bauer, W., Cardinaux, F., Closse, A., Hauser, D., and Huguenin, R. (1977) A synthetic enkephalin analogue with prolonged parenteral and oral analgesic activity. *Nature* **268**, 547–549.

Roques, B. P., Fournie-Zaluski, M.-C., Soroca, E., Lecomte, J. M., Malfroy, B., Llorens, C., and Schwartz, J.-C. (1980) The enkephalinase inhibitor thiorphan shows antinociceptive activity in mice. *Nature* **288**, 286–288.

Roques, B. P., Lucas-Soroca, E., Chaillet, P., Costentin, J., and Fournie-Zaluski, M.-C. (1983) Complete differentiation between enkephalinase and angiotensin-converting enzyme inhibition by retro-thiorphan. *Proc. Natl. Acad. Sci. USA* **80**, 3178–3182.

Ruprecht, J., Ukponmwan, O. E., Admiraal, P. V., and Dzolijic, M. R. (1983) Effect of phosphoramidon—a selective enkephalinase inhibitor—on nociception and behavior. *Neurosci. Lett.* **41**, 331–335.

Sandyk, R. (1985) The endogenous opioid system in neurological disorders of the basal ganglia. *Life Sci.* **37**, 1655–1663.

Schick, R. and Schusdziarra, V. (1985) Physiological, pathophysiological and pharmacological aspects of exogenous and endogenous opiates. *Clin. Physiol. Biochem.* **3**, 43–60.

Schmauss, C. and Emrich, H. M. (1985) Dopamine and the action of opiates: A reevaluation of the dopamine hypothesis of schizophrenia with special consideration of the role of endogenous opioids in the pathogenesis of schizophrenia. *Biol. Psychiatry* **20**, 1211–1231.

Schmauss, C. and Yaksh, T. L. (1984) In vivo studies on spinal opiate receptor systems mediating antinociception. II. Pharmacological profiles suggesting a differential association of μ, δ and κ receptors with visceral chemical and cutaneous thermal stimuli in the rat. *J. Pharmacol. Exp. Ther.* **228**, 1–12.

Schmauss, C., Shimohigashi, Y., Jensen, T. S., Rodbard, D., and Yaksh, T. L. (1985) Studies on spinal opiate receptor pharmacology. III. Analgetic effects of enkephalin dimers as measured by cutaneous-thermal and visceral-chemical evoked responses. *Brain Res.* **337**, 209–215.

Schultzberg, M., Hokfelt, T., Lundberg, J. M., Terenius, L., Elfrin, L., and Elde R. (1978) Enkephalin-like immunoreactivity in nerve terminals in sympathetic ganglia and adrenal medulla and in adrenal medullary gland cells. *Acta Physiolog. Scand.* **103**, 475–477.

Schuman, C. D., Gmerek, D. E., Mosberg, H. I., Rice, K. C., Jacobson, A. E., and Woods, J. H. (1987) Tail flick and analgesia following intracerebroventricular administration of opioids in the rat. I. Direct involvement of mu but not delta receptors. *J. Pharmacol. Exp. Ther.* (submitted).

Schwartz, J. C., Costentin, J., and Lecomte, J. M. (1985) Pharmacology of enkephalinase inhibitors. *Trends Pharm. Sci.* **6**, 472–476.

Scott, W. L., Mendelsohn, L. G., Cohen, M. L., Evans, D. A., and Frederickson, R. C. A. (1985) Enantiomers of [R,S]-thiorphan: Dissociation of analgesia from enkephalinase A inhibition. *Life Sci.* **36,** 1307–1313.

Seizinger, B. R., Liebisch, D. C., Gramsch, C., Herz, A., Weber, E., Evans, C. J., Esch, F. S., and Bohlen, P. (1985) Isolation and structure of a novel C-terminally amidated opioid peptide, amidorphin, from bovine adrenal medualla. *Nature* **313,** 57–62.

Shimohigashi, Y., Costa, T., Chen, H.-C., and Rodbard, D. (1982) Dimeric tetrapeptide enkephalins display extraordinary selectivity for the δ opiate receptor. *Nature* **297,** 333–335.

Smyth, D. G. (1983) β-Endorphin and related peptides in pituitary, brain, pancreas and antrum. *Br. Med. Bull.* **39,** 25–30.

Smyth, D. G., Massey, D. E., Zakarian, S., and Finnie, M. D. A. (1979) Endorphins are stored in biologically active and inactive forms: Isolation of α-N-acetyl peptides. *Nature* **279,** 252–254.

Spampinato, S. and Candeletti, S. (1985) Characterization of dynorphin A-induced antinociception at spinal level. *Eur. J. Pharmacol.* **110,** 21–30.

Stern, A. S., Jones, B. N., Shively, J. E., Stanley, S., and Udenfriend, S. (1981) Two adrenal opioid polypeptides: Proposed intermediates in the processing of proenkephalin. *Proc. Natl. Acad. Sci. USA* **78,** 1962–1966.

Stern, A. S., Lewis, R. V., Kimua, S., Rossier, J., Gerber, L. D., Brink, L., Stein, S., and Udenfriend, S. (1979) Isolation of the opioid heptapeptide Met-enkephalin[Arg^6, Phe^7] from bovine adrenal medullary granules and striatum. *Proc. Natl. Acad. Sci. USA* **76,** 6680–6683.

Takagi, H., Satoh, M., Akaike, A., Shibata, T., Yajima, H., and Ogawa, H. (1978) Analgesia by enkephalins injected into the nucleus reticularis gigantocellularis of rat medulla oblongata. *Eur. J. Pharmacol.* **49,** 113–116.

Tortella, F. C., Cowan, A., and Adler, M. W. (1981) Comparison of the anticonvulsant effects of opioid peptides and etorphine. *Life Sci.* **29,** 1039–1045.

Tortella, F. C., Long, J. B., and Holaday, J. W. (1985) Endogenous opioid systems: Physiological role in the self-limitation of seizures. *Brain Res.* **332,** 174–178.

Tseng, L.-F. (1981) Comparison of analgesic and body temperature responses to intrathecal β-endorphin and D-Ala^2-D-Leu$_5$-enkephalin. *Life Sci.* **29,** 1417–1424.

Tseng, L.-F. and Fujimoto, J. M. (1985) Differential actions of intrathecal naloxone on blocking the tail-flick inhibition induced by intra-ventricular β-endorphin and morphine in rats. *J. Pharmacol. Exp. Ther.* **232,** 74–79.

Tseng, L.-F., Wei, E. T., Loh, H. H., and Li, C. H. (1980) β-Endorphin: Central sites of analgesia, catalepsy and body temperature changes in rats. *J. Pharmacol. Exp. Ther.* **214,** 328–332.

Tsong, S. D., Phillips, D., Halmi, N., Liotta, A. S., Margioris, A., Bardin, C. W., and Krieger, D. T. (1982) ACTH and β-endorphin-related peptides are present in multiple sites in the reproductive tract of the male rat. *Endocrinology* **110,** 2204–2206.

Tung, A. S. and Yaksh, T. L. (1982) In vivo evidence for multiple opiate receptors mediating analgesia in the rat spinal cord. *Brain Res.* **247,** 75–83.

Turner, A. J., Matsas, R., and Kenny, A. J. (1985) Are there neuropeptide-specific peptidases? *Biochem. Pharmacol.* **34**, 1347–1356.

Tyers, M. B. (1980) A classification of opiate receptors that mediate antinociception in animals. *Br. J. Pharmacol.* **69**, 503–512.

Vaught, J. L. and Barrett, R. (1987) Modulation of Morphine Analgesia by Opioid Peptides: Implications for Antinociceptive Processes, in *Advances in Pain and Headache Research: Neurotransmitters and Pain* (Akil, H., ed.) Karger (in press).

Vaught, J. L., Rothman, R. B., and Westfall, T. C. (1982) μ and δ receptors: Their role in analgesia and in the differential effects of opioid peptides on analgesia. *Life Sci.* **30**, 1443–1455.

VonVoigtlander, P. F., Lahti, R. A., and Ludens, J. H. (1983) U-50,488: A selective and structurally novel (κ) opioid agonist. *J. Pharmacol. Exp. Ther.* **224**, 7-12.

Walker, J. M., Akil, H., and Watson, S. J. (1980) Evidence for homologous actions of pro-opiocortin products. *Science* **210**, 1247–1249.

Walker, J. M., Moises, H. C., Coy, D. H., Baldrighi, G., and Akil, H. (1982) Nonopiate effects of dynorphin and des-tyr-dynorphin. *Science* **218**, 1136–1138.

Ward, S. J. and Takemori, A. E. (1983) Relative involvement of μ, κ and δ receptor mechanisms in opiate-mediated antinociception in mice. *J. Pharmacol. Exp. Ther.* **224**, 525–530.

Watkins, L. R. and Mayer, D. J. (1982) Organization of endogenous opiate and nonopiate pain control systems. *Science* **216**, 1185–1192.

Watson, S. J., Akil, H., Richard, III, C. W., and Barchas, J. D. (1978) Evidence for two separate opiate peptide neuronal systems. *Nature* **275**, 226–228.

Watson, S. J., Khachaturian, H., Akil, H., Coy, D. H., and Goldstein, A. (1982) Comparison of the distribution of dynorphin systems and enkephalin systems in brain. *Science* **218**, 1134–1136.

Weber, E., Evans, C. J., and Barchas, J. D. (1981) Acetylated and nonacetylated forms of endorphin in pituitary and brain. *Biochem. Biophys. Res. Commun.* **103**, 982–989.

Weber, E., Evans, C. J., and Barchas, J. D. (1982a) Predominance of the amino-terminal octapeptide fragment of dynorphin in rat brain regions. *Nature* **299**, 77–79.

Weber, E., Evans, C. J., Chang, J.-K., and Barchas, J. D. (1982b) Brain distributions of α-neo-endorphin: Evidence for regional processing differences. *Biochem. Biophys. Res. Comm.* **108**, 81–88.

Weber, E., Evans, C. J., Chang, J.-K., and Barchas, J. D. (1982c) Antibodies specific for α-N-acetyl β-endorphins: Radioimmunoassays and detection of acetylated β-endorphins in pituitary extracts. *J. Neurochem.* **38**, 436–477.

Weber, E., Roth, K. A., and Barchas, J. D. (1982d) Immunohistochemical distribution of α-neo-endorphin/dynorphin neuronal systems in rat brain: Evidence for colocalization. *Proc. Natl. Acad. Sci. USA* **79**, 3062–3066.

Weber, E., Esch, F. S., Bohlen, P., Barchas, J. D., and Evans, C. J. (1983a) Metorphamide: Isolation, structure and biologic activity of a novel amidated opioid actapeptide from bovine brain. *Proc. Natl. Acad. Sci. USA* **80**, 7362–7366.

Weber, E., Evans, C. J., and Barchas, J. D. (1983b) Multiple endogenous ligands for opioid receptors. *Trends. Neurosci.* **6**, 333–336.

Wen, H. L., Mehal, Z. D., Ong, B. H., Ho, W. K. K., and Wen, D. Y. K. (1985) Intrathecal administration of β-endorphin and dynorphin-(1-13) for the treatment of intractable pain. *Life Sci.* **37**, 1213–1220.

Wood, P. L., Rackam, A., and Richard, J. (1981) Spinal analgesia, comparison of the mu agonist morphine and the kappa agonist ethylketocylclazocine. *Life Sci.* **28**, 2119–2125.

Woolf, C. J. (1980a) Analgesia and hyperalgesia produced in the rat by intrathecal naloxone. *Brain Res.* **189**, 593–597.

Woolf, C. J. (1980b) Intracerebral naloxone and the reaction to thermal noxious stimulation in the rat. *Brain Res.* **190**, 578–583.

Wuster, M., Schulz, R., and Herz, A. (1979) Specificity of opioids towards the μ, δ and ε opiate receptors. *Neurosci. Lett.* **15**, 193–198.

Wuster, M., Schulz, R., and Herz, A. (1980) Opiate activity and receptor selectivity of dynorphin $_{1-13}$ and related peptides. *Neurosci. Lett.* **20**, 79–83.

Wybran, J. (1985) Enkephalins and endorphins as modifiers of the immune system: Present and future. *Fed. Proc.* **44**, 92–94.

Xie, G. X., Han, J. S., and Hollt, V. (1983) Electroacupuncture analgesia blocked by microinjection of anti-β-endorphin antiserum into periaqueductal gray of the rat. *Int. J. Neurosci.* **18**, 287–292.

Xu, S.-F., Lu, W.-X., Zhou, K.-R., He, X.-P., Niu, S.-F., Xu, W.-M., Zhang, A.-L., Weber, E., and Chang, J. K. (1985) The analgesic and respiratory depressant actions of metorphamide in mice and rabbits. *Neuropeptides* **6**, 121–131.

Yaksh, T. L. (1983) In vivo studies on spinal opiate receptor systems mediating antinociception I. μ and δ receptor profiles in the primate. *J. Pharmacol. Exp. Ther.* **226**, 303–316.

Yaksh, T. L. (1984) Multiple opioid receptor systems in brain and spinal cord. 2. *Eur. J. Anesthesiol.* **1**, 201–243.

Yaksh, T. L. and Elde, R. P. (1981) Factors governing release of methionine enkephalin-like immunoreactivity from mesencephalon and spinal cord of the cat in vivo. *J. Neurophysiol.* **46**, 1056–1075.

Yaksh, T. L. and Harty, G. J. (1982) Effects of thiorphan on the antinociceptive actions of intrathecal [D-Ala^2,Met^5] enkephalin. *Eur. J. Pharmacol.* **79**, 293–300.

Yaksh, T. L. and Henry, J. L. (1978) Antinociceptive effects of intrathecally administered human β endorphin in the rat and cat. *Can. J. Physiol. Pharmacol.* **56**, 754–759.

Yaksh, T. L. and Noueihed, R. (1985) The physiology and pharmacology of spinal opiates. *Ann. Rev. Pharmacol. Toxicol.* **25**, 433–462.

Yaksh, T. L., Huang, S. P., Rudy, T. A., and Frederickson, R. C. A. (1977) The direct and specific opiate-like effect of Met^5-enkephalin and analogues on the spinal cord. *Neuroscience* **2**, 593–596.

Yaksh, T. L., Gross, K. F., and Li, C. H. (1982) Studies on the intrathecal effect of β-endorphin in primate. *Brain Res.* **241**, 261–269.

Yaksh, T. L., Terenius, L., Nyberg, F., Jhamandas, K., and Wang, J-Y. (1983) Studies on the release by somatic stimulation from rat and cat spinal cord of active materials which displace dihydromorphine in an opiate-binding assay. *Brain Res.* **268**, 119–128.

Yang, H.-Y.-T., Panula, P., Tang, J., and Costa, E. (1983) Characterization and location of met^5-enkephalin-arg^6-phe^7 stored in various rat brain regions. *J. Neurochem.* **40,** 969–976.

Yen, S. S. C., Quigley, M. E., Reid, R. L., Ropert, J. F., and Cetel, N. S. (1985) Neuroendocrinology of opioid peptides and their role in the control of gonadotropin and prolactin secretion. *Am. J. Obstet. Gynecol.* **152,** 485–493.

Zajac, J-M., Gacel, G., Petit, F., Dudey, P., Rossignol, P., and Roques, B. P. (1983) Tyr-D-Thr-Gly-Phe-Leu-Thr: A new highly potent and fully specific agonist for opiate δ receptors. *Biochem. Biophys. Res. Commun.* **111,** 390–397.

Zakarian, S. and Smyth, D. (1979) Distribution of active and inactive forms of endorphins in rat pituitary and brain. *Proc. Natl. Acad. Sci. USA* **76,** 5972–5976.

Zakarian, S. and Smyth, D. G. (1982) β-Endorphin is processed differently in specific regions of rat pituitary and brain. *Nature* **296,** 250–252.

Zamir, N., Weber, E., Palkovits, M., and Brownstein, M. (1984) Differential processing of prodynorphin and proenkephalin in specific regions of the rat brain. *Proc. Natl. Acad. Sci. USA* **81,** 6886–6889.

Zlokovic, B. V., Begley, D. J., and Chain-Eliash, D. G. (1985) Blood–brain barrier permeability to leucine-enkephalin, D-Alanine^2-D-Leucine^5-enkephalin and their N-terminal amino acid (tyrosine). *Brain Res.* **336,** 125–132.

SECTION 2
CHARACTERIZATION OF OPIOID
RECEPTOR BINDING SITES

Chapter 3

Early Studies of Opioid Binding

Gavril W. Pasternak

1. Introduction

The complexity of opioid binding studies in recent years has increased dramatically as a result of the identification of multiple subclasses of receptors. Early studies performed prior to the report of multiple binding sites, however, identified a number of interesting features of opioid binding. Although the interpretations of this early work need to be reexamined, much of it is still relevant. This chapter will review some of the early studies in light of our current knowledge.

2. Early Attempts To Demonstrate Opiate Binding Sites

The pharmacological concept of receptors, based upon the observation of rigid structure–activity relationships, stereospecificity, and the observation of maximal pharmacological responses, goes back to the turn of the century (Langley, 1909; Ehrlich, 1913; Clark, 1933; Gaddum, 1937). Opioid structure–activity relationships established for literally thousands of semisynthetic and synthetic compounds (de Stevens, 1965; Jacobson et al., 1970; Janssen et al., 1960, 1966) revealed very rigid requirements for activity, including strict stereospecificity (Portoghese, 1966, 1970). Furthermore, both in vivo testing and bioassays clearly fulfilled the other criteria expected of a receptor-mediated action, including cross tolerance and dependence. Based upon these observations, Beckett and Casey even attempted to map an opioid receptor binding site (Beckett and Casey, 1965, 1954a,b; Beckett, 1955; Beckett et al., 1956a,b).

With such strong pharmacological evidence in favor of a receptor mechanism of action, it is not surprising that many groups attempted to label it biochemically prior to 1973 without success (Chernov and Woods, 1965; Ingoglia and Dole, 1970; van Praag and Simon, 1966; Berkowitz and Way, 1971; Clouet and Williams, 1973; Hug and Oka, 1971; Navon and Lajtha, 1970; Seeman et al., 1972; Goldstein et al., 1971). Most groups used the concept of stereospecificity; i.e., looking at differences in the ability of the active and inactive stereoisomers to compete binding (Goldstein et al., 1971). The most common difficulty encountered was the high nonspecific binding resulting from drug concentrations that were too high and specific radioactivities that were too low. Estimates of morphine concentrations within the brain during analgesia were between 0.1 and 1 μM and most investigators assumed similar K_d values. Nanomolar affinities were not expected. With the benefit of hindsight, we now know that opioid concentrations in the low nanomolar range are needed to obtain favorable ratios of specific to nonspecific binding.

3. Identification and Characterization of Opiate Binding Sites

In 1973 three laboratories reported the biochemical demonstration of opioid binding sites using ^{3}H-labeled naloxone (Pert and Snyder, 1973), dihydromorphine (Terenius, 1973), or etorphine (Simon et al., 1973). The success of these three groups rested primarily upon their ability to examine low ligand concentrations with compounds of high specific activity. These reports fulfilled the major criteria required to document a relevant binding site. These binding sites demonstrated the same stereospecificity observed pharmacologically, and unlabeled compounds inhibited binding with the same relative potency observed in bioassays and in vivo (Table 1). Furthermore, compounds without opioid-like

TABLE 1
Inhibition of [^{3}H]Naloxone Binding
by a Series of Opioids

Compound	IC$_{50}$, nM^a
(−)-Etorphine	0.3
(−)-Levallorphan	1
(−)-Levorphanol	2
(−)-Nalorphine	3
(−)-Morphine	7
(−)-Cyclazocine	10
(−)-Naloxone	10
(−)-Hydromorphone	20
(−)-Methadone	30
(±)-Pentazocine	50
(+)-Methadone	300
(±)-Meperidine	1000
(±)-Propoxyphene	1000
(+)-3-Hydroxy-N-allylmorphinan	7000
dextrorphan	8000
(−)-Codeine	20,000
(−)-Oxycodone	30,000

^{a}IC$_{50}$ values were determined by log probit analysis and are taken from Snyder et al., 1975. Note that dextrorphan is the (+)-isomer of levorphanol and (+)-3-hydroxy-N-allylmorphinan is the (+)-isomer of levallorphan.

activity in standard pharmacological assays did not inhibit binding at concentrations under 10 μM (Table 2). For the most part, these initial reports were labeling mu binding sites. [^{3}H]Naloxone and ^{3}H-dihydromorphine used in these early studies are relatively mu selective, but naloxone is an antagonist, whereas dihydromorphine is an agonist. The agonist etorphine, however, is less selective among the opioid receptors and labels a variety of subtypes in addition to mu.

Saturation studies from all initial reports implied a single class of receptor with an affinity constant in the nanomolar range. Subsequent studies established the importance of both protein and phospholipid integrity (Simon et al., 1973; Pasternak and Snyder, 1974, 1975b). Trypsin and chymotrypsin both effectively lowered binding, whereas DNAase, RNAase, neuraminidase, and phospholipase C were all without effect. Although Pasternak and Snyder (1974) found a dramatic lowering of binding with phospholipase A, Simon and coworkers (Simon et al., 1973) did not. This difference might have resulted from different sources of

TABLE 2
Drugs Ineffective in Altering [³H] Dihydromorphine Binding[a]

Acetyl-β-methylcholine	Epinephrine	Ornithine
Acetylsalicylic acid	Ethosoximide	Orphenadrine
γ-Aminobutyric acid	Fenfluramine	Oxytropane
Arecoline	Glutamic acid	Pargyline
Atropine	Glycine	Peganone
Bicuculline	Hemicholinium-3	Pentylenetetrazole
Bretylium	Histamine	Phenelzine
Brocresine	Hydroxyamphetamine	Phenobarbital
Bromodiphenhydramine	Hydroxychloroquine	Phenylpropanolamine
3α-(5H-Dibenzo[a,d]-	Hydroxyzine	Pilocarpine
cyclohepten-S-yl)	Hyoscine	Promethazine
Bulbocapnine	Imipramine	Serotonin
Butylcholine	3-Iodo-L-tyrosine	Taurine
Caffeine	Iprindole	Tetrabenazine
Carbamylcholine	Isoproteronol	Δ-Tetrahydrocanna-
Carbinoxamine	Leucine	binol
Chlordiazepoxide	Mecamylamine	β-(2-Thienyl)-
Chlorpheniramine	Methergine	isopropylamine
Cobefrin	Methdilazine	Threonine
Colchicine	3-Methoxytyramine	Tranylcypromine
Cycramine	3-Methoxy-4-hydroxy-	Trifluoperazine
Decamethonium	mandelic acid	Triprolidine
Desipramine	α-Methyldopa	Tryptamine
Diethylpropion	Neostigmine	Tryptophan
Doxepin	Nialamide	Urecholamine
Dopamine	Nicotine	Valine
Ecolid	Nortriptyline	
Ephedrine	Octopamine	

[a]Drugs at a final concentration of 3 μM were preincubated with rat brain homogenate in a standard binding assay using [³H]dihydromorphine. None of the listed compounds produces significant inhibition of stereospecific binding (from Snyder et al.,
1975).

enzyme. However, the inactivity of phospholipase A in the study
from Simon might be explained by inadequate levels of calcium,
and more recently, Simon and coworkers have suggested that the
fatty acids generated by phospholipase A are responsible for the
lowered binding (Lin et al., 1981).

Subcellular studies revealed an association of the binding
sites with synaptosomes (Hitzeman and Loh, 1974; Pert et al.,
1973, 1974a) consistent with its postulation as a transmitter receptor. Following lysis of the synaptosomes, binding was associated
with the synaptic membranes. Injection of ³H-etorphine in vivo

revealed an association of radiolabel with synaptic membrane fractions (Mule et al., 1975).

Regional studies documented dramatic differences in the levels of binding in various brain structures (Table 3; Kuhar et al., 1973; Hiller et al., 1973; Lee et al., 1975; Wong and Horng, 1976). In these homogenate studies, high levels of binding were noted in areas associated with the limbic system, brain regions known to be important in opioid action (Pert and Yaksh, 1974, 1975). No significant specific opioid binding was detected in white matter, again implying an association with neuronal elements. Autoradiographic studies labeling sites in vivo or in vitro provided a more detailed distribution (Pert et al., 1975, 1976; Schubert et al., 1975; Atweh and Kuhar, 1977a,b,c), which will be discussed in detail in a later chapter.

Early studies identified binding sites both pre- and postsynaptically. Lamotte et al. (1976) addressed the issue by lesioning dorsal roots and then measuring binding within the cord. In brief, they found approximately 50% decreases in binding, implying the presence of sites both pre- and postsynaptically. Autoradiographic approaches are more suited to this type of question. Atweh and Kuhar (1977a) found binding sites situated along the vagus nerve. In a later series of experiments (Young et al., 1980), Kuhar again reported the presence of opioid binding sites on the vagus nerve. In addition, they examined the effects of litgation of the nerve and observed axoplasmic flow of the binding sites. Other investigators using electrophysiological approaches, however, implied postsynaptic localizations as well (Ziegelgansberger and Fry, 1976).

The developmental appearance of these sites (Coyle and Pert, 1976; Garcin and Coyle, 1976; Clendeninn et al., 1976) and their phylogenetic distribution (Pert et al., 1974b) also have been investigated. Developmentally, these sites show their greatest rate of increase during the first 3 wk after birth. Interestingly, Coyle and Pert found a caudal to rostral development of regions. Zhang and Pasternak (1981) examined the appearance of high-affinity (mu_1) and low affinity (mu_2, delta, kappa) binding sites. Overall, they reported a similar appearance for total binding, but noted significant differences between the high-affinity (mu_1) site and the others. Whereas the others had appreciable levels at birth (approximately 40% of adult levels), the density of the high-affinity (mu_1) sites was quite low. Over the first 2 wk after birth, the density of the mu_1 sites increased rather dramatically in contrast to the others, which stayed relatively constant.

TABLE 3
Opioid–Receptor Binding in Regions of Monkey Brain[a]

	Stereospecific [³H]dihydromorphine binding, fmol/mg protein	
Cerebral hemispheres		
Frontal pole	11.9 ± 1.4	(4)[b]
Superior temporal gyrus	10.8 ± 2.5	(3)
Middle temporal gyrus	7.1	(1)
Inferior temporal gyrus	6.0	(1)
Precentral gyrus	3.4	(2)
Postcentral gyrus	2.8	(2)
Occipital pole	2.3 ± 0.5	(4)
White matter areas		
Corpus callosum	<2	(2)
Corona radiata	<2	(2)
Anterior commissure	5.4	(2)
Fornix	<2	(2)
Optic chiasm	<2	(2)
Limbic cortex		
Anterior amgydala	65.1 ± 21	(4)
Posterior amgydala	34.1 ± 4.2	(4)
Hippocampus	12.5 ± 2.2	(4)
Hypothalamus		
Medial hypothalamus	24.2 ± 3.2	(4)
Anterior hypothalamus	24.3 ± 3.7	(3)
Posterior hypothalamus	24.7 ± 1.4	(3)
Hypothalamus	32.2	(1)
Mammillary bodies	5.0	(1)
Thalamus		
Medial thalamus	24.6 ± 1.6	(3)
Lateral thalamus	7.8	(2)

(continued)

Phylogenetically, opioid binding sites have been reported in a wide range of species. In general, ontogeny recapitulates phylogeny. Initial studies by Snyder's group suggested low levels in invertebrates. Among the vertebrates, binding generally increased progressively in higher animals. It should be kept in mind, however, that these early studies used radioligands relatively selective for mu sites. More recent studies utilizing radiolabeled enkephalin analogs have reported opioid binding sites in

TABLE 3 *(continued)*
Opioid–Receptor Binding in Regions of Monkey Brain[a]

	Stereospecific [³H]dihydromorphine binding, fmol/mg protein	
Extrapyramidal areas		
Caudate nucleus (head)	19.4 ± 2.3	(4)
Caudate nucleus (body)	9.0 ± 1.2	(3)
Caudate nucleus (tail)	8.9 ± 3.0	(3)
Putamen	11.7 ± 1.9	(6)
Globus pallidus	7.7	(2)
Internal capsule	5.4	(2)
Midbrain		
Superior colliculi	10.6 ± 2.0	(3)
Inferior colliculi	6.7 ± 0.7	(3)
Interpeduncular nucleus area	13.7 ± 1.5	(4)
Raphe area	8.2	(2)
Periaqueductal gray	31.1 ± 4.6	(4)
Cerebellum-lower brain stem		
Pons (ventral)	1.4	(2)
Cerebellar cortex	<2	(2)
Dentate nucleus	1.9	(2)
Floor of fourth ventricle	6.3 ± 1.3	(3)
Pyramidal tract	3.0	(2)
Lower medulla	5.8	(2)
Spinal cord (thoracic)		
Dorsal column (white)	3.1	(2)
Lateral cord (white)	3.3	(1)
Gray matter	8.8	(2)

[a]From Kuhar et al., 1973.
[b]Numbers in parentheses represent replications.

insects (Stefano and Scharrer, 1981) and in a mollusk (Stefano et al., 1982). In addition these early reports did not distinguish between mu subtypes. Evidence now suggests that mu_1 sites are present only in higher species since they cannot be detected in fish (Buatti and Pasternak, 1981). Finally, binding levels can also vary significantly among different strains of a single species, and these levels correlate quite well with the sensitivity of the strains to opioids (Shuster et al., 1975).

4. Correlating Opiate Binding Sites with Opiate Actions

Establishing the relevancy of these binding sites was a major objective in these early studies. The demonstration of stereospecificity and the correlation of binding and pharmacological potency provided the first bit of evidence. This was supported by the localization of the binding sites to brain regions known to be important for opioid action and the association of binding sites with neural tissue, more specifically synaptic membranes.

Perhaps the strongest evidence correlating binding activity with pharmacological actions comes from studies by Creese and Snyder (1975). Pert and Snyder (1973) reported the presence of binding sites on the nerve plexus of the ileum. Creese and Snyder extended these observations. First they demonstrated the relationship between binding in the brain and in the guinea pig ileum. They then compared the relative potency of the agents in the ileum binding assay with their activity in the ileum contraction assay and found an excellent correlation.

With our current knowledge of multiple classes of receptors, it might seem simply fortuitous that they found such a good correlation. Keep in mind, however, that the investigators were using a radiolabeled mu ligand, and that mu receptors were responsible for the opioid actions in the guinea pig ileum. The correlation was improved by examining binding in the presence of sodium, which markedly decreases the affinity of agonists to a far greater degree than antagonists (see below). They reasoned that this correlation was more appropriate since sodium was normally present. This concept is still controversial since we do not really know yet the "physiological condititions" associated with binding. Since many receptors extend through the membrane, the inside and outside portions of the binding site may actually be exposed to entirely different conditions.

5. Discrimination of Agonist and Antagonist Binding

One of the major advantages of the opioid system is the availability of a number of useful radiolabeled agonists and antagonists. Using these compounds, differences in the effects of a number of treatments on agonist and antagonist binding were identified, including monovalent and divalent cations, enzymes, reagents, and temperature.

The ability of sodium ions to enhance antagonist binding and lower agonist binding was first reported in 1973 (Pert et al., 1973). Indeed, this observation was based upon an interesting series of events. After noting in December of 1972 that Na_2EDTA doubled the binding of the antagonist [³H]naloxone, I suggested to Adele Snowman, a technician working in the laboratory, that she try it in her assays with the agonist [³H]dihydromorphine. She tried it several times and reported that the Na_2EDTA consistently destroyed her binding. We argued back and forth, each convinced of the reproducibility of our own observations. Several weeks later, when she tested both ³H-ligands together, we realized that the actions of Na_2EDTA reflected the agonist and antagonist properties of the two ligands. We then established that the sodium used to make the salt was responsible for these actions. The studies were then extended to include several radiolabeled opioid agonists and antagonists (Table 4).

The development of the sodium shift to evaluate unlabeled compounds turned out to be a very important aspect of these studies. IC_{50} values of the compound to be tested were determined against [³H]naloxone binding in the presence and absence of sodium chloride (100 mM). Since agonist binding was depressed by sodium, the IC_{50} value of agonists was shifted to the right in the presence of sodium, yielding a ratio of IC_{50} values

TABLE 4
Effect of Sodium Ions on Radiolabeled Opioid Agonists
and Antagonists[a]

³H-Labeled drug	Change in binding by sodium chloride, 100 mM
Agonists	
Dihydromorphine	−70%
Oxymorphone	−44%
Levorphanol	−28%
Antagonists	
Nalorphine	+45%
Naloxone	+141%
Levallorphan	+29%

[a]Binding of each radioligand was assessed in the presence and absence of sodium chloride (100 mM) (from Pert et al., 1973).

(presence of sodium/absence of sodium) of greater than one (Table 5). Antagonists retain their potency in the presence of sodium and have ratios of approximately one. Partial agonists have shifts intermediate between pure agonists and antagonists. The actual shifts are dependent upon the assay conditions and the concentration of [^{3}H]naloxone, and therefore can vary from study to study. Thus, the interpretation of sodium shifts requires the inclusion of internal controls, such as naloxone and morphine, to provide a reference for the unknown compounds. This technique has proven extremely valuable in the classification of new opioids.

Several reagents also discriminate between the binding of agonists and antagonists (Table 6; Wilson et al., 1975; Pasternak et al., 1975a,b). In brief, treatment of tissue with a wide variety of reagents lowered the binding of radiolabeled agonists far more effectively than antagonists. Equally interesting was the relationship between the actions of these reagents and sodium. Although some of the reagents did differentiate between agonists and antagonists in the absence of sodium, its presence markedly potentiated the differences in binding. Further studies examining the sensitivity of binding to sodium in treated and untreated tissue clearly revealed a shift to the left of the sodium inhibition curve.

TABLE 5
Sodium Shifts of Opioids on [^{3}H]Naloxone Binding

| Opioid | IC$_{50}$, nM[a] | | |
	Control	NaC1 100 mM	Sodium shift
Naloxone	1.5	1.5	1.0
Naltrexone	0.5	0.5	1.0
Diprenorphine	0.5	0.5	1.0
Cyclazocine	0.9	1.5	1.7
Levallorphan	1.0	2.0	2.0
Nalorphine	1.5	4.0	2.7
Pentazocine	15.0	50.0	3.3
Etorphine	0.5	6.0	12
Meperidine	3,000	50,000	17
Levorphanol	1.0	15	15
Oxymorphone	1.0	30	30
Dihydromorphine	3.0	140	47
Propoxyphene	200	12,000	60
Phenazocine	0.6	80	133

[a]IC$_{50}$ values for each compound against [^{3}H]naloxone was determined in the presence and absence of sodium chloride (100 mM), and the ratio determined (from Pert et al., 1973).

TABLE 6

Effects of Reagents, Enzymes, and Cations on the Binding
of Opioid Agonists and Antagonists[a]

Treatment	Change in binding			
	Assayed with NaCl, 100 mM		Assayed without NaCl	
	[³H]Naloxone	[³H]Dihydro-morphine	[³H]Naloxone	[³H]Dihydro-morphine
Reagent				
N-ethylmaleimide (100 μM)	−15%	−91%	−25%	−47%
Iodoacetamide (5 mM)	−10%	−90%	−15%	−55%
Mersalyl acid (10 μM)	−24%	−77%	−41%	−65%
1-Ethyl-3-(3-dimethylamino-propyl) carbodiimide (1 mM)	−19%	−70%	−11%	−48%
5,5'-Dithiobis-(2-nitrobenzoic acid) (0.1 mM)	0	−79%	0	−16%
p-Chloromercuribenzoate (10 μM)	−10%	−75%	−40%	−45%
Enzyme				
Trypsin (1 μg/mL)	−21%	−95%	−35%	−63%
Chymotrypsin (10 μg/mL)	−29%	−55%	−38%	−46%
Phospholipase A (50 ng/mL)	−50%	−85%	−81%	−77%
Divalent cation				
Manganese chloride (1 mM)	+8%	+105%	−1%	+17%
Magnesium chloride (1 mM)	+17%	+58%	−1%	+24%
Calcium chloride (10 mM)	−15%	+28%	−23%	−9%
Nickel chloride (20 μM)	−3%	+63%	+6%	+22%
Copper chloride (10 μM)	−27%	−79%	−56%	−63%
Ferrous chloride (0.01 mM)	−34%	−96%	−50%	−64%

[a]Tissue was assayed with either [³H]dihydromorphine or [³H]naloxone either after treatments with the stated reagent or enzyme or in the presence and absence of the indicated divalent cation with or without sodium. All enzymes and reagents were washed from the tissue prior to the assay (from Pasternak et al., 1975a,b).

Other treatments also discriminated between agonist and antagonist binding. Enzymatic treatments lowered agonist binding more effectively than that of antagonists (Table 6; Pasternak et al., 1975b). As noted with reagents, sodium dramatically enhanced the differential effect. Lowering the temperature of the binding assay to 0°C enhances antagonist binding while lowering agonist binding (Creese et al., 1975).

Not all treatments preferentially lower agonist binding. Divalent cations, for example, can enhance agonist binding relatively selectively (Table 6; Pasternak et al., 1975a). A variety of anions, including chloride, sulfate, fluoride, bromide, iodide, thiocyanate, perchlorate, and formate had no effect. Manganese and magnesium were the most interesting, although nickel also produced a similar effect. Our current understanding of the role of opioid binding sites with nucleotide binding proteins (N_s and N_i) now provides a better understanding of these interactions. As with the earlier studies, these actions are interrelated with those of sodium. In studies directly measuring the ability of sodium to inhibit the binding of [^{3}H]dihydromorphine, manganese and magnesium shift the inhibition dose–response curve for sodium up to fivefold to the right.

In the same manner in which sodium shifts can be determined for opioids, manganese shifts can also be examined (Table 7). In effect, this type of approach examines the ability of manganese to "reverse" the effects of sodium. Antagonists have shifts close to one, whereas agonist shifts are greater.

Chelator studies are consistent with the above divalent studies. As expected, EDTA potentiated the ability of sodium to inhibit agonist binding. This effect was reversible, since subsequent addition of manganese or magnesium restored binding to normal levels.

6. Membrane Lipids and Opiate Binding

The sensitivity of opioid binding to phospholipase A strongly suggested a role for phospholipids (Pasternak and Snyder, 1974, 1975b; Abood et al., 1978). Exposing brain membranes to phosphatidylserine enhanced opioid binding to brain membranes (Abood et al., 1978). In addition, Abood and coworkers reported the reversal of phospholipase A inhibition of binding with phosphatidylserine, implying an important role of phosphatidylser-

TABLE 7
Manganese Shifts of Opioids on [³H]Naloxone Binding[a]

| | IC$_{50}$ value, nM | | | | Manganese shift, |
| | Assayed with NaCl | | Assayed without NaCl | | |
Opiate	Control	MnCl$_2$	Control	MnCl$_2$	with NaCl
Methadone	65	11	4.5	1.9	5.9
Oxymorphone	19	4.2	2.0	1.0	4.5
Morphine	29	7	2.5	0.6	4.1
Levorphanol	6.4	2.5	0.9	0.5	2.7
Pentazocine	95	35	16	18	2.7
Nalorphine	11	6.6	3.9	2.2	1.7
Levallorphan	1.5	1.2	0.75	0.57	1.2

[a]Tissue was assayed with or without sodium chloride (100 mM) or manganese chloride (1 mM) using [³H]naloxone. The manganese shift is the ratio of the IC$_{50}$ values of the compounds in the presence of sodium divided by the IC$_{50}$ value in the presence of both sodium and manganese (from Pasternak et al., 1975a).

ine in the vicinity of the binding site. Furthermore, phosphatidyl-serine decarboxylase, which converts phosphatidylserine to phos-phatidylethanolamine, also inhibits binding.

Much work has been reported on the role of cerebroside sul-fate in opioid binding. In studies reported soon after the initial reports of opioid binding, Loh and his group reported the ability of cerebroside sulfate to bind opioids saturably and stereospecifi-cally (Loh et al., 1974, 1975; Cho et al., 1976; Loh and Law, 1980). Equally important, cerebroside sulfate also bound opioids with a rank order of potency similar to their pharmacological actions. Additional studies revealed that agonists and antagonists inter-acted with cerebroside sulfate differentially (Cho et al., 1976, 1979), and the interactions were influenced by sodium (Cho et al., 1979). On the other hand, there is no correlation between the re-gional distribution of cerebroside sulfate and opioid binding sites within the brain. However, in view of the low density of opioid binding sites, one would not expect that a large proportion of cerebroside sulfate would be associated with opioid receptors. In-deed, hydrolysis of only 2% of cerebroside sulfate by cerebroside sulfatase lowers ^3H naloxone binding by approximately 50% (Law et al., 1979). All these early studies examined predominently mu ^3H-ligands. Many questions regarding the potential role of cere-broside sulfate in the various opioid binding subtypes remain.

7. Binding Heterogeneity

Martin first raised the issue of receptor multiplicity with his pro-posal of "Receptor Dualism" in 1967 (Martin, 1967). However, the early reports of opioid binding did not reveal evidence of binding heterogeneity (Pert and Snyder, 1973; Terenius, 1973; Simon et al., 1973; Pasternak and Snyder, 1974). When radiolabeled opi-oids of even higher specific activity became available, our labora-tory identified a novel, very-high-affinity binding component that was very sensitive to sodium (Pasternak and Snyder, 1975b). Whereas sodium increased the number of high-affinity [^3H]nalox-one binding sites, it eliminated the high-affinity binding of [^3H]dihydromorphine. This high-affinity binding component ex-hibited the same stereospecificity and rank order potency of the earlier sites. Interestingly, the number of these high-affinity bind-ing components was far less than the number of the lower-affinity binding sites. At the time, we assumed a single binding site and proposed that the high- and low-affinity components represented agonist and antagonist conformations of a single site. Subsequent studies indicate that this is almost certainly not the case, as discussed in greater detail in a subsequent chapter. In brief, this high-affinity site, which we recently termed the mu_1 site, is a distinct site that differs from the morphine- and enkephalin-selective sites (Pasternak and Wood, 1986). In vivo pharmacological studies utilizing novel affinity antagonists naloxonazine and naloxazone have correlated this site with analgesia and a number of other opioid actions, firmly establishing its relevancy.

8. Conclusion

The opioid field has evolved quite rapidly in the decade since the identification of opioid binding sites within the brain. The discovery of several subtypes of opioid receptors has complicated the interpretation of many of the earlier binding studies. However, many of these earlier studies reported important observations that should be reexamined in light of our current knowledge of the various subtypes.

References

Abood, L. G., Salem, N., MacNeil, M., and Butler, M. (1978) Phospholipid changes in synaptic membranes by lipolytic enzymes and subsequent restoration of opiate binding with phosphoserine. *Biochim. Biophys. Acta* **530**, 35–46.

Atweh, S. F. and Kuhar, M. J. (1977a) Autoradiographic localization of opiate receptors in rat brain. I. Spinal cord and lower medulla. *Brain Res.* **124**, 53–67.

Atweh, S. F. and Kuhar, M. J. (1977b) Autoradiographic localization of opiate receptors in rat brain. II. The brain stem. *Brain Res.* **129**, 1–12.

Atweh, S. F. and Kuhar, M. J. (1977c) Autoradiographic localization of opiate receptors in rat brain. III. The telencephalon. *Brain Res.* **134**, 393–405.

Beckett, A. H. (1955) Analgetics and their antagonists: Some steric and chemical considerations. *J. Pharm. Pharmacol.* **8**, 848–859.

Beckett, A. H. and Casy, A. F. (1954a) Stereochemistry of certain analgesics. *Nature* **173**, 1231–1232.

Beckett, A. H. and Casy, A. F. (1954b) Synthetic analgetics: Stereochemical considerations. *J. Pharm. Pharmacol.* **6**, 986–1001.

Beckett, A. H. and Casy, A. F. (1965) Analgesics and Their Antagonists: Biochemical Aspects and Structure–activity Relationships, in *Progress in Medicinal Chemistry* (Ellis, G. P. and West, G. B., eds.) Butterworth, London, England.

Beckett, A. H., Casy, A. F., Harper, N. J., and Phillips, P. M. (1956a) Analgetics and their antagonists: Some steric considerations. *J. Pharm. Pharmacol.* **8**, 874–889.

Beckett, A. H., Casy, A. F., Harper, N. J. and Phillips, P. M. (1956b) Analgesics and their antagonists: Some steric and chemical considerations. *J. Pharm. Pharmacol.* **8**, 860–873.

Berkowitz, B. A. and Way, E. L. (1971) Analgesic activity and central nervous system distribution of the optical isomers of pentazocine in the rat. *J. Pharm. Exp. Ther.* **177**, 500–508.

Buatti, M. C. and Pasternak, G. W. (1981) Multiple opiate receptors: Phylogenetic differences. *Brain Res.* **218**, 400–405.

Chernov, H. I. and Woods, L. A. (1965) Central nervous system distribution and metabolism of ^{14}C-morphine during morphine-induced feline mania. *J. Pharm. Exp. Ther.* **149**, 146–155.

Cho, T. M., Cho, J. S., and Loh, H. H. (1976) ^{3}H-Cerebroside sulfate redistribution induced by cations, opiate or phosatidylserine. *Life Sci.* **19**, 117–124.

Cho, T. M., Loh, H. H., and Way, E. L. (1979) Effects of monovalent cations on cerebroside sulfate binding to opiate agonists and antagonists. International Narcotic Conference, North Falmouth, Massachusetts.

Clark, A. J. (1933) *The Mode of Action of Drugs on Cells* Williams and Wilkins, Baltimore.

Clendeninn, N. J., Petraitis, M., and Simon, E. J. (1976) Ontological development of opiate receptor in rodent brain. *Brain Res.* **118**, 157–160.

Clouet, D. H. and Williams, N. (1973) Localization in brain particulate fractions of narcotic analgesic drugs administered intracisternally to rats. *Biochem. Pharm.* **22**, 1283–1293.

Coyle, J. T. and Pert, C. B. (1976) Ontogenetic development of ^{3}H-naloxone binding in rat brain. *Neuropharmacology* **15**, 555–560

Creese, I. and Snyder, S. H. (1975) Receptor binding and pharmacological activity in the guinea pig intestine. *J. Pharm. Exp. Ther.* **194**, 205–219.

Creese, I., Pasternak, G. W., Pert, C. B., and Snyder, S. H. (1975) Discrimination by temperature of opiate agonist and antagonist receptor binding. *Life Sci.* **16**, 1837–1842.

de Stevens, G. (1965) *Analgetics* vol. 5, Academic, New York, p. 475

Ehrlich, P. (1913) Chemotherapeutics: Scientific principles, methods and results. *Lancet* **2**, 445–451.

Gaddum, J. H. (1937) The quantitative effects of antagonistic drugs. *J. Physiol.* **89**, 7p–9p.

Garcin, F. and Coyle, J. T. (1976) Ontogenetic Development of ^{3}H-Naloxone Binding and Endogenous Morphine-Like Factor in Rat Brain, in *Opiates and Endogenous Opioid Peptides* (Kosterlitz, H. W., ed.) Elsevier/North Holland Biomedical Press, Amsterdam.

Goldstein, A., Lowney, L. I., and Pal, B. K. (1971) Stereospecific and nonspecific interactions of the morphine congener levorphanol in subcellular fractions of mouse brain. *Proc. Natl. Acad. Sci USA* **68**, 1742–1747.

Hiller, J. M., Pearson, J., and Simon, E. J. (1973) Distribution of stereospecific binding of the potent narcotic analgesic etorphine in human brain: Predominance in the limbic system. *Res. Commun. Chem. Pathol. Pharmacol.* **6**, 1052–1062.

Hitzeman, R. J. and Loh, H. H. (1974) Characteristics of the binding of ^{3}H-naloxone in the mouse brain. *Proc. Soc. Neurosci.* **3**, 350.

Hug, C. C. and Oka, T. (1971) Uptake of ^{3}H-dihydromorphine by synaptosomes. *Life Sci.* **10**, 201–213.

Ingoglia, N. A. and Dole, V. P. (1970) Localization of *d*- and *l*-methadone after intraventricular injection into rat brains. *J. Pharm. Exp. Ther.* **175**, 84–87.

Jacobson, A. E., May, E. L., and Sargent, L. J. (1970) Analgetics, in *Medicinal Chemistry* part II, 3rd Ed. (Burger, A., ed.) Wiley Interscience, New York.

Janssen, P. A. J., Hellerback, J., Schnider, O., Besendorf, L. T., and Pellmont, B. (1960) Diphenylpropylamines, Morphinans, in *Synthetic Analgesics* part I, Pergamon, New York.

Janssen, P. A. J., Hellerback, J., Schnider, O., Besendorf, L. T., and Pellmont, B. (1966) Diphenylpropylamines, Morphinans, in *Synthetic Analgesics* part II, Pergamon, New York.

Kuhar, M. J., Pert, C. B., and Snyder, S. H. (1973) Regional distribution of opiate receptor binding in monkey and human brain. *Nature* **245**, 447–451.

Lamotte, C., Pert, C. B., and Snyder, S. H. (1976) Opiate receptor binding in primate spinal cord: Distribution and changes after dorsal root section. *Brain Res.* **112**, 407–416.

Langley, J. N. (1909) On the contraction of muscle, chiefly in relation to the presence of "receptive" substances. IV. The effect of curare and of some other substances on the nicotine response of the sartorius and gastrocnemius muscles of the frog. *J. Physiol.* **39**, 235–295.

Law, P.Y., Fischer, G., Loh, H. H., and Herz, A. (1979) Inhibition of specific opiate binding to synpatic membranes by cerebroside sulfatase. *Biochem. Pharmacol.* **28**, 2557–2562.

Lee, C. Y., Akera, T., Stolman, S., and Brody, T. M. (1975) Saturable binding of dihydromorphine and naloxone to rat brain tissue in vitro. *J. Pharm. Exp. Ther.* **194**, 583–592.

Lin, H. K., Holland, M. J., and Simon, E. J. (1981) Characterizational phospholipase A inhibition of stereospecific opiate bindings and its reversal by bovine serum albumin. *J. Pharmacol. Exp. Ther.* **216**, 149–155.

Loh, H. H., and Law, P. Y. (1980) The role of membrane lipids in receptor mechanisms. *Ann. Rev. Pharmacol.* **20**, 201–234.

Loh, H. H., Cho, T. M., Wu, Y. C., Harris, R. A., and Way, E. L. (1975) Opiate binding to cerebroside sulfate: A model system for opiate-receptor interactions. *Life Sci.* **16**, 1811–1818.

Loh, H. H., Cho, T. M., Wu, Y. C., and Way, E. L. (1974) Stereospecific binding of narcotics to brain cerebrosides. *Life Sci.* **14**, 2231–2245.

Martin, W. R. (1967) Opioid antagonists. *Pharmacol. Rev.* **19**, 463–521.

Mule, S. J., Casella, G., and Clouet, D. H. (1975) The specificitity of binding of the narcotic agonist etorphine in synaptic membranes of rat brain in vivo. *Psychopharmacologia* (Berl.) **44**, 125–129.

Navon, S. and Lajtha, A. (1970) Uptake of morphine in particulate fractions from rat brain. *Brain Res.* **24**, 534–536.

Pasternak, G. W. and Snyder, S. H. (1974) Opiate receptor binding: Effects of enzymatic treatments. *Mol. Pharmacol.* **10**, 183–193.

Pasternak, G. W. and Snyder, S. H. (1975a) Opiate receptor binding: Enzymatic treatments discriminate between agonist and antagonist interactions. *Mol. Pharmacol.* **11**, 478–484.

Pasternak, G. W. and Snyder, S. H. (1975b) Identification of novel high affinity opiate receptor binding in rat brain. *Nature* **253**, 563–565.

Pasternak, G. W. and Wood, P. L. (1986) Multiple mu opiate receptors. *Life Sci.* **38**, 1889–1898.

Pasternak, G. W., Snowman, A., and Snyder, S. H. (1975a) Selective enhancement of ³H-opaite agonist binding by divalent cations. *Mol. Pharmacol.* **11**, 735–744.

Pasternak, G. W., Wilson, H. A., and Snyder, S. H. (1975b) Differential effects of protein-modifying reagents on receptor binding of opiate agonists and antagonists. *Mol. Pharmacol.* **11**, 340–351.

Pert, C. B. and Snyder, S. H. (1973) Opiate receptor: Demonstration in nervous tissue. *Science* **179**, 1011–1014.

Pert, A. and Yaksh, T. L. (1975) Sites of morphine induced analgesia in the primate brain: Relation to pain pathways. *Brain Res.* **80**, 135–140.

Pert, A. and Yaksh, T. L. (1975) Localization of the antinociceptive action of morphine in primate brain. *Pharmacol. Biochem. Behav.* **3**, 733–738.

Pert, C. B., Pasternak, G. W., and Snyder, S. H. (1973) Opiate agonists and antagonists discriminated by receptor binding in brain. *Science* **182**, 1359–1361.

Pert, C. B., Snowman, A. M., and Snyder, S. H. (1974a) Localization of opiate receptor binding in synaptic membranes of rat brain. *Brain Res.* **70**, 184–188.

Pert, C. B., Aposhian, D., and Snyder, S. H. (1974b) Phylogenetic distribution of opiate receptor binding. *Brain Res.* **75**, 356–361.

Pert, C. B., Kuhar, M. J., and Snyder, S. H. (1976) Opiate receptor: Autoradiographic localization in rat brain. *Proc. Natl. Acad. Sci. USA* **73**, 3729–3733.

Pert, C. B., Kuhar, M. J., and Snyder, S. H. (1975) Autoradiographic localization of the opiate receptor in rat brain. *Life Sci.* **16**, 1849–1854.

Portoghese, P. S. (1966) Stereochemical factors and receptor interactions associated with narcotic analgesics. *J. Pharm. Sci.* **55**, 865–887.

Portoghese, P. S. (1970) Relationships between stereostructure and pharmacological activity. *Ann. Rev. Pharmacol.* **10**, 51–76.

Schubert, P., Hollt, V., and Herz, A. (1975) Autoradiographic evaluation of the intracerebral distribution of ³H-etorphine in the mouse brain. *Life Sci.* **16**, 1855–1856.

Seeman, P., Chan-Wong, M., and Moyyen, S. (1972) The membrane binding of morphine, diphenylhydantoin and tetrahydrocannabinol. *Can. J. Physiol. Pharm.* **5**, 1181–1192.

Shuster, L., Baran, A., and Eleftherion, B. E. (1975) Opiate receptors and analgesic response in mice: Basis for genetic differences. *Fed. Proc.* **34**, 713.

Simon, E. J., Hiller, J. M., and Edelmand, I. (1973) Stereospecific binding of the potent narcotic analgesic ^{3}H-etorphine to rat brain homogenates. *Proc. Natl. Acad. Sci. USA.* **70**, 1947–1949.

Snyder, S. H., Pasternak, G. W., and Pert, C. B. (1975) Opiate Receptor Mechanisms, in *Handbook of Psychopharmacology* vol. 5 (Iverson, L., Iverson, S., and Snyder, S. H., eds.) Plenum, New York.

Stefano, G. B. and Scharrer, B. (1981) High affinity binding of an enkephalin analog in the cerebral ganglion of the insect *Eucophaea maderae (blattaria)*. *Brain Res.* **225**, 107–114.

Stefano, G. B., Zukin, R. S., and Kream, R. M. (1982) Evidence for the presynaptic localization of a high affinity opiate binding site on dopamine neurons in the pedal ganglia of *Mytilus edulis (Bivalvia)*. *J. Pharmacol. Exp. Ther.* **222**, 759–763.

Terenius, L. (1973) Characteristics of the "receptor" for narcotic analgesics in synaptic plasma membrane fractions from rat brain. *Acta Pharmacol. Toxicol.* **33**, 377–384.

van Praag, D. and Simon, E. J. (1966) Studies on the intracellular distribution and tissue binding of dihydromorphine-7, 8-^{3}H in the rat. *Proc. Soc. Exp. Biol.* **122**, 6–11.

Wilson, H. A., Pasternak, G. W., and Snyder, S. H. (1975) Differentiation of opiate agonist and antagonist receptor binding by protein modifying reagents. *Nature* **253**, 448–450.

Wong, D. T. and Horng, J. S. (1976) Effect of Sodium on Specific Binding of ^{3}H-Dihydromorphine to and ^{3}H-Naloxone to Striatal Membranes of Rat Brain, in *Tissue Responses to Addictive Drugs* (Ford, D. H., and Clouet, D. H., eds.) Spectrum, New York.

Young, W. S., Wamsley, J. K., Zarbin, M. A., and Kuhar, M. J. (1980) Opioid receptors undergo axonal flow. *Science* **210**, 76–78.

Ziegelgansberger, W. and Fry, J. P. (1976) Actions of Enkephalin on Cortical and Striatal Neurons of Naive and Morphine Tolerant/Dependent Rats, in *Opiates and Endogenous Opioid Peptides* (Kosterlitz, H. W., ed.) Elsevier/North-Holland Biomedical, Amsterdam.

Zhang, A.-Z. and Pasternak, G. W. (1981) Ontogeny of opioid pharmacology and receptors: High and Low affinity site differences. *Eur. J. Pharmacol.* **73**, 29–40.

Chapter 4

Multiple Opioid Binding Sites

Yossef Itzhak

1. Introduction

The conceptual role of multiple subtypes of neurotransmitter receptors in our understanding of their actions has become more important in recent years. The acetylcholine and norepinephrine receptor systems provided some of the earliest examples with the proposal of muscarinic and nicotinic acetylcholine receptor subtypes and alpha and beta norepinephrine receptors. More recently, the alpha and beta receptors have been subdivided even further into alpha-1 and alpha-2 and beta-1 and beta-2 subtypes, which have been well characterized both functionally and in binding studies. Indeed, the concept of multiple receptor subtypes appears to be the general rule rather than the exception, as typified by the D_1 and D_2 dopamine receptors and H_1 and H_2 histamine receptors, to name a few.

    In the early 1950s, the determination of the structural requirements of opiates for the production of analgesia led to the hypothesis that they interacted with specific binding sites (Beckett and Casy, 1954; Beckett et al., 1956; Portoghese, 1965). The synthesis of the specific pure antagonists naloxone and naltrexone, as well as the mixed agonist-antagonist nalorphine, and their ability to reverse opiate analgesia and respiratory depression, also provided strong evidence for a receptor mechanism of action. The development of the guinea pig ileum bioassay provided a simpler system to examine the action of these drugs in which the opiates inhibited neurotransmission with potencies similar to their analgesic actions (Paton, 1957; Kosterlitz and Watt, 1968; Kosterlitz and Waterfield, 1975). Naloxone and naltrexone also antagonized opiate actions in this bioassay. The major development in the field of opiate receptor research, however, was the demonstration of stereospecific opiate binding sites in mammalian central nervous system (CNS).

The attempts by Goldstein and coworkers (Goldstein et al., 1971) to demonstrate the existence of specific binding sites for opiates were unsuccessful, probably because of the low specific activity of the radiolabeled opiates available at that time. In these studies the level of specifically bound [^{3}H]levorphanol was only 2% of the total labeling. Only 2 yr later, three laboratories independently reported the stereospecific binding of radiolabeled opiates in brain (Pert and Snyder, 1973; Terenius, 1973; Simon et al., 1973). These opioid binding sites were extensively characterized, as discussed in the chapter entitled Early Studies of Opioid Binding, in this volume. In brief, the binding of all three ^{3}H-opiates (naloxone, etorphine, and dihydromorphine) is highly sensitive to proteolytic enzymes, sulfhydryl reagents (Simon et al., 1973; Pasternak and Snyder, 1974, 1975a; Simon and Groth, 1975), and phospholipase A (Pasternak and Snyder, 1974; Lin and Simon, 1978, 1981). These results, along with others (Loh et al., 1974, 1975), implicated a role for both protein and lipid components in the opiate binding site.

Martin (1967) first proposed the existence of multiple types of opioid receptors on the basis of the interactions of morphine and nalorphine, as well as detailed structure–activity relationship studies (Portoghese, 1965, 1966). Later, in a series of pharmacological studies, Martin and coworkers (Martin et al., 1976; Gilbert and Martin, 1976a,b) documented different pharmacological profiles for a series of opiate alkaloids and noted that they did not substitute for each other in the prevention of withdrawal symptoms in dogs chronically treated with another of the drugs. They then suggested the existence of three types of opiate receptors: mu for morphine, kappa for ketocyclazocine, and sigma for N-allynormetazocine (SKF 10, 047). The biochemical demonstration of these sites appeared shortly after the discovery of the enkephalins, two endogenous pentapeptides with opiate activity (Hughes et al., 1975; Terenius and Whalstrom, 1975; Pasternak et al.,

1975a, 1976). Although the enkephalins had many properties similar to those of the classical alkaloids, Kosterlitz's group noted different rank orders of potency between the enkephalins and morphine in the guinea pig ileum and the mouse vas deferens bioassays, leading them to postulate the presence of a distinct receptor selective for the enkephalins, termed delta (Lord et al., 1977). Furthermore, the sensitivity of these two bioassays to reversal by naloxone, as measured by pA_2 values, also indicated major differences in pharmacological selectivity. This chapter will focus upon the binding evidence for the heterogeneity of opiate binding sites. Table 1 provides a tentative list of the various types of opioid receptors that will be discussed in this chapter. Pharmacological studies will be reviewed elsewhere in this volume.

2. Ligand–Receptor Binding Assays

Receptor–ligand interactions differ significantly from those between an enzyme and its substrate. Whereas an enzyme converts the substrate to a product, ligands bind to a receptor and dissociate unchanged. Under most conditions, it is assumed that the interaction between a ligand (L) and its receptor (R) to form the ligand–receptor complex (LR) obeys simple reversible mass action laws:

$$L + R \rightleftharpoons LR$$

where

$$K_d = \frac{[L][R]}{[LR]} = \frac{1}{K_{eq}}$$

This assumption is consistent with experimental results for most systems and has been used in the development of sophisticated computer analysis programs of binding isotherms, but evidence is mounting that this may be a simplistic interpretation of the actual events associated with ligand binding. Receptors may undergo conformational changes to different affinity states and may associate with other entities, such as nucleotide binding proteins and/or effector systems. From a practical viewpoint, however, the assumptions of simple mass law are very useful in understanding

TABLE 1
Tentative List of Opioid Receptor Types

Receptor subtype	Prototypic ligand
Mu	
Mu$_1$	Morphine and enkephalins
Mu$_2$	Morphine
Delta	Enkephalins
Kappa	Ketocyclazocine and dynorphin
Epsilon	β-Endorphin
Sigma	(+)-N-Allylnormetazocine (SKF 10,047)

ligand–receptor interactions. One very important assumption is that the binding sites are finite in number and therefore saturable, whereas nonspecific binding over the concentration range of radioligand used is not saturable. Thus, unlabeled compounds lower specific, saturable binding, but not nonspecific binding, and the difference represents specific binding.

Binding studies are routinely carried out under steady-state conditions. This permits the estimation of dissociation constants (K_d) and inhibition constants (K_i). Alternatively, dissociation constants can be estimated from the ratios of the association and dissociation rate constants of the ligand ($K_d = k_{-1}/k_1$). A number of technical issues need to be addressed before formalizing a binding assay. Some of these issues include linearity with tissue, estimation of the percentage of radioligand bound, determination of ligand and receptor stability under the assay conditions, and so on. Most important, however, is the relevance of the binding site being examined. Within the opiate system, much evidence is placed upon stereospecificity, since this is a well-established pharmacological observation. The levorotatory (−)-isomer of a number of alkaloids often competes binding 1000-fold more effectively than the (+)-isomer. This is not always the case, however. Some compounds, such as methadone, possess significant flexibility that lowers the difference in potency between the two stereoisomers (Pert and Snyder, 1973). In other situations, it may not be able to separate the optical isomers sufficiently well. An isomer has to be at least 99.9% pure to see a 1000-fold difference between active and inactive isomers.

In binding studies, the affinity of a ligand and the number of binding sites are usually the most important issues to be evaluated. When examining a radioligand, saturation analysis will yield both values. Although most investigators still use the

Scatchard (Rosenthal) plot (Scatchard, 1949) to demonstrate the data, nonlinear regression analysis is now used most effectively to calculate the actual values from the data (Munson and Rodbard, 1980). When a ligand is not available in radioactive form, its characteristics are evaluated through competition studies. The affinity of an unlabeled ligand to a binding site can be estimated either as an IC_{50} or a K_i and, in fact, they are related by the following equation (Cheng and Prusoff, 1973):

$$K_i = \frac{IC_{50}}{1 + \frac{[L]}{K_d}}$$

where [L] is the concentration of radioligand, IC_{50} is the concentration of unlabeled compound that lowers the binding by 50%, and K_d is the dissociation constant of the radiolabeled ligand. Whereas the K_i of a ligand is independent of the radioligand used and its concentration, IC_{50} values are dependent upon the specific radioligand used and its concentration. Obviously, comparisons of K_i values provide a more accurate assessment, provided that the radioligand is labeling a single site and all the assumptions regarding mass law hold. IC_{50} values, on the other hand, require no assumptions. It is also routine to determine the "Hill coefficient" of inhibition for the unlabeled compound (Hill, 1910). Originally proposed to examine cooperative effects with enzymatic reactions, these plots are most suitable to assess binding site heterogeneity in competition studies. Values under 1 raise the possibility that the radioligand is labeling more than one site. A value of 1, on the other hand, is consistent with a single site, but does not prove it.

3. Multiple Opioid Binding Sites

3.1. Mu and Delta Binding Sites

Separate receptors selective for either the enkephalins or morphine were first identified in bioassays comparing the guinea pig ileum and mouse vas deferens (Lord et al., 1977). These peripheral actions of the alkaloids and the peptides are discussed in detail in the chapter in this volume entitled Peripheral Actions Mediated by Opioid Receptors. Much binding evidence supports the presence of these selective sites. Initial studies focused upon competitive interactions between the enkephalins and morphine-like compounds. They were soon expanded to include regional, protection, and biochemical studies, which are discussed later in this chapter. Autoradiography provided the most convincing evidence, however, revealing the presence of these two receptor subtypes in different brain regions. These results are presented in the chapter entitled Regional Distribution of Opioid Receptors, in this volume.

Distinct mu and delta sites were demonstrated in competitive binding assays by comparing labeled enkephalins and opiate alkaloids (Lord et al., 1977; Chang and Cuatrecasas, 1979). Kosterlitz and coworkers (Lord et al., 1977) compared the ability of a series of compounds to compete with [^{3}H][Leu^5]enkephalin and [^{3}H]naloxone binding in guinea pig brain membranes. In brief, they found that morphine and naloxone inhibited the binding of [^{3}H]naloxone more effectively than [^{3}H][Leu^5]enkephalin, whereas [Met^5]enkephalin and [Leu^5]enkephalin competed [^{3}H]-[Leu^5]enkephalin binding more potently than [^{3}H]naloxone. Chang and Cuatrecasas (1979) addressed these issues by labeling delta sites with [^{125}I][D-Ala^2-D-Leu^5]enkephalin (DADL) and mu sites with [^{3}H]naloxone and described the ability of various opioid

TABLE 2
Discrimination Between Mu and Delta Binding Sites
in Rat Central Nervous System

	IC$_{50}$ values, nM[a]		Ratio, delta/mu
	Delta	Mu	
Butorphanol	1.4	1.0	1.4
Morphine	35	0.5	70
Naloxone	15	0.8	19
Meperidine	3000	300	10
Pentazocine	30	10	3
Oxilorphan	1.0	0.7	1.4
[Met^5]enkephalin	4	10	0.4
[D-Ala^2,Met^5] enkephalin	1.5	6	0.25
[Leu^5]enkephalin	3.2	25	0.14
[D-Ala^2,Leu^5] enkephalin	1.5	6	0.25

[a]Apparent IC$_{50}$ values were estimated from displacement curves of the unlabeled compound on the binding of [^{125}I] [D-Ala^2,D-Leu^5] enkephalin and [^{3}H]naloxone, which label delta and mu sites, respectively (adapted from Chang and Cuatrecasas, 1979).

compounds to discriminate between these two sites (Table 2). Differences between delta and mu sites were present in a wide variety of species and could be demonstrated with a number of radio-labeled mu and delta ligands (Terenius, 1977; Law and Loh, 1978; Simantov et al., 1978; Chang et al., 1979, 1980; Simon et al., 1980).

The major difficulty with the naturally occurring enkephalins is their sensitivity to proteolytic enzymes and their rapid degradation. In an effort to overcome this disadvantage, literally thousands of analogs have now been synthesized and tested. In general, substitution of a D-alanine at the 2-position for glycine greatly enhances stability. Other substitutions, including those at the 5-position, also increase stability as well as changing the pharmacological profile of the compound. For example, amidation of the C-terminal carboxyl group of [Met^5]enkephalin retains the delta activity of the derivative while increasing the mu component, yielding a compound with actions at both mu and delta sites. Several peptides relatively selective for mu sites with little delta activity have been reported. Studies with these compounds support the previous studies. Although the analogs were often more potent, reflecting their resistance to degradation, they also demonstrated the presence of morphine- and enkephalin-selective sites (Kosterlitz et al., 1980; Romer et al., 1977; Chang and Cuatrecasas, 1979). Table 3 provides a listing of some of the endogenous and synthetic opioid peptides. Often, the most complicating issue with the interpretation of opiate binding is the large number of enkephalin analogs and their selectivity. Table 4 describes the receptor classification of some opiates and opioid peptides.

The selectivity of the peptides and alkaloids is an important consideration in the interpretation of binding studies. Frequently, compounds thought to be specific have turned out not to be as selective as originally proposed. This is probably most evident for the kappa compounds, many of which are "universal" ligands, labeling several binding subtypes with relatively high affinity. Etorphine, ethylketocyclazocine, Mr2034, bremazocine, and diprenorphine, for example, display similar high affinities in the nanomolar range to all three major types of opioid receptors (mu, delta, and kappa) (Kosterlitz et al., 1981; Magnan et al., 1982; James and Goldstein, 1984; Wolozin et al., 1982; Johnson and Pasternak, 1983; Pasternak, 1980). Even dihydromorphine and naloxone, which are considered mu ligands and label mu sites approximately 20-fold more potently than delta sites (Gillan et al., 1980; Leslie et al., 1980; Pfeiffer and Herz, 1981), are not as selective as normorphine and DAMPGO, which display mu selectivi-

TABLE 3

Amino Acid Sequences of Selected Endogenous and Synthetic Opioid Peptides[a]

Endogenous opioid peptides	
[Leu⁵]enkephalin	H-**TYR-GLY-GLY-PHE**-*Leu*-OH
[Met⁵]enkephalin	H-**TYR-GLY-GLY-PHE**-*Met*-OH
β-Endorphin	H-**TYR-GLY-GLY-PHE**-*Met*-Thr-Ser-Glu-Lys-Ser-Gln-Thr-Pro-Leu-Val-Thr-Leu-Phe-Lys-Asn-Ala-Ile-Lys-Asn-Ala-Tyr-Lys-Lys-Gly-Glu-OH
Dynorphin A	H-**TYR-GLY-GLY-PHE**-*Leu*-Arg-Arg-Ile-Arg-Pro-Lys-Leu-Lys-Trp-Asp-Asn-Gln-OH
Dynorphin B	H-**TYR-GLY-GLY-PHE**-*Leu*-Arg-Arg-Gln-Phe-Lys-Val-Val-Thr
α-Neo-endorphin	H-**TYR-GLY-GLY-PHE**-*Leu*-Arg-Lys-Tyr-Pro-Lys-OH
Exogenous opioid peptides	
β-Casomorphan	H-Tyr-Pro-Phe-Pro-Gly-Pro-Ile-OH

Synthetic opioid peptides: enkephalin analogs

[D-Ala^2,Met^5]-enkephalinamide	DAMEA	H-Tyr-D-Ala-Gly-Phe-Met-CONH$_2$
[D-Ala^2,D-Leu^5]-enkephalin	DADL	H-Tyr-D-Ala-Gly-Phe-D-Leu-OH
FK 33-824		H-Tyr-D-Ala-Gly-Phe(N-CH$_3$)-Met(O)ol
Morphiceptin		H-Tyr-Pro-Phe-Pro-CONH$_2$
Metkephamid		H-Tyr-D-Ala-Gly-Phe(N-CH$_3$)-Met-CONH$_2$
[D-Pen^2,D-Pen^5]-enkephalin	DPDPE	H-Tyr-D-Pen-Gly-Phe-D-Pen
[D-Ser^2, Leu^5]enkephalin-Thr^6	DSLET	H-Tyr-D-Ser-Gly-Phe-Leu-Thr
[D-Ala^2,MePhe^4,Gly-(ol)^5]enkephalin	DAMPGO or DAGO	H-Tyr-D-Ala-Gly-MePhe-Gly(ol)

[a]Amino acid sequences of selected endogenous and synthetic opioid peptides. Exact sequences of longer natural peptides will vary with different species. Bolded portions represent the four amino acids common to all opioid peptides occurring within the central nervous system.

TABLE 4
Receptor Classification of Opiates and Opioid Peptides[a]

Receptor subtype	Agonist	Antagonist
Mu	Morphine Dihydromorphine Oxymorphone DAMPGO Morphiceptin β-Casomorphin PL017	Naloxone Naltrexone
Delta	Met-enkephalin Leu-enkephalin DADLE DSLET DAMEA DPDPE	ICI 154129
Kappa	Ketocyclazocine[b] Ethylketocyclazocine[b] Tifluadome[b] Bremazocine[b] U50488H Mr2034[b] Dynorphin	Mr2266[b]
Sigma	(+)-N-allylnormetazocine (SKF 10,047)	
Nonselective	Etorphine Cyclazocine	Diprenorphine

[a]This data summarizes the relative affinity of selected opioids for the various opioid receptor types.
[b]Although potent at kappa sites, these ligand also label mu and delta sites.

ties of 70- and 200-fold, respectively (Handa et al., 1981; Kosterlitz and Paterson, 1981). Selectivity is not always correlated with potency. Morphiceptin, a relatively weak opioid peptide, is one of the most mu-selective compounds available (Chang et al., 1981). Also, a novel analgesic phencyclidine analog, PCP-4-Ph-4-OH, unexpectedly displayed 60- and 300-fold higher affinity to mu sites than to delta and kappa sites, respectively, in binding assays (Itzhak and Simon, 1984).

Of the delta-selective ligands, DADL has been used most extensively. Yet this peptide labels delta sites only three- to ten-fold more potently than the morphine-selective mu sites (Chang et al., 1979; Gillan et al., 1980; Wolozin and Pasternak, 1981; James and

Goldstein, 1984). Several compounds with far greater selectivity for delta sites are now available. DSTLE, for example, is at least 20-fold more potent at the delta than at the mu sites and is now available in tritiated form with high specific activity (Gacel et al., 1980; James and Goldstein, 1984). Several *bis*-penicillamide enkephalin analogs were described as highly selective delta ligands (Mosberg et al., 1983). Among these, DPDPE and DPLPE demonstrated delta selectivities of between 170- and 370-fold in binding assays and approximately 1000-fold in the mouse vas deferens and guinea pig ileum bioassays (Corbett et al., 1984).

3.1.1. Cross-Protection Studies

Cross-protection studies provided further evidence for the existence of separate mu and delta binding sites. Robson and Kosterlitz (1979) used the nonspecific irreversible agent phenoxybenzamine to inactivate either mu or delta sites in guinea pig brain. They reported that dihydromorphine protected [^{3}H]dihydromorphine binding sixfold more potently than DADL, but dihydromorphine was far less active against [^{3}H]DADL binding, consistent with distinct mu and delta binding sites.

Studies with N-ethylmaleimide (NEM) yielded similar results (Smith and Simon, 1980). In this study, morphine protected the mu binding of [^{3}H]naltrexone eight times more potently than the delta binding of [^{3}H]DADL. Conversely, unlabeled DADL protected [^{3}H]DADL more efficiently than [^{3}H]naltrexone binding in rat brain membranes (Table 5).

The irreversible inhibition of opioid binding produced by phenoxybenzamine and NEM is not opioid-specific (Cicero et al., 1974, 1975; Simon and Groth, 1975; Simon et al., 1975a). To confirm these findings, it was important to utilize opioid ligands that selectively inactivate the various subtypes of opioid receptors. Portoghese and coworkers (Portoghese et al., 1979; Caruso et al., 1979) synthesized several potential receptor alkylating agents. The mustard derivative of naltrexone and oxymorphone, β-chlornaltrexamine (β-CNA) and β-chloroxymorphamine (β-COA), irreversibly inactivated opioid binding sites, but did not discriminate well among the various subtypes. The fumarate methylester derivative of naltrexone, β-funaltrexamine (β-FNA), alkylates only the mu sites, but reacts reversibly with delta and kappa receptors (Ward et al., 1982). The corresponding derivative of oxymorphone (β-FOA) reacts reversibly with all opioid receptor types (Portoghese et al., 1980).

TABLE 5

Protection of Mu and Delta Binding from N-ethymaleimide[a]

Protecting ligand	Concentration of ligand, nM, to protect binding 50%		Ratio, DADL/naltrexone
	[³H]Naltrexone	[³H]DADL	
Morphine	100	800	8
Naltrexone	3	60	20
[D-Ala², Met⁵]enkephalin	300	10	0.03
[D-Ala², Leu⁵]enkephalin	400	60	0.15
[D-Ala², Met⁵]enkephalin-amide	70	40	0.6

[a]The values given represent the concentration (nM) of protecting ligands required to produce 50% of the maximal protection achieved for each labeled ligand (modified from Smith and Simon, 1980).

The lack of selectivity of β-CNA as an alkylating agent provided a useful approach in cross-protection studies, however. James et al. (1982) have reported a method of preparing brain membranes containing a single subtype of binding site using cross-protection from β-CNA inactivation. In their procedure, sufentanil protects mu sites, leaving the others to be eliminated by the β-CNA, whereas DADL can selectively protect delta sites.

3.2. Multiple Mu Receptors: Mu_1 and Mu_2 Sites

Early studies using [^{3}H]dihydromorphine and [^{3}H]naloxone of high specific activity reported the existence of curvilinear Scatchard (Rosenthal) plots that were resolved into high- and low-affinity binding components (Pasternak and Snyder, 1975b). The lower-affinity binding components corresponded to the previously reported binding, whereas the higher-affinity component, with K_d values under 1 nM, had not been previously described. With the subsequent discovery of the enkephalins and delta receptors, the relationship of these high- and low-affinity components with mu and delta sites became a crucial question. Recent evidence suggests that the lower-affinity sites, with K_d values between 1 and 10 nM, correspond to the morphine-selective (mu_2) and enkephalin-preferring (delta) sites, whereas the high-affinity component represents a unique, common site for opiates and opioid peptides, termed the mu_1 site (Wolozin and Pasternak, 1981; Fig. 1). Extensive computerized analysis of saturation studies has confirmed the presence of these two binding components (Lutz et al., 1984; Fischel and Medzihradsy, 1981).

Two unique affinity labels, naloxazone and naloxonazine, greatly facilitated studies of this mu_1 site and provided the first evidence for a common very-high-affinity opiate and enkephalin binding site (Pasternak and Hahn, 1980; Hahn et al., 1982). Both compounds irreversibly eliminated the high-affinity binding observed with a large series of mu (dihydromorphine and morphine), kappa (ethylketocyclazocine and Mr2034), and sigma [($\pm$)-SKF 10,047]opiates, enkephalins ([Met^5]enkephalin, [Leu^5]-enkephalin, [D-Ala^2-D -Leu^5]enkephalin, [D-Ala^2-Met^5]en kephalinamide, β-endorphin, and opiate antagonists (naloxone and naltrexone) (Pasternak et al., 1980a,b, 1981; Pasternak, 1980, 1981; Wolozin and Pasternak, 1981; Zhang and Pasternak, 1981a; Hazum et al., 1981; Hahn and Pasternak, 1982; Hahn et al., 1982; Johnson and Pasternak, 1983). The similar loss of the high-affinity

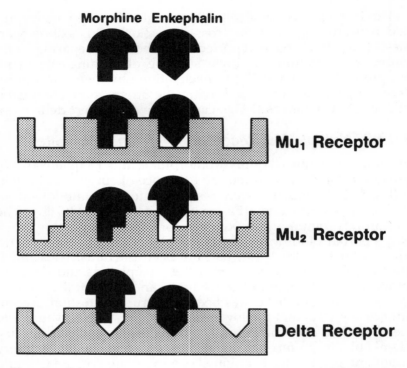

Morphine Enkephalin

Mu₁ Receptor

Mu₂ Receptor

Delta Receptor

Fig. 1.   Schematic representation of mu₁, mu₂, and delta binding.

site for all classes of opiates, enkephalins, and β-endorphin raised
the possibility that the radioligands were labeling the same site.
Equally important, the elimination of the high-affinity site for
both agonists and antagonists suggested that the high- and low-
affinity sites did not correspond simply to agonist/antagonist conformations.

Competition experiments provided additional support for
the mu₁ concept. Morphine inhibits radiolabeled enkephalin
binding biphasically, implying that the radioligand was labeling
both mu and delta sites (Chang and Cuatrecasas, 1979). A small
portion of binding, typically 25–35%, was competed by morphine
at concentrations under 1 nM, whereas the remainder required
far greater concentrations. Based upon this sensitivity, the morphine-sensitive portion was felt to be mu, whereas the larger remainder corresponded to delta sites. Treating tissue with either
naloxazone or naloxonazine eliminated the morphine-sensitive,

or mu, binding seen in these competition studies (Wolozin and Pasternak, 1981; Zhang and Pasternak, 1981a; Hazum et al., 1981; Pasternak, 1981; Pasternak, 1982; Nishimura et al., 1984). Thus, the morphine-sensitive radiolabeled enkephalin binding in competition studies and the high-affinity binding radiolabeled enkephalin binding component in saturation experiments both possessed similar sensitivities toward both naloxonazine and naloxazone. Reciprocal studies employing radiolabeled dihydromorphine and unlabeled enkephalins revealed analogous results (Figs. 2 and 3).

The idea that the high-affinity binding component of radiolabeled enkephalin binding corresponded to a mu site could be tested directly by including a low concentration of morphine in a radiolabeled enkephalin saturation experiment. When such experiments were performed, the low morphine concentrations inhibited the higher-affinity enkephalin binding component far more effectively than the lower one (Nishimura et al., 1984). Similarly, low [D-Ala^2-D-Leu^5]enkephalin concentrations competed

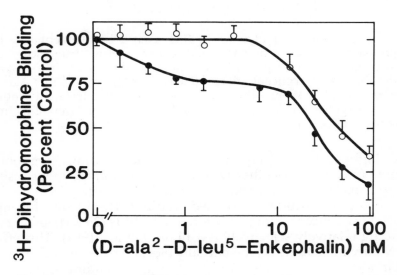

Fig. 2.   Inhibition of [^{3}H]dihydromorphine binding by DADL. Rat brain membranes were prepared and treated with no drug (closed circles) or naloxazone (2 μM) (open circles), washed, and then assayed with 1 nM of [^{3}H]dihydromorphine and increasing concentrations of unlabeled DADL (modified from Wolozin and Pasternak, 1981).

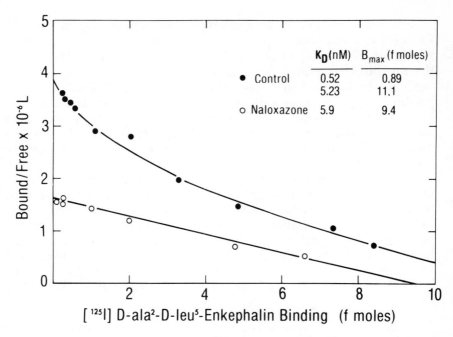

Fig. 3. Scatchard plots of $[^{125}I][D\text{-}Ala^2\text{-}D\text{-}Leu^5]$enkephalin. Rat brain mambranes were prepared and treated with no drug (closed circles) or naloxazone (2 μM) (open circles), washed, and then assayed with increasing concentrations (0.06–13 nM) of $[^{125}I][D\text{-}Ala^2\text{-}D\text{-}Leu^5]$enkephalin. From saturation experiments Scatchard (Rosenthal) plots were generated. Only specific binding is presented (modified from Hazum et al., 1981).

the higher-affinity $[^3H]$dihydromorphine binding component more effectively. Together with the earlier studies, these results were consistent with a common high-affinity site.

Protection studies provided additional evidence for mu_1 sites. Low concentrations of N-ethylmaleimide (25 μM) lower mu_1 binding relatively selectively (Nishimura et al., 1984). This effect of N-ethylmaleimide can be partially blocked by preincubating the membranes with opiates, thus protecting the binding sites. As expected, morphine partially reversed the inhibition of $[^3H]$dihydromorphine binding by N-ethylmaleimide. $[D\text{-}Ala^2,D\text{-}LeuLe5]$enkephalin, however, also protected $[^3H]$dihydromorphine as effectively as morphine. On the surface, these results seem to conflict with those reported earlier. The mu_1 studies used very low N-ethylmaleimide concentrations, however, that did not affect the selective mu_2 or delta sites appreciably. The earlier studies used concentrations of reagents sufficient to markedly inhibit the selective sites and thus showed no cross-protection.

Together the above investigations were consistent with a common high-affinity binding site for both opiates and enkephalins. The next question that needed to be resolved was the characterization of the lower-affinity sites and how all these binding sites fit with the previously established mu/delta concept. In naloxazone-treated tissue that contained no high-affinity, or mu_1, sites, the lower-affinity [^{3}H]dihydromorphine binding (K_d approximately 3 nM) was inhibited far more effectively by morphine-like compounds than the enkephalins, whereas [^{3}H][D-Ala^2-Leu^5]enkephalin labeled an enkephalin-selective site (K_d approximately 5 nM; Wolozin and Pasternak, 1981). Thus, the lower-affinity [^{3}H]dihydromorphine binding site corresponded to the classical morphine-selective mu receptor, termed mu_2, whereas the lower-affinity enkephalin binding site corresponded to the enkephalin-preferring delta site.

The interaction of a more selective delta ligand, DSTLE, with mu_1 sites was recently examined (Itzhak and Pasternak, 1987). Approximately 20% of [^{3}H]DSTLE binding was readily inhibited by low concentrations of the mu-selective enkephalin DAMPGO (1–5 nM), and 15–25% of [^{3}H]DAMPGO binding was inhibited by low concentrations (<10 nM) of DSTLE. Naloxonazine pretreatment eliminated the inhibition of [^{3}H]DSTLE binding by DAMPGO and the inhibition of [^{3}H]DAMPGO binding by the delta ligands, supporting their interactions with mu_1 sites. Furthermore, Scatchard (Rosenthal) analysis of [^{3}H]DSTLE binding revealed a biphasic plot. Naloxonazine treatment abolished the high-affinity binding sites (K_d 0.3 nM). These results suggested that even more relatively selective delta ligands still display high affinity to mu_1 sites. This does not necessarily mean, however, that every delta-selective ligand must label mu_1 sites. Indeed, some evidence now suggests that DPDPE retains its high affinity for delta sites without appreciably labeling mu_1 sites (Clark et al., 1986).

The pharmacological significance of mu_1 sites was evaluated extensively using naloxazone and naloxonazine, as discussed in a later chapter. In brief, treatment of either rats or mice with either agent eliminated the high-affinity binding of a series of radiolabeled opiates and enkephalins, as discussed above. This loss of binding was associated with a dramatic shift of the analgesic dose–response curve to the right, implying that mu_1 sites mediated analgesia. This does not mean, however, that other receptor subtypes are not involved in opioid analgesia. Indeed, much evidence implicates both delta and kappa sites. The data do suggest that mu_1 sites are responsible for supraspinal analgesia (Ling and Pasternak, 1983). Binding and morphine's analgesic potency both returned to control values after 3 d, showing a good correlation. On the other hand, mu_1 blockade did not alter morphine's respiratory depression (Ling et al., 1983, 1985) or most of the signs associated with morphine dependence (Ling et al., 1984).

Throughout the above studies, naloxonazine has proven to be a very important ligand for the characterization of mu_1 sites. Recent studies suggest that the compound is not acting through a bivalent mechanism and may be forming covalent linkages (Hahn et al., 1985a,b). Direct studies of the binding of [^{3}H]naloxonazine revealed that about 40% of specific binding is resistant to multiple washes or to inhibition by levallorphan (1 μM) added 60 min after [^{3}H]naloxonazine (Johnson and Pasternak, 1984). The authors suggested that this portion of binding, which is not freely reversible, may indicate covalent binding to mu_1 sites.

3.3. Kappa Binding Sites

Neuropharmacological evidence supporting the existence of distinct kappa sites has been growing in recent years. In vivo studies revealed that monkeys reacted very differently to benzomorphans like ethylketocyclazocine or bremazocine when compared to morphine effects (Woods et al., 1979). Also, the withdrawal symptoms in morphine-addicted monkeys were not suppressed by benzomorphans. In drug-discriminative studies, rats trained to recognize bremazocine generalized to ethylketocyclazocine, cyclazocine, and SKF 10,047, but not fentanyl or morphine (Sherman and Herz, 1981). In bioassay studies, certain benzomorphans, including ethylketocyclazocine, inhibited the electrically induced contractions of the mouse vas deferens quite poorly, whereas they were potent inhibitors in the guinea pig ileum. Moreover, their inhibitory actions in the guinea pig ileum required naloxone concentrations from three- to seven-fold greater than required to antagonize morphine (Hutchinson et al., 1975).

Attempts to identify the kappa receptors in binding experiments were initially unsuccessful. [^{3}H]Ethylketocyclazocine binding in rat brain membranes was very similar to that of mu and delta ligands (Hiller and Simon, 1980; Pasternak, 1980). The inability of these assays to identify distinct kappa sites probably reflected their low level in rat brain relative to mu and delta sites (Maurer, 1982). Using guinea pig brain, however, Kosterlitz and coworkers (Kosterlitz and Paterson, 1980; Kosterlitz et al., 1981; Magnan et al., 1982) clearly demonstrated kappa binding sites. In these studies mu (DAMPGO) and delta (DADL) enkephalins inhibited [³H]ethylketocyclazocine binding in a biphasic manner, suggesting that a portion of [³H]ethylketocyclazocine binding corresponded to a combination of mu and delta sites, whereas the remainder, which was resistant to the two peptides, represented binding to kappa sites. Thus, [³H]ethylketocyclazocine labels all three subtypes of opioid binding sites.

Saturation studies [³H]ethylketocyclazocine binding revealed biphasic Scatchard (Rosenthal) plots (K_d 0.8 and 1.6 nM). In the presence of DAMPGO and DADL, however, the Scatchard (Rosenthal) plots were linear (K_d 0.74 nM) with a B_{max} value approximately one half of the original number of sites (6 and 13 pmol/g tissue, respectively) (Magnan et al., 1982). Thus, they concluded that about 40% of the opioid binding sites in the guinea pig brain correspond to kappa sites. The concentrations of DAMPGO and DADL (100 nM each) used to block mu and delta sites labeled by [³H]ethylketocyclazocine are about 100-fold higher than the K_i values of DAMPGO and DADL for mu and delta sites, respectively, and have little effect on the binding to kappa sites. These mu and delta blocking concentrations of DAMPGO and DADL also lower by approximately 50% the binding of tritiated bremazocine and etorphine. The residual binding represented kappa sites (Table 6; Itzhak et al., 1984a).

Recently, Robson et al. (1984) reported that 80–90% of opioid binding to guinea pig cerebellum membranes corresponds to kappa sites. Similar results were observed with [³H]bremazocine, [³H]ethylketocyclazocine, and [³H]etorphine binding in this tissue in which mu and delta blockers lowered binding by 11–15%. (Itzhak et al., 1984a). Also, binding levels of [³H]DAMPGO and [³H]DADL to guinea pig cerebellum represented only 4–5% of their binding to rat brain membranes (Table 6). Other compounds with known kappa activity had high affinity for these guinea pig cerebellum binding sites (Table 7; Itzhak et al., 1984b). One report also described the presence of kappa sites on a neuroblastoma-glioma hybrid cell line (McLawhon et al., 1981).

Tifluadom, a benzodiazepine compound synthesized by Romer et al. (1982), labeled kappa sites approximately 100-fold

TABLE 6
Kappa Binding of a Series of ^{3}H-labeled Opioids to Guinea Pig Brain and Cerebellar Membranes[a]

	^{3}H-Opioid-specific binding, fmol/mg protein				
	Etorphine	EKC	Bremazocine	DAMPGO	DADL
Brain membranes					
Total specific binding	186 ± 12	75 ± 4	210 ± 11	31 ± 3	42 ± 3
Kappa binding	92 ± 4	32 ± 5	101 ± 8	ND[b]	ND
Percentage kappa	49%	43%	48%		
Cerebellum membranes					
Total specific binding	115 ± 10	37 ± 5	108 ± 3	1.5 ± 1	1.7 ± 1
Kappa binding	98 ± 6	33 ± 4	92 ± 2	ND	ND
Percentage kappa	85%	89%	85%		

[a]Specific binding of ^{3}H-opioid ligands (2 nM) was determined in the absence (total specific) and the presence (kappa) of DAMPGO and DADL (100 nM each). The results represent the mean ± SEM of three experiments (modified from Itzhak et al., 1984a).
[b]ND, none detected.

TABLE 7
Affinity of Various Opioid Ligands
for Kappa Binding Sites
in the Guinea Pig Cerebellum
Membranes

Ligand	K_i, nM[a]
Bremazocine	0.2 ± 0.02
Tifluadom	0.9 ± 0.4
EKC	1.4 ± 0.28
Etorphine	2.0 ± 0.12
U50488	40.0 ± 5.7
DAGO	>10000
DSLET	>10000

[a] K_i values were calculated from IC_{50} values determined in competition studies using [³H]bremazocine. Data represent the mean $\pm$ SEM of three experiments (modified from Itzhak et al., 1984b).

more selectively than mu and delta sites (James and Goldstein, 1984). Similarly, James and Goldstein (1984) reported that U50488 (*trans*-3,4-dichloro-*N*-methyl-*N*-[2-(1-pyrrolidinyl) cyclohexyl] benzenacetamide) (Piercey et al., 1982) was 1300-fold more potent at kappa than mu and delta sites.

The endogenous ligands for delta binding sites clearly are [Met⁵]enkephalin and [Leu⁵]enkephalin. Dynorphin has been suggested as the endogenous ligand for kappa receptors (Chavkin and Goldstein, 1981a,b; Chavkin et al., 1982). Dynorphin (1-13), purified from porcine pituitary extracts, was about 700-fold more potent than [Leu⁵]enkephalin in the guinea pig ileum and far less sensitive to naloxone antagonism (Goldstein et al., 1979). These results suggested that dynorphin receptors are distinct from mu and delta sites (Goldstein et al., 1979). In binding assays dynorphin (1-9) displays about 10-fold higher affinity for kappa sites compared to mu and delta sites (Corbett et al., 1982). Dynorphin (1-13) and dynorphin (1-17) are less selective for kappa sites, and their cross reactivity with mu and delta sites is higher than dynorphin (1-9). In addition, dynorphin (1-13) and dynorphin (1-17) are relatively resistant to enzymatic degradation and have long duration of action in vitro. Dynorphin (1-8) and dynorphin (1-9) are readily degraded and have short durations of action. Thus, it was suggested that dynorphin (1-8) and dynorphin (1-9) may be considered transmitters or modulators at the kappa sites, whereas dynorphin (1-13) and dynorphin (1-17) may act as hormones (Corbett et al., 1982).

3.3.1. Cross-Protection Studies

In order to further characterize the various opioid receptor types, it became important to obtain a system that contains only one type of binding site. One approach has been described by James et al. (1982). Opioid receptors were inactivated by alkylation with the irreversible opioid antagonist β-chlornaltrexamine (β-CNA) (Portoghese et al., 1979; Caruso et al., 1979) in the presence of relatively selective opioid ligands to protect one type of receptors. Treatment of guinea pig brain membranes with β-CNA in the presence of dynorphin (1-13) protected approximately 40% of the kappa-selective high-affinity [^{3}H]ethylketocyclazocine binding sites but not the binding of [^{3}H]dihydromorphine or [^{3}H]DADL from inactivation by β-CNA. These results provided further evidence that dynorphin (1-13) may be the endogenous peptide for kappa receptors. In similar studies, sufentanil (a selective mu ligand) and DADL selectively protected mu and delta binding sites, respectively.

Using this method, James and Goldstein (1984) evaluated the binding selectivity of a large number of opioid alkaloids and peptides for mu, delta, and kappa opioid receptors. The method of site-directed alkylation in the presence of a protecting ligand for one type of the opioid receptors was also employed to characterize the pharmacological selectivity of various opioid agonists in isolated preparations such as the mouse vas deferens and the guinea pig ileum (Goldstein and James, 1984). Together these findings may provide further evidence for the concept that mu, delta, and kapp receptors are not interconvertible sites.

3.4. Sigma [(+)-N-Allylnormetazocine]-Specific Binding Sites

The hypothesis of distinct receptors for N-allylnormetazocine (SKF 10,047) was initially supported by behavioral studies in which the unique behavior effects of SKF 10,047 and related benzomorphans such as pentazocine, and cyclazocine in dogs (Martin et al., 1976; Gilbert and Martin, 1976a,b), was thought to be related to psychotomimetic activity in man (Keats and Telford, 1964). Recent studies suggest that some of the behavioral effects elicited by psychotomimetic benzomorphans may be activated preferentially by their dextrorotatory (+)-isomers (Brady et al., 1982; Holtzman, 1982; Shannon, 1981, 1983). Attempts to eluci- date the mode of action of phenyclidine (PCP), which induces acute psychotic syndromes in humans (Luby et al., 1960), re- vealed a pharmacological profile very similar to that of SKF 10,047 in the chronic spinal dog (Jasinski et al., 1981). In drug discrimina- tion tests, monkeys and rats generalized between (+)- or (±)-SKF 10,047 and PCP, but not between (−)-SKF 10,047 and PCP (Brady et al., 1982). Both in vivo and in vitro studies support the involvement of the opioid system in the effects elicited by PCP. The analgesic effect of PCP in mice and its actions in the guinea pig ileum are both partially reversed by naloxone, and PCP derivatives compete for radiolabeled opioid binding (Itzhak et al., 1981a,b). These results, together with the demonstration that specific [^{3}H]PCP binding to rat brain membranes (Vincent et al., 1979; Zukin and Zukin, 1979) is inhibited by PCP analogs and also by several benzomorphans (Zukin and Zukin, 1979; Quirion et al., 1981; Zukin et al., 1984), suggested the existence of com- mon binding sites for psychotomimetic benzomorphans and PCP.

Providing direct biochemical evidence for distinct SKF 10,047 binding sites has proven difficult, however. Binding studies show considerable cross-reactivity of (±) [^{3}H]SKF 10,047, binding with mu, kappa, and delta binding sites in rat brain (Pasternak et al., 1981). Nevertheless, using (+)-[^{3}H]SKF 10,047 and in HEPES- KOH buffer (10 mM), high-affinity binding sites (K_d of 20 nM and B_{max} of 260 fmol/mg of protein) were demonstrated in rat brain membranes (Fig. 4; Itzhak et al., 1985). The rank order of potency among opioid-benzomorphans and phencyclidine analogs for these sites was (+)-SKF 10,047 = 1-[1(3-hydroxyphenyl)cyclo- hexyl]pip eridine > (+)-cyclazocine > N-ethylphenyl- cyclo- hexylamine > PCP > (−)-cyclazocine > (−)-SKF 10,047 > (−)-le- vorphanol. Other opioid ligands such as morphine (mu), DAMPGO (mu), DADL (delta), tifluadom (kappa), U50488 (kappa), etorphine, and naloxone all did not lower (+)-[^{3}H]SKF 10,047 binding at a concentration of 1 μM. Thus, this study sup- ported the view that PCP and dextrorotatory isomers of psychoto- mimetic benzomorphans may act at a common sigma/PCP recog- nition site in rat central nervous system.

The concept of multiple subtypes of sigma/PCP receptors has emerged only recently. Evidence for this concept appeared from studying the binding properties of one of the most potent ana- logs of PCP: [^{3}H]1[1-(3-hydroxypheny)-cyclohexyl]piperidine

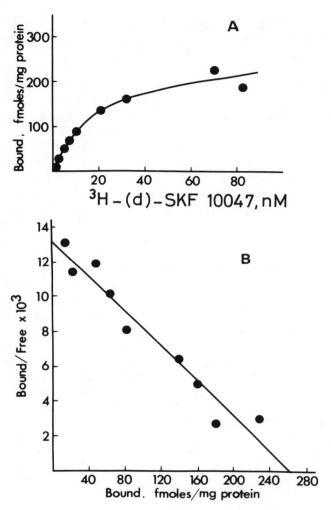

Fig. 4.   Saturation curve (A) and Scatchard (Rosenthal) plot (B) of specific [³H](d)-SKF 10,047 binding. Rat brain membranes were prepared and incubated for 35 min at 25°C with various concentrations (1–80 n*M*) of [³H](d)-SKF 10,047. Specific binding was assessed in the absence andpresence of 10 μ*M* of either (d)-SKF 10,047 or 3-hydroxy-phencyclidine, all of which resulted in similar levels of nonspecific binding for a given concentration of [³H](d)-SKF 10,047. The binding data were analyzed by the program (MED 58) described by Munson and Rodbart (1980) and resulted in selection of one-site fit as the best fit ($p < 0.05$; $r = 0.88$) (modified from Itzhak et al., 1985).

([^{3}H]PCP-3-OH; Itzhak, 1986). Binding of [^{3}H]PCP-3-OH in guinea pig brain membranes indicated the labeling of two distinct binding components. High-affinity [^{3}H]PCP-3-OH binding sites (K_d = 0.5 nM) display pharmacological selectivity very similar to that described for (+)-[H^3]SKF 10,047 binding sites (Itzhak et al., 1985), whereas low-affinity [^{3}H]PCP-3-OH binding sites (K_d = 20 nM) display preferential selectivity only for phencyclidine analogs. Sigma/PCP binding sites are discussed in detail in the chapter entitled The σ Receptor, in this volume.

3.5. β-Endorphin Binding Sites

The sensitivity of the rat vas deferens toward β-endorphin coupled with the insensitivity of other isolated organ systems led to the suggestion of distinct receptors for β-endorphin, which were termed epsilon (Lemnair et al., 1978; Schultz et al., 1979). Receptor binding studies have also suggested differences in the binding profile of [^{3}H]β-endorphin compared to other opioid ligands (Ferrara et al., 1979; Houghten et al., 1980; Hammonds and Li, 1981; Ho et al., 1983). In a detailed study, Pasternak and coworkers (Johnson et al., 1982; Houghten et al., 1984) reported that [^{3}H]β-endorphin labeled a distinct epsilon site and the mu$_1$ site with similar affinity (K_d < 1 nM). In their report, they found that a portion of [^{3}H]β-endorphin binding was sensitive to low concentrations (<5 nM) of morphine and DADL, as well as naloxonazine, suggesting that this sensitive binding component may represent binding to mu$_1$ sites. The binding remaining in the presence of both morphine and DADL, however, did not correspond to either mu or delta sites on the basis of detailed competition studies. It has been reported that some benzomorphans may also interact with β-endorphin binding sites (Chang et al., 1984). It seems, however, that the development of other opioid ligands more selective for the putative epsilon sites is required in order to support further the existence of these sites.

4. Regional Distribution of Opioid Binding Sites Within the Brain

Early studies investigating the regional distribution of opioid receptors in mammalian CNS did not distinguish between the various subtypes of opioid receptors. Binding of [^{3}H]etorphine to regions of the human brain (Hiller et al., 1973) and [³H]DHM to regions of monkey brain (Kuhar et al., 1973) revealed high levels of specific binding in areas associated with the limbic system, such as the amygdala, thalamus, hypothalamus, caudet nucleus, and periaqueductal gray. Binding was low in the cerebellum and the cortex, except in the frontal lobe. More recent studies examining mu and delta sites revealed different regional distributions (Chang et al., 1979; Simon et al., 1980). The thalamus contained predominately mu sites, whereas delta sites predominated in the frontal cortex. In cow brain, the ratio of mu to delta binding, measured with [³H]morphine and [³H]DADL, respectively, varied by as much as 10-fold (Ninkovik et al., 1981). Similar results were obtained in rat brain, with high ratios of mu to delta binding in the thalamus and substantia nigra. Low rations of mu to delta binding were noted in the frontal cortex and hippocampus. The distribution of mu and delta sites in human brain revealed a similar pattern to that seen in other mammalians (Bonnet et al., 1981; Pfeiffer et al., 1982). Of particular note was the high density of mu sites in the thalamus found using competition studies. Autoradiography studies in the rat brain (Goodman et al., 1980) demonstrated also differential distribution of mu and delta sites. These findings, which are described in detail in the chapter entitled Regional Distribution of Opioid Receptors, in this volume, were in agreement with results obtained from in vitro binding to homogenates of brain regions.

The distribution of naloxazone-sensitive, or mu_1, sites was also studied in rat brain (Zhang and Pasternak, 1980). Naloxazone treatment lowered [³H][D-Ala²-Met⁵]enkephalinamide binding in hypothalamus and spinal cord the most, whereas that in the corpus striatum and thalamus was less sensitive. Binding in membranes from the frontal cortex, midbrain, and pons medulla was relatively insensitive to naloxazone inhibition. Studies with [³H]naloxonazine provided more direct evidence for differences in the regional distribution of mu_1 sites (Johnson and Pasternak, 1984). The hypothalamus contained the highest percentage of mu_1 binding (60%), measured as that binding not freely reversible, whereas the brainstem had the lowest (18%). Moderate levels were reported in the frontal cortex and striatum (27–35%).

Autoradiography provided the first evidence of the regional distribution of kappa sites in the guinea pig brain (Goodman and Snyder, 1982). Kappa sites were selectively labeled by using [³H]ethylketocyclazocine or [³H]bremazocine in the presence of high concentrations of morphine and DADL to block mu and delta sites. Layers V and VI of the cerebral cortex and the pyriform cortex contained the highest density of kappa sites. Low levels were detected in the caudate nucleus and the nucleus accumbens. Recent radioreceptor binding assays demonstrated very high levels of kappa binding sites with little mu or delta binding in the cerebellum of the guinea pig (Robson et al., 1984; Itzhak et al., 1984a) it was concluded that 85–90% of opioid binding to cerebellar membranes of the guinea pig corresponds to binding to kappa sites.

A comparison of the distribution of kappa and mu sites in seven regions of the human brain revealed the highest density of kappa binding in the hypothalamus, followed by the parietal cortex, hippocampus, and cingulate gyrus, as defined by the residual [^{3}H]bremazocine binding in presence of mu and delta blockers (Table 8; Itzhak et al., 1982). The thalamus, a region with high levels of mu and low density of delta sites, had the lowest levels of kappa binding. Using ($\pm$)-[^{3}H]SKF 10,047 to assess sigma binding sites, the authors reported that mu and delta blockers lowered binding in the hypothalamus only 34%. Residual ($\pm$)-[^{3}H] SKF 10,047 binding was inhibited by 3-hydroxy-PCP, whereas the residual binding of [^{3}H]bremazocine, which corresponded to kappa sites, was not affected. Therefore, the hypothalamus of human brain contained a combination of kappa and SKF 10,047 binding sites. The one difficulty with this study was the use of the racemic ^{3}H-ligand. More recent studies in the rat using (+)-[^{3}H]SKF 10,047 revealed high levels of binding in the hippocampus (101 fmol/mg protein) with moderate levels in the midbrain, frontal cortex, and caudate (50–55 fmol/mg protein) and low levels in the cerebellum and nonfrontal cortex (25–30 fmol/mg protein (Itzhak et al., 1985). These findings were very similar to those reported for the distribution of [^{3}H]PCP binding in rat brain (Zukin and Zukin, 1979).

Autoradiographic studies also suggested the presence of distinct β-endorphin binding sites (Goodman et al., 1983). In these studies, the pattern of labeling with [^{3}H]β-endorphin in the striatum, nucleus accumbens, lamina IV of the cortex, hippocampus, and dorsal raphe presented a different pattern than that of either [^{3}H]dihydromorphine or [^{3}H]DADL. Although quite suggestive, this study suffered from the absence of mu and delta blockers. Thus, the overall labeling of the [^{3}H]β-endorphin consisted of several binding subtypes.

TABLE 8
Assessment of Benzomorphan Binding Sites in Human Brain Regions[a]

Brain region	[³H]Naloxone	[³H]DHM	[³H]Bremazocine	(±)[³H]SKF 10,047
Hypothalamus				
Total specific binding	23 ± 2	14 ± 2	152 ± 4	35 ± 4
Benzomorphan binding	10 ± 1	2 ± 1	97 ± 5	23 ± 2
Percentage	41%	14%	64%	60%
Parietal				
Total specific binding	20 ± 2	11 ± 0.2	114 ± 4	30 ± 3
Benzomorphan binding	7 ± 0.4	0.3	49 ± 3	19 ± 2
Percentage	35%	3%	43%	63%
Hippocampus				
Total specific binding	29 ± 6	19 ± 1	105 ± 13	54 ± 4
Benzomorphan binding	8 ± 2	1.5 ± 0.4	50 ± 5	29 ± 1
Percentage	27%	8%	48%	54%
Frontal cortex				
Total specific binding	28 ± 1	14 ± 2	129 ± 3	29 ± 8
Benzomorphan binding	8 ± 1	2 ± 1	53 ± 3	14 ± 5
Percentage	29%	14%	41%	48%

Cingulate				
Total specific binding	20 ± 2	11 ± 0.5	91 ± 8	18 ± 4
Benzomorphan binding	5 ± 0.5	1 ± 0.4	44 ± 5	8 ± 0.4
Percentage	25%	9%	48%	44%
Caudate				
Total specific binding	45 ± 6	33 ± 2	140 ± 20	56 ± 1
Benzomorphan binding	9 ± 1	1 ± 0.7	45 ± 8	19 ± 2
Percentage	20%	3%	32%	34%
Thalamus				
Total specific binding	58 ± 6	45 ± 5	140 ± 13	54 ± 5
Benzomorphan binding	9 ± 0.4	3 ± 1	32 ± 1	15 ± 2
Percentage	15%	7%	23%	28%

[a]Specific binding (fmol/mg protein) of ^{3}H-opioids (1 nM) in the absence (total specific) and presence (benzomorphan binding) of DAMPGO and DADL (100 nM each) was determined in seven regions of human brain. Results from 3–5 experiments are expressed as mean ±SEM (modified from Itzhak et al., 1982).

5. Biochemical Properties of Opioid Binding Sites

5.1. Physical and Chemical Properties

Opioid binding is highly sensitive to proteolytic enzymes and reagents. Sulfhydryl reagents such as N-ethylmaleimide, iodacetate, and others all inhibit opioid binding (Simon et al., 1973; Pasternak and Snyder, 1974, 1975a; Pasternak et al., 1975a; Simon and Groth, 1975). These effects are prevented in the presence of unlabeled opiates, which presumably protect the binding site (Pasternak et al., 1975a; Simon and Groth, 1975). Results from these studies suggested the involvement of protein component(s) in the specific binding of opioids and the proximity of sulfhydryl groups near the active site. Of the various binding subtypes, the mu_1 sites were the most sensitive to trypsin and N-ethylmaleimide (Nishimura et al., 1984). Virtually all the mu_1 binding of [^{3}H]dihydromorphine and [^{3}H]DADL was eliminated by these two treatments at 5 μg/mL and 50 μM, respectively.

Several studies suggest the involvement of lipids in the binding of opioids to their receptors. Phospholipase A, but not C and D, potently lowers binding (Pasternak and Snyder, 1974). It was also reported that phosphatidylserine stimulates opioid binding (Abood et al., 1977). Interestingly, bovine serum albumin has been reported to reverse the inhibition of opioid binding by phospholipase A (Lin and Simon, 1978, 1981). Possible involvement of cerebroside sulfate in the binding of opioids has also been suggested (Loh et al., 1974, 1975). The sensitivity of solubilized opioid binding sites to heat denaturation, proteases, N-ethylmaleimide, phospholipase A, and phosphatidylserine decarboxylase provides further evidence for the protein and lipid nature of the opioid binding sites (Bidlack and Abood, 1980; Ruegg et al., 1981; Simonds et al., 1980; Itzhak et al., 1984a).

Solubilized binding sites provided evidence for a glycoprotein component. Digitonin-solubilized binding sites are retained on a wheat germ agglutinin column and are specifically eluted by N-acetylglucosamine (Gioannini et al., 1982; Howells et al., 1982).

5.2. Effect of Ions and Nucleotides

The ability of sodium to discriminate between agonist and antagonist binding was one of the earliest discoveries in the opioid field (Pert et al., 1973; Simon et al., 1975a,b). Similar effects were observed with LiCl. The divalent cation manganese reversed in large part the actions of sodium on agonist binding, restoring binding levels almost to normal levels (Pasternak et al., 1975b). Sodium and managanese ions had similar actions on the binding of opioid peptides such as $[^3H][Leu^5]$enkephalin and $[^3H][Met^5]$-enkephalin (Morin et al., 1976; Meunier and Moisand, 1977; Simantov et al., 1978). In contrast to opioid alkaloids and enkephalins, the binding of $[^3H]\beta$-endorphin was inhibited by divalent ions such as manganese, magnesium, and calcium (Ferrara et al., 1979; Akil et al., 1980; Ferrara and Li, 1980). These results suggested that the binding sites for β-endorphin are different from those for the enkephalins (Hazum et al., 1979).

Mixed agonist/antagonists are less sensitive to sodium ions compared to morphine-like compounds (Kosterlitz and Leslie, 1978). The effects of ions on the binding of $[^3H]$ethylketocyclazocine may be more complex, however. In rat brain assays using Tris buffer, sodium ions clearly lowered $[^3H]$ethylketocyclazocine binding (Pasternak, 1980), whereas studies using potassium phosphate buffer reported increased binding (Hiller and Simon, 1980). Although the discrepancy between these two reports has not been conclusively resolved, most groups now report a decrease in $[^3H]$ethylketocyclazocine binding with sodium ions. It is important to remember, however, that under these conditions, $[^3H]$ethylketocyclazocine is labeling predominently mu and delta sites in the rat brain.

In a recent study, the effects of a series of cations on $[^3H]$ethylketocyclazocine binding in rat brain, in which most of the binding corresponded to mu and delta sites (Maurer, 1982), and in guinea pig cerebellum, in which the binding reflected kappa sites (Robson et al., 1984), were compared (Itzhak and Pasternak, 1986). Unlike $[^3H]$ethylketocyclazocine binding in rat brain, which was reduced by 64 to 61% by 100 mM sodium or lithium chloride, respectively, binding in the guinea pig cerebellum was unaffected. Moreover, manganese and calcium ions lowered binding in the cerebellum by 25% without affecting binding in the rat brain assay (Table 9). Similar results were obtained using either Tris or potassium phosphate buffers and in the absence or presence of mu and delta blockers in the cerebellar assay.

Guanine nucleotides also differentially effect the binding of opioid agonists and antagonists. GTP (50 μM) lowers the binding of radiolabeled dihydromorphine, $[Leu^5]$enkephalin, and $[Met^5]$-enkephalin binding by 40–50%, whereas $[^3H]$naloxone binding is virtually unaffected. Addition of sodium ions to GTP greatly

TABLE 9
Effect of Ions and Nucleotides on [^{3}H]Ethylketocyclazocine Binding
to Rat Brain and Guinea Pig Cerebellum Membranes[a]

| | | Specific binding, percent control . | | |
| | | Guinea pig cerebellum | | Rat brain |
Addition	mM	Kappa binding	Total binding	Total binding
NaCl	50	115 ± 3	101 ± 2	46 ± 4
	100	102 ± 6	97 ± 3	36 ± 6
LiCl	50	98 ± 2	102 ± 2	50 ± 3
	100	105 ± 3	104 ± 2	40 ± 5
KCl	50	101 ± 2	98 ± 2	74 ± 4
	100	99 ± 2	101 ± 3	65 ± 3
MgCl$_2$	1	91 ± 3	100 ± 2	99 ± 6
	3	96 ± 4	101 ± 3	102 ± 4
MnCl$_2$	1	79 ± 1	78 ± 2	103 ± 3
	3	80 ± 4	82 ± 4	93 ± 2
CaCl$_2$	1	75 ± 6	74 ± 2	103 ± 3
	3	74 ± 4	76 ± 3	100 ± 3
GDP	0.1	97 ± 5	98 ± 2	76 ± 3
+ NaCl	50	63 ± 3	60 ± 3	27 ± 1
GTP	0.1	95 ± 5	94 ± 3	78 ± 3
+ NaCl	50	62 ± 3	58 ± 4	24 ± 2
Gpp NH p	0.1	100 ± 4	98 ± 4	71 ± 7
+ NaCl	50	60 ± 2	57 ± 4	25 ± 2

[a]Binding of [^{3}H]ethylketocyclazocine (2 nM) to guinea pig cerebellum homogenate
and rat brain homogenates. Total binding represents total opiate-specific binding,
whereas kappa binding was assessed in the presence of both DAMPGO and DADL
(both 100 nM) (modified from Itzhak and Pasternak, 1986).

increases the inhibition of agonist binding to 80–90%. Again,
[^{3}H]naloxone binding is not altered (Childers and Snyder, 1978,
1980). Similar effects on the binding of [^{3}H]Leu^5-enkephalin to
NG108-15 cells were reported (Blum, 1978). These interactions are
discussed in greater detail in the chapter entitled Opioid-Coupled
Second Messenger Systems.

The sensitivity of kappa sites to guanyl nucleotides differs
from mu and delta sites (Itzhak and Pasternak, 1986). Guanosine
5-triphosphate (GTP), guanosine 5-diphosphate (GDP), or the
stable analog 5-guanylyimidodiphosphate [Gpp(NH)p] at concentrations of 100 μM in the presence of sodium chloride lowered
[^{3}H]ethylketocyclazocine binding by only 36–40% in guinea pig
cerebellar membranes. Guanosine 5-monophosphate (GMP) and
adenosine 5-triphosphate (ATP) had no effect on cerebellar bind-

ing in the absence or presence of NaCl. Under similar conditions, GTP, Gpp(NH)p, or GDP in the presence of NaCl lowered the binding of [³H]ethylketocyclazocine to rat brain membranes by 75–80% (Table 9). Ethylketocyclazocine is a kappa agonist in the guinea pig ileum (Hutchinson et al., 1975), and its binding in rat brain to mu and delta sites reveals an agonist-like sensitivity to monovalent cations and nucleotides (Pasternak, 1980). Thus, the insensitivity of [³H]ethylketocyclazocine binding in guinea pig cerebellum to monovalent cations and nucleotides cannot be explained by simply considering the compound an antagonist. In view of the association of guanyl nucleotide and sodium ion sensitivity with N (or G) proteins, the differences between kappa sites and mu and delta sites raise the possibility of a different effector system other than cyclase for the kappa sites.

On the basis of the sensitivity of opioid binding sites to GTP, Pert and Taylor (1980) have suggested the existence of two types of opiate and enkephalin binding sites: type 1 sites, which are sensitive to GTP, and type 2 sites, which are insensitive to GTP. The authors have studied the regional distribution of these sites in rat brain, and claimed that type 1 sites may correspond to mu receptors, and type 2 to delta receptors.

5.3. Effect of Alcohols and Detergents

The sensitivity of binding to phospholipase A, discussed earlier, raised the question of the role of lipids in opioid binding. Other agents that influence membrane fluidity also affect binding. Alcohols lower [³H]DADL binding with potencies increasing with chain length (Hiller et al., 1981, 1984). This inhibition correlates with a decrease in affinity, an accelerated dissociation rate, and no change in B_{max}. Delta sites are more sensitive to these alcohol effects. Binding of labeled dihydromorphine and naloxone was not affected by these alcohols. Based upon this differential sensitivity, the authors suggested that delta sites were more sensitive to changes in membrane fluidity.

Detergents such as Triton X-100, digitonin, CHAPS, and others were used in order to solubilize the opioid binding sites. All of these detergents may, however, inhibit opioid specific binding. Low concentrations of the nonionic detergent digitonin (0.01–0.1%) lower agonist binding ([³H]etorphine) to a greater extent than antagonist binding ([³H]diprenorphine) (Itzhak et al., 1984c). Sodium chloride (100 mM) protects antagonist binding, but not agonist binding. The inhibition of opioid binding by these low concentrations of digitonin is reversible and results from an increase in the dissociation rate of the ligand–receptor complex. The mechanism by which the detergent acts to inhibit opioid binding is still not clear. The differential sensitivities of opiate agonist and antagonist binding, however, coupled with the protective effect of sodium ions on antagonist binding suggest that agonist and antagonist conformations are differentially affected (Pasternak and Snyder, 1975a; Pasternak et al., 1975c; Simon et al., 1975b; Simon and Hiller, 1978). These findings are quite similar to the variety of treatments that distinguish between agonist and antagonist binding discussed in the chapter entitled Early Studies of Opioid Binding.

Solubilization of the various types of opioid receptors with digitonin also differs among the binding subtypes. Digitonin solubilizes mu and delta sites in rat brain in high yields only in the presence of high concentrations of sodium chloride ($1M$) (Howells et al., 1982; Gioannini et al., 1982; Itzhak et al., 1984a). In contrast, kappa sites in the guinea pig cerebellum are solubilized in good yields by digitonin, even in the absence of NaCl (Itzhak et al., 1984b). Similarly, kappa opioid binding sites present in the toad brain (Simon et al., 1982) were solubilized in high yields in the absence of NaCl (Ruegg et al., 1981). Solubilization and purification of receptors are discussed in greater detail in a later chapter. These findings further supported the hypothesis that kappa sites may represent molecular species different from mu and delta sites.

6. Developmental Appearance of Opioid Binding Sites

Specific [3H]naloxone and [3H]naltrexone binding can be detected in brains of rat fetuses at embryonic d 14. Binding levels increase rapidly until 21 d after birth and then more slowly until adulthood (Clendeninn et al., 1976; Coyle and Pert, 1976; Garcin and Coyle, 1976; Messing et al., 1980). These changes reflect increases in receptor number without changes in affinity, as revealed by saturation analysis (Clendeninn et al., 1976). Studying the development of opioid binding sites in various regions of rat brain, it has been shown that increases in receptor density vary among regions, with greater changes in the cortex than in the striatum or pons and medulla (Garcin and Coyle, 1976; Bardo et al., 1981).

Binding capacity of $[^3H][Met^5]$enkephalin in forebrain increased by fivefold between the fifth and 20th day after birth. Binding in brainstem homogenates increased at a similar rate until the fifth day, but by the 20th day returned to the levels of newborn rats (Tsang and Ng, 1980; Tsang et al., 1982). Several investigators have reported differences in the development of the various types of opioid receptors. Wohltman et al., (1982) found that mu sites in rat brain appear before delta sites postnatally. Autoradiographic approaches, which are discussed in greater detail in a later chapter, revealed similar findings (Kent et al., 1982). Sites labeled by $[^3H]$naloxone first appeared in the striatum of 14-d-old rats, and their density increased rapidly by adulthood. $[^3H]$DADL binding to striatum appeared at a later stage of development and gradually increased into an homogenous adult pattern. Recently, Spain et al. (1985) compared the ontogeny of mu, delta, and kappa receptors. The authors found that immediately after birth the density of mu sites, labeled by $[^3H]$DAMPGO, declined for several days and then increased rapidly over the next 2 wk with a final increase of twofold by adulthood. Delta sites labeled by $[^3H]$DADL in the presence of 10 mM of DAMPGO to block mu binding appeared in the second week postnatally and increased by eightfold during the next 2 wk. Levels of kappa sites labeled by $[^3H]$EKC in the presence of DAMPGO and DADL were relatively low at birth and increased slowly by only twofold by adulthood. They concluded that mu and kappa sites are present at birth, whereas delta sites appear only in the second week.

Zhang and Pasternak examined the postnatal appearance of mu_1, mu_2, and delta sites (Pasternak 1980c; Zhang and Pasternak, 1981b). At 2 d of age, levels of mu_1 sites were only 22% of the adult levels, but increased rapidly so that by 14 d of age the density had increased to greater than 50% compared to those of adult levels. In contrast, levels of mu_2 and delta sites remained relatively constant between 2 and 14 d at approximately 50% of adult levels. The authors concluded that mu_1 sites have a later developmental appearance than either mu_2, delta, or kappa sites. These results are consistent with phylogenetic studies from the same laboratory that found mu_2 and delta sites in lower species, such as goldfish, but not mu_1 sites, which appeared in higher species (Buatti and Pasternak, 1981).

Studies of morphine analgesia in the developmental study revealed a close correlation of the appearance of mu_1 sites with analgesic potency. At 2 d of age, when the density of mu_1 sites was quite low, the ED_{50} of morphine in the tailflick assay was 56

mg/kg. By 14 d of age, the ED_{50} had decreased to 1.4 mg/kg. Of
course, many developmental changes occur during this period,
making the interpretation of these results difficult. This association of mu_1 sites with analgesia is in agreement, however, with
other studies using the mu_1-selective antagonists naloxazone and
naloxonazine (Pasternak et al., 1980a,b; Pasternak, 1981; Ling and
Pasternak, 1983; Pasternak, 1980; Zhang and Pasternak, 1981a).
The authors concluded that mu_1 sites have a later appearance, in
rat brain, then either mu_2 or delta sites.

7. Opiate Binding in Pathological States

Clearly, one question is the issue of changes of opioid binding
sites in pathological states. Their high density in limbic structures
and striatum, along with their association with dopamine, norepinephrine, and acetylcholine systems, raises specific questions regarding schizophrenia, Parkinson's disease, and Alzheimer's disease. To date, only a handful of studies have suggested changes
in binding in these diseases. One major difficulty with studies of
this type is the long delay between death and autopsy and the
potential problems of receptor loss because of autolysis of brain
tissue. Careful controls are usually included in the experiments,
but questions will always remain. To date, these autopsy studies
remain the best method to address these issues, but the recent advances in positron emission tomography may offer the potential
of examining receptor number in vivo.

Reisine and coworkers (Reisine et al., 1979, 1980; Reisine and
Soubrie, 1982) have reported that [^{3}H]naloxone binding in caudate nuclei obtained from schizophrenic patients and Parkinson's
disease patients was decreased by 44% and 65%, respectively.
This decrease in binding was related to reduction in the number
of opioid binding sites, and no change in the affinity of [^{3}H]nalox-
one was observed. Binding to other brain regions, such as the putamen, was unchanged compared to controls. These results suggest a change in mu binding sites, since naloxone, at low
concentrations, will label predominantly mu receptors. The question of changes in specific subtypes remains.

A more recent study examined binding in patients with Alzheimer's disease and age-matched controls (Hiller et al., 1987).
The most consistent observation was an elevation in kappa binding in all five areas of the limbic system examined (caudate,

amygdala, temporal cortex, putamen, and hippocampus). Kappa binding to the putamen and caudate was increased 114 and 53%, respectively. In addition, the overall binding of [^{3}H]bremazocine, reflecting binding to mu, kappa, and delta sites, increased an average of 85% over controls. Mu ([^{3}H]DAMPGO) and delta ([^{3}H]DADL) binding was 41 and 55% lower, respectively, in the amygdala of the Alzheimer patients. Mu and delta binding in frontal cortex, caudate, and hippocampus of Alzhemier brains were unchanged from control levels. The authors suggested that the increase in kappa binding may result from up-regulation secondary to a decrease in dynorphin levels.

8. Concluding Remarks

Evidence from binding experiments and pharmacological studies accumulated during the last several years all indicate the existence of multiple types of opioid binding sites. The understanding of how many opioid receptor types exist and how they differ from each other is crucial for the definition of their functions. The physiological significance of each type of opioid receptor has still to be further elucidated. Such studies may allow researchers to design highly selective ligands for each of the receptor types, compounds which will elicit desired pharmacological response relatively devoid of undesired side effects.

Acknowledgment

The author greatly appreciates the helpful remarks of Dr. G. W. Pasternak.

References

Abood, L. C., Salem, N., MacNeil, M., Bloom, L., and Abood, M. E. (1977) Enhancement of opiate binding by various molecular forms of phosphatidylserine and inhibition by other unsaturated lipids. *Biochem. Biopsy. Acta* **468**, 51–62.

Akil, H., Hewlett, W. A., Barchas, J. D., and Li, C. H. (1981) Binding of ^{3}H-β-endorphin to rat brain membranes: Characterization of opiate properties and interaction with ACTH. *Eur. J. Pharmacol.* **64**, 1–8.

Bardo, M. T., Bhatgart, R. K., and Gebhart, G. F. (1981) Opiate receptor ontogeny and morphine induced effects: Influence of chronic footshock
stress in preweanling rats. *Dev. Brain Res.* **1**, 487–495.

Beckett, A. H. and Casy, A. F. (1954) Synthetic analgesics: Stereochemical
considerations. *J. Pharmacol.* **6**, 986.

Beckett, A. H., Casy, A. F., and Harper, N J. (1956) Analgesics and their
antagonists: Some steric and chemical considerations. The influence of
the basic group on biological response. *J. Pharm. Sci.* **8**, 874–884.

Bidlack, J. M. and Abood, L. G. (1980) Solubilization of opiate receptor. *Life
Sci.* **27**, 331–340.

Blum, A. J. (1978) Opiate binding to membrane preparations of neuroblastoma × glioma hybrid cells Ng108-15; Effects of inos and nucleotides.
Life Sci. **22**, 1843–1852.

Bonnet, K. A., Groth, J., Gioannini, T., Cortes, M., and Simon, E. J. (1981)
Opiate receptor heterogeneity in human brain regions. *Brain Res.* **221**,
437–440.

Brady, K. T., Balster, R. L., and May, E. L. (1982) Stereoisomers of N-allylnormetazocine, phencyclidine-like behavioral effects in squirrel monkeys and rats. *Science* **215**, 178–180.

Buatti, M. C. and Pasternak, G. W. (1981) Multiple opiate receptors: Phylogenetic differences. *Brain Res.* **218**, 400–405.

Caruso, J. P., Takemori, A. E., Larson, D. L., and Portoghese, P. S. (1979)
Chloroxymorphamine, an opioid receptor site directed alkylating agent
having narcotic agonist activity. *Science* **204**, 316–318.

Chang, K. -J. and Cuatrecasas, P. (1979) Multiple opiate receptors: Enkephalins and morphine bind to receptors of different specificity. *J. Biol.
Chem.* **254**, 2610–2618.

Chang, K. -J., Killian, A., Hazum, E., and Cuatrecasas, P. (1981) Morphiceptin: A potent and specific agonist for morphine (mu) receptor. *Science* (Washington, DC), **212**, 75–77.

Chang, K. -J., Blanchard, S. G., and Cuatrecasas, P. (1984) Benzomorphan
sites are ligand recognition sites for putative epsilon receptor. *Mol.
Pharmacol.* **26**, 484–488.

Chang, K. -J., Cooper, B. R., Hazum, E., and Cuatrecasas, P. (1979) Multiple opiate receptors: Different regional distribution in the brain and differential binding of opiates and opioid peptides. *Mol. Pharmacol.* **16**,
91–104.

Chang, K. -J., Hazum, E., and Cuatrecasas, P. (1980) Possible role of distinct
morphine and enkephalin receptors in mediating actions of benzomorphan drugs (putative kappa and sigma agonists). *Proc. Natl. Acad. Sci.
USA* **77**, 4469–4473.

Chavkin, C. and Goldstein, A. (1981a) Demonstration of a specific dynorphin receptor in the guinea pig ileum myenteric plexus. *Nature* (Lond.)
291, 591–593.

Chavkin, C. and Goldstein, A. (1981b) Specific receptor for the opioid peptide dynorphin: Structure activity relationships. *Proc. Natl. Acad. Sci.
USA* **78**, 6543–6547.

Chavkin, C., James, I. F., and Goldstein, A. (1982) Dynorphin is a specific
endogenous ligand of the kappa opiate receptors. *Science* **215**, 413–415.

Cheng, Y.-.C. and Prusoff, W. H. (1973) Relationship between the inhibition constant (Ki) and the concentration of inhibitor which causes 50%

inhibition (IC50) of an enzymatic reaction. *Biochem. Pharmocol.* **22**, 3099–3108.

Childers, S.R. and Snyder, S. H. (1978) Guanine nucleotides differentiate agonist and antagonist interactions with opiate receptors. *Life Sci.* **23**, 759–762.

Childers, S. R. and Snyder, S. H. (1980) Differential regulation by guanine nucleotides of opiate agonist and antagonist receptor interaction. *J. Neurochem.* **34**, 583–593.

Cicero, T. J., Wilcox, C. E. and Meyer, E. R. (1974) Effect of α-adrenergic blockers on naloxone binding in brain. *Biochem. Pharmacol.* **23**, 2349–2352.

Cicero, T. J., Wilcox, C. E., Meyer, E. R., and Michael, H. (1975) Influence of cathecholaminergic agents on narcotic binding in brain. *Arch. Int. Pharmacodyn. Ther.* **218**, 221–230.

Clark, J. A., Itzhak, Y. Hruby, V. J., Yamamura, H. I., and Pasternak, G. W. (1986) [D-Pen^2, D-Pen^5]enkephalin (DPDPE): A delta-selective enkephalin with low affinity for μ_1 opiate binding sites. *Eur. J. Pharmacol.* **128**, 303–304.

Clendeninn, N. J., Petraitis, M., and Simon, E. J. (1976) Ontological development of opiate receptors in rodent brain. *Brain Res.* **118**, 157–160.

Corbett, A. D., Gillam, M. G. C., Kosterlitz, H. W., McKnight, A. T., Paterson, S. J., and Robson, L. E. (1984) Selectivities of opioid peptide analogs as agonists and antagonists at the delta receptor. *Br. J. Pharmacol.* **83**, 271–279.

Corbett, A. D., Paterson, S. J., McKnight, A. T., Magnan, J., and Kosterlitz, H. W. (1982) Dynorphin 1-8 and dynorphin 1-9 are ligands for kappa subtype of opiate receptor. *Nature* (Lond.) **299**, 79–81.

Coyle, J. T. and Pert, C. B. (1976) Ontogenic development of 3H-naloxone binding in rat brain. *Neuropharmacology* **15**, 555–560.

Ferrara, P. and Li, C. H. (1980) β-Endorphin: Characteristics of binding sites in rabbit spinal cord. *Proc. Natl. Acad. Sci. USA* **77**, 5746–5748.

Ferrara, P., Houghten, R., and Li, C. H. (1979) β-Endorphin: Characteristics of binding sites in the rat. *Biochem. Biophys. Res. Commun.* **89**, 786–792.

Fischel, S. V. and Medzihradsy, F. (1981) Scatchard analyses of opiate receptor binding. *Mol. Pharmacol.* **20**, 269–279.

Gacel, G., Fournie-Zaluski, M.-.C., and Roques, B. P. (1980) Try-D-Ser-Gly-Phe-Leu-Thr, a highly preferential ligand for delta opiate receptors. *FEBS Lett.* **118**, 245–247.

Garcin, F. and Coyle, J. T. (1976) Ontogenic Development of 3H-Naloxone Binding and Endogenous Morphine-Like Factor in Rat Brain, in *Opiates and Endogenous Opioid Peptides* (Kosterlitz, H. W., ed.) Elsevier, North Holland Biomedical Press, Amsterdam.

Gilbert, P. E. and Martin, W. R. (1976a) Sigma effects of nalorphine in the chronic spinal dog. *Drug Alcohol Depend.* **1**, 373–376.

Gilbert, P. E. and Martin, W. R. (1976b) The effects of morphine and nalorphine-like drugs in the nondependent, morphine-dependent, and cyclalzocine-dependent chronic spinal dog. *J. Pharmacol. Exp. Ther.* **198**, 66–82.

Gillan, M. G. C., Kosterlitz, H. W., and Paterson, S. J. (1980) Comparison of the binding characteristics of tritiated opiates and opioid peptides. *Br. J. Pharmacol.* **70**, 481–490.

Gioannini, T., Foucaud, B., Hiller, J. M., Hatten, M. E., and Simon, E. J. (1982) Lectin binding of solubilized opiate receptors: Evidence for their glycoprotein nature. *Biochem. Biophys. Res. Commun.* **105**, 1128–1134.

Goldstein, A. and James, I. F. (1984) Site-directed alkylation of multiple opioid receptors: Pharmacological selectivity. *Mol. Pharmacol.* **25**, 343–348.

Goldstein, A., Lowney, L. I., and Pal, B. K. (1971) Stereospecific and nonspecific interactions of the morphine congener levorphanol in subcellular fractions of mouse brain. *Proc. Natl. Acad. Sci. USA* **68**, 1742–1747.

Goldstein, A., Tachibana, S., Lowney, L. I., Hunkapiller, M., and Hood, L. (1979) Dynorphin-(1-13), an extraordinarily potent opioid peptide. *Proc. Natl. Acad. Sci. USA* **76**, 6666–6670.

Goodman, R. R. and Snyder, S. H. (1982) Kappa opiate receptors localized by autoradiography deep layers of cerebral cortex: Relation to sedative effects. *Proc. Natl. Acad. Sci. USA* **79**, 5703–5707.

Goodman, R. R., Snyder, S. H., Kuhar, M. J., and Young, W. S. (1980) Differentiation of delta and mu opiate receptor localizations by light microscopic autoradiography. *Proc. Natl. Acad. Sci. USA* **77**, 6239–6243.

Goodman, R. R., Houghten, R. A., and Pasternak, G. W. (1983) Autoradiography of 3H-β-endorphin binding in brain. *Life Sci.* **288**, 334–337.

Hahn, E. F., and Pasternak, G. W. (1982) Naloxonazine, a potent, long-acting inhibitor of opiate binding sites. *Life Sci.* **31**, 1385–1388.

Hahn, E. F., Carroll-Buatti, M., and Pasternak, G. W. (1982) Irreversible opiate agonists and antagonists: The 14-hydroxydihydromorphine azines. *J. Neurosci.* **2**, 572–576.

Hahn, E. F., Nishimura, S., Goodman, R. R., and Pasternak, G. W. (1985a) Irreversible opiate agonists and antagonists: II. Evidence against a bivalent mechanism of action for opiate azines and diacylhydrazones. *J. Pharmacol. Exp. Ther.* **235**, 839–845.

Hahn, E. F., Itzhak, Y., Nishimura, S., Johnson, N., and Pasternak, G. W. (1985b) Irreversible opiate agonists and antagonists: III. Phenylhydrazone derivatives of naloxone and oxymorphone. *J. Pharmacol. Exp. Ther.* **235**, 846–850.

Hammonds, R. G. and Li, C. H. (1981) Human β-endorphin: Specific binding in neuroblastoma N18TG2 cells. *Proc. Natl. Acad. Sci. USA* **78**, 6764–6765.

Handa, B. K., Lane, A. C., Lord, J. A. H., Morgan, B. A., Rance, M. J., and Smith, C. F. C. (1981) Analogs of B-LPH61-64 possessing selective agonist activity at mu opiate receptors. *Eur. J. Pharmacol.* **70**, 531–540.

Hazum, E., Chang, K.-J., and Cuatrecasas, P. (1979) Interaction of iodinated human (D-Ala2-B-endorphin with opiate receptors. *J. Biol. Chem.* **254**, 1765–1767.

Hazum, E., Chang, K.-J., Cuatrecasas, P., and Pasternak, G. W. (1981) Naloxazone irreversibly inhibits the high affinity binding of [125I]-DAla2-D-Leu5enkephalinβ. *Life Sci.* **28**, 2973–2979.

Hill, A. V. (1910) The possible effects of the aggregation of the molecules of haemoglobin on its dissociation curves. *J. Physiol. (Lond.)* **40**, iv–viii.

Hiller, J. M. and Simon, E. J. (1980) Specific high affinity 3H-ethylketocyclazocine binding in rat central nervous system: Lack of evidence for kappa receptors. *J. Pharmacol. Exp. Ther.* **214**, 516–519.

Hiller, J. M., Angel, L. M., and Simon, E. J. (1981) Multiple opiate receptors: Alcohol selectively inhibits binding to delta receptors. *Science* **214**, 468–469.

Hiller, J. M., , Angel, L. M., and Simon, E. J. (1984) Characterization of the selective inhibition of the delta subclass of opioid binding sites by alcohols. *Mol. Pharmacol.* **25**, 249–255.

Hiller, J. M., Itzhak, Y., and Simon, E. J. (1987) Selective changes in the binding levels of mu, delta and kappa opioid ligands in limbic regions of the brain in Alzheimer's Disease Patients. *Brain Res.* **406**, 17–23.

Hiller, J. M., Pearson, J., and Simon, E. J. (1973) Distribution of stereospecific binding of the potent narcotic analgesic etorphine in the human brain: Predominance in limbic system. *Res. Commun. Pathol. Pharmacol.* **6**, 1052–1062.

Ho, C. L., Hammonds, R. G., and Li, C. H. (1983) β-Endorphin; characteristics of binding sites in rabbit cerebellar brain membranes. *Biochem. Biophys. Res. Commun.* **111**, 1096–1104.

Holtzman, S. G. (1982) Phencyclidine-like discriminative stimulus properties of opioids in squirrel monkey. *Psychopharmacology* **77**, 29–300.

Houghten, R. A., Chang, W. C., and Li, C. H. (1980) Human β-endorphin: Synthesis and characterization of iodinated and tritiated analogs. *Int. J. Peptide Protein Res.* **16**, 311–320.

Houghten, R. A., Johnson, N., and Pasternak, G. W. (1984) 3H-β-Endorphin binding in rat brain. *J. Neurosci.* **4**, 2460–2465.

Howells, R. D., Gioannini, T., Hiller, J. M., and Simon, E. J. (1982) Solubilization and characterization of active opiate binding sites from mammalian brain. *J. Pharmacol. Exp. Ther.* **222**, 629–634.

Hughes, J., Smith, T. W., Kosterlitz, H. W., Fothergill, L. A., Morgan, B. A., and Morris, H. R. (1975) Identification of two related pentapeptides from the brain with potent opiate agonist activity. *Nature* **258**, 577–579.

Hutchinson, M., Kosterlitz, H. W., Leslie, F. M., Waterfield, A. A., and Terenius, L. (1975) Assessment in the guinea pig ileum and mouse vas deferens of benzomorphans which have strong antinociceptive activity but do not substitute for morphine in the dependent monkey. *Br. J. Pharmacol.* **55**, 541–546.

Itzhak, Y. (1986) High and Low Affinity Psychotomimetic Opioid Binding Sites: Characterization by a Novel [³H]-PCP-Analog, in *The International Narcotic Research Conference*. July 6–11, 1986, San Francisco, California.

Itzhak, Y. and Pasternak, G. W. (1987) Interaction of [D-Ser², Leu⁵]Enkephalin-Thr⁶ (DSLET), a relatively selective delta ligand, with mu₁ opioid binding sites. *Life Sci.* **40**, 307–311.

Itzhak, Y. and Pasternak, G. W. (1986) Kappa opiate binding to rat brain and guinea pig cerebellum: Sensitivity towards ions and nucleotides. *Neurosci. Lett.* **64**, 81–84.

Itzhak, Y. and Simon, E. J. (1984) A novel phencyclidine analog selectively interacts with mu opioid receptors. *J. Pharmacol. Exp. Ther.* **230**, 383–386.

Itzhak, Y., Bonnet, K. A., Groth, J., Hiller, J. M., and Simon, E. J. (1982) Multiple opiate binding sites in human brain regions: Evidence for kappa and sigma sites. *Life Sci.* **31**, 1363–1366.

Itzhak, Y., Hiller, J. M., and Simon, E. J. (1985) Characterization of specific binding sites for (+)N-allylnormetazocine in rat brain membranes. *Mol. Pharmacol.* **27,** 46–52.

Itzhak, Y., Kalir, A., Weissman, B. A., and Cohen, S. (1981a) Receptor binding and antinociceptive properties of phencyclidine opiate-like derivatives. *Eur. J. Pharmacol.* **72,** 305–311.

Itzhak, Y., Kalir, A., and Sarne, Y. (1981b) On the opioid nature of phencyclidine and its 3-hydroxy derivative. *Eur. J. Phamacol.* **73,** 229–233.

Itzhak, Y., Hiller, J. M., and Simon, E. J. (1984a) Solubilization and characterization of mu, delta and kappa opioid binding sites from guinea pig brain: Physical separation of kappa receptors. *Proc. Natl. Acad. Sci. USA* **81,** 4217–4221.

Itzhak, Y., Hiller, J. M., and Simon, E. J. (1984b) Solubilization of kappa opioid binding sites from guinea pig cerebellum. *Neuropeptides* **5,** 201–204.

Itzhak, Y., Hiller, J. M., Gionnanini, T. L., and Simon, E. J. (1984c) Effect of digitonin on the binding of opiate agonists and antagonists to membrane bound and soluble opioid binding sites. *Brain Res.* **291,** 309–315.

James, I. F. and Goldstein, A. (1984) Site-directed alkylation of multiple opioid receptors: Binding selectivity. *Mol. Pharmacol.* **25,** 337–342.

James, I. F., Chavkin, C., and Goldstein, A. (1982) Preparation of brain membranes containing a single type of opioid receptor highly selective for dynorphin. *Proc. Natl. Acad. Sci. USA* **79,** 7570–7574.

Jasinski, D. R., Shannon, H. E., Cone, E. J., Vaupel, D. B., Risner, M. E., McQuinn, R. L., Su, T. P., and Pickworth, W. B. (1981) Interdisciplinary Studies on Phencyclidine, in *PCP (Phencyclidine): Historical and Current Perspectives* (Domino E. F., ed.) NPP Books, Ann Arbor.

Johnson, N. and Pasternak, G. W. (1983) The binding to rat brain homogenates of Mr2034, a universal opiate. *Life Sci.* **33,** 985–991.

Johnson, N. and Pasternak, G. W. (1984) Binding of 3H-naloxonazine to rat brain membranes. *Mol. Pharmacol.* **26,** 477–483.

Johnson, N., Houghten, R., and Pasternak, G. W. (1982) Binding of 3H-β-endorphin in rat brain. *Life Sci.* **31,** 1381–1384.

Keats, A. S. and Telford, J. (1964) Narcotic Antagonists as Analgesic: Clinical Aspects, in *Molecular Modification in Drug Design: Advances in Chemistry* (R. F. Gould, ed.) American Chemical Society, Washington, DC.

Kent, J. L., Pert, C. B., and Herkenham, M. (1982) Ontogeny of opiate receptors in rat forebrain: Visualization by in vitro autoradiography. *Dev. Brain Res.* **2,** 487–504.

Kosterlitz, H. W. and Leslie, F. M. (1978) Comparison of the receptor binding characteristics of opiate agonists interacting with μ or κ receptors. *Br. J. Pharmacol.* **64,** 607–614.

Kosterlitz, H. W. and Paterson, S. J. (1980) Characterization of opioid receptors in nervous tissue. *Proc. R. Soc. Lond.* **210,** 113–122.

Kosterlitz, H. W. and Paterson, S. J. (1981) Tyr-D-Ala-Gly-MePhe-NH-(CH3)OH is selective ligand for the mu opiate binding sites. *Br. J. Pharmacol.* **73,** 299p.

Kosterlitz, H. W. and Waterfield, A. A. (1975) In vitro models in the study of structure–activity relationships of narcotic analgesics. *Ann. Rev. Pharmacol.* **15,** 29–47.

Kosterlitz, H. W. and Watt, A. J. (1968) Kinetic parameters of narcotic agonists and antagonists with particular reference to N-allynoroxymorphone (naloxone). *Br. J. Pharmacol.* **33**, 266–276.

Kosterlitz, H. W., Lord, J. A. H., Paterson, S. J., and Waterfield, A. A. (1980) Effect of changes in the structure of enkephalins and of narcotic analgesic drugs on their interaction with mu and delta receptors. *Br. J. Pharmacol.* **68**, 333–342.

Kosterlitz, H. W., Paterson, S. J., and Robson, L. E. (1981) Characterization of the kappa-subtype of the opiate receptor in the guinea-pig brain. *Br. J. Pharmacol.* **73**, 939–949.

Kuhar, M. J., Pert, C. B., and Snyder, S. H. (1973) Regional distribution of opiate receptor binding in monkey and human brain. *Nature* **245**, 447–451.

Law, P. Y., and Low, H. H. (1978) 3H-Leu-enkephalin specific binding to synaptic membranes, comparison with 3H-dihydromorphine and 3H-naloxone. *Res. Commun. Chem. Pathol. Pharmacol.* **21**, 409–434.

Lemnaire, S., Magnan, J., and Regoli, D. (1978) Rat vas deferens: A specific bioassay for endogenous opioid peptides. *Br. J. Pharmacol.* **64**, 327–329.

Leslie, F. M., Chavkin, C., and Cox, B. M. (1980) Opioid binding properties of brain and peripheral tissues: Evidence for heterogeneity in opiate ligand binding sites. *J. Pharmacol. Exp. Ther.* **214**, 395–402.

Lin, H.-.K., and Simon, E. J. (1981) Characterization of phospholipase A inhibition of stereospecific opiate binding and its reversal by bovine serum albumin. *J. Pharmacol. Exp. Ther.* **216**, 149–155.

Lin, H.-.K., and Simon, E. J. (1978) Phospholipase A inhibition of opiate receptor binding can be prevented by albumin. *Nature* (Lond.) **271**, 383–384.

Ling, G. S. F. and Pasternak, G. W. (1983) Spinal and supraspinal analgesia in the mouse: The role of subpopulations of opioid binding sites. *Brain. Res.* **271**, 152-156.

Ling, G. S. F., Macleod, J. M., Lee, S., Lockhart, S., and Pasternak, G. W. (1984) Separation of morphine analgesia from physical dependence. *Science* **226**, 462–464.

Ling, G. S. F., Spiegel, K., Lockhart, S. H., and Pasternak, G. W. (1985) Separation of opioid analgesia from respiratory depression: Evidence for different receptor mechanisms. *J. Pharmacol. Exp. Ther.* **232**, 149–155.

Ling, G. S. F., Spiegel, K., Nishimura, S., and Pasternak, G. W. (1983) Dissociation of morphine's analgesic and respiratory depressant actions. *Eur. J. Pharmacol.* **86**, 487–488.

Loh, H. H., Cho, T. M., Wu, Y.-C., Harris, R. A., and Way, E. L. (1975) Opiate binding to cerebroside sulphate: A model system for opiate receptor interaction. *Life Sci.* **16**, 1881–1887.

Loh, H. H., Cho, T. M., Wu, Y.-C., and Way, E. L. (1974) Stereospecific binding of narcotics to brain cerebrosides. *Life Sci.* **14**, 2231–2245.

Lord, J. A. H., Waterfield, A. A., Hughes, J., and Kosterlitz, H. W. (1977) Endogenous opioid peptides: Multiple agonists and receptors. *Nature* (Lond.) **267**, 495–499.

Luby, E. D., Gottlieb, J. S., Cohen, D. D., Rosenbaum, G., and Domino, E. F. (1960) Model psychoses and schizophrenia. *Am. J. Psychiat.* **119**, 61–67.

Lutz, R. A., Cruciani, R. A., Costa, T., Munson, P. J., and Robard, D. (1984) A very high affinity opioid binding site in rat brain: Demonstration by computer modeling. *Biochem. Biophys. Res. Comm.* **122**, 265–269.

Magnan, J., Paterson, S. J., Tavani, A., and Kosterlitz, H. W. (1982) The binding spectrum of narcotic analgesic drugs with different agonist and antagonist properties. *Naunyn Schmiedebergs Arch. Pharmacol.* **319**, 197–205.

Martin, W. R. (1967) Opioid antagonists. *Pharmacol. Rev.* **19**, 463–521.

Martin, W. R., Eades, C. G., Thompson, J. A., Huppler, R. E., and Gilbert, P. E. (1976) The effects of morphine- and nalorphine-like drugs in the nondependent and morphine-dependent chronic spinal dog. *J. Pharmacol. Exp. Ther.* **197**, 517–532.

Maurer, R. (1982) Multiplicity of opiate receptors in different species. *Neurosci. Lett.* **30**, 303–307.

McLawhon, R. W., West, R. E., Jr., Miller, R. J., and Dawson, G. (1981) Distinct high affinity binding sites for benzomorphan drugs and enkephalin in a neuroblastom-brain hybrid cell line. *Proc. Natl. Acad. Sci. USA* **78**, 4309–4313.

Messing, R. B., Vasquez, B. J., Spiehler, V. R., Martinez, J., Jensen, R. A., Rigter, H., and McGaugh, J. L. (1980) 3H-dihydromorphine binding in brain regions of young and aged rats. *Life Sci.* **26**, 921–927.

Meunier, J.-.C. and Moisand, D. (1977) Binding of Leu-enkephalin and Met-enkephalin to particulate fraction from rat cerebrum. *FEBS. Lett.* **77**, 209–213.

Morin, O., Caron, M. G., DeLean, A., and Labrie, F. (1976) Binding of the opiate-like pentapeptide Met-enkephalin to a particulate fraction from rat brain. *Biophys. Res. Commun.* **73**, 940–946.

Mosberg, H. I., Hurst, R., Hruby, V. J., Gee, K., Yamamura, H. I., Galligan, J. J., and Burks, T. F. (1983) Bispenicillamine enkephalins possess highly improved specificity towards delta opioid receptors. *Proc. Natl. Acad. Sci. USA* **80**, 5871–5874.

Munson, P. J., and Rodbard, D. (1980) Ligand: A versatile computerized approach for characterization of ligand-binding systems. *Anal. Biochem.* **107**, 220–239.

Ninkovik, M., Hunt, S. P., Emson, P. C., and Iverson, L. L. (1981) The distribution of multiple opiate receptors in bovine brain. *Brain Res.* **214**, 163–167.

Nishimura, S. L., Recht, L. D., and Pasternak, G. W. (1984) Biochemical characterization of high affinity 3H-opioid binding: Further evidence for mu1 sites. *Mol. Pharmacol.* **25**, 29–37.

Pasternak, G. W. (1980) Multiple opiate receptors: [^{3}H]Ethylketocyclazocine receptor binding and ketocyclazocine analgesia. *Proc. Natl. Acad. Sci. USA* **77**, 3691–3694.

Pasternak, G. W. (1981) Opiate, enkephalin and endorphin analgesia: Relations to a single subpopulation of opiate receptors. *Neurology* **31**, 1311–1315.

Pasternak, G. W. (1982) High and low affinity opioid binding sites: Relationship to mu and delta sites. *Life Sci.* **31**, 1303–1306.

Pasternak, G. W. and Hahn, E. F. (1980) Long acting opiate agonists and antagonists: 14-Hydroxydiphydromorphinone hydrazone. *J. Med. Chem.* **23**, 674–676.

Pasternak, G. W. and Snyder, S. H. (1974) Opiate receptor binding: Effects of enzymatic treatments. *Mol. Pharmacol.* **10**, 183–193.

Pasternak, G. W. and Snyder, S. H. (1975a) Opiate receptor binding: Enzymatic treatments and discrimination between agonists and antagonists. *Mol. Pharmacol.* **11**, 478–484.

Pasternak, G. W. and Snyder, S. H. (1975b) Identification of novel high affinity opiate receptor binding in rat brain. *Nature* **253**, 563–565.

Pasternak, G. W., Carrol-Buatti, M., and Spiegel, K. (1981) The binding and analgesic properties of a sigma opiate, SKF10,047. *J. Pharmacol. Exp. Ther.* **219**, 192–198.

Pasternak, G. W., Childers, S. R., and Snyder, S. H. (1980a) Naloxazone, a long-acting opiate antagonist: Effects on analgesia in intact animals and on opiate receptor binding in vitro. *J. Pharmacol. Exp. Ther.* **214**, 455–462.

Pasternak, G. W., Childers, S. R., and Snyder, S. H. (1980b) Opiate analgesia: Evidence for mediation by a subpopulation of opiate receptors. *Science* **208**, 514–516.

Pasternak, G. W., Zhang, A.-.Z., and Tecott, L. (1980c) Developmental differences between high and low affinity opiate binding sites: Their relationship to analgesia and respiratory depression. *Life Sci.* **27**, 1185–1190.

Pasternak, G. W., Goodman, R., and Snyder, S. H. (1975a) An endogenous morphine-like factor in mammalian brain. *Life Sci.* **16**, 1765–1769.

Pasternak, G. W., Wilson, H. A., and Snyder, S. H. (1975b) Differential effects of protein-modifying reagents on receptor binding of opiate agonists and antagonists. *Mol. Pharmacol.* **11**, 340–351.

Pasternak, G. W., Snowman, A., and Snyder, S. H. (1975c) Selective enhancement of 3H-opiate agonist binding by divalent actions. *Mol. Pharmacol.* **11**, 735–744.

Pasternak, G. W., Simantov, R., and Snyder, S. H. (1976) Characterization of an endogenous morphine-like factor (enkephalin) in mammalian brain. *Mol. Pharmacol.* **12**, 504–513.

Paton, W. D. M. (1957) The interaction of morphine and related substances on contraction and on acethylcholine output or coaxially stimulated guinea pig ileum. *Br. J. Pharmacol. Chemother.* **12**, 119–127.

Pert, C. B. and Snyder, S. H. (1973) Opiate receptor: Demonstrated in nervous tissue. *Science* **179**, 1011–1014.

Pert, C. B. and Taylor, D. (1980) Type 1 and type 2 Opiate Receptors: A Subclassification Scheme Based on GTP'S Differential Effects on Binding, in *Endogenous and Exogenous Opiate Agonists and Antagonists* (Way, E. L., ed.) Pergamon, New York.

Pert, C. B., Pasternak, G. W., and Snyder, S. H. (1973) Opiate agonists and antagonists discriminated by receptor binding in brain. *Science* **182**, 1359–1361.

Pfeiffer, A. and Herz, A. (1981) Demonstration and distribution of an opiate binding site in rat brain with high affinity for ethylketocyclazocine and SKF 10,047. *Biochem. Biophys. Res. Comm.* **101**, 38–44

Pfeiffer, A., Pasi, A., Mehraein, P., and Herz, A. (1982) Opiate receptor binding sites in human brain. *Brain Res.* **248**, 87–96.

Piercey, M. F., Lahti, R. A., Schroeder, L. A., Einspaher, F. J., and Brasuhn, C. (1982) U50488H, a pure kappa receptor agonist with spinal analgesia loci in the mouse. *Life Sci.* **31**, 1197–1200.

Portoghese, P. S. (1965) A new concept on the mode of interaction of narcotic analgesics with receptors. *J. Med. Chem.* **8**, 609.

Portoghese, P. S. (1966) Stereochemical factors and receptor interactions associated with narcotic analgesics. *J. Pharm. Sci.* **55**, 865–887.

Portoghese, P. S., Larson, D. L., Jiang, J. B., Caruso, T. P., and Takemori, A. E. (1979) Synthesis and pharmacologic characterization of alkylating analogue (chlornaltrexamine) of naltrexone with ultralong-lasting narcotic antagonist properties. *J. Med. Chem.* **22**, 168–173.

Portoghese, P. S., Larson, D. L., Sayre, L. M., Fries, D. S., and Takemori, A. E. (1980) A novel opioid receptor site directed alkylating agent with irreversible narcotic antagonistic and reversible agonistic activities. *J. Med. Chem.* **23**, 233.

Quirion, R., Hammer, R., Herkenham, M., and Pert, C. B. (1981) A phencyclidine/sigma opiate receptor: Its visualization by tritium-sensitive film. *Proc. Natl. Acad. Sci. USA* **78**, 5881–5885.

Reisine, T., and Soubrie, P. (1982) Loss of rat cerebral cortical opiate receptors following chronic desimipramine treatment. *Eur. J. Pharmacol.* **77**, 39–44.

Reisine, T. D., Rossor, M., Iversen, L. L., and Yamamura, H. I. (1979) Alteration in brain opiate receptors in Parkinson's Disease. *Brain Res.* **173**, 378–382.

Reisine, T. D., Rossor, M., Spokes, E., Iversen, L. L., and Yamamura, H. I. (1980) Opiate and Neuroleptic Receptor Alterations in Human Schizophrenic Brain Tissue, in (Pepeu, M., Kuhar, M. J., and Enna, S. J., eds.) *Receptors for Neurotransmitter and Peptide Hormones* Raven, New York.

Robson, L. E. and Kosterlitz, H. W. (1979) Specific protection of the binding sites of D-Ala^2-D-leu ^{5}-enkephalin (delta-receptors) and dihydromorphine (mu-receptors). *Proc. R. Soc. Lond.* **205**, 425–432.

Robson, L. E., Foote, R. W., Maurer, R., and Kosterlitz, H. W. (1984) Opioid binding sites of the kappa-type in guinea pig cerebellum *Neuroscience* **12**, 621–627.

Romer, D., Buscher, H. H., Hill, R. C., Pless, J., Bauer, W., Cardinaux, F., Closse, A., Hauser, D., and Huguenin, R. (1977) A synthetic enkephalin analog with prolonged parenteral and oral analgesic activity. *Nature* (Lond.) **268**, 547–549.

Romer, D., Buscher, H. H., Hill, R. C., Maurer, R., and Petcher, T. J. (1982) An opioid bemzpdoazepine, *Nature* (Lond.) **298**, 759–760.

Rosenthal, H. E. (1967) Graphic method for the determination and presentation of binding parameters in a complex system. *Anal. Biochem.* **20**, 525–532.

Ruegg, U. T., Cuenod, S., Hiller, J. M., Gionnini, T., Howells, R. D., and Simon, E. J. (1981) Characterization and partial purification of solubilized active opiate receptors from toad brain. *Proc. Natl. Acad. Sci. USA* **78**, 4635–4638.

Scatchard, G. (1949) The attraction of proteins for small molecules and ions. *Annuals NY Acad. Sci.* **51**, 660–674.

Schulz, R., Faase, E., Wuster, M., and Herz, A. (1979) Selective receptors for β-endorphin on the rat vas deferens. *Life Sci.* **24**, 843–850.

Shannon, H. E. (1981) Evaluation of phencyclidine analogs on the basis of their discriminative stimulus properties in the rat. *J. Pharmacol. Exp. Ther.* **216**, 543–551.

Shannon, H. E. (1983) Pharmacological evaluation of N-allylnormetazocine (SKF 10,047) on the basis of its discriminative stimulus properties in the rat. *J. Pharmacol. Exp. Ther.* **225**, 144–152.

Sherman, G. T. and Herz, A. (1981) Discriminative stimulus properties of bremazocine in the rat. *Neuropharmacology* **20**, 1209–1213.

Simantov, R., Childers, S. R., and Snyder, S. H. (1978) The opiate receptor binding interactions of 3H-methionine enkephalin, an opiate peptide. *Eur. J. Pharmacol.* **47**, 319–331.

Simon, E. J. and Groth, J. (1975) Kinetics of opiate receptor inactivation by sulfhydryl reagents: Evidence for conformational change in the presence of sodium ions. *Proc. Natl. Acad. Sci. USA* **72**, 2404–2407.

Simon, E. J. and Hiller, J. M. (1978) The opiate receptor. *Ann. Rev. Pharmacol. Toxicol.* **18**, 371–394.

Simon, E. J., Bonnet, K. A., Crain, S. M., Groth, J., Hiller, J. M., and Smith, J. R. (1980) Recent Studies on Interaction Between Opioid Peptides and Their Receptors, in *Advances in Biochemical Psychopharmacology* (Costa, E. and Trabucchi, M., eds.) Raven, New York.

Simon, E. J., Hiller, J. M., and Edelman, I. (1973) Stereospecific binding of the potent narcotic analgesic 3H-etorphine to rat brain homogenates. *Proc. Natl. Acad. Sci. USA* **70**, 1947–1949.

Simon, E. J., Hiller, J. M., Edelman, I., Groth, J., and Stahl, K. D. (1975a) Opiate receptors and their interaction with agonists and antagonists. *Life Sci.* **16**, 1795–1800.

Simon, E. J., Hiller, J. M., Groth, J., Edelman, I. (1975b) Further properties of stereospecific opiate binding sites in rat brain: On the nature of the sodium effect. *J. Pharmacol. Exp. Ther.* **192**, 531–537.

Simon, E. J., Hiller, J. M., Groth, J., Itzhak, Y., Holland, M. J., and Beck, S. G. (1982) The nature of opiate receptors in toad brain. *Life Sci.* **31**, 1367–1370.

Simonds, W. F., Koski, G., Streaty, R. A., Hjelmeland, L. M., and Klee, W. A. (1980) Solubilization of active opiate receptors. *Proc. Natl. Acad. Sci USA* **77**, 4623–4627.

Smith, J. R. and Simon, E. J. (1980) Selective protection of stereospecific enkephalin and opiate binding against inactivation by N-ethylmaleimide: Evidence for two classes of opiate receptors. *Proc. Natl. Acad. Sci. USA* **77**, 281–284.

Spain, W., Roth, B. L., and Coscia, C. J. (1985) Differential ontogeny of multiple opioid receptors. *J. Neurosci.* **5**, 584–588.

Terenius, L. (1973) Characteristics of the "receptor" for narcotic analgesics in synaptic plasma membrane fractions from rat brain. *Acta Pharmacol. Toxicol.* **33**, 377–384.

Terenius, L. (1977) Opioid peptides and opiates differ in receptor selectivity. *Psychoneuroendocrinology* **2**, 53–58.

Terenius, L. and Whalstrom, A. (1975) Search for an endogenous ligand for the opiate receptor. *Acta Physiol. Scand.* **94**, 74–81.

Tsang, D. and Ng, S. C. (1980) Effect of antenatal exposure to opiates on the development of opiate receptors in rat brain. *Brain Res.* **188**, 199–206.

Tsang, D., Ng, S. C., Ho, K. P., and Ho, W. K. K. (1982) Ontogenesis of opiate binding sites and radioimmunoassayable β-endorphin and enkephalin in regions of rat brain. *Dev. Brain Res.* **5**, 257–261.

Vincent, J. P., Kartalovski, B., Genest, P., Kamenka, J. M., and Lazdunski, M. (1979) Interaction of phencyclidine (angel dust) with a specific receptor in rat brain membranes. *Proc. Natl. Acad. Sci. USA* **76**, 4678–4682.

Ward, S. J., Portoghese, P. S., and Takemori, A. E. (1982) Improved assays for the assessment of kappa and delta properties of opioid ligands. *Eur. J. Pharmacol.* **85**, 163–170.

Wohltman, M., Roth, B. L., and Coscia, C. J. (1982) Differential postnatal development of mu and delta opiate receptors. *Dev. Brain Res.* **3**, 679–684.

Wolozin, B. L. and Pasternak, G. W. (1981) Classification of multiple morphine and enkephalin binding sites in the central nervous system. *Proc. Natl. Acad. Sci. USA* **78**, 6181–6185.

Wolozin, B. L., Nishimura, S. L., and Pasternak, G. W. (1982) The binding of kappa and sigma opiates in rat brain. *J. Neurosci.* **2**, 708–713.

Woods, J. H., Smith, C. B., Medzihradsky, F., and Swain, H. H. (1979) Preclinical Testing of New Analgesic Drugs, in *Mechanisms of Pain and Analgesic Compounds* (Beers, R. F. and Basset, E. G., eds.) Raven, New York.

Zhang, A.-.Z. and Pasternak, G. W. (1981a) Opiates and enkephalins: A common binding site mediates their analgesic actions in rats. *Life Sci.* **29**, 843–857.

Zhang, A.-.Z. and Pasternak, G. W. (1981b) Ontogeny of opioid pharmacology and receptors: High and low affinity site differences. *Eur. J. Pharmacol.* **73**, 29–40.

Zhang, A.-.Z. and Pasternak, G. W. (1980) Mu and delta opiate receptors: Correlation with high and low affinity opiate binding sites. *Eur. J. Pharmacol.* **67**, 323–324.

Zukin, S. R. and Zukin, R. S. (1979) Specific [³H]phencyclidine binding in rat central nervous system. *Proc. Natl. Acad. Sci. USA* **76**, 5372–5376.

Zukin, S. R., Brady, K. T., Slifer, B. L., and Balser, R. L. (1984) Behavioral and biochemical stereoselectivity of sigma opiate/PCP receptors. *Brain Res.* **294**, 174–177.

Chapter 5

The σ Receptor

R. Suzanne Zukin and
Stephen R. Zukin

1. Introduction

The psychotropic actions of opiates and opioid peptides are mediated by interaction with μ, δ, and κ opioid receptors and the related σ receptor. The μ receptor is operationally defined as the high-affinity site at which morphine-like opioids produce analgesia and other classical opioid effects. The δ receptor is operationally defined as the receptor that is found in peripheral tissues such as the mouse vas deferens (Lord et al., 1977) as well as in the CNS (Chang et al., 1979), and that exhibits a higher affinity for the naturally occurring enkephalins (shorter opioid peptides) than for morphine. The κ receptor is the receptor at which ketocyclazocine-like opioids produce analgesia as well as their unique ataxic and sedative effects (Gilbert and Martin, 1976; Martin et al., 1976). More recently it has been defined as a receptor highly selective for dynorphin, a 17-amino acid opioid peptide (Chavkin et al., 1982). Actions at all three of these sites are reversible by the specific opioid antagonist naloxone, with decreasing sensitivity going from μ to δ to κ receptors.

The σ receptor was proposed to be the site at which the psychotomimetic and stimulatory effects of N-allylnormetazocine

(SKF 10,047), cyclazocine, and related opioids are mediated (Martin et al., 1976; Zukin and Zukin, 1981). σ Opioids differ from classical opioids in displaying psychotomimetic effects in humans and unique behavioral effects in animals (Haertzen, 1970; Holtzman, 1974). The complex actions of such drugs vary with the dose administered. At low doses they produce actions resembling those of morphine, such as analgesia (Lasagna et al., 1964), as well as antagonist actions such as precipitation of withdrawal in morphine-addicted subjects (Haertzen, 1974). At high doses, they produce a combination of sedation, "drunkenness," and psychosis differing from any morphine effect (Gilbert and Martin, 1976; Martin et al., 1976). Most behavioral effects of σ opioids observed in animals are not reversible by naloxone or naltrexone (Teal and Holtzman, 1980a; Vaupel, 1983; Vaupel et al., 1986).

It now appears that σ opioids interact (in addition to possible interactions with μ, δ, and κ opioid receptors) with two distinct binding sites, neither of which is naloxone-sensitive. One is the phencyclidine (PCP) or PCP/σ receptor, which mediates the psychotomimetic effects of PCP and related drugs. The PCP/σ receptor is highly selective for PCP derivatives, σ opioids, dioxolanes, and other drugs that elicit PCP-like or SKF 10,047-like behavioral effects (Vincent et al., 1979; Zukin and Zukin, 1979; Holtzman, 1980, 1982; Quirion et al., 1981; Hampton et al., 1982; Mendelsohn et al., 1984). This site was shown to be a pharmacologically relevant receptor on the basis of behavioral, electrophysiological, neurochemical, and neuroanatomical evidence (see below). It can be labeled by [^{3}H]PCP, by the potent PCP derivative N-(1-[2-thienyl]cyclohexyl)[^{3}H]piperidine ([^{3}H]TCP) (Vignon et al., 1983; Sircar and Zukin, 1985), or by radiolabeled σ opioids in the presence of μ and δ blockers (Zukin and Zukin, 1981; Zukin et al., 1986) or by (+)-^{3}H-SKF 10,047 (Itzhak et al., 1985; Sircar et al., 1986; Largent et al., 1986). The ligand selectivity pattern, neuroanatomical distribution, and functional significance of this site are well-characterized.

The other site that has been termed a σ site is relatively insensitive to PCP, but is very sensitive to haloperidol, a butyrophenone neuroleptic, and to the putative dopamine autoreceptor ligand (+)-[^{3}H]3-(3-hydroxyphenyl)-N-(1-propyl)piperidi ne. This site can be labeled with (+)-[^{3}H]SKF 10,047 (Su, 1981, 1982; Tam, 1983; Gundlach et al., 1985; Largent et al., 1986) or with (+)-[^{3}H]3-(3-hydroxyphenyl)-N-(1-propyl)piperidine (Largent et al., 1984). To date no specific behavioral or physiological function has been demonstrated for the haloperidol-sensitive σ binding site, and thus the question of whether it could represent a receptor mediating some component of σ opioid psychotropic action remains unresolved.

2. The PCP/σ Receptor

The existence of a common receptor for the σ class of opioids and PCP-like drugs is no longer surprising. These two classes of drugs share commonalities at the behavioral, cellular, and molecular levels. In 1979, SKF 10,047, the prototypic σ opioid, was the first opioid shown to produce PCP-like effects in the discriminative stimulus assay in rats (H. E. Shannon, personal communication). Since then, in rodents (Holtzman, 1980), primates (Holtzman, 1982), and pigeons (Herling and Woods, 1981), σ opioids, but not non-σ opioids, have been found to elicit the PCP-appropriate response in PCP-trained animals, and vice versa. In the spinal dog preparation, the paradigm in which σ opioid properties were originally defined, the behavioral effects of SKF 10,047 and those of PCP were found to be indistinguishable (Vaupel, 1983). PCP and SKF 10,047 also reveal strikingly similar effects upon unconditioned behaviors, including stimulation of locomotion, sniffing, head and mouth stereotypy, and ataxia (Greenberg and Segal, 1985). In electrophysiological studies, PCP and the prototypic σ opioid cyclazocine have been shown to produce identical effects upon Purkinje cells of the cerebellum (Wang et al., 1986). Sigma opioids compete for the binding of [^{3}H]PCP, and PCP-like drugs compete for [^{3}H]SKF 10,047 binding (see below). Perhaps most importantly, sigma opioids have been demonstrated to bind to the same solubilized receptor proteins from rat brain as does PCP (Haring et al., 1986). Together, these findings provide strong evidence for a common receptor mediating the common actions of σ opioids and PCP-like drugs.

2.1. PCP/σ Receptors Labeled with [^{3}H]PCP

Phencyclidine [N-1-(phenylcyclohexyl) piperidine; PCP] exhibits a wide spectrum of neurobehavioral effects, including psychotomimetic, anesthetic, analgesic, stimulant, and depressant actions (Johnstone et al., 1959; Luby et al., 1959). In humans, a single very low subanesthetic dose of PCP can rapidly produce a transient psychotic state closely resembling schizophrenia, with symptoms including hallucinations and thought disorder (Luby et al., 1959; Davies and Beech, 1960). In remitted schizophrenics, the same single small dose causes a prompt, highly specific, and long-lasting rekindling of the schizophrenic illness (Luby et al., 1959). Such findings raised the question of how, on the molecular level, PCP exerts its unique psychotropic effects.

The existence of high-affinity [³H]PCP binding sites in rat brain was reported independently in 1979 by two groups (Vincent et al., 1979; Zukin and Zukin, 1979). Since then, others have confirmed these findings and provided further characterization of these sites (including Vincent et al., 1980; Quirion et al., 1981; Hampton et al., 1982; Vignon et al., 1982, 1983; Zukin et al., 1983; Sircar and Zukin, 1985; Sircar et al., 1986). Together, these studies showed that [³H]PCP binding is inhibited by a series of more than 30 PCP analogs in the same rank order of potency as is observed for their PCP-like behavioral effects (in the discriminative stimulus and rotarod paradigms). Non-PCP like hallucinogens and multiple known neurotransmitters proved inactive in the [³H]-PCP binding assay. Binding was of high affinity ($K_d = 1.5$–$2.5 \times 10^{-7} M$ in 50 mM Tris-HCl buffer or 4–$8 \times 10^{-8} M$ in 5 mM Tris-HCl buffer). The [³H]PCP binding sites exhibited a heterogeneous distribution across tissues and brain regions, as well as subcellularly. Moreover, these sites displayed the required characteristics for a protein receptor, including stereospecificity (Vincent et al., 1980; Hampton et al., 1982; Zukin et al., 1983, 1984).

Confirmatory evidence regarding [³H]PCP binding was obtained by utilization of experimental methodologies not involving the use of filters. Quirion et al. (1981) confirmed the presence of [³H]PCP receptors in a study using [³H]PCP binding to slide-mounted sections of brain. We detected specific, saturable [³H]-PCP binding to rat brain homogenates with a centrifugation assay (Zukin et al., 1983).

In order to establish the pharmacological relevance of the PCP/σ receptor, it is important to demonstrate that the potencies of drugs in the receptor binding assay parallels their potencies in eliciting PCP-like behaviors. PCP derivatives inhibit specifically bound [³H]PCP in rank order of potency strictly corresponding to their rank orders of potency in the mouse rotarod ($r = 0.81$; $p < 0.05$) and the rat discriminative stimulus ($r = 0.92$, $p < 0.001$) tests (Zukin and Zukin, 1979). Several classes of drugs not structurally related to PCP exert PCP-like behavioral and receptor-binding actions. These include the dioxolane derivatives dexoxadrol and etoxadrol (Zukin, 1982; Slifer and Balster, 1985), benz-f-isoquinolines (Mendelsohn, 1984), and σ opioids. Table 1 summarizes the potencies of a series of benzomorphans for inhibition of specifically bound [³H]PCP from rat brain membranes. These drugs display approximately a 200-fold range of potency from cyclazocine (most potent) to nalorphine and levallorphan (least potent), in agreement with their potencies in the discriminative stimulus paradigm (Holtzman, 1980; Shannon, 1982).

The anatomical localization of the PCP/σ receptor in rat brain was determined by light microscopy autoradiography using [³H]PCP (Quirion et al., 1981) and quantitatively with the more specific ligand [³H]TCP (Sircar and Zukin, 1985) (Table 2). Anterior forebrain areas including neocortex and olfactory structures were heavily labeled. Highest selective localization of sites was observed in dentate gyrus and hippocampal fields CA_1 and CA_2. Levels of [³H]TCP binding were generally low in midbrain/pontine areas. White matter areas including corpus callosum and anterior commisure, and gray matter areas including globus pallidus, ventral tegmental area, and some pontine and thalamic nuclei were essentially devoid of [³H]TCP binding. The distribution pattern of PCP receptors is distinctly different from those of opioid receptors. Autoradiographic localization of μ opioid receptors in rat brain has shown highest densities in the nucleus accumbens, medial habenula, interpeduncular nucleus, patchy areas of the caudate-putamen, presubiculum, amygdala, and stria terminalis (Atweh and Kuhar, 1977; Herkenham and Pert, 1980). High levels of δ opioid receptors have been reported in laminae II, III, and V of the cerebral cortex, amygdala, nucleus accumbens, and olfactory tubercle (Goodman et al., 1980). Certain areas of the brain, such as locus ceruleus, dentate gyrus, and superior colliculus, and some regions of the cerebral cortex shown to contain high levels of PCP/σ receptors have elevated densities of several receptor types. These areas have been termed receptor "hot spots" (Kuhar, 1982).

2.2. Receptors Labeled with (−)-[³H]SKF 10,047

The PCP/σ receptor has been characterized also using the prototypic σ opioid SKF 10,047. An early study showed that binding of (±)-[³H]SKF 10,047 to rat brain membranes was biphasic

TABLE 1

IC$_{50}$ Values for Drugs Competing Against Various ^{3}H-Ligands for σ and PCP Receptor Binding Sites[a,b]

			IC$_{50}$		
Drug	(+)-[^{3}H]3-PPP, nM	(+)-[^{3}H]SKF 10,047 (+2 μM TCP), nM	(+)-[^{3}H]SKF 10,047, nM	(+)-[^{3}H]SKF 10,047 (+5 μM haloperidol), nM	[^{3}H]TCP, nM
(+)-SKF 10,047	365 ± 33	55 ± 20	75 ± 20	375 ± 30	405 ± 7
(−)-SKF 10,047	1440 ± 110	690 ± 134	895 ± 175	530 ± 25	821 ± 17
(±)-Pentazocine	25 ± 2	40 ± 15	286 ± 47	1520 ± 220	2820 ± 120
(+)-3-PPP	32 ± 2	45 ± 5	49 ± 6[c]	≥100,000	≥100,000
Haloperidol	2 ± 0.4	8 ± 0.9	5 ± 1.3[c]	≥50,000	≥50,000
PCP	758 ± 84	625 ± 182	311 ± 34	48 ± 12	66 ± 4
Dexoxadrol	2000 ± 510	1050 ± 120	569 ± 143	46 ± 9	41 ± 3
Levoxadrol	2220 ± 490	2340 ± 980	3790 ± 70	10,700 ± 2400	16,900 ± 1400
TCP	3720 ± 1130	6200 ± 1900	265 ± 52	19 ± 4	11 ± 1
m-NH$_2$-PCP	3690 ± 430	1800 ± 260	360 ± 86	32 ± 10	31 ± 5

[a]Values given are the mean (nanomolar) ± SEM for three to eight determinations and were determined from the data using a computer-assisted iterative curve-fitting program, EBDA. Rat brain membranes (7.5 mg of original wet weight tissue) were incubated with 1–3 nM (+)-[^{3}H]3-PPP, 7–10 nM (+)-[^{3}H]SKF 10,047 (+2 μM TCP or 5 μM haloperidol), or 1–3 nM [^{3}H]TCP with 10–12 concentrations of unlabeled drug in duplicate for 90 min [(+)-[^{3}H]3-PPP] or 30 min [(+)-[^{3}H]SKF 10,047 and [^{3}H]TCP] at room temperature. Non-specific binding of (+)-[^{3}H]3-PPP, (+)-[^{3}H]SKF 10,047 (+2 μM TCP), (+)-[^{3}H]SKF 10,047, (+)-[^{3}H]SKF 10,047 (+5 μM haloperidol), and [^{3}H]TCP was defined as that in the presence of 5 μM (±)-pentazocine, 1 μM haloperidol, 100 μM PCP, 10 μM PCP, and 100 μM (+)-SKF 10,047, respectively.

[b]Largent et al. (1986).

[c]Values represent the IC$_{50}$ value for the portion (~60%) of total specific binding inhibited by these drugs.

TABLE 2
Densities of Receptors Labeled by [³H]TCP, (+)-[³H]SKF-10,047,
and [³H]3-PPP

Region	Receptor Densities, fmol/mg tissue		
	[³H]TCP sites[a]	(+)-[³H]SKF 10,047 sites[b]	[³H]3-PPP sites[c]
Hippocampus			
CA1	104	200	—
CA2	105	217	—
CA3	66	173	—
Stratum pyramidale	—	—	144
Stratum radiatum	—	—	146
Dentate	111	200	126
Subiculum	84	—	144
Frontal cortex	83	134	85
Superior colliculus	65	134	159
Nucleus accumbens	52	100	70
Cerebellum	47	145	330 (Purkinje layer)
Locus ceruleus	46	140	241
Amygdala	42	—	107 (central nucleus)
Dorsomedial hypothalamus	40	162	134
Central gray	26	167	268
Substantia nigra	14	145	172
Pontine reticular nucleus	8	84	373
Globus pallidus	0	—	77
Corpus callosum	0	6	—

[a]Sircar and Zukin (1985).
[b]Sircar et al. (1986).
[c]Gundlach et al. (1986).

(Pasternak et al., 1981). The higher-affinity site was naloxone-sensitive, but the sites were not further identified. Subsequently, an important strategy to target σ receptors was developed in several laboratories (Zukin and Zukin, 1981; Zukin et al., 1986). This method involves the use of radiolabeled σ drugs after suppression of their interactions with μ and δ receptors. We used [³H]cyclazocine (Zukin and Zukin, 1981) in the presence of selective μ and δ blockers to demonstrate the presence of σ receptors in rat brain homogenates. We showed the σ receptor to differ from the other opioid receptors, but to resemble the PCP receptor on the basis of four criteria: (1) rank order of potencies of opioids in competition analyses; (2) kinetic parameters; (3) sensitivity to sodium and N-ethylmaleimide; and (4) distribution throughout the CNS.

We (Zukin et al., 1986) used (−)-[³H]SKF 10,047 to characterize central σ receptors in rat brain homogenates. Normorphine (relatively selective μ ligand) and [D-Ala², D-Leu⁵]enkephalin (selective δ ligand) were included to suppress interaction of the radiolabeled drug with μ and δ receptors and to direct its binding to σ sites. Homogenate binding studies were used to characterize σ-directed (−)-[³H]SKF 10,047 receptor binding biochemically and light-microscopic autoradiography was used to visualize quantitatively neuroanatomical patterns of these binding sites on thaw-mounted sections of frozen rat brain. Binding of (−)-[³H]SKF 10,047 to rat brain membranes was shown to be of high affinity, saturable, and reversible. Saturation experiments revealed the apparent interaction of this drug with two distinct binding sites characterized by apparent affinities of 0.03 and 75 nM (in 5 mM Tris-HCl buffer, pH 7.4 at 4°C). The high-affinity (−)-[³H]SKF 10,047 binding site, revealed using normorphine as the definition of nonspecific binding, was found to display selectivity characteristics of the μ opioid receptor. The rank order of potency (levorphanol = etorphine > FK 33-824 = (−)cyclazocine = cyclorphan > naloxone > dihydromorphine > (+)-SKF 10,047 > PCP) of drugs at this site was similar both to that reported for [³H]dihydromorphine binding and for high-affinity [³H]ethylketazocine binding to μ receptors (Eghbali et al., 1987). The lower-affinity (K_d = 75 nM) (−)-[³H]SKF 10,047 site, labeled by (−)-[³H]SKF 10,047 after suppression of its binding to μ and δ receptors with 40 nM normorphine and 100 nM DADLE, was also characterized pharmacologically. In this case, the rank order of potency was (−)cyclazocine = cyclorphan > (−)-SKF 10,047 > PCP > levorphanol = dextrorphan > (+)-SKF 10,047. Dihydromorphine, naloxone, and DADLE were essentially inactive at this site. These results are generally consistent with the pattern of opioids that bind to [³H]PCP receptors (Zukin et al., 1983), as well as with the pattern of opioids that generalizes to PCP in animal behavioral studies (Holtzman, 1980; Brady and Balster, 1982; Brady et al., 1982; Shannon, 1982; Herling and Woods, 1981;

Shearman and Herz, 1982). Such evidence is consistent with the concept of a common receptor for the σ opioids and for PCP.

In vitro autoradiography was utilized to visualize neuroanatomical patterns of receptors labeled using $(-)$-[^{3}H]SKF 10,047 in the presence of normorphine and [D-Ala^2, D-Leu^5]enkephalin to block μ and δ interactions, respectively. Labeling patterns differ markedly from those for μ, δ, or κ receptors. The highest densities (determined by quantitative autoradiography) are found in the medial portion of the nucleus accumbens, amygdaloid nucleus, hippocampal formation, central gray, locus ceruleus, and parabrachial nuclei. Receptors in those structures could account for the stimulatory, mood-altering, and analgesic properties of σ drugs. Although not the most selective σ ligand, $(-)$-[^{3}H]SKF 10,047 binds to σ receptors in brain, and this interaction can be readily distinguished from its interactions with other classes of brain opioid receptors.

3. The Haloperidol-Sensitive non-PCP σ Site

Several studies indicated that σ opioids could also interact with a site distinct from the PCP receptor. This site was first identified by Su (1981, 1982) using $(\pm)$-[^{3}H]SKF 10,047 in the presence of excess nonlabeled etorphine to block classical opioid receptors. That technique yielded a low percentage of specific binding of $(\pm)$-[^{3}H]SKF 10,047. Subsequently, it was shown that the same sites could be labeled with $(+)$-[^{3}H]SKF 10,047 (Tam, 1983, 1985; Martin et al., 1984; Gundlach et al., 1985; Largent et al., 1986; Tam and Cook, 1984; Sircar et al., 1986), $(\pm)$- and $(+)$-[^{3}H]ethylketocyclazocine (Tam, 1983, 1985), and [^{3}H]haloperidol (Largent et al., 1984; Tam and Cook, 1984). These studies demonstrated that the haloperidol-sensitive σ binding site differed in both its ligand selectivity and regional distribution from the PCP/σ receptor.

3.1. Sites Labeled with (+)-[^{3}H]SKF 10,047

The lack of interaction of the $(+)$-isomer of SKF 10,047 with classical opioid receptors suggested that $(+)$-[^{3}H]SKF 10,047 might be an ideal specific ligand for studying PCP/σ receptors. We found that $(+)$-[^{3}H]SKF 10,047 bound saturably and reversibly to membranes of both rat and mouse brain (Sircar et al., 1986). Rosenthal (Scatchard) analysis, however, yielded curvilinear plots in both species and in all brain regions examined. Computer-assisted analysis (Munson and Rodbard, 1980) indicated that the best fit of the data was to a two-site model; a valid fit to a one-site model could not be obtained. Analysis on the basis of a two-site model yielded apparent K_d and B_{Max} values of 3.6 nM, 40 fmol/mg protein, and 153 nM, 1.6 pmol/mg protein, for the apparent high- and low-affinity sites, respectively.

In order to test the hypothesis that the curvilinear Rosenthal analysis resulted from the interaction of $(+)$-[³H]SKF 10,047 with two independent binding sites, the pharmacological characteristics of the two apparent sites were tested. Measurement of $(+)$-[³H]SKF 10,047 binding in the presence of 100 nM haloperidol yielded a Rosenthal plot in which the density of the apparent high-affinity sites was decreased by >90% relative to the value obtained in the absence of haloperidol, whereas the density of the apparent low-affinity binding sites showed little alteration. Ligand selectivity analysis provided further support for the concept of two independent $(+)$-[³H]SKF 10,047 binding sites. The rank order of potency (PCE > dexoxadrol > PCP > ketamine > pentazocine > levoxadrol) (Table 1) of ligands for displacement of 100 nM $(+)$-[³H]SKF 10,047 from the predominant lower-affinity sites in the presence of 100 nM haloperidol was similar to that reported for the displacement of [³H]PCP from its receptors (Zukin and Zukin, 1979; Zukin et al., 1983). By contrast, the rank order of potency of drugs inhibiting the binding of $(+)$-[³H]SKF 10,047 to the higher-affinity site (haloperidol > dexoxadrol > pentazocine > PCP > levoxadrol) (Table 1) proved distinct from the pattern for PCP receptors. Thus, we found $(+)$-[³H]SKF 10,047 to label both the σ/PCP receptor and the haloperidol-sensitive, non-PCP σ binding site.

Our findings are consistent with other published studies of $(+)$-[³H]SKF 10,047 binding (Largent et al., 1986; Gundlach et al., 1986). These studies also showed that $(+)$-[³H]SKF 10,047 interacts with two sites in brain: (1) a high-affinity, low-density site sensitive to haloperidol and (2) a lower-affinity, high-density site with the pharmacological characteristics of the PCP receptor. The higher-affinity site was shown to be the same site as had been previously identified using $(+)$-[³H]3-(3-hydroxyphenyl)-N-(1-propyl)piperidine [$(+)$-[³H]3-PPP]. Radioligand binding to this higher-affinity $(+)$-[³H]SKF 10,047 site was potently inhibited by $(+)$-3-PPP, haloperidol, and pentazocine. In contrast, binding of $(+)$-[³H]SKF 10,047 to its lower-affinity binding site was inhibited by TCP and other PCP analogs, but not by (+)-3-PPP, haloperidol, or pentazocine.

It is now clear that the distinctive PCP-like behavioral properties of SKF 10,047 are mediated at the (+)-[³H]SKF 10,047 binding site of lower affinity. This conclusion is based upon the findings that animals trained to discriminate PCP from vehicle generalize to (+)-SKF 10,047 and other σ opioids (Brady and Balster, 1982; Brady et al., 1982; Shannon, 1982), and that animals trained to discriminate σ opioids from vehicle generalize to PCP and related arylcyclohexylamines (Teal and Holtzman, 1980a,b; Holtzman, 1982). Moreover, the ligand selectivity pattern revealed by the drug-discrimination experiments generally agrees with that observed for binding to the haloperidol-insensitive, but not the haloperidol-sensitive, (+)-[³H]SKF 10,047 binding sites. That the PCP-like behavioral actions of σ opioids are *not* mediated by the higher-affinity haloperidol-sensitive σ site is indicated by two additional findings. First, haloperidol is unable to block specifically or to potentiate PCP in the drug discrimination paradigm (Browne and Welch, 1982). Second, in rats trained to discriminate 10 mg/kg (+)-SKF 10,047 from vehicle, generalization to PCP derivatives is observed, but haloperidol neither specifically antagonizes nor augments the (+)-SKF 10,047 cue. It is of particular interest that (+)-ketocyclazocine (a potent ligand of the haloperidol-sensitive σ sites in binding experiments) up to 60 mg/kg is inactive (R. Balster, personal communication). The apparent dominance of the haloperidol-insensitive sites labeled by (+)-[³H]SKF 10,047 in determining the behavioral profile of the drug may stem from their much greater abundance relative to the haloperidol-sensitive sites.

3.2. Sites Labeled with (+)-[³H]3-(3-hydroxyphenyl)-N-(1-propyl)piperidine [(+)-[³H]3-PPP]

The site labeled by the putative dopamine autoreceptor agonist (+)-[³H]3-(3-hydroxyphenyl)-N-(1-propyl)piperidine [(+)-[³H]3-PPP] has a pharmacological profile essentially identical with that of the haloperidol-sensitive σ site labeled by (+)-[³H]SKF 10,047 (Table 1). The neuroanatomical distribution of the haloperidol-sensitive σ binding site was determined using (+)-[³H]3-PPP (Table 2) and shown to be similar to that determined for the higher-affinity (+)-[³H]SKF 10,047 site. The highest density of those sites is found in the spinal cord (particularly the ventral horn and dorsal root ganglia), the pons-medulla (associated with the cranial-nerve and pontine nuclei and the reticular formation); the cerebellum (over the Purkinje cell layer), the midbrain (particularly the central gray and red nucleus); the hippocampus, and basal ganglia, and parts of the thalamus. Other areas including hypothalamus and cortex exhibit moderate grain densities. Lesion studies have been carried out in order to determine upon which neuronal elements the haloperidol-sensitive non-PCP σ binding sites reside. Gundlach et al. (1986) showed, in studies involving quinolinic acid-induced lesions of the hippocampus, that $(+)$-[^{3}H]3-PPP labels hippocampal pyramidal cells and granule cells of the dentate gyrus. Those sites are relatively unaffected by 6-hydroxydopamine injection into striatum, a finding that suggests that they are unlikely to be located on striatal dopaminergic terminals.

To date, no unique physiological or behavioral function has been clearly associated with the haloperidol-sensitive, non-PCP σ binding sites. Their role in mediating some component of the psychotropic actions of sigma opioids or of other drugs remains to be determined.

4. A Biological Function of σ Receptors

It is now known that a consequence of ligand binding to the PCP/σ receptor is the modulation of the CNS effects of N-methyl D-aspartic acid (NMDA). NMDA is the prototypic agonist of the N-type excitatory amino acid (glutamate) receptor. PCP derivatives, σ opioids, and benz-f-isoquinolines stereospecifically and potently antagonize NMDA-induced excitation of spinal (Anis et al., 1983; Lodge et al., 1983, 1984; Berry et al., 1984) and cerebral cortical neurons (Thomson and Lodge, 1985; Thomson et al., 1985; Lacey and Henderson, 1986). This effect is specific in that PCP-like drugs fail to modulate the excitatory responses of neurons to quisqualate or kainate, prototypic agonists of the Q- and K-type excitatory amino acid receptors, respectively. PCP/σ-type drugs also specifically antagonize NMDA-induced neurotransmitter release from brain slices (Snell and Johnson, 1985, 1986). Each of these effects is stereospecific, and the potencies of drugs in modulating such NMDA effects correlate well with their potencies in binding to PCP/σ receptors (Anis et al., 1983; Berry et al., 1984). The antagonism of NMDA receptors by PCP/σ drugs in those studies has been shown to be noncompetitive; slopes of dose–response curves were not parallel to those for direct NMDA antagonists such as D-(−)-2-amino-5-phosphonovaleric acid [D-(−)-AP5] (Martin and Lodge, 1985).

The biochemical mechanism of the interaction between PCP/σ and NMDA receptors has been the focus of several recent studies. Loo et al. (1986) reported that [^{3}H]TCP binding is dependent upon the level of glutamate in the incubation medium, but did not determine the mechanism of this effect. We (Javitt et al., 1987) have shown that the direct NMDA antagonist D-(−)-AP5 significantly decreases the apparent B_{Max} of [^{3}H]TCP binding without altering the K_d. In addition, we determined that stimulation of [^{3}H]TCP binding by NMDA agonists represents an increase in receptor number without change in the affinity of [^{3}H]TCP binding. Such findings suggest that PCP receptors and NMDA-type excitatory amino acid receptors may be functionally, and even structurally, related, perhaps as components of a supramolecular complex.

5. The Question of Endogenous Ligands

The finding of PCP/σ receptors in the mammalian CNS raises the possibility of the existence of endogenous ligands with PCP-like pharmacological properties. Following the demonstration and characterization of receptors for opioids, a series of structurally related endogenous opioid ligands were discovered (Hughes et al., 1975; Li and Chung, 1976; Guillemin et al., 1976; Goldstein et al., 1979, James et al., 1982). These and subsequently discovered endogenous opioid ligands have been shown to be neuropeptides. Their existence suggests the presence of as yet unidentified peptides in brain that function as endogenous ligands for other drug receptor systems.

Quirion et al. (1984) reported the partial isolation of a factor from porcine brain that could compete with PCP in the [^{3}H]PCP binding assay. Specificity was demonstrated in that the factor was inactive in assays for several other known neuroreceptors. The regional distribution of the active material paralleled that of PCP/σ receptors; highest levels occurred in hippocampus and frontal cortex. The active fraction was sensitive to proteolytic enzymes, a finding that suggests that it is a peptide. When injected unilaterally directly into the substantia nigra, the factor mimics PCP in its effect on rat rotational behavior. In addition, the factor depresses spontaneous activity in cortical and hippocampal neurons in a manner similar to PCP. Although the molecular basis of PCP effects in the two bioassay systems used in this study are unknown, the results are consistent with those expected for a partially purified endogenous ligand of the PCP/σ receptor.

We (Zukin et al., 1987) have identified and characterized a substance in partially purified extracts of bovine brain that exhibited not only the receptor-binding properties, but also the specific biological effects of PCP/σ-like drugs. The partially purified endogenous factor shows dose-dependent inhibition of [³H]TCP binding. Moreover, the active fractions mimics the actions of PCP and σ opioids upon neurotransmitter release. HPLC fractions active in the [³H]TCP binding assay, in contrast to fractions inactive in the [³H]TCP binding assay, potently elicit stimulation of spontaneous [³H]dopamine efflux and NMDA-stimulated [³H]dopamine and [¹⁴C]acetylcholine release from striatal slices. Furthermore, these actions are dose-dependent. An aliquot of active fractions corresponding to 0.001 hippocampus was similar in potency in the bioassays to 100 pmol of PCP. Furthermore, the slopes of the dose–effect curves were parallel to those obtained for PCP. Taken together, these results provide evidence that the partially purified bovine hippocampal extract exhibit specific PCP-like actions both at the receptor-binding level and in terms of biological effects. Our results would appear to be consistent with those of Quirion et al. (1984).

Finally, there has been a recent report of a possible endogenous ligand for the haloperidol-sensitive, non-PCP σ binding site (Su et al., 1986). Guinea pig brain extract was fractionated by gel filtration chromatography. Two fractions were identified that showed activity in the halperidol-sensitive σ binding assay. The same fractions were inactive in the [³H]PCP binding assay, a finding that indicated specificity for the non-PCP type of σ site.

No group has yet purified to homogeneity and characterized an endogenous σ ligand. Knowledge of the structure and physiological actions of such a ligand would be very helpful to our understanding of the physiological functions of the σ sites. It is possible that the PCP/σ endogenous ligand may serve as the endogenous modulator of NMDA receptor-mediated mechanisms in the limbic system. In the case of the haloperidol-sensitive, non-PCP σ binding site, the availability of an endogenous ligand might finally clarify the issue of its functional significance.

TABLE 3
PCP/σ vs non-PCP/σ Sites: Summary of Characteristics

Site	Sensitivity to haloperidol	Ligand potencies[a]	Modulation of NMDA	Radioligands
PCP/σ	0	dexoxadrol >> levoxadrol PCE > PCP PCP >> pentazocine	+	[^{3}H]PCP, [^{3}H]TCP, 100 nM (+)-[^{3}H]SKF 10,047 in presence of haloperidol
non-PCP/σ	+	dexoxadrol > levoxadrol PCE < PCP pentazocine >> PCP	0	(+)-[^{3}H]3-PPP, [^{3}H]haloperidol, [^{3}H]EKC in presence of naloxone, (±)-[^{3}H]-SKF 10,047 in presence of etorphine, (+)-[^{3}H]SKF 10,047

[a]PCE, N-ethyl-1-phenylcyclohexylamine.

6. Nomenclature

Considerable evidence thus indicates the presence of two distinct σ sites in mammalian brain. Their properties are summarized in Table 3. What should these sites be called? If sensitivity to naloxone is to be accepted as a necessary criterion for opioid character (Hughes, 1985), then neither of the entities that have been termed σ sites should be termed "opiate" or "opioid." It is now known that W. R. Martin's "σ opiate receptor" (Martin et al., 1976) is not sensitive to naloxone (Vaupel, 1983; Vaupel et al., 1986). The question arises of whether this should be renamed. On the basis of the behavioral and biochemical studies that support the concept of the commonality of the PCP receptor with Martin's "σ opiate" receptor, it would seem appropriate to utilize the term "PCP/σ receptor." This receptor is, by definition, the entity at which PCP derivatives and σ opioids exert their common pharmacological effects in the chronic spinal dog, in the discriminative stimulus paradigm, and in their noncompetitive antagonism of NMDA-mediated neurotransmission. We suggest the use of the term "haloperidol-sensitive σ binding site" or "(+)-3-PPP-sensitive σ binding site" to refer to the σ site that is distinct from PCP/σ receptors and does not modulate NMDA receptors. It is especially important that the same unmodified "σ" term not be used to refer to two distinct entities. The crucial point is that the terminology should be self-descriptive and unambiguous.

Acknowledgments

The work in the authors' laboratories was supported in part by PHS grants from the National Institute on Drug Abuse DA02587 and DA03383 to S.R.Z. and DA01843 and DA00069 to R.S.Z.; by NSF grant BNS-8607398 to S.R.Z.; and by the Department of Psychiatry, Albert Einstein College of Medicine/Montefiore Medical Center, Herman M. van Praag, MD, PhD, Chairman.

References

Anis, N. A., Berry, S. C., Burton, N. R. and Lodge, D. (1983) The dissociative anaesthetics ketamine and phencyclidine selectively reduce excitation of central mammalian neurones by N-methyl-aspartate. *Br. J. Pharmacol.* **79,** 565–575.

Atweh, S. F. and Kuhar, M. J. (1977) Autoradiographic localization of opiate receptors in rat brain. III. The telencephalon. *Brain Res.* **134,** 393–405.

Berry, S. C., Dawkins, S. L., and Lodge, D. (1984) A comparison of sigma and kappa opiate receptor ligands as excitatory amino acid antagonists. *Br. J. Pharmacol.* **83**, 179–185.

Brady, K. T. and Balster, R. L. (1982) Discriminative stimulus properties of stereoisomers of cyclazocine in phencyclidine-trained squirrel monkeys. *Life Sci.* **31**, 541–549.

Brady, K. T., Balster, R. L., and May, E. L. (1982) Stereoisomers of N-allylnormetazocine: Phencyclidine-like behavioral effects in squirrel monkeys and rats. *Science* **215**, 178–180.

Browne, R. G. and Welch, W. M. (1982) Stereoselective antagonism of phencyclidine's discriminative properties by adenosine receptor agonists. *Science* **217**, 1157–1159.

Chang, K.-J. Cooper, B. R., Hazum, E., and Cuatrecasas, P. (1979) Multiple opiate receptors: Different regional distribution in the brain and differential binding of opiates and opioid peptides. *Mol. Pharmacol.* **16**, 91–104.

Chavkin, C., James, I. F., and Goldstein, A. (1982) Dynorphin is a specific endogenous ligand of the κ opioid receptor. *Science* **215**, 413–415.

Davies, B. M. and Beech, H. R. (1960) The effects of l-arylcyclohexylamine (Sernyl) on twelve normal volunteers. *J. Ment. Sci.* **106**, 912–924.

Eghbali, M., Tempel, A., Henriksen, S., and Zukin, R. S. (1987) Characterization and visualization of brain kappa opiate receptors: Evidence for a conformational change, submitted for publication.

Gilbert, P. E. and Martin, W. R. (1976) The effects of morphine and morphine-like drugs in the nondependent and cyclazocine-dependent chronic spinal dog. *J. Pharmacol. Exp. Ther.* **198**, 66–82.

Goldstein, A., Tachibana, S., Lowney, L. I., Hunkapiller, M., and Hood, L. (1979) Dynorphin-(1-13): An extraordinarily potent opioid peptide. *Proc. Natl. Acad. Sci. USA* **76**, 6666–6670.

Goodman, R. R., Snyder, S. H., Kuhar, M. J., and Young, W. S., III (1980) Differentiation of delta and mu receptor localizations by light microscopic autoradiography. *Proc. Natl. Acad. Sci. USA* **77**, 6239–6243.

Greenberg, B. D. and Segal, D. S. (1985) Acute and chronic behavioral interactions between phencyclidine (PCP) and amphetamine: Evidence for a dopaminergic role in some PCP-induced behaviors. *Pharmacol. Biochem. Behav.* **23**, 99–105.

Guillemin, R., Ling, N., and Burgus, R. (1976) Endorphins, peptides d'origine hypothalamique et neurohypophysaire d'activite morphinomimetique. Isolement et structure moleculaire d'alpha-endorphine, C.R. *Hebd. Seances Acad. Sci.* ser. D **282**, 783–785.

Gundlach, A. L., Largent, B. L., and Snyder, S. H. (1985) Phencyclidine and sigma opiate receptors in brain: Biochemical and autoradiographical differentiation. *Eur. J. Pharmacol.* **113**, 465–466.

Gundlach, A. L., Largent, B. L., and Snyder, S. H. (1986) Autoradiographic localization of sigma receptor binding sites in guinea pig and rat central nervous system with $(+)^3$H-3-(3-Hydroxyphenyl)-N-(1-propyl)piperidine *J. Neurosci.* **6**, 1757–1770.

Haertzen, C. A. (1970) Subjective effects of narcotic antagonists cyclazocine and nalorphine on the Addiction Research Center Inventory (ARCI). *Psychopharmacologia* **18**, 366–367.

Haertzen, C. A. (1974) Advances in Biochemical Psychopharmacology, in *Subjective Effects of Narcotic Antagonists* vol. 8 (Brande, M., Harris, L., May, E., Smith, J. P., and Villereal, J., eds.) Raven, New York.

Hampton, R. Y., Medzihradsky, F., Woods, J. H., and Dahlstrom, P. J. (1982) Stereospecific binding of [^{3}H]-phencyclidine in brain membranes. *Life Sci.* **30**, 2147–2154.

Haring, R., Kloog, Y., and Sokolovsky, M. (1986) Identification of polypeptides of the phencyclidine (PCP) receptor of rat hippocampus by photoaffinity labeling with [^{3}H]azidophencyclidine. *Biochemistry* **25**, 612–620.

Herkenham, M. and Pert, C. B. (1980) In vitro autoradiography of opiate receptors in rat brain suggest loci of "opiatergic" pathways. *Proc. Natl. Acad. Sci. USA* **77**, 5532–5536.

Herling, S. and Woods, J. H. (1981) Discriminative stimulus effects of narcotics: Evidence for multiple receptor mediated actions. *Life Sci.* **28**, 1571–1584.

Holtzman, S. G. (1974) Narcotic Antagonists as Stimulants of Behavior in the Rat: Specific and Nonspecific Effects, in *Advances in Biochemical Psychopharmacology* vol. 8: *Narcotic Antagonists* (Braude, M. C., Harris, L. S., May, E. L., Smith, J. P., and Villarreal, J. E., eds.) Raven, New York.

Holtzman, S. G. (1980) Phencyclidine-like discriminative effects of opioids in the rat. *J. Pharmacol. Exp. Ther.* **214**, 614–619.

Holtzman, S. G. (1982) Phencyclidine-like discriminative stimulus properties of psychotomimetic opioids. *Ann. NY Acad. Sci.* **398**, 230–240.

Hughes, J. (1985) Opioid Peptides-Families of Receptors and Neurotransmitters, in *Neurotransmitters in Action* (Bousefield, D., ed.) Elsevier, New York.

Hughes, J., Smith, T. W., Kosterlitz, H. W., Fothergill, L. A., Morgan, B. A., and Morris, H. R. (1975) Identification of two related pentapeptides from the brain with potent opiate agonist activity. *Nature* **258**, 577–579.

Itzhak, Y., Hiller, J. M., and Simon, E. J. (1985) Characterization of specific binding sites for [^{3}H] (d)-N-allylnormetazocine in rat brain membranes. *Mol. Pharmacol.* **27**, 46–52.

James, I., Chavkin, C., and Goldstein, A. (1982) Selectivity of dynorphin for κ opioid receptors. *Life Sci.* **31**, 1331–1334.

Javitt, D. C., Jotkowitz, A., Sircar, R., and Zukin, S. R. (1987) Noncompetitive regulation of PCP receptors by the NMDA receptor antagonist D($-$)AP5. *Neurosci. Lett.*, in press.

Johnstone, M., Evans, V., and Baigel, S. (1959) Sernyl (CI-395) in clinical anesthesia. *Br. J. Anaesth.* **31**, 433–439.

Kuhar, M. J. (1982) Localization of Drug and Neurotransmitter Receptors in Brain by Light Microscopic Autoradiography, in *Handbook of Psychopharmacology* vol. 15 (Iverson, L. L., Iverson, S. D., and Snyder, S. H., eds.) Plenum, New York.

Lacey, M. G. and Henderson, G. (1986) Actions of phencyclidine on rat locus coeruleus neurones in vitro. *Neuroscience* **2**, 485–494.

Largent, B. L., Gundlach, A. L., and Snyder, S. H. (1984) Psychotomimetic opiate receptors labeled and visualized with (+)-[^{3}H]-(3-hydroxyphenyl)-N-(1-propyl)piperidphe *Proc. Natl. Acad. Sci. USA* **81**, 4983–4987.

Largent, B. L., Gundlach, A. L, and Snyder, S. H. (1986) Pharmacological and autoradiographic discrimination of sigma and phencyclidine receptor binding sites in brain with (+)-[^{3}H] SKF 10,047, (+)-[^{3}H]-3-[3-hydroxyphenyl]-N-(1-propyl)piperidine and [^{3}H]-1-[1-(2-thienyl)cyclohexyl]piperidine. *J. Pharmacol. Exp. Ther.* **238,** 739–748.

Lasagna, L., Dekornfeld, T. J., and Pearson, J. W. (1964) The analgesic efficacy and respiratory effects in man of a benzomorphan "narcotic antagonist." *J. Pharmacol. Exp. Ther.* **144,** 12–16.

Li, C. H. and Chung, D. (1976) Isolation and structure of an untriakontapeptide with opiate activity from camel pituitary glands. *Proc. Natl. Acad. Sci. USA* **73,** 1145–1148.

Lodge, D., Anis, N. A., Berry, S. C., and Burton, N. R. (1983) Arylcyclohexamines Selectively Reduce Excitation of Mammalian Neurones by Aspartate-Like Amino Acids, in *Phencyclidine and Related Arylcyclohexamines: Present and Future Applications* (Kamenka, J.-M., Domino, E. F., and Geneste, P., eds.) NPP, Ann Arbor, Michigan.

Lodge, D., Berry, S. C., Church, J., Martin, D., McGhee, A., Lai, H. M., and Thomson, A. M. (1984) Isomers of cyclazocine as excitatory amino acid antagonists. *Neuropeptides* **5,** 245–248.

Loo, P., Braunwalder, A., Lenmann, J., and Williams, M. (1986) Radioligand binding to central phencyclidine recognition sites is dependent on excitatory amino acid receptor antagonists. *Eur. J. Pharmacol.* **123,** 467–468.

Lord, J. A. H., Waterfield, A. A., Hughes, J., and Kosterlitz, H. W. (1977) Endogenous opioid peptides: Multiple agonists and receptors. *Nature* (Lond.) **267,** 495–500.

Luby, E. D., Cohen, B. D., Rosenbaum, G., Gottlieb, J., and Kelly, R. (1959) Study of a new schizophrenomimetic drug—sernyl. *AMA Arch. Neurol. Psychiat.* **81,** 363–369.

Martin, B. R., and Lodge, D. (1985) Ketamine Acts as a non-competitive N-methyl-D-aspartate antagonist on frog spinal cord in vitro. *Neuropharmacology* **24,** 999–1003.

Martin, W. R., Eades, C. G., Thompson, J. A., Huppler, R. E., and Gilbert, P. E. (1976) The effects of morphine- and nalorphine-like drugs in the nondependent and morphine-dependent chronic spinal dog. *J. Pharmacol. Exp. Ther.* **197,** 517–532.

Martin, B. R., Katzen, J. S., Woods, J. A., Tripathi, H. L., Harris, L. S., and May, E. L. (1984) Stereoisomers of [^{3}H]-N-allylnormetazocine bind to different sites in mouse brain. *J. Pharmacol. Exp. Ther.* **231,** 539–544.

Mendelsohn, L. G., Karchner, G. A., Kalra, V., Zimmerman, D. M., and Leander, J. D. (1984) Phencyclidine receptors in rat brain cortex. *Biochem. Pharmacol.* **33,** 3529–3535.

Munson, P. J. and Rodbard, D. (1980) Ligand: A versatile computerized approach for characterization of ligand-binding systems. *Anal. Biochem.* **107,** 220–226.

Pasternak, G. W., Carroll-Buatti, M., and Spiegel, K. (1981) The binding and analgesic properties of a sigma opiate, SKF-10,047. *J. Pharmacol. Exp. Ther.* **219,** 192–198.

Quirion, R., Jr., Hammer, R. P., Herkenham, M., and Pert, C. B. (1981) A phencyclidine/sigma opiate receptor: Its visualization by tritium-sensitive film. *Proc. Natl. Acad. Sci. USA* **78,** 5881–5885.

Quirion, R., DiMaggio, D. A., French, E. D., Contreras, P. C., Shiloch, J., Pert, C. B., Everist, H., Pert, A., and O'Donohue, T. L. (1984) Evidence for an endogenous peptide ligand for the phencyclidine receptor. *Peptides* **5**, 967–973.

Shannon, H. E. (1982) Pharmacological analysis of the phencyclidine-like discriminative stimulus properties of narcotic derivatives in rats. *J. Pharmacol. Exp. Ther.* **216**, 543–551.

Shearman, G. T. and Herz, A. (1982) Non-opioid psychotomimetic-like discriminative stimulus properties of N-allylnormetazocine (SKF 10,047) in the rat. *Eur. J. Pharmacol.* **82**, 167–172.

Sircar, R. and Zukin, S. R. (1985) Visualization of [³H]TCP binding in rat brain by quantitative light-microscopy autoradiography. *Brain Res.* **344**, 142–145.

Sircar, R., Nichtenhauser, R., Ieni, J. R., and Zukin, S. R. (1986) Characterization and autoradiographic visualization of [³H](+)SKF-10,047 binding in rat and mouse brain: Further evidence for phencyclidine/"sigma opiate" receptor commonality. *J. Pharmacol. Exp. Ther.*, **237**, 681–688.

Slifer, B. L. and Balster, R. L. (1985) Phencyclidine-like discriminative stimulus properties of the stereoisomers of dioxadrol. *Subst. Alcohol Actions Misuse* **5**(6), 273–280.

Snell, L. D. and Johnson, K. M. (1985) Antagonism of N-methyl-D-aspartate-induced transmitter release in the rat striatum by phencyclidine-like drugs and its relationship to turning behavior. *J. Pharmacol. Exp. Ther.* **235**, 50–57.

Snell, L. D. and Johnson, K. M. (1986) Characterization of the inhibition of excitatory amino acid-induced transmitter release in the rat striatum by phencyclidine-like drugs. *J. Pharmacol. Exp. Ther.* **238**, 938–946.

Su, T.-P. (1981) Psychotomimetic opioid binding: Specific binding of [³H]SKF-10047 to etorphine-inaccessible sites in guinea-pig brain. *Eur. J. Pharmacol.* **75**, 81–91.

Su, T.-P. (1982) Evidence for sigma opioid receptor: Binding of [³H]SKF 10,047 to etorphine-accessible sites in guinea-pig brain. *J. Pharmacol. Exp. Ther.* **223**, 284–290.

Su, T.-P., Weissman, A. D., and Yeh, S. Y. (1986) Endogenous ligands for sigma opioid receptors in the brain ("sigmaphin"): Evidence from binding assays. *Life Sci.* **24**, 2199–2210.

Tam, S. W. (1983) Naloxone-inaccessible receptor in rat central nervous system. *Proc. Natl. Acad. Sci. USA* **80**, 6703–6707.

Tam, S. W. (1985) (+)-[³H]SKF 10,047, (+)-[³H]ethylketocyclazocine, μ, κ, δ and phencyclidine bindings sites in guinea pig brain membranes. *Eur. J. Pharmacol.* **109**, 33–41.

Tam, S. W. and Cook, L. (1984) σ Opiates and certain antipsychotic drugs mutually inhibit (+)-[³H]SKF 10,047 and [³H]haloperidol binding in guinea pig brain membranes. *Proc. Natl. Acad. Sci. USA* **80**, 5618–5621.

Teal, J. J. and Holtzman, S. G. (1980a) Discriminative stimulus effects of cyclazocine in the rat. *J. Pharmacol. Exp. Ther.* **212**, 368–376.

Teal, J. J. and Holtzman, S. G. (1980b) Discriminative stimulus effects of prototype opiate receptor agonists in monkeys. *Eur. J. Pharmacol.* **68**, 1–10.

Thompson, A. M. and Lodge, D. (1985) Selective blockade of an excitatory synapse in rat cerebral cortex by the sigma opiate cyclazocine: An intracellular, in vitro study. *Neurosci. Lett.* **54**, 21–26.

Thompson, A. M., West, D. C., and Lodge, D. (1985) An N-methylaspartate receptor-mediated synapse in rat cerebral cortex: A site of action of ketamine? *Nature* (Lond.) **313**, 479–481.

Vaupel, B. (1983) Naloxone fails to antagonize the σ effects of PCP and SKF 10,047 in the dog. *Eur. J. Pharmacol.* **92**, 269–274.

Vaupel, D. B., Risner, M. E., and Shannon, H. E. (1986) Pharmacologic and reinforcing properties of phencyclidine and the enantiomers of N-allylnormetazocine in the dog. *Drug Alcohol Depend.* **18**, 173–194.

Vignon, J., Vincent, J. P., Bidard, J. N., Kamenka, J. M., Geneste, P., Monier, S., and Lazdunski, M. (1982) Biochemical properties of the brain phencyclidine receptor. *Eur. J. Pharmacol.* **81**, 531–543.

Vignon, J., Chicheportiche, R., Chicheportiche, M., Kamenka, J.-M., Geneste, P., and Lazdunski, M. (1983) [³H]TCP: A new tool with high affinity for the PCP receptor in rat brain. *Brain Res.* **280**, 194–197.

Vincent, J. P., Kartalovski, B., Geneste, P., Kamenka, J. M., and Lazdunski, M. (1979) Interaction of phencyclidine ("angel dust") with a specific receptor in rat brain membranes. *Proc. Natl. Acad. Sci. USA* **76**, 4678–4682.

Vincent, J. P., Vignon, J., Kartalovski, B., and Lazdunski, M. (1980) Compared properties of central and peripheral binding sites for phencyclidine. *Eur. J. Pharmacol.* **68**, 79–82.

Wang, Y., Palmer, M. R., Freedman, R., Rice, K. C., Lessor, R. A., Jacobson, A. E., and Hoffer, B. J. (1986) Electrophysiological interactions of isomers of cyclazocine with the phencyclidine antagonist metaphit in rat cerebellar Purkinje neurons. *J. Neurosci.* **11**, 3189–3196.

Zukin, S. R. (1982) Differing stereospecificites distinguish opiate receptor subtypes. *Life Sci.* **31**, 1307–1310.

Zukin, R. S. and Zukin, S. R. (1981) Demonstration of [³H]-cyclazocine binding to multiple opiate receptor sites. *Mol. Pharmacol.* **20**, 246–254.

Zukin, S. R. and Zukin, R. S. (1979) Specific [³H]-phencyclidine binding in rat central nervous system. *Proc. Natl. Acad. Sci. USA* **76**, 5372–5376.

Zukin, S. R., Fitz-Syage, M. L., Nichtenhauser, R., and Zukin, R. S. (1983) Specific binding of [³H]-phencyclidine in rat central nervous tissue: Further characterization and technical considerations. *Brain Res.* **258**, 277–284.

Zukin, S. R., Brady, K. T., Slifer, B. L., and Balster, R. L. (1984) Behavioral and biochemical stereoselectivity of sigma opiate/PCP receptors. *Brain Res.* **294**, 174–177.

Zukin, S. R., Tempel, A., Gardner, E. L., and Zukin, R. S. (1986) Interaction of [³H] (−)-SKF-10,047 with brain σ receptors: Characterization and autoradiographic visualization. *J. Neurochem.* **46**, 1032–1041.

Zukin, S. R., Zukin, R. S., Vale, W., Rivier, J., Nichtenhauser, R., Snell, L. D., and Johnson, K. M. (1987) An endogenous ligand of the brain σ/PCP receptor antagonizes NMDA-induced neurotransmitter release. *Brain Res.*, in press.

Chapter 6

Solubilization and Purification of Opioid Binding Sites

Eric J. Simon and Jacob M. Hiller

1. Introduction

This chapter will summarize the state of the art of the isolation in soluble form and purification of opioid receptors. One may well ask why investigators would want to undertake such a tedious and difficult task. Even if successful, the danger exists that the purified receptor will in no way resemble the membrane-bound receptor. This apprehension goes back to the early days of enzymology, when scientists were concerned that enzymes in broken-cell preparations or in purified form would behave very differently from their counterparts in intact cells. This fear has fortunately proven to be relatively unfounded. An enormous amount of information has been gained from isolated crude and purified enzymes as well as receptors. To the extent that changes do occur, these can be studied by reconstituting the isolated macromolecule into an environment resembling its original milieu. In the case of membrane proteins, such as receptors, this has been done by reconstitution into both artificial and natural membranes.

Purification to homogeneity has been achieved for only a small number of membrane receptors, of which the best known are the low-density lipoprotein (LDL), acetylcholine, and insulin receptors. A perusal of the literature on these receptors provides an idea of what can be learned from purification. The subunit structure of the receptor can be studied. Antibodies can be produced to various epitopes in the receptor molecule. Such antibodies can help in elucidating the distribution and function of the receptors. With the use of molecular biological techniques it becomes possible to obtain the complete amino acid sequence for all receptor polypeptide chains. Information regarding the presence and nature of other moieties, such as lipids and carbohydrates, and posttranslational modifications, such as phosphorylation, sulfatation, or methylation, also become accessible to study. For receptors that exist in multiple types, as is the case for opioid receptors, it becomes possible to prove which types represent different conformers of the same molecule and which are separate molecular entities. The relationship between binding proteins and accessory coupled proteins, such as G proteins and adenylate cyclase, can be studied by reconstitution into artificial and natural membranes. Much can be learned about the nature of the binding site and about receptor function by the production of site-specific mutations in the gene or cDNA that codes for the receptor. These are some of the rewards in store for investigators if success is achieved in the isolation and purification of opioid receptors.

2. Solubilization

2.1. Prebound Opioid Binding Sites

Opioid receptors are tightly attached to cell membranes. The first step in any purification procedure is to detach the molecule from the membrane and put it in aqueous solution. This proved to be a difficult procedure, since opioid receptors are very sensitive to many of the conditions and reagents used for membrane protein solubilization. Attempts to solubilize opioid receptors were initiated in our laboratory shortly after their discovery (Simon et al., 1973; Terenius, 1973; Pert and Snyder, 1973).

Exposure of brain cell membranes to high salt concentrations, low pH, or sonication were tried without success. The use of a large number of detergents, ionic and nonionic, did not yield soluble binding sites that retained their opiate binding activity in solution. These disappointing results led us to try to obtain a prebound ligand–receptor complex in solution. Using the nonionic detergent BRIJ 36T, in 1975 our laboratory (Simon et al., 1975) succeeded in solubilizing a macromolecular complex of [^{3}H]etorphine from rat brain. This complex did not sediment when centrifuged for 60 min at 100,000g, had an apparent molecular weight of approximately 400,000, and exhibited properties consistent with its being a receptor–etorphine complex. Thus, binding was stereospecific, i.e., formation of soluble complex was blocked by opiates, but not their inactive enantiomers, and the complex was sensitive to heat, proteolytic enzymes, and sulfhydryl reagents. All attempts to dissociate the etorphine–receptor complex and obtain opiate binding to soluble receptor were unsuccessful. Solubilization of prebound receptor was a useful first step, but a receptor that retained its binding activity in solution was not obtained until 4 years later.

Zukin and Kream (1979) confirmed this early work and demonstrated that a macromolecular complex of [D-Ala^2]Leu-enkephalin (DALE) could also be solubilized with BRIJ 36T. In a more recent study (Ruegg et al., 1982), we showed that prebound opioid binding sites can be solubilized by a variety of detergents. The highest yield, up to 80%, was obtained with lysolecithin or digitonin. A similar yield was obtained with the enzyme phospholipase A from bee venom, when used in the presence of the synergistically acting peptide, melittin. In none of these experiments, carried out on rat brain membranes, was it possible to solubilize active binding sites.

In recent years prelabeled receptors, solubilized in this manner, have proved very useful. For example, they have been used by Meunier and collaborators (Puget et al., 1980) to study their hydrodynamic properties on sucrose density gradients and gel filtration columns. [^{3}H]Etorphine was the most frequently employed ligand because of its very slow rate of dissociation from the receptor. The antagonist diprenorphine was also used. For receptors solubilized from rabbit cerebellum (largely mu type), these workers (Jauzac et al., 1983) found a physical separation of the agonist (etorphine-bound) and antagonist (diprenorphine-bound) forms of the receptor on a sucrose density gradient.

2.2. Active Opioid Binding Sites in Solution

In collaboration with Dr. Urs Ruegg (Ruegg et al., 1980, 1981) we succeeded in solubilizing active opioid receptors from the brain of the toad *Bufo marinus*. The reason a nonmammalian species was tried was based on a reading of the literature on the isolation of β-adrenergic receptors, in which, up to that time, active receptors had been solubilized from turkey and frog erythrocytes, but not from mammalian sources. Solubilization of active opioid receptors from toad brain was achieved by the use of digitonin, but not with several other detergents tried, again very analogous to the reports on adrenergic receptors. The solubilized opioid receptors strongly resembled the membrane-bound receptors, indicating that detergent treatment and removal of receptors from their membrane environment did not significantly damage the binding site. Binding activity in solution represented a yield of 50–60% of membrane-bound receptors. The method worked equally well for receptors from frog brain and somewhat less well for chicken brain. It did not work for solubilization of receptors from mammalian brain, except in minute yields (3–5%).

During the time this work was in progress Bidlack and Abood (1980) reported the solubilization of active opioid receptors from rat brain by the use of Triton X-100. The detergent was removed with Bio-beads SM-2, yielding a supernatant able to bind opiates.

Simonds et al. (1980) reported the solubilization of active opioid receptors from the neuroblastoma-glioma hybrid cell line NG108-15. This was accomplished with a novel detergent called CHAPS, a zwitterionic derivative of cholate, synthesized by Hjelmeland (1980). Some success was also achieved with this method for receptors from rat brain.

Solubilization of active opioid receptors from mammalian brain was achieved in good yield in our laboratory (Howells et al., 1982) by a modification of the technique used for toad brain receptors. The addition of high concentrations of sodium chloride (0.5–1.0M) to the extraction medium permitted the solubilization by digitonin or glycodeoxycholate of active receptors from various mammalian brains. Yields ranged from 20 to 50%. The requirement was shown to be specific for sodium salts, since substitution of a variety of other salts did not work. The nature of the effect of sodium is not completely understood. It may help keep the receptor in a conformation that is stable in the presence of detergent. Dr. Itzhak in our laboratory demonstrated that sodium protects antagonist, but not agonist, binding against inhibition by digitonin (Itzhak et al., 1984c). In fact, the disadvantage of this solubilization procedure is that although the soluble receptors bind antagonists with high affinity, they will bind agonists with very low affinity, except after special, rather tedious treatments (see below). Optimal conditions for recovery of active opioid binding sites after solubilization require the presence of sodium chloride during extraction and binding, as well as dilution of the extract to reduce the digitonin concentration to 0.1% or lower.

Several other methods of solubilization should be mentioned. Cho et al. (1981) reported the solubilization of opioid binding activity from rat brain membranes by long periods of sonication (twice for 9 min). It was never clearly shown, however, that this technique did not result in tiny, nonsedimentable membrane fragments with high lipid content. This possibility received support from work in our laboratory demonstrating that receptors so solubilized had a molecular weight of several million daltons (Lin and Simon, unpublished results). In their more recent studies, Loh and coworkers have used sonication plus treatment with Triton X-100 (Cho et al., 1983).

Ilien et al. (1982) have reported the solubilization of active opioid receptors with lysolecithin. Their binding measurements were done with [^{3}H]lofentanil, which the authors recommend as a very useful ligand because of its potency and slow rate of dissociation. Competition studies indicated that affinities of various ligands to the soluble receptors were about 5–20-fold lower than those to membrane-bound receptors. The authors attribute at least a portion of this discrepancy to differences in incubation conditions. There was good correlation between the rank order of affinities to the soluble receptor and pharmacological potencies of the eight ligands tested.

A more recent paper by Demoliou-Mason and Barnard (1984) recommends a modification of the digitonin procedure (Howells et al., 1982). Solubilization was carried out in Tes-KOH buffer, pH 7.5, containing EGTA-K$^+$ (1 mM) and MgSO$_4$ (10 mM) and a number of protease inhibitors. The resulting soluble receptors were found to bind mu, delta, and kappa ligands, including peptides.

Before leaving the subject of solubilization, a word is in order on how binding is assayed in such preparations. The filtration and centrifugation techniques used with membrane preparations are clearly not applicable. The earliest methods used were columns, such as XAD-2, which retain free ligands via hydrophobic bonds, but allow ligand bound to proteins to pass through, or Sephadex G-50 or G-25, which separate free and bound ligand by size. These methods, although very useful, tend to be too slow for running large numbers of samples. More rapid, commonly used methods include precipitation of the ligand–receptor complex by polyethyleneglycol in the presence of a protein carrier, first developed by Cuatrecasas (1972), and a more recent method (Bruns et al., 1983) of filtration on glass fiber filters pretreated with polyethylenimine. Methods that have been used less frequently are ammonium sulfate precipitation of bound ligand, removal of free ligand by charcoal, and the method of Hummel and Dreyer (1962).

2.3. Characteristics of Solubilized Opioid Receptors

Space permits the mention of only some of the work on the characterization of the crude soluble receptors. In general, the solubilization step results in little or no purification, i.e., the amount of protein extracted is comparable to the amount of binding activity extracted from the membranes. In most laboratories, binding affinities to soluble receptors were found to be similar or only slightly lower than those to their membrane-bound counterparts. There were some exceptions. In the case of our digitonin procedure, this was restricted to antagonist binding (including bremazocine, a kappa agonist that seems to be a mu and delta antagonist). The results of Ilien et al. (1982), in which affinities for soluble receptors were 1–2 orders of magnitude lower, have been discussed. Loh and associates (Cho et al., 1983) found that high binding affinity in their soluble preparations required the addition of a lipid fraction, but still remained 1–2 orders of magnitude below that of membrane-bound receptors.

Molecular weights of soluble nondenatured receptors varied between 1 and 5×10^5. These values should be interpreted with great caution since they are not corrected for the presence of detergent micelles.

An important result that had not been obtainable with membranes was the demonstration that opioid receptors are glycoproteins. This was done by determining whether soluble receptors are retained by immobilized plant (and some animal) lectins, which have high affinity for specific sugars. Of nine agarose-bound lectins tried, we (Gioannini et al., 1982) found that significant numbers of opioid receptors were retained on beads containing wheat germ agglutinin (WGA), a lectin that specifically binds the sugar N-acetylglucosamine. Specific elution was achieved with this sugar. This result indicates the presence of carbohydrate in the receptor molecule. Other sugars are likely to be present, but may not be sufficiently exposed to be bound by the lectin columns. The lectin binding site of the receptor is geographically and functionally separate from the opioid binding site. This is shown by the finding that prebound and free receptors are retained equally well by WGA beads and by the inability of even very high concentrations of free WGA to inhibit opioid binding.

2.4. Separation of Opioid Receptor Types

There is considerable evidence in support of the existence of the three major types of opioid receptors, mu, delta, and kappa, but very little that permits distinction between the hypotheses that they are separate molecular species or different conformers of a single receptor. Such evidence requires the physical separation of various receptor types. Some progress has been made in this direction. The separation of polypeptide constituents derived from denatured receptors will be discussed in the sections on crosslinking and purification. Here we shall discuss separation of native receptor types. Several laboratories have succeeded in separating kappa receptors from the other major types. To date the separation of native mu and delta receptors from each other has not been achieved.

Chow and Zukin (1983) applied prelabeled, CHAPS-solubilized receptors to a column of Sepharose CL-6B for molecular exclusion chromatography. They found that the peak of [^{3}H]bremazocine binding, carried out in the presence of 40 nM normorphine and 100 nM [D-Ala^2,D-Leu^5]enkephalin (DADLE) to saturate mu and delta sites, eluted 20 mL behind the major peak for [^{3}H]dihydromorphine binding. The kappa nature of the bremazocine binding peak was supported by competition experiments in which only kappa ligands exhibited high affinity.

In our laboratory (Itzhak et al., 1984a) the separation was achieved in the following manner. Guinea pig brain membranes were solubilized with digitonin in the presence of NaCl (1.0M). To improve the affinity of agonist binding, the extract was centrifuged into a sucrose density gradient devoid of sodium and containing a low concentration (0.02%) of digitonin. When binding was assayed with the "universal" ligand [^{3}H]bremazocine in the fractions obtained after density centrifugation, two distinct, well-separated peaks of binding activity were observed. When [^{3}H]bremazocine was bound in the presence of saturating concentrations of mu and delta ligands, [D-Ala^2,MePhe^4,Gly-ol^5]enkephalin (DAGO) and DADLE, only the first peak of binding activity was found and was undiminished in size, suggesting that this peak contained largely kappa (and possibly sigma) receptors. The second peak was found to bind both [^{3}H]DAGO and [^{3}H]DADLE with high affinity, suggesting that it is a mixture of mu and delta sites. [^{3}H]Bremazocine binding in the first peak, on the other hand, was not sensitive to competition even by high concentrations of mu or delta ligands, but was readily decreased by kappa ligands such as EKC and bremazocine. Further confirmation for the kappa nature of the binding activity in the first peak came from the finding that only one peak of binding activity was obtained when a digitonin extract of guinea pig cerebellum was centrifuged on the same sucrose gradient. The peak was identical in position and binding properties to the first peak from guinea pig brain. The guinea pig cerebellum has been shown by Robson et al. (1984) to contain 80–90% kappa sites.

It should be noted here that solubilization of kappa sites from guinea pig cerebellum by digitonin does not require the presence of sodium chloride (Itzhak et al., 1984b). This is similar to our earlier finding for the solubilization of opioid receptors from toad brain, which were also found to be largely of the kappa type (Simon et al., 1982). It therefore appears that kappa sites are more resistant to the harmful effects of digitonin and do not require the protection afforded by high concentrations of sodium, quite unlike what we have found for mu and delta sites. This result further supports the notion that kappa receptors are distinct molecular species different from mu and delta sites.

A more recent study by J. Simon et al. (1984) in Hungary, using similar techniques, showed separation of kappa from mu and delta sites in digitonin extracts of frog brain membranes.

All of these results provide strong evidence that kappa sites can be physically separated from other opioid receptor types and suggest that kappa sites represent a distinct class of molecules. Whether the difference resides in the polypeptide or the carbohydrate portion of the molecule is not known.

3. Covalent Labeling

The conventional method of receptor identification involves reversible binding of labeled agonists and antagonists to intact cells or cell membranes. However, when the resultant receptor–ligand complex is subjected to biochemical purification techniques, such as electrophoresis and chromatography, the inherent drawback of the lability of the receptor–ligand complex becomes a special concern. This problem has been broached by the use of techniques that result in the formation of covalent linkages between receptor protein and ligand, which have enabled investigators to identify binding site polypeptides biochemically. In addition, if multiple binding sites are separate molecules, the use of suitable competitive ligands may permit identification of specific polypeptides involved in each of the multiple sites.

Numerous approaches have evolved for biospecific (affinity) labeling procedures. All essentially involve the formation of covalent linkages between binding site and labeled ligand. One method involves the synthesis of molecules closely related to the ligand, but containing an additional active chemical group able to form a covalent bond with functional groups at or near the active binding site of the receptors. An exception to the rule that affinity labels depend on the formation of covalent linkages for their characteristic irreversibility is the case in which a ligand possesses very high affinity (K_d in the picomolar range) and yet maintains its receptor selectivity. An example of this type of ligand is α-bungarotoxin (Changeux et al., 1970), which remains firmly attached to nicotinic acetylcholine receptors even days after labeling procedures have been carried out.

A second related method, known as photoaffinity labeling, involves ligand molecules containing photolabile groups that react with the active site in the usual reversible manner, but that will form covalent bonds with functional groups in the binding site when irradiated with uv or visible light.

A third method, affinity crosslinking, involves the addition of an exogenous bifunctional crosslinking reagent to a preexisting ligand–receptor complex to effect covalent linkage.

3.1. Affinity Labeling

Affinity labeling reagents do not require activation and can therefore be used for both in vitro and in vivo labeling. Because these reagents contain groups that are intrinsically reactive toward many proteins, the ligand analog must retain high affinity and selectivity for the binding site in order to be an effective probe. Many attempts have been made to prepare site-directed irreversible probes for opioid receptors from opiate agonists and antagonists as well as opioid peptides.

The nitrogen mustard derivative of the agonist oxymorphone, β-chloroxy-morphamine (β-COA), which has the nitrogen mustard group at the 6-beta position of the opiate, possesses potent nonequilibrium narcotic agonist properties. This alkylating agent is an irreversible agonist in the guinea pig ileum and binds irreversibly to opioid receptor sites in brain membranes (Caruso et al., 1979, 1980a). The fumarate methyl ester derivative of oxymorphone, β-fuoxymorphamine (β-FOA), was synthesized to determine whether the fumarate ester moiety of this Michael acceptor analog could interact covalently with the receptor site. In the guinea pig ileum, however, β-FOA acted as a reversible agonist (Takemori et al., 1981).

β-Chlornaltrexamine (β-CNA), a nitrogen mustard derivative of naltrexone, was the first successful antagonist affinity label synthesized (Portoghese et al., 1978, 1979). The binding of ^{3}H-naloxone or ^{3}H-naltrexone is irreversibly inhibited by this potent affinity label. This alkylating reagent also produced irreversible antagonism in both the guinea pig ileum and mouse vas deferens preparations (Caruso et al., 1979; Ward et al., 1982a). β-CNA irreversibly blocks all opioid receptor types, but with differing efficacy, i.e., mu > kappa > delta. This selectivity reflects the multiple opioid receptors' affinities for the parent compound naltrexone. The suggestion that covalent bonding of β-CNA also occurs in vivo is supported by the finding that a single icv injection of this compound will inhibit the development of physical dependence on morphine for at least 72 h and can antagonize the analgesic effect of morphine for at least 13 d (Caruso et al., 1980a). By use of selective protection techniques first used by Robson and Kosterlitz (1979) and Smith and Simon (1980), in which membrane preparations are preincubated with unlabeled ligands highly selective for various types of opioid receptors, followed by β-CNA, preparations enriched in a specific type of receptor can be produced. James and Goldstein (1984) selected sufentanil, DADLE, and dynorphin A as their protective agents for mu, delta, and kappa binding, respectively, against β-CNA inactivation and were thereby able to achieve significant enrichment of the desired receptor. A better estimate of ligand selectivity for the various types of receptors was obtained using such enriched tissues.

[^{3}H]β-CNA has been used in attempts to isolate a receptor complex from membranes (Caruso et al., 1980b). The solubilized complex was chromatographed on an Ultrogel AcA 22 column and the elution profile showed a portion of the complex migrating in a major peak of 590 kdalton.

The aziridium ion generated by β-CNA, which is responsible for the alkylation of opioid receptors, has a very high reactivity, and thus renders this molecule unable to distinguish among the various receptor types. Therefore electrophilic groups with less reactivity were sought for attachment to the C-6 position of naltrexone. The fumarate methyl ester derivative of naltrexone, β-funaltrexamine (β-FNA), was synthesized and found to have increased selectivity (Portoghese et al., 1980). Based on its actions in the guinea pig ileum and mouse vas deferens, β-FNA appears to be a reversible kappa agonist and an irreversible mu antagonist and to have little or no antagonist effect against delta agonists (Ward et al., 1982a,b). Results from opiate binding studies (Ward et al., 1985) showed reduced binding capacity for [^{3}H]morphine and [^{3}H]naltrexone following treatment with β-FNA in mouse brain membranes. The binding of [^{3}H]Met-enkephalin, [^{3}H]DADLE, and [^{3}H]ethylketocyclazocine was decreased in this preparation, but to a lesser extent. Brain membranes from mice treated with β-FNA showed a 50% reduction in ^{3}H-morphine binding, but no effect on [^{3}H]Met-enkephalin binding. Binding competitions against the reversible binding of [^{3}H]β-FNA gave a profile similar to that of competitions against [^{3}H]ethylketocyclazocine.

In a further quest for selective, site-directed alkylating agents, Rice et al. (1982) synthesized the isothiocyanate derivatives of fentanyl (FIT) and etonitazine (BIT) and the fumaramido derivative of endoethenotetrahydrooripavine (FAO). Using rat brain membranes and membranes from NG108-15 cells, FIT and FAO were found to be highly selective alkylators of delta receptors and BIT was shown to be highly selective toward mu receptors. Interestingly, all these compounds have antinociceptive potencies similar to morphine (Burke et al., 1984), even though FIT and FAO are delta selective in vitro. Using the tritiated form of fentanyl isothiocyanate [^{3}H]FIT, Klee et al. (1982) labeled NG108-15 membranes irreversibly in the presence and absence of competing opioid ligands at alkaline pH. After extensive washing, membranes were subjected to SDS-PAGE followed by autoradiography. One protein of M_r 58 kdalton, labeled in the presence of dextrorphan, but not in the presence of active opioids such as levorphanol, [D-Ala^2,Met^5]enkephalinamide, buprenorphine, or naloxone, was thought likely to be a component of the delta receptor.

Rice et al. (1977), taking another approach to the formation of covalent linkage between receptor and ligand, synthesized N(2,4,5-trihydroxyphenethyl)normetazocine. The mechanism for the activation *in situ* was the biooxidation of the trihydroxyphenethyl moiety to an electrophilic intermediate that would react covalently with the receptor. This compound, however, displayed very low affinity for the receptors and was much less active than codeine in antinociceptive assays.

Maryanoff et al. (1982) modified the propionyl group and the amino substituent of fentanyl, 3-methylfentanyl, sufentanil, and lofentanil. They examined mainly α-halocarbonyl, α-diazocarbonyl, β-chlorophenethyl, and *p*-azidophenethyl derivatives. Some irreversible attachment was achieved with α-diazoamide and aryl azide derivatives.

Koolpe et al. (1984) synthesized a 6-desoxy-6-spiro-α-methylene-γ-lactone derivative of naltrexone. At a concentration of 5 nM, this compound produced a 50% inhibition in the membrane binding of [^{3}H]naltrexone. The major portion of this inhibition (30%) was irreversible. Based on their data, the authors suggested that a receptor nucleophile, perhaps a sulfhydryl group, is accessible to react with the α-β-unsaturated carbonyl system of this compound. Following up on this work, this group (Koolpe et al., 1985) synthesized 6-desoxy-6-substituted lactone, epoxide, and glycidate ester derivatives of naltrexone and oxymorphone. Although many of these analogs demonstrated good binding affinities, none showed irreversible effects. The authors concluded from this that the α-methylene-γ-lactone functional group is required for irreversible binding in this series since the saturated lactone analog and the endocyclic α, β-unsaturated lactone were reversible ligands. The fact that the fused α-methylene-γ-lactones showed no irreversible effects demonstrated the extreme sensitivity of covalent ligand–opioid receptor interactions to small structural changes.

The bromomercurio derivative of 6,16-endo-ethenotetrahydrothebaine, called Hybromet, was synthesized by Archer et al. (1985) with the idea that it could be used as a site-directed alkylating agent. Hybromet manifested a modest preference for mu over delta sites. Binding experiments suggested that covalent binding of Hybromet to mu receptors had occurred.

The nonequilibrium binding of the 14-hydroxydihydromorphinone hydrazones (naloxazone, oxymorphazone, and naltrexazone) has been suggested to be the result of the formation of their azines (Hahn et al., 1982). Naloxonazine, naltrexonazine, and oxymorphonazine irreversibly block opiate binding 20- to 40-fold more potently than their corresponding hydrazones. The mechanism for irreversible inhibition of opiate binding by azine derivatives remains to be elucidated.

An affinity labeling agent derived from enkephalin has also been synthesized. The peptide Tyr-D-Ala-Gly-Phe-Leu-CH₂Cl, (DALECK) was first synthesized by Pelton et al. (1980) and subsequently by Venn and Barnard (1981) and Szucs et al. (1983). The binding of this chloromethylketone derivative of DADLE (100 nM) at alkaline pH led to irreversible blockade of 40% of delta sites in rat brain homogenate. At higher concentrations of DALECK, 95% of enkephalin binding sites were irreversibly blocked, whereas [³H]etorphine binding was reduced by only 50% (Venn and Barnard, 1981). Bioassays of this drug showed conflicting results. DALECK caused irreversible inhibition of the electrically stimulated contractions in mouse vas deferens (Venn and Barnard, 1981), whereas naloxone was able to reverse DALECK inhibition of electrically stimulated contractions in the guinea pig ileum (Pelton et al., 1980), as well as the analgesic effect of intracisternally administered DALECK in the rat tail withdrawal test (Szucs et al., 1983). An explanation of these results put forward by some of these groups (Szucs et al., 1983; Venn and Barnard, 1981) was that DALECK binds irreversibly to delta receptors, but reversibly to mu receptors. Upon further examination, the Barnard group (Newman and Barnard, 1984) reversed their earlier conclusion and stated that DALECK is a mu-selective peptide. This was based on their new findings that exposure of membranes at pH 8.1 to DALECK (30 µM) and subsequent assays of remaining active sites showed a permanent reduction (30%) in the number of high-affinity DAGO binding sites with little effect on the affinity of these sites. The Rosenthal plot for the binding of [³H]DADLE was unchanged by the DALECK pretreatment. Newman and Barnard (1984) alkylated purified synaptic membranes with [³H]DALECK and analyzed the solubilized membrane components on SDS-PAGE. A major labeled band of 58 kdalton was present on the gel. The authors suggested that this represents a subunit of the mu type of the opioid receptor.

3.2. Photoaffinity Labeling

The elegant technique of photoaffinity labeling developed by Westheimer and colleagues (Singh et al., 1962) has been utilized in attempts to identify the membrane components comprising the opioid receptors. The first attempted photoaffinity labeling of opioid receptors was carried out by Winter and Goldstein (1972). A derivative of levorphanol, [^{3}H]N-β-(p-azidophenyl)ethyl norlevorphanol, synthesized by these investigators, had potent opiate-like pharmacological activity in mice and in the isolated guinea pig ileum. Following photolysis in the presence of brain homogenate, radioactivity was irreversibly incorporated into the particulate matter of this homogenate. However, this incorporation was not specific since stereospecific blocking could not be demonstrated.

With the discovery of the endogenous opioid peptides, efforts were initiated to equip the enkephalin series of peptides with photoactivatable groups. Hazum et al. (1979) prepared a lysine[6] derivative of DALE that was subsequently chemically modified by the addition of a nitro-azidophenyl group to the epsilon-amino group of the lysine. The iodinated derivative of this compound retained high binding affinity, as reflected in its apparent K_d of 2.1 nM. Following photoactivation of this iodinated compound, the authors reported that covalent binding to brain membrane preparations had been achieved. However, the data are not unequivocal since the known sensitivity of the receptor itself to the effect of UV light was not controlled for.

Using a similar approach, Lee et al. (1979) synthesized an arylazide enkephalin derivative [D-Ala^2,Met^5] enkephalin-Tyr-N-(2-nitro-4-azidophenyl)ethylenediamine (ETN). Binding competitions of ETN in NG108-15 cell membranes against [^{3}H]enkephalinamide showed a K_i of 7 nM. Photolysis of ETN in the presence of cell membranes caused an irreversible inactivation of enkephalin binding. Addition of enkephalin to the incubation mixture protected the receptors from inactivation. The concentration of enkephalin needed to protect 50% of the binding was 3 nM. Selectivity of this ligand for mu, delta, and kappa binding sites was not examined.

Smolarsky and Koshland (1980) investigated the binding characteristics of a series of azide enkephalin analogs in bovine caudate nucleus. A nitrocinnamylamine group was introduced into either position 4 or 5 of enkephalin. The nitro group and the double bond were reduced and the resulting amino group was converted to the azide. [^{3}H]Etorphine, which has almost equal affinity to all types of opioid receptors, was used to assess the degree of inactivation of binding caused by these analogs. Because of the use of this "universal" ligand to label binding sites, selectivity of the potential photoaffinity labels for the various receptor types was not established.

More recently Zioudrou et al. (1983) synthesized two derivatives of DALE in which a 2-nitro-4-azidophenyl group was linked to the carboxyl group of the enkephalin by means of an ethylenediamine or ethylenediamine β-alanine spacer. Both peptides bound to opioid receptors with affinities in the nanomolar range. They also inhibited the electrically stimulated contractions of the mouse vas deferens, as well as adenylate cyclase activity in NG108-15 cells, both in a naloxone reversible manner. In contrast to earlier studies, irradiation with visible light was made possible by the presence of a nitro moiety on the ligand. This change prevented problems of UV-induced loss of binding activity. Following irradiation by visible light (540 nm) in the presence of rat brain or NG108-15 membranes, irreversible losses of about 50 and 80% of binding sites, respectively, were noted. However, direct binding and irradiation of the tritiated form of the photolyzable peptide containing the β-alanine spacer showed that the labeling of brain membranes was by no means specific, since nonspecific binding accounted for 72% of total binding.

In an effort to prepare photolabile peptide derivatives that exhibit greater selectivity, Garbay-Jaureguiberry et al. (1983) chose to introduce azido groups into the Phe residue of the highly mu-selective peptide, DAGO, and the selective delta peptide, Thr-Gly-Phe-Leu-Thr (DTLET). Although little loss in selectivity was noted for the azido-DAGO derivative, a sixfold increase in the K_i value for this compound was seen against [^{3}H]DAGO and a fivefold increase in the K_i value against [^{3}H]DTLET. More promising results were seen with azido-DTLET (AZ-DTLET), which also showed little loss in selectivity and only a 2.5-fold increase in K_i against [^{3}H]DTLET (from 1.3 to 3.8 nM). Irradiation in the UV range of rat brain membranes in presence of AZ-DTLET led to a 70–80% loss of delta binding sites without significant changes in the level of [^{3}H]DAGO binding. Addition of 7.5 nM DTLET prior to incubation with AZ-DTLET and irradiation provided complete protection against the loss of specific delta binding. If the tritiated form of AZ-DTLET proves to retain its high selectivity for delta binding sites, it will be extremely useful in the further characterization of this site.

Another technique of photoaffinity labeling, called energy transfer photoaffinity labeling, has been developed by Hirth and Goeldner at the Center for Neurochemistry, Strasbourg, France, and shows great promise for highly specific covalent labeling of enzymes and receptors (Kieffer et al., 1981). This new method is contingent on the presence of a fluorescent amino acid, usually tryptophan, at or near the binding site of the receptor protein. A photolabile derivative of the ligand is synthesized, which is stable at the excitation wavelength of tryptophan (290 nm) and is an efficient tryptophan fluorescence quencher. Most importantly, it must be photosensitive at the emission wavelength of tryptophan (340 nm). The reactive photo-decomposition product is able to form a covalent bond with groups at or near the active site of the protein. Since photoactivation depends on energy transfer from a nearby tryptophan, unbound molecules are not photodecomposed. It is therefore possible to obtain highly specific covalent labeling with ligands of low affinity in the presence of a large excess of unbound ligand.

Aryldiazonium salts, especially those substituted in the *para* position with electron donating groups (NH_2, OCH_3, amido), have been found to be very suitable for energy transfer affinity labeling (Goeldner et al., 1980). These workers have successfully applied this technique to the nicotinic acetylcholine receptor (Kotzyba-Hibert et al., 1985). A number of diazonium salts of opiates, in particular of fentanyl and its analogs, have been prepared by this group and are being tested for use in opioid receptor labeling by this technique (Hirth, Goeldner, Galzi, Hiller and Simon, unpublished results).

3.3. Affinity Crosslinking

The structural characterization of mu and delta opioid binding sites by affinity crosslinking technology has been carried out in our laboratory (Howard et al., 1985) with the high-affinity probe, human ^{125}I-labeled β-endorphin ([125]I $β_h$-end). The recent commercial availability of highly purified [125]I-$β_h$-end with high specific activity presents one with an excellent ligand for receptor labeling studies and at the same time with a probe that is amenable to reaction with bifunctional crosslinking reagents. $β_h$-end is unique among its homologs isolated from various species in that a tyrosine moiety is present at position 27. Radioiodination of Tyr^{27}, in contrast to Tyr^1, can be carried out without loss of binding affinity. Separation of the two iodinated species has been achieved by HPLC. $β_h$-end exhibits high affinity at both mu and delta sites, but only very low affinity binding at kappa sites.

Different crosslinking reagents may react with amino groups or sulfhydryl groups, or may have photoreactive properties. The bifunctionality of the reagent may be of a homo- or hetero-type, and with some reagents may form a cleavable linkage. Specific crosslinking of ^{125}I β_h-end to opioid receptors is best accomplished with BSCOES, *bis*[2-(succinimidooxycarbonyloxy)ethyl] sulfone, which is a homo-bifunctional reagent that reacts with amino groups present in both ligand and receptor. SDS-PAGE followed by autoradiography of ^{125}I-β_h-end-crosslinked SDS or digitonin-solubilized rat brain membranes, revealed the presence of four reproducible bands or areas of approximate molecular weights of 65, 53, 41, and 38 kdalton. All labeled bands seemed to be opioid-receptor-related, since they were eliminated when binding was carried out in an excess of various opiates. The evidence obtained using tissues that vary in their relative content of mu and delta sites, such as rat whole brain (delta = mu), rat thalamus (mostly mu), bovine frontal cortex (delta:mu = 2:1), and the neuroblastoma-glioma hybrid cell line, NG108-15 (only delta), demonstrates that different labeling patterns are obtained when mu and delta sites are crosslinked. The pattern obtained on SDS-PAGE from crosslinked mu sites contains a major (heavily labeled) component of 65 kdalton, whereas patterns from delta sites contain a major labeled component of 53 kdalton. This 53-kdalton band appears clearly in extracts from NG108-15 cells and bovine frontal cortex, although in rat whole brain a diffusely labeled region is present between 55 and 41 kdalton.

Further and more convincing evidence demonstrating that mu and delta opioid binding sites contain major peptide subunits that differ in molecular size was obtained in our laboratory (Howard et al., 1986). This was accomplished by selective competition for binding and crosslinking of ^{125}I β_h-end using highly selective mu and delta ligands. Covalent labeling of the 65-kdalton peptide was selectively reduced or eliminated by the highly selective mu ligand, DAGO, but not by the highly selective delta ligand [D-penicillamine^2,D-penicillamine^5]enkephalin (DPDPE), whereas radioactivity in the 53-kdalton peptide band was selectively reduced by DPDPE, but not by DAGO. When DAGO and DPDPE were added together, the disappearance of the labeled peptides was more pronounced than expected from the additive effects of these ligands. Although this phenomenon is not understood, it could be interpreted as providing evidence for an allosteric relationship between mu and delta receptors, as has been previously suggested (Rothman and Westfall, 1982). The labeling of the 41- and 38-kdalton peptide bands was reduced by either DAGO or DPDPE. The 41-kdalton peptide is seen only in bovine caudate and guinea pig whole brain, whereas the 38-kdalton species is seen to some extent in every brain tissue studied. Some of the explanations for bands suppressed by both mu- and delta-selective ligands include the following. They may represent binding subunits common to mu and delta receptors, or they could represent the binding site subunits of other receptors that have been postulated to have affinity for both mu and delta ligands, such as mu_1 (Nishimura et al., 1984) or epsilon (Chang et al., 1984) receptors. Further evidence that the labeling of all four peptides was pharmacologically relevant was provided by the finding that sodium (100 mM) and GTP (50 μM), when added during binding either separately or together, decreased or prevented the labeling of these four bands.

The earliest use of crosslinking to form covalent opioid receptor–ligand complexes was reported by Zukin and Kream (1979). Labeled derivatives of enkephalin were bound to rat brain synaptosomal/mitochondrial (P_2) fraction, solubilized with BRIJ 36T, and crosslinked with dimethyl suberimidate. The resultant macromolecular complex had a molecular weight of 380 kdalton on gel filtration and 35 kdalton on SDS-PAGE. No information was presented as to which type of opioid receptor this labeled complex may represent.

4. Purification

4.1. Partial Purification

There has been considerable progress in the purification of active opioid binding sites. At least partial purification has been achieved in several laboratories. In every case the major purification step involved affinity chromatography. This work will be summarized here.

The earliest partial purification was reported by Bidlack et al. (1981). Receptors solubilized from rat brain with Triton X-100 were purified on an affinity gel prepared by coupling a newly synthesized ligand, 14-β-bromoacetamidomorphine to aminohexyl-Sepharose. After removal of nonspecific proteins with buffer, receptor proteins were eluted with 1 μM levorphanol or etorphine. Dihydromorphine bound to the eluted receptor with high affinity (K_d = 3.8 nM) and its binding was readily inhibited by other opiates and by methionine-enkephalin. The purified receptor was found to bind 40 pmol of dihydromorphine per mg of protein. This represents only about 200–400-fold purification over membrane preparations. However, when SDS-PAGE was performed on purified receptor, only three protein bands of molecular weight 43, 35, and 23 kdalton were obtained. The authors suggest that the apparent discrepancy between the relatively modest purification and only three bands on the gels might be the result of partial inactivation of binding sites during purification.

A partial purification was reported from our laboratory (Gioannini et al., 1982), using wheat germ agglutinin-agarose (WGA-agarose). These lectin beads retain opioid receptors, indicating that they are glycoproteins (see above). A single passage of digitonin-solubilized receptors through a WGA-agarose column resulted in 25–35-fold purification, as determined from the specific binding of [³H]diprenorphine.

More recently, we reported (Gioannini et al., 1984) substantially improved purification using affinity chromatography. A newly synthesized derivative of naltrexone, β-naltrexyl-6-ethyl-enediamine (NED) was coupled to CH-Sepharose 4B, an agarose gel equipped with spacers ending in free carboxyl groups. Digitonin-solubilized receptors from the brains of rats, cows, and toads were efficiently retained by this column and could be eluted in yields of 20–25% with naloxone (1–3 μM). Purification achieved was 300–450-fold (specific binding of 0.5 nM ³H-diprenorphine was approximately 100 pmol/mg protein).

Cho et al. (1983) utilized another affinity gel and found that reconstitution of a protein and a lipid fraction was necessary to obtain stereospecific binding. The ligand, 6-succinylmorphine, was prepared and coupled to aminohexyl Sepharose as described by Simon et al. (1972). Attempts to elute binding sites from the column with either morphine or naloxone at concentrations up to 0.1 mM were not successful. High concentration of NaCl (a linear gradient of Tris buffer and Tris containing 1M NaCl) was therefore used for elution. The eluted protein exhibited very little binding of ³H-dihydromorphine inhibitable by unlabeled ligand, but, when combined with an acidic lipid fraction, eluted in a later peak from the same column, it showed stereospecific binding. Opiates of the mu type bound to this protein/lipid mixture with an order of affinities closely paralleling those to membrane-bound receptors, but 1–2 orders of magnitude lower. Binding of delta, kappa, and sigma ligands was much less. In a recent report these workers (Cho et al., 1985) were able to elute from the same affinity column an opiate-binding fraction in a single peak. This fraction contained both protein and acidic lipid and resembled the earlier reconstituted protein/lipid mixture very closely. This elution was achieved by using Tris buffer containing naloxone, NaCl, and CHAPS. Based on the protein content of this isolated opioid receptor, a 3200-fold purification over the original brain P_2 fraction had been achieved.

A partial purification of mu opioid receptors has been reported by Maneckjee et al. (1985). Opioid binding sites were solubilized from rat brain mitochondrial/synaptosomal (P_2) membranes using the zwitterionic detergent CHAPS. Purification was carried out on an affinity matrix made by attaching a newly synthesized compound named Hybromet to Affigel 401, an agarose derivative containing sulfhydryl groups. Hybromet, an analog of thebaine with a large substituent in the 7 position carrying an HgBr group, can bind tightly to the SH groups of Affigel 401. Elution of mu opioid receptors was accomplished with the selective mu ligand normorphine (1 μM). The degree of purification reported was 506-fold with an overall yield of 0.6%. The fold purification was based on the activity of the highly unstable CHAPS extract 5 d following solubilization. The B_{max} of the purified preparation was 2800 fmol/mg of protein, which is only about 20-fold higher than the B_{max} for etorphine binding in rat brain membranes. These workers have recently succeeded in stabilizing their CHAPS extracts and have combined their affinity chromatographic step with a hydroxyapatite column to obtain considerably higher purification (Zukin, personal communication). They have also compiled considerable evidence that their isolated binding site is derived from mu receptors, with little or no contamination from delta and kappa sites. Electrophoresis of purified protein on native polyacrylamide gels (PAGE) yielded a band with a M_r of 300–350 kdalton. Under denaturing conditions (SDS-PAGE), a major band of M_r 94 kdalton and minor bands at M_r 44 and 35 kdalton were seen.

Another report of partial purification of active opioid binding sites has come from Fujioka et al. (1985). This group constructed an affinity matrix by coupling DALE to AH-Sepharose (agarose containing amino sidechains). Solubilization was carried out by the digitonin method (Howells et al., 1982), as modified by

Demoliou-Mason and Barnard (1984). Binding sites were eluted from the affinity beads with 0.1 mM DALE in a batchwise procedure. The eluate was concentrated and then fractionated on Sepharose G-75. The purification reported was 450-fold. Rosenthal analysis of ^{3}H-DADLE binding gave a K_d of 34 nM and a B_{max} of 200 pmol/mg of protein. SDS-PAGE analysis yielded major bands at M_r 62 and 39 kdalton. Since delta-preferring ligands were used for purification and binding, the 62-kdalton band may represent a subunit of the delta receptor, in good agreement with the crosslinked polypeptide of M_r 58 kdalton of Klee et al. (1982). The crosslinked delta binding protein reported from our laboratory (Howard et al., 1985) is somewhat smaller (53 kdalton), possibly reflecting differences in the experimental conditions used.

4.2. Purification to Homogeneity

Purification of opioid binding proteins to apparent homogeneity has been reported to date from only two laboratories, one for an active binding subunit derived from mu receptors, the other for an affinity-labeled polypeptide derived from delta receptors.

Our laboratory (Gioannini et al., 1985) has recently succeeded in the purification to virtual homogeneity from bovine striatal membranes of a polypeptide of M_r 65 kdalton, which appears to be a binding component of mu receptors. The purification of digiton-solubilized receptors was accomplished in two steps (Table 1): affinity chromatography on NED-agarose, followed by lectin affinity chromatography on WGA-agarose. In an earlier report, discussed above (Gioannini et al., 1984), the purification achieved by affinity chromatography on NED-agarose was 300– 450-fold. By improvements in washing and elution procedures, as well as in the precision of measuring very small amounts of protein, the degree of purification achieved in a single passage through NED-agarose was improved to 3000–7000-fold. When the NED-eluate was further purified on WGA-agarose, a total purification of 65,000–75,000-fold was obtained (B_{max} for the binding of ^{3}H]bremazocine of approximately 13,000 pmol/mg protein), with an overall yield of approximately 6%. Theoretical purification, assuming a single binding site per 65,000 daltons, is 77,000-fold. When the purified material was run on SDS-PAGE, after light iodination with ^{125}I, a single protein band of M_r 65,000 was seen by autoradiography. The same protein band can also be visualized by silver staining when sufficient protein is put on the

TABLE 1
Purification of an Opioid Binding Protein from Bovine Striata Membranes[a,b]

Preparation	Protein, mg	Activity,[c] pmol	Step yield%		Overall yield%		Specific activity, B_{max} pmol/mg	Purification factor, x-fold
			Protein	Activity[c]	Protein	Activity[c]		
Membrane homogenate	3270	667	100	100	100	100	0.20	—
Digitonin extract	1308	258	40	38	40	38	0.19	1
Eluate from NED-Sepharose	0.070[d]	64	<0.001	24.8	<0.001	9.6	914	4570
Eluate from WGA-Agarose	0.003[e]	39	4.3	60.9	<0.001	5.8	13,000	65,000

[a]Data are from a typical experiment in which ~50 g of tissue was homogenized and solubilized with digitonin.
[b]From Gioannini et al., 1985.
[c]Measured by [^{3}H]bremazocine binding at 1.5 nM and B_{max} calculated from saturation curves at identical conditions (0.5 M NaCl, 0.05% digitonin). Values shown represent specific binding at saturation.
[d]Determined by densitometric scanning of Coomassie blue-stained SDS-PAGE gels using bovine serum albumin and carbonic anhydrase as calibration standards.
[e]Determined by amino acid analysis.

gel. The following evidence suggests that this purified protein represents a binding component of mu receptors: (1) bovine striatum contains very few delta receptors (<10%), (2) the matrix used has a preference for mu over kappa sites, (3) the 65-kdalton polypeptide has the same molecular size as the mu polypeptide crosslinked with β_h-end, (4) β_h-end can be crosslinked to the purified binding site, and (5) binding of [^{3}H]bremazocine to the purified receptor can be competed for by the highly mu-selective ligand, DAGO.

The other report of purification to apparent homogeneity comes from the laboratory of Klee (Simonds et al., 1985). As discussed earlier, this group had identified a binding subunit of delta opioid receptors from NG108-15 cells (Klee et al., 1982). This was a glycoprotein with a M_r value of 58,000 that had been affinity labeled with [^{3}H]FIT. For purification these workers used a more potent tritiated delta-selective analog, [^{3}H]3-methylfentanylisothiocyanate, named [^{3}H]superFIT. Purification was accomplished in five steps (Table 2): (1) labeling of opioid receptors in NG108-15 membranes with [^{3}H]superFIT; (2) solubilization in a mixture of lubrol and CHAPS; (3) adsorption to and elution from a WGA-agarose column; (4) immunoaffinity chromatography on a column of anti-FIT antibodies coupled to Sepharose 4B; and (5) preparative SDS-PAGE. This final step yielded a protein that was purified 30,000-fold with an overall yield of 2–3%. It migrated as a single component on SDS-PAGE with a M_r value of near 58,000. The material contained 1 mol of labeled superFIT per mol of protein, corresponding to 21,000 pmol per mg of protein, close to the theoretical specific activity for pure receptor.

5. Conclusions

As can be seen from this review, it took about 12 years before concrete progress was achieved in the purification of opioid receptors. This progress has been confined to the binding site portion of the receptors and has not so far been extended to other components of the receptor complex. The reason it took so long was not a lack of interest (attempts at isolation began shortly after their biochemical demonstration), but can be attributed in large part to the difficulty of this endeavor. Opioid receptors present a very small portion (approximately 0.001%) of the total cell membrane proteins. No enriched source for these receptors, equivalent to

TABLE 2
Purification of ^{3}H-super-FIT-Labeled Opiate Receptors[a]

Step	Vol, mL	Protein, μg	^{3}H, pmol	Specific activity		Recovery, %
				pmol per mg of protein	Range	
Detergent extract	1000	1270×10^3	889	0.7	0.6–2.1 ($n = 7$)	100
WGA-agarose eluate	13.5	22×10^3	807	37	21–58 ($n = 7$)	91
Anti-FIT-agarose						
FIT/lysine eluate	0.15	49	87	1,790	1,790–6,480 ($n = 6$)	10
Propionate eluate	0.15	16.2	70	4,320	2,140–4,320 ($n = 2$)	8
NaDodSO$_4$/PAGE eluate	0.17	0.385	8	20,800	20,800–22,700 ($n = 2$)	2

[a]From Simonds et al., 1985.

the electric organ of electric fish for acetycholine receptors, has yet been discovered. Nor is there a natural, tightly binding, highly specific probe similar to the snake toxins, such as α-bunga-rotoxin, that have proved so useful for the isolation of cholinergic receptors. A further obstacle was the remarkable sensitivity of opioid receptors to detergents, even those of the nonionic variety.

These obstacles have finally been overcome, and there are two reports of purification to homogeneity of opioid binding proteins, reviewed in the previous section. One appears to be a binding component of mu, the other of delta, receptors. In both cases the amino terminal was found to be blocked. It therefore becomes necessary to purify relatively large quantities of receptor (in the nanomole range) in order to facilitate fragmentation and purification of polypeptide fragments with free N-terminals for sequencing. This is a tedious task and new problems arise when a purification procedure is scaled up. There is reason for hope, however, that in the near future some amino acid sequence data will be available. Such sequences can then be used to prepare oligonucleotide probes for detection and isolation of cDNA complementary to receptor message from an appropriate cDNA library. This would permit total sequencing of the cDNA and thus yield the total amino acid sequence of the receptor protein.

Another area of research that has already begun to show results, but will now be greatly accelerated, is the production of antibodies to opioid receptor proteins. The availability of antibodies should further facilitate the distinction of opioid receptor types, speed receptor purification, and provide the means for detailed immunohistochemical mapping of the various types of opioid receptors. Such studies will complement the autoradiographic distribution studies already carried out and may shed some light on the mysterious discrepancies between the distribution of receptors and their putative natural opioid peptide ligands. Finally, reconstitution experiments of purified opioid binding sites and other receptor components (G protein, adenylate cyclase) into artificial or natural membranes should aid in the elucidation of the steps triggered by receptor–ligand interaction and in our understanding of the functions of the endogenous opioid system.

References

Archer, S., Michael, J., Osei-Gyimah, P., Seyed-Mozaffari, A., Zukin, R. S., Maneckjee, R., Simon, E. J., and Gioannini, T. L. (1985) Hybromet: A ligand for purifying opioid receptors. *J. Med. Chem.* **28,** 1950–1953.

Bidlack, J. M. and Abood, L. G. (1980) Solubilization of the opiate receptor. *Life Sci.* **27,** 331–340.

Bidlack, J. M., Abood, L. G., Osei-Gyimah, P., and Archer, S. (1981) Purification of the opiate receptor from rat brain. *Proc. Natl. Acad. Sci. USA* **78,** 636–639.

Bruns, R. F., Lawson-Wendling, K., and Pugsley, T. A. (1983) A rapid filtration assay for soluble receptors using polyethylenimine-treated filters. *Anal. Biochem.* **132,** 74–81.

Burke, T. R., Jr., Bajwa, B. S., Jacobson, A. E., Rice, K. C., Streaty, R. A., and Klee, W. A. (1984) Probes for narcotic receptor mediated phenomena. 7. Synthesis and pharmacological properties of irreversible ligands specific for mu and delta opiate receptors. *J. Med. Chem.* **27,** 1570–1574.

Caruso, T. P., Takemori, A. E., Larson, D. L., and Portoghese, P. S. (1979) Chloroxymorphamine, an opioid receptor site-directed alkylating agent having narcotic agonist activity. *Science* **204,** 316–318.

Caruso, T. P., Larson, D. L., Portoghese, P. S., and Takemori, A. E. (1980a) Pharmacological studies with an alkylating narcotic agonist chloroxymorphamine and antagonist, chlornaltrexamine. *J. Pharmacol. Exp. Ther.* **213,** 539–544.

Caruso, T. P., Larson, D. L., Portoghese, P. S., and Takemori, A. E. (1980b) Isolation of selective ^{3}H-chlornaltrexamine-bound complexes, possible opioid receptor components in brains of mice. *Life Sci.* **27,** 2063–2069.

Chang, K-J., Blanchard, S. G., and Cuatrecasas, P. (1984) Benzomorphan sites are ligand recognition sites of putative epsilon-receptors. *Mol. Pharmacol.* **26,** 484–488.

Changeux, J. P., Kasai, M., and Lee, C. Y. (1970) Use of a snake toxin to characterize the cholinergic receptor protein. *Proc. Natl. Acad. Sci. USA* **67,** 1241–1247.

Cho, T. M., Yamato, C., Cho, J. S., and Loh, H. H. (1981) Solubilization of membrane bound opiate receptors from rat brain. *Life Sci.* **28,** 2651–2657.

Cho, T. M., Ge, B. L., Yamato, C., Smith, A. P., and Loh, H. H. (1983) Isolation of opiate binding components by affinity chromatography and reconstitution of binding activities. *Proc. Natl. Acad. Sci. USA* **80,** 5176–5180.

Cho, T. M., Ge, B-L., and Loh, H. H. (1985) Isolation and purification of morphine receptor by affinity chromatography. *Life Sci.* **36,** 1075–1085.

Chow, T. and Zukin, R. S. (1983) Solubilization and preliminary characterization of mu and kappa opiate receptor subtypes from rat brain. *Mol. Pharmacol.* **24,** 203–212.

Cuatrecasas, P. (1972) Isolation of the insulin receptor of liver and fat-cell membranes. *Proc. Natl. Acad. Sci. USA* **69,** 318–322.

Demoliou-Mason, C. D. and Barnard, E. A. (1984) Solubilization in high yield of opioid receptors retaining high-affinity delta, mu and kappa binding sites. *FEBS Lett.* **170,** 378–382.

Fujioka, T., Inoue, F., and Kuriyama, M. (1985) Purification of opioid-binding materials from rat brain. *Biochem. Biophys. Res. Comm.* **131,** 640–646.

Garbay-Jaureguiberry, C., Robichon, A., and Roques, B. P. (1983) Selective photoinactivation of delta-opiate binding sites by azido DTLET: Tyr-D-Thr-Gly-pN₃PHE-Leu-Thr. *Life Sci.* **33,** (suppl. I), 247–250.

Gioannini, B., Foucaud, B., Hiller, J. M., Hatten, M. E., and Simon, E. J. (1982) Lectin binding of solubilized opiate receptors: Evidence for their glycoprotein nature. *Biochem. Biophys. Res. Comm.* **105,** 1128–1134.

Gioannini, T. L., Howard, A., Hiller, J. M., and Simon, E. J. (1984) Affinity chromatography of solubilized opioid binding sites using CH-Sepharose modified with a new naltrexone derivative. *Biochem. Biophys. Res. Comm.* **119,** 624–629.

Gioannini, T. L., Howard, A. D., Hiller, J. H., and Simon, E. J. (1985) Purification of an active opioid-binding protein from bovine striatum. *J. Biol. Chem.* **260,** 15117–15121.

Goeldner, M. P. and Hirth, C. G. (1980) Specific photoaffinity labeling induced by energy transfer. Application to the irreversible inhibition of acetylcholinesterase. *Proc. Natl. Acad. Sci. USA* **77,** 6439–6442.

Hahn, E. F., Carrol-Buatti, M., and Pasternak, G. W. (1982) Irreversible opiate agonists and antagonists: The 14-hydroxydihydromorphonone azines. *J. Neurosci.* **2,** 572–576.

Hazum, E., Chang, K-J., Shecter, Y., Wilkinson, S., and Cuatrecasas, P. (1979) Fluorescent and photo-affinity enkephalin derivatives: Preparation and interaction of opiate receptors. *Biochem. Biophys. Res. Comm.* **88,** 841–846.

Hjelmeland, L. (1980) A nondenaturing zwitterionic detertegent for membrane biochemistry: Design and synthesis. *Proc. Natl. Acad. Sci. USA* **77,** 6368–6370.

Howard, A. D., de la Baume, S., Gioannini, T. L., Hiller, J. M., and Simon, E. J. (1985) Covalent labeling of opioid receptors with radioiodinated human beta-endorphin. *J. Biol. Chem.* **260,** 10833–10839.

Howard, A. D., Sarne, Y., Gioannini, T. L., Hiller, J. M., and Simon, E. J. (1986) Identification of distinct binding site subunits of mu and delta opiate receptors. *Biochemistry* **25,** 357–360.

Howells, R. D., Gioannini, T. L., Hiller, J. M., and Simon, E. J. (1982) Solubilization and characterization of active opiate binding sites from mammalian brain. *J. Pharmacol. Exp. Ther.* **222,** 629–634.

Hummel, J. P. and Dreyer, W. J. (1962) Measurement of protein-binding phenomena by gel filtration. *Biochim. Biophys. Acta* **63,** 530–532.

Ilien, B., Gommeren, W., Leysen, J. E., and Laduron, P. M. (1982) Solubilized opiate receptors labeled with ³H-Lofentanil. *Arch. Int. Pharmacodyn. Ther.* **258,** 313–316.

Itzhak, Y., Hiller, J. M., and Simon, E. J. (1984a) Solubilization and characterization of mu, delta and kappa opioid binding sites from guinea pig brain: Physical separation of kappa receptors. *Proc. Natl. Acad. Sci. USA* **81,** 4217–4221.

Itzhak, Y., Hiller, J. M., and Simon, E. J. (1984b) Solubilization and characterization of kappa opioid binding sites from guinea pig cerebellum. *Neuropeptides* **5,** 201–204.

Itzhak, Y., Hiller, J. M., Gioannini, T. L., and Simon, E. J. (1984c) Effect of digitonin on the binding of opiate agonists and antagonists to membrane-bound and soluble opioid binding sites. *Brain Res.* **291,** 309–315.

James, I. F. and Goldstein, A. (1984) Site directed alkylation of multiple opioid receptors. I. Binding selectivity. *Mol. Pharmacol.* **25,** 337–342.

Jauzac, P., Puget, A., and Meunier, J. C. (1983) Physical separation of agonist and antagonist forms of a mu receptor? *Life Sci.* **33,** (suppl. I), 195–198.

Kieffer, B. L., Goeldner, M. P., and Hirth, C. G. (1981) Aryl diazonium salts as photo-affinity labeling reagents for proteins. *J. Chem. Soc. Chem. Commun.* 398–399.

Klee, W. A., Simonds, W. F., Sweat, F. W., Burke, T. R., Jr., Jacobson, A. E., and Rice, K. C. (1982) Identification of a M_r 58000 glycoprotein subunit of the opiate receptor. *FEBS Lett.* **150,** 125–128.

Koolpe, G. A., Nelson, W. L., Gioannini, T. L., Angel, L., and Simon, E. J. (1984) Diastereomeric 6-desoxy-6-spiro-alpha-methylene-gamma-butyrola cton derivatives of naltrexone and oxymorphone. Selective irreversible inhibition of naltrexone binding in an opioid receptor preparation by a conformationally restricted Michael acceptor ligand. *J. Med. Chem.* **27,** 1718–1723.

Koolpe, G. A., Nelson, W. L., Gioannini, T. L., Angel, L., Appelmans, N., and Simon, E. J. (1985) Opioid agonists and antagonists. 6-Desoxy-6-substituted lactone, epoxide, and glycidate ester derivatives of naltrexone and oxymorphone. *J. Med. Chem.* **28,** 949–957.

Kotzyba-Hibert, F., Langenbuch-Cachet, J., Jaganathen, A., Goeldner, M., and Hirth, C. G. (1985) Aryldiazonium salts as photoaffinity labels of the nicotinic acetylcholine receptor PCP binding site. *FEBS Lett.* **182,** 297–301.

Lee, T. T., Williams, R. E., and Fox, C. F. (1979) Photoaffinity inactivation of the enkephalin receptor. *J. Biol. Chem.* **254,** 11787–11790.

Maneckjee, R., Zukin, R. S., Archer, S., Michael, J., and Osei-Gyimah, P. (1985) Purification and characterization of the mu opiate receptor from rat brain using affinity chromatography. *Proc. Natl. Acad. Sci. USA* **82,** 594–598.

Maryanoff, B. E., Simon, E. J., Gioannini, T., and Gorissen, H. (1982) Potential affinity labels for the opiate receptor based on fentanyl and related compounds. *J. Med. Chem.* **25,** 913–919.

Newman, E. L. and Barnard, E. A. (1984) Identification of an opioid receptor subunit carrying the mu binding site. *Biochemistry* **23,** 5385–5389.

Nishimura, S. L., Recht, L. D., and Pasternak, G. W. (1984) Biochemical characterization of high-affinity ^{3}H-opioid binding. Further evidence for mu$_1$ sites. *Mol. Pharmacol.* **25,** 29–37.

Pelton, J. T., Johnson, R. B., Balk, J. L., Schmidt, C. J., and Roche, E. B. (1980) Synthesis and biological activity of chloromethylketones of leucine enkephalin. *Biochem. Biophys. Res. Comm.* **97,** 1391–1398.

Pert, C. B. and Snyder, S. H. (1973) Opiate receptor: Demonstration in nervous tissue. *Science* **179,** 1011–1014.

Portoghese, P. S., Larson, D. L., Jiang, J. B., Takemori, A. E., and Caruso, T. P. (1978) 6-β-[*N,N*-bis(2-chloroethyl)amino]-17(cyclopropylmethyl)-4,5α-epoxy-3,14-dihydroxymorphinan   (chlornaltrexamine),   a   potent opioid receptor alkylating agent with ultralong narcotic antagonist activity. *J. Med. Chem.* **21,** 598–599.

Portoghese, P. S., Larson, D. L., Jiang, J. B., Caruso, T. P., and Takemori, A. E. (1979) Synthesis and pharmacologic characterization of an alkylating analogue (chlornaltrexamine) of naltrexone with ultralong-lasting narcotic antagonist properties. *J. Med. Chem.* **22,** 168–173.

Portoghese, P. S., Larson, D. L., Sayre, L. M., Fries, D. S., and Takemori, A. E. (1980) A novel opioid receptor site directed alkylating agent with irreversible narcotic antagonistic and reversible agonistic activities. *J. Med. Chem.* **23,** 233–234.

Puget, A., Jauzac, P., and Meunier, J. C. (1980) Hydrodynamic properties of a ^{3}H-etorphine macromolecular complex from rat brain. *FEBS Lett.* **122,** 199–202.

Rice, K. C., Shiotani, S., Creveling, C. R., Jacobson, A. E., and Klee, W. A. (1977) N-(2,4,5-trihydroxyphenethyl)normetazocine, a potential irreversible inhibitor of the narcotic receptor. *J. Med. Chem.* **20,** 673–675.

Rice, K. C., Jacobson, A. E., Burke, T. E., Jr., Bajwa, B. S., Streaty, R. A., and Klee, W. A. (1982) Irreversible ligands with high selectivity toward delta and mu opiate receptors. *Science* **220,** 314–316.

Robson, L. E. and Kosterlitz, H. W. (1979) Specific protection of the binding site of D-Ala^2- D-Leu^5-enkephalin (delta receptors) and dihydromorphine (mu-receptors). *Proc. R. Soc. Lond. (Biol.)* **205,** 425–432.

Robson, L. E., Foote, R. W., Maurer, R., and Kosterlitz, H. W. (1984) Opioid binding sites of the kappa-type in guinea pig cerebellum. *Neuroscience* **12,** 621–627.

Rothman, R. B. and Westfall, T. C. (1982) Allosteric coupling between morphine and enkephalin receptors in vitro. *Mol. Pharmacol.* **21,** 548–557.

Ruegg, U. T., Hiller, J. M., and Simon, E. J. (1980) Solubilization of an active opiate receptor from *Bufo marinus. Eur. J. Pharmacol.* **64,** 367–368.

Ruegg, U. T., Cuenoud, S., Hiller, J. M., Gioannini, T., Howells, R. D., and Simon, E. J. (1981) Characterization and partial purification of solubilized active opiate receptors from toad brain. *Proc. Natl. Acad. Sci. USA* **78,** 4635–4638.

Ruegg, U. T., Cuenoud, S., Fulpius, B. W., and Simon, E. J. (1982) Inactivation and solubilization of opiate receptors by phospholipase A2. *Biochim. Biophys. Acta* **685,** 241–248.

Simon, E. J., Dole, W. P., and Hiller, J. M. (1972) Coupling of a new, active morphine derivative to Sepharose for affinity chromatography. *Proc. Natl. Acad. Sci. USA* **69,** 1835–1837.

Simon, E. J., Hiller, J. M., and Edelman, I. (1973) Stereospecific binding of the potent narcotic analgesic ^{3}H-etorphine to rat brain homogenate. *Proc. Natl. Acad. Sci. USA* **70,** 1947–1949.

Simon, E. J., Hiller, J. M., and Edelman, I. (1975) Solubilization of a stereospecific opiate-macromolecular complex from rat brain. *Science* **190,** 389–390.

Simon, E. J., Hiller, J. M., Groth, J., Itzhak, Y., Holland, M. J., and Beck, S. G. (1982) The nature of opiate receptors in toad brain. *Life Sci.* **31,** 1367–1370.

Simon, J., Benyhe, S., Borsodi, A. Szucs, M., and Wollemann, M. (1984) Separation of kappa-opioid receptor subtype from brain. *FEBS Lett.* **183,** 395–397.

Simonds, W. F., Koski, G., Streaty, R. A., Hjelmeland, L. M., and Klee, W. A. (1980) Solubilization of active opiate receptors. *Proc. Natl. Acad. Sci. USA* **77,** 4623–4627.

Simonds, W. F., Burke, T. R., Jr., Rice, K. C., Jacobson, A. E., and Klee, W. A. (1985) Purification of the opiate receptor of NG108-15 neuroblastoma glioma hybrid cells. *Proc. Natl. Acad. Sci. USA* **82,** 4974–4978.

Singh, A., Thornton, E. R., and Westheimer, F. H. (1962) The photolysis of diazoacetyl chymotrypsin. *J. Biol. Chem.* **237,** 3006–3008.

Smith, J. R. and Simon, E. J. (1980) Selective protection of stereospecific enkephalin and opiate binding against inactivation by N-ethylmaleimide: Evidence for two classes of opiate receptors. *Proc. Natl. Acad. Sci. USA* **77,** 281–284.

Smolarsky, M. and Koshland, D. E., Jr. (1980) Inactivation of the opiate receptor in bovine caudate nucleus by azide enkephalin analogs. *J. Biol. Chem.* **255,** 7244–7249.

Szucs, M., Benyhe, S., Borsodi, A., Wolleman, M., Jancso, G., Szecsi, J., and Medzihradsky, K. (1983) Binding characteristics and analgesic activity of D-ala^2-leu^5-enkephalin chloromethyl ketone. *Life Sci.* **32,** 2777–2784.

Takemori, A. E., Larson, D. L., and Portoghese, P. S. (1981) The irreversible narcotic antagonistic and reversible agonist properties of the fumarate methyl ester derivative of naltrexone. *Eur. J. Pharmacol.* **70,** 445–451.

Terenius, L. (1973) Stereospecific interaction between narcotic analgesics and a synaptic plasma membrane fraction of rat cerebral cortex. *Acta Pharmacol. Toxicol.* **32,** 317–320.

Venn, R. F. and Barnard E. A. (1981) A potent peptide affinity reagent for the opiate receptor. *J. Biol. Chem.* **256,** 1529–1532.

Ward, S. J., Portoghese, P. S., and Takemori, A. E. (1982a) Pharmacological profiles of beta-funaltrexamine (beta-FNA) and beta-chlornaltrexamine (beta-CNA) on the mouse vas deferens preparation. *Eur. J. Pharmacol.* **80,** 377–384.

Ward, S. J., Portoghese, P. S., and Takemori, A. E. (1982b) Improved assays for the assessment of kappa- and delta-properties of opioid ligands. *Eur. J. Pharmacol.* **85,** 163–170.

Ward, S. J., Fries, D. S., Larson, D. L., Portoghese, P. S., and Takemori, A. E. (1985) Opioid receptor binding characteristics of the nonequilibrium mu antagonist, beta-funaltrexamine (beta-FNA). *Eur. J. Pharmacol.* **107,** 323–330.

Winter, B. A. and Goldstein, A. (1972) A photochemical affinity-labeling reagent for the opiate receptor(s). *Mol. Pharmacol.* **8,** 601–611.

Zioudrou, C., Varoucha, D., Loukas, S., Nicolaou, N., Streaty, R. A., and Klee, W. A. (1983) Photolabile opioid derivatives of D-ala^2-leu^5-enkephalin and their interactions with the opiate receptor. *J. Biol. Chem.* **258,** 10934–10937.

Zukin, R. S. and Kream, R. M. (1979) Chemical crosslinking of a solubilized enkephalin macromolecular complex. *Proc. Natl. Acad. Sci. USA* **76,** 1593–1597.

SECTION 3
LOCATION OF
OPIOID RECEPTORS

Chapter 7

Regional Distribution of Opioid Receptors

Robert R. Goodman, Benjamin A. Adler, and Gavril W. Pasternak

1. Introduction

The development of biochemical techniques to quantitatively determine the interaction of drugs or neurotransmitters with their receptor site(s) was understandably met with enthusiasm by the scientific community. Homogenate binding studies provided a wealth of biochemical information, but only a limited amount of neuroanatomical data. The major problem was the limited resolution associated with macroscopic dissections, which resulted in only very general localizations of drug and neurotransmitter receptors. The development of autoradiography with its microscopic resolution was a major advance. Technical issues as well as the identification of various subtypes of opioid receptors have greatly complicated the interpretation of autoradiographic studies over the past decade. Initially, most investigators assumed the presence of a single class of receptor, as suggested by standard homogenate binding assays. To facilitate their studies, investigators chose radioligands upon the basis of their potency and technical factors, such as the ratio of specific to nonspecific binding, not aware that some compounds nonselectively labeled a variety of opioid receptor subtypes, whereas others were relatively selective. It soon became apparent that the various opioid receptor subtypes mediated different actions, underscoring the importance of establishing the differential distributions of subtypes of opiate binding sites.

As the pharmacology of opiate actions advanced, so did many technical aspects of autoradiography. Early studies were simply descriptive. The subsequent development of in vitro labeling approaches offered several advantages, such as comparing virtually identical adjacent sections under different binding conditions. The next milestone was the availability of tritium-sensitive film. Instead of tedious grain counting, accurate and rapid quantification could be obtained with computerized densitometry. Soon computerized image digitization with full quantification was expected for all publications. Recently potential sources of small, but potentially important, systematic errors were reported, including the differential quenching of tritium (Alexander et al., 1981; Herkenham and Sokoloff, 1984; Kuhar and Unnerstall, 1985). White matter, by virtue of its higher density, absorbs more β emissions from tritium than gray matter. Therefore, given equal levels of radioactivity, the density of autoradiographic grains in white matter is lower than in gray. If brain regions contained solely gray or white matter, this obstacle could easily be overcome by simply including two sets of standards. Most regions contain varying mixtures of white and gray tissue, however, greatly complicating results. Defatting the tissue will eliminate differential quenching, but the procedure also greatly lowers opioid binding, eliminating any simple solutions (Kuhar and Unnerstall, 1982). Although this factor complicates the comparison of binding among various regions, much of the information used to differentiate multiple receptor subtypes is not altered by this phenomenon since it involves comparisons of different ligands within the same region with a relatively constant amount of quenching for each. Furthermore, variability among different animals is usually far greater than the effects of differential quenching. Together, however, these issues require great caution in the interpretation of absolute levels of binding and most studies should be considered to be semiquantitative.

Cross binding of ligands among various receptor subtypes has also created difficulties. Virtually no ligand will label a single site. Thus, analysis of receptor subtypes must be indirect, utilizing selective displacement of one or more subpopulations of sites. In some circumstances, such as the distribution of mu_1 sites, complex subtraction approaches needed to be employed in order to establish a regional distribution. These last issues may soon be overcome, however, as more selective agents continue to be synthesized.

2. Early Autoradiographic Studies

2.1. In Vivo Autoradiography

Early homogenate binding studies revealed high levels of binding in limbic areas (medial thalamus, amygdala, and hippocampus) and the caudate nucleus, with very low binding in other areas, such as the cerebellum (Kuhar et al., 1973; LaMotte et al., 1978). Using [^{3}H]diprenorphine, an antagonist with high affinity for opiate binding sites, Kuhar's group developed the first autoradiographic techniques used to localize opiate receptors at the light microscopic level, permitting far more detailed studies (Pert et al., 1975, 1976). Following the systemic administration of a radiolabeled ligand, they fixed and sectioned the brain and then exposed the sections to emulsion-coated slides. This approach quickly revealed unique distributions of binding that could not be appreciated with homogenate binding experiments: dense clusters of binding sites within the striatum, a subcallosal streak consisting of a thin, dense band of grains just ventral to the corpus callosum, as well as high levels within the amygdala, interpeduncular nucleus, substantia gelatinosa of the spinal cord, locus ceruleus, and zona compacta of the substantia nigra. The cerebellum and white matter areas contained few binding sites. Since the multiplicity of receptors was not appreciated, radioligands were chosen on the basis of their affinities and other technical factors. [^{3}H]Diprenorphine is relatively nonspecific and labels several different classes of binding sites with high affinity. Thus, its autoradiograms reflect the summation of several receptor subtypes, although we can now appreciate their predominantly "mu" pattern. Similar findings were reported by Pearson and coworkers (1980). Duka et al. (1981a,b) reported similar distributions of [^{3}H]etorphine, an agonist with a selectivity similar to that of diprenorphine.

Shortly thereafter, Atweh and Kuhar (1977a,b,c) published a detailed description of the distribution of [^{3}H]diprenorphine binding throughout the central nervous system, providing an excellent correlation between regions capable of mediating the various opiate actions and those containing receptors (Table 1). Areas implicated in opioid analgesia, such as layers I and II of the spinal cord, the periaqueductal and periventricular gray regions, certain raphe nuclei, and intralaminar and medial thalamic nuclei, all possess high levels of binding. Other localizations were not anticipated, however, including high levels of opioid receptors in parts of the limbic system (nucleus accumbens, lateral septal nucleus, hippocampus, olfactory tubercle, amygdala, and several hypothalamic nuclei) and various other sensory processing areas (inferior and superior colliculi, layers I and III of the neocortex,

TABLE 1
Correlation of Opiate Action with Receptor Localization[a]

Opioid action	Receptor localization
Analgesia	
Spinal, body	Laminae I and II of spinal cord
Trigeminal, face	Substantia gelatinosa of trigeminal nerve
Supraspinal	Periaqueductal gray, medial thalamic nuclei, intralaminar thalamic nuclei
Autonomic reflexes	
Cough suppression, orthostatic hypotension, inhibition of gastric secretion	N. tractus solitarius, commisuralis, ambiguus, and locus ceruleus
Respiratory depression	N. tractus solitarius, parabrachial nuclei
Nausea and vomiting	Area postrema
Meiosis	Superior colliculus, pretectal nuclei
Endocrine effects	
Inhibition of vasopressin release	Posterior pituitary
Hormonal effects	Hypothalamic infundibulum, hypothalamic nuclei, accessory optic system, ? amygdala
Behavioral and mood effects	Amygdala, N. stria terminalis, hippocampus, cortex, medial thalamic nuclei, N. accumbens, ? basal ganglia
Motor rigidity	Striatum

[a]Adapted from Atweh and Kuhar, 1983.

the parabrachial nuclei, vestibular nuclei, the dorsal cochlear nucleus, and the accessory optic tract). The cranial parasympathetic nuclei (e.g., Edinger-Westphal and vagal nuclei) also contained moderate densities of binding sites.

Other distributions of opiate binding sites correlated well with their pharmacology, such as the association of opiate respiratory depression with opiate receptors in the nucleus tractus solitarius and the dorsal motor nucleus of the vagus nucleus. Similarly, hypothalamic receptors located in the paraventricular and other nuclei might play a role in the actions of opiates on feeding or on the release of hypothalamic releasing hormones. Receptors located in the preoptic, anterior, and medial basal hypothalamus probably mediate most of these effects. Opioid receptors in the pretectal area, superior colliculus, and accessory optic nuclei may be responsible for miosis. Antitussive actions might be caused by modulation of the sensory input from the throat at the level of the nucleus tractus solitarius, whereas emesis is probably associated with receptors in the area postrema. Thus, the autoradiographic localization of opiate receptors has greatly enhanced our understanding of opiate physiology and pharmacology.

2.2. In Vitro Autoradiography

The in vivo approach provided several advances, as detailed above, but drawbacks prompted Young and Kuhar (1979) to develop an in vitro labeling technique. Comparing adjacent sections separately in vitro offered many advantages over in vivo techniques, particularly allowing the accurate comparison of different subtypes of opiate receptors. Other advantages include the ability to (1) compare multiple radioligands, (2) examine the effects of different conditions, (3) use lipophobic and lower-affinity ligands, and (4) study large animals (e.g., primates). Furthermore, the method was applicable to human tissue. The technique was based upon that of Roth et al. (1974) and consisted of binding the radioligands to thin sections mounted on gelatin-coated slides, after which they were dried and exposed to emulsion for varying periods of time, depending upon the levels of radioactivity in the section. The coverslips were developed and the sections stained. This approach (Young and Kuhar, 1979) yielded results very similar to those obtained in the in vivo technique and identified two areas that had not previously been noted to have significant opiate receptor densities (layer I of the cerebral cortex and the pyriform cortex). Subsequent studies in monkey brain determined opioid receptor localization in the primate CNS (Wamsley et al., 1982; Wise and Herkenham, 1982). The similarity to localizations in the rat was striking, but of particular note were both the lack of clusters in the corpus striatum and the marked variations throughout the cerebral cortex.

Next came quantification using tritium standards to generate standard curves, permitting the determination of tissue levels of radioactivity (Unnerstall et al., 1982; Rainbow et al., 1982). It quickly became apparent that the time of exposure and concentration of radioactivity are critical factors in determining the grain density produced and that the relationships are not simply linear. Differential quenching between gray and white matter was also noted, as discussed above (Herkenham and Sokoloff, 1984).

The development of tritium-sensitive film and the ability to use a single sheet of film for dozens of sections at once greatly simplified autoradiography (Palacios et al., 1981; Penny et al., 1981). The large size of the film also permitted studies of sections larger than standard slides. Most important, film allowed computerized microdensitometry for a more practical quantification of binding levels. The coverslip technique with its superior resolution and more precise anatomical alignment, however, still has an important place in autoradiography.

Despite the large amount of information available from quantitative autoradiography at the light level (*see* review by Wamsley, 1983), little is known about their ultrastructural localization, which requires resolution at the level of electron microscopy. Recently, Hamel and Beaudet (1984) used electron microscopic techniques with probability analysis to examine opiate receptors in the rat neostriatum and noted a relatively low percentage of receptors associated with synaptic junctions.

3. Ontogeny of Opioid Receptors

The ontogeny of opioid receptors in homogenate binding assays revealed a relatively late appearance of sites at embryonic day 14 and large increases in binding densities postnatally (Coyle and Pert, 1976; Garcin and Coyle, 1976; Clendenin et al., 1976; Pasternak et al., 1980; Zhang and Pasternak, 1981). Early in vitro autoradiographic studies using the relatively mu-selective antagonist [^{3}H]naloxone detected binding by day 14–15 of gestation, whereas [^{3}H]DADL binding was not seen until embryonic day 18

(Kent et al., 1982). Unlike the striatal [^{3}H]naloxone binding, the increase in [^{3}H]DADL binding in the medial septum and frontal neocortex was more gradual, findings which were confirmed by Recht et al. (1985).

Postnatal studies reported the presence of [^{3}H]dihydromorphine binding in the hippocampus as early as day 2 (Unnerstall et al., 1983). The time course of receptor appearance and clustering in the pyramidal cell layer of the hippocampus prompted the authors to suggest that these receptors are located on Golgi type II inhibitory neurons in this layer. Differences in the distribution of receptors in the olfactory bulb were noted between day 2, when high levels of binding in the external plexiform layer were seen, and in the adult (day 21) when the granule cell layer and glomeruli were heavily labeled. Both binding site density and distribution in the striatum, neocortex, and olfactory tubercle in this mu agonist study were similar to those of Kent et al. (1982), supporting the mu character of labeling seen with the mu antagonist [^{3}H]naloxone.

4. Presynaptic and Postsynaptic Localization of Opioid Binding Sites

Opiate binding sites have been localized both pre- and postsynaptically. The spinal cord, in which sensory input can be easily disrupted by dorsal rhizotomy, and the striatum, in which both presynaptic distributions on dopamine terminals and postsynaptic distributions on intrinsic neurons can be examined, have been studied most extensively.

4.1. Striatum and Limbic System

The distribution of opioid binding sites between intrinsic neurons and afferent nerve terminals has been studied extensively. Either intracerebroventricular 6-hydroxydopamine (6-OHDA) or electrolytic lesions of the substantia nigra decrease both [^{3}H]naloxone and [^{3}H][Leu^5]enkephalin binding, suggesting that both mu and delta receptors are present presynaptically on dopaminergic nerve terminals in the striatum (Pollard et al., 1977a,b, 1978). Comparisons between the two ligands, however, is difficult since one is an agonist, whereas the other is an antagonist. The ability of kainic acid to reduce [^{3}H][Leu^5]enkephalin binding by 45% implied that intrinsic neurons also contain opioid receptors. Similarly, destruction of dopamine cell bodies in the ventral tegmental area reduced [³H]naloxone binding in the septum and nucleus accumbens. Others have also observed decreases in [³H]naloxone binding following 6-OHDA lesions. Reisine et al. (1979) reported a 28% decrease on the denervated side, but also found a 26% increase in [³H]naloxone binding in the frontal cortex. In their hands, striatal kainate lesions did not alter [³H]naloxone binding, perhaps reflecting a combined loss of receptors on intrinsic neurons with an increase of presynaptic sites.

The localization of the 6-OHDA lesion within the substantia nigra may play an important role on the effects on binding (Gardner et al., 1980). Lesions placed medially, characterized by contraversive rotational behavior after systemic apomorphine, decreased [³H][D-Ala²-Met⁵]enkephalin (DALA) binding in the striatum and amygdala, whereas laterally placed lesions, characterized by ipsiversive rotations, increased [³H]DALA binding. These results led the authors to speculate that the lesion of the lateral substantia nigra produced a denervation supersensitivity or upregulation, whereas the loss of [³H]DALA binding with medial lesions reflected the loss of receptors located presynaptically on dopaminergic nerve terminals in the striatum. The effects of 6-OHDA and kainic acid lesions on [³H]diprenorphine binding has also been reported (Murrin et al., 1980). Kainate lesions of the striatum decreased [³H]diprenorphine binding 83% in striatal clusters. Medial forebrain bundle lesions and intrastriatal 6-OHDA reduced the diffuse striatal [³H]diprenorphine binding 22 and 28%, respectively, with much smaller effects on the cluster binding. They concluded that the majority of opioid receptors in the striatum is localized postsynaptically on intrinsic neurons. Parenti et al. (1983) localized [³H][D-Ala²-Met⁵]enkephalinami binding sites in rat striatum after transection of the nucleus raphe dorsalis (NRD) or intraventricular 5,6-dihydroxytryptamine and noted a significant decrease in the striatum after NRD transection, suggesting the presence of opioid receptors on serotonin nerve terminals ending in the striatum.

Abou-Khalil et al. (1984) studied [³H]DADL and [³H]naloxone binding autoradiographically in rat striatum, globus pallidus, and substantia nigra after unilateral kainate lesions. The lesions reduced [³H]DADL and [³H]naloxone binding 70–80 and 20–35%, respectively, in the striatum. Caution must be exercised in interpreting the differences between the two ligands since one is an agonist, and the other is an antagonist. The reduction of [³H]DADL binding by 31 and

41% in the globus pallidus and substantia nigra, respectively, supports the hypothesis that striatal efferent fibers represent another central nervous system pathway containing opioid receptors presynaptically.

4.2. Spinal Cord

Sectioning dorsal roots consistently decreased binding in the dorsal horn of the spinal cord, suggesting the presence of some binding sites on primary afferent nerve terminals. LaMotte et al. (1976) noted a decrease in [^{3}H]naloxone binding in layers I–III of the monkey dorsal horn, whereas others reported a 40% decrease in [^{3}H]diprenorphine binding in the dorsal horn (Jessell et al., 1979). Autoradiographic approaches revealed similar findings in the rat spinal cord, with a 40% reduction in layers I and II (Ninkovic et al., 1981, 1982). Sectioning the sciatic nerve, which contains both motor and sensory fibers, reduces both [^{3}H]morphine and [^{3}H]DADL binding, suggesting that small diameter primary afferents contain both mu and delta binding sites (Fields et al., 1980). In subsequent studies, Csillik et al. (1982) examined [^{3}H]diprenorphine binding following peripheral nerve transection and found a shift of [^{3}H]diprenorphine binding sites in the dorsal horn, with a decrease over nerve fibers and an increase over nerve cell bodies in layers I, II, and III.

Neonatal capsaicin treatment provides another experimental approach to the localization of binding sites by inducing a degeneration of small fiber sensory neurons. Capsaicin lowered [^{3}H]diprenorphine binding by 37%, a result quite similar to sectioning studies and consistent with the presence of binding sites on small, chemosensitive primary sensory neurons (Gamse et al., 1979). The interpretation of these findings is not entirely certain since the effects of early lesions on development of pathways are not understood.

4.3. Other Studies

Other investigations also supported presynaptic opioid binding sites. Atweh et al. (1978) reported a decrease in [^{3}H]diprenorphine binding in the rat vagus nerve and accessory optic system following vagotomy and enucleation, respectively. Vagotomy also reduced the number of opioid receptors associated with the nucleus of the solitary tract and nucleus ambiguus. Herkenham

and Pert (1980) compared the distribution of [³H]naloxone binding sites autoradiographically with that of known neuronal
pathways determined by tracing injected ³H-amino acids. They
reported two major pathways. The first described fibers travers-
ing from the bed nucleus of the stria terminalis to the medial
habenula, whereas the second demonstrated a pathway from the
medial habenula to the median raphe and interpeduncular nucleus. Interestingly, the bed nucleus of the stria terminalis, the
medial habenula, the median raphe, and the interpeduncular nucleus all contain high or very high concentrations of opioid receptors. Another area with high levels of opioid receptors is the
amygdala, which has projections to the bed nucleus of the stria
terminalis. These findings support the concept that known
neuroanatomical pathways may, at least in part, be "opioidergic"
(Herkenham and Pert, 1980).

5. Localization of Multiple Opioid Receptor Subtypes

5.1. Mu and Delta Receptors

Autoradiographic studies using delta and mu iodinated enkephalins in the rat central nervous system (Goodman et al., 1980; Duka
et al., 1981a,b; Gulya et al., 1985; Quirion et al., 1983) confirmed
the biochemical and pharmacological studies suggesting distinct
mu and delta receptors (Lord et al., 1977; Chang and Cuatrecasas,
1979; Chang et al., 1979). Mu receptors were densely localized in
the clusters of the striatum, the subcallosal streak, layers I and IV
of cerebral cortex, certain thalamic areas, hypothalamus, interpeduncular nucleus, pyramidal cell layer of the hippocampus, and
periaqueductal gray. In contrast, delta receptors appeared more
localized to layers II, III, and V of the cerebral cortex, the amygdala, olfactory tubercle, and pontine nuclei, and diffusely in the
striatum with an increasing dorsomedial to ventrolateral gradient,
nucleus accumbens, and hippocampus. Many regions contained
both mu and delta sites, including the nucleus ambiguus, nucleus
tractus solitarius, substantia gelatinosa of the spinal cord and trigeminal tract, and layer VI of the cerebral cortex. The existence
of multiple classes of receptors raised the question of which
subtypes mediated the various aspects of opioid actions. The relative concentration of mu receptors in many areas associated with

the transmission of nociceptive stimuli supported the involvement of mu receptors in antinociception. Similarly, the relative density of delta receptors in many limbic areas raised the possibility of an association of these sites with behavioral and mood effects.

Studies of mu and delta localizations in other species have also proven important. In monkey cortex, mu receptors increase in density toward more intricate sensory processing areas, whereas delta receptors maintain a constant density throughout the cortex (Lewis et al., 1981). The distributions in mouse brain are quite similar to those in the rat (Moskowitz and Goodman, 1984). Unanticipated observations included high levels of mu receptors relative to delta receptors in the claustrum, the subthalamic nucleus, medial and lateral mammillary nuclei, and ventral pallidum. High levels of delta receptors relative to mu receptors were reported in mouse amygdala, substantia nigra-pars reticulata, pyriform cortex, and hippocampus. Many areas of the mouse brain contained similar levels of mu and delta receptors, including the interstitial nucleus of the stria terminalis, raphe nuclei, dorsal motor nucleus of the vagus, and globus pallidus.

5.2. Mu$_1$ Receptors

The mu$_1$ receptor is one of the newest subdivisions of opioid receptors, and is unique since it has similar, very high affinities for opiates, enkephalins, and β-endorphin (Wolozin and Pasternak, 1981; Pasternak and Wood, 1986). Its association with certain pharmacological actions, including supraspinal analgesia, but not others such as respiratory depression, emphasizes its importance. Homogenate studies have suggested a distinct localization in the brain using both competition approaches and selective mu$_1$ antagonists (Goodman et al., 1985; Zhang and Pasternak, 1980; Johnson and Pasternak, 1984; Hahn et al., 1982). A unique anatomical localization of the high-affinity mu$_1$ opioid receptor now has been demonstrated in mouse brain, using a grain-counting technique (Moskowitz and Goodman, 1985a,b), and in rat brain, using a computerized digital subtraction approach (Goodman and Pasternak, 1985).

The lack of suitable mu$_1$-selective radioligands made these studies difficult. Identifying mu$_1$ sites therefore rested upon the ability of compounds such as [³H]dihydromorphine and [³H][D-Ala²-D-Leu⁵]enkephalin (DADL) to label both mu$_1$ and either mu$_2$ or delta sites, respectively. Total specific binding then reflects two different classes of sites (mu_1 + mu_2 or mu_1 + delta). The mu_1 binding is then selectively inhibited, leaving only mu_2 or delta binding, and the difference corresponds to mu_1 sites. Unlabeled DADL inhibited the mu_1 component of [^{3}H]dihydromorphine binding, whereas morphine eliminated the mu_1 binding of [^{3}H]DADL. The mouse studies (Moskowitz and Goodman, 1985a,b) used grain counting to quantitate binding in regions and then subtracted binding with, from that without, mu_1 competition to determine levels of mu_1 sites. The rat studies (Goodman and Pasternak, 1985) also utilized this type of subtraction technique, but had the computer perform pixel-by-pixel subtractions of the two superimposable images and then generate an image of the competed mu_1 binding. In the mouse, the ventral periaqueductal gray and layers I and II of the spinal cord, two areas intimately concerned with the transmission of pain impulses, contain high levels of mu_1 receptors. Of particular interest, the dorsal motor nucleus of the vagus and the nucleus of the solitary tract, regions involved in the control of respiration, contain few mu_1 sites. Although the general distributions of the two mu receptors are similar, the ratio of mu_1/mu_2 sites varied markedly from region to region, supporting the concept of a discrete mu_1 receptor (Table 2).

In an effort to correlate mu_1 receptors with analgesia, Moskowitz and Goodman also compared the densities of the binding subtypes in two strains of mice that varied in their sensitivity to mor-

TABLE 2
Regional Distribution of Mu$_1$, Mu$_2$, and Delta Binding in the Mouse[a]

Region	Mu$_1$	Mu$_2$	Delta	Mu$_1$/mu$_2$	Mu$_1$/delta
Frontal cortex					
Lamina I	17.1	5.6	39.7	3.05	0.43
Lamina II/III	ND[b]	7.0	39.7	0	0
Lamina IV	9.9	2.8	43.7	3.54	0.23
Lamina V	8.5	2.8	63.8	3.04	0.13
Lamina VI	8.5	2.8	35.7	3.04	0.24
Temporal cortex					
Lamina I	ND	17.0	27.7	0	0
Lamina II/III	ND	9.8	59.8	0	0
Lamina IV	ND	21.2	31.7	0	0
Lamina V	ND	21.2	23.7	0	0
Pyriform cortex					
pyramidal layer	7.1	12.7	27.7	0.56	0.26

(continued)

TABLE 2 (*continued*)
Regional Distribution of Mu$_1$, Mu$_2$, and Delta Binding in the Mouse[a]

Region	Mu$_1$	Mu$_2$	Delta	Mu$_1$/mu$_2$	Mu$_1$/delta
Olfactory tubercle pyriform layer	ND	11.3	47.7	0	0
Interstitial N. of stria terminalis	14.5	64.4	71.8	0.23	0.20
Striatum					
Patches	59.3	32.7	ND	1.81	0
Diffuse, caudal	ND	17.0	47.7	0	0
Ventral pallidum	53.5	38.5	55.7	1.39	0.96
Globus pallidus	ND	15.5	15.7	0	0
Claustrum	ND	41.3	35.7	0	0
N. accumbens					
Rostral	ND	25.5	23.7	0	0
Caudal	103.1	50.0	55.7	2.06	1.85
Hippocampus					
MCA3	7.2	15.5	31.7	0.46	0.23
PCA3	ND	7.0	27.7	0	0
Amygdala					
Central	23.0	24.1	51.7	0.95	0.44
Medial	ND	45.7	43.7	0	0
Cortical	7.2	15.5	75.9	0.46	0.09
Hypothalamus: preoptic	10.1	45.7	58.8	0.22	0.17
Thalamus: medial	18.8	77.5	63.8	0.24	0.29
Superior colliculus	5.8	21.2	15.7	0.27	0.29
Periaqueductal gray					
Dorsal	7.1	18.4	23.7	0.39	0.30
Ventral	18.6	14.1	23.7	1.32	0.78
Raphe nucleus	5.7	15.5	19.7	0.37	0.29
Interpeduncular nucleus	ND	67.4	31.7	0	0
Dorsal N. of vagus	12.9	18.4	31.7	0.7	0.41
N. of solitary tract	ND	12.7	15.7	0	0
Spinal cord					
Laminae I/II	53.5	32.7	59.8	1.64	0.89
Lamina V	8.6	9.8	19.7	0.88	0.44

[a]Adapted from Moskowitz and Goodman, 1985a.
[b]ND, no statistically significant binding.

phine analgesia. The CXBK strain is relatively insensitive to morphine analgesia, and in homogenate binding studies they have 30% fewer sites. In view of the association of mu_1 sites pharmacologically with supraspinal analgesia and their localization in regions of the brain closely associated with pain modulation, Moskowitz and Goodman (1985b) compared the density of mu_1 sites in CXBK mice with control mice more sensitive to morphine analgesia (Table 3). Compared to the control mice, the CXBK strain contained low levels

TABLE 3
Comparison of Opioid Binding in Control and CXBK Mice[a]

Region	Ratio of binding, CXBK/C57[b]		
	Mu_1	Mu_2	Delta
Frontal cortex			
Lamina I	0.33	1.00	1.00
Lamina IV	0.71	2.00	1.28
Lamina V	0.66	1.00	1.00
Olfactory tubercle plexiform layer	1.00	0	1.8
Striatum: patches	0.75	0.61	
Nucleus accumbens, caudal	0.50	0.48	1.28
Hippocampus MCA3	1.00	0.72	1.25
Amygdala			
Central nucleus	1.00	1.00	1.00
Basal nucleus	0	1.00	0.80
Mammillary nucleus			
Medial	1.00	1.00	0.37
Lateral mammillary	0	1.00	1.00
Thalamus, medial	0.52	0.78	1.00
Superior colliculus	1.00	1.00	1.00
Periaqueductal gray			
Dorsal	1.00	1.00	1.33
Ventral	0.45	1.00	1.67
N. of the spinal tract of V:			
substantia gelatinosa	0.56	1.00	1.00
Spinal cord			
Lamina I/II	0	1.22	0.79
Lamina V	0	1.00	1.51

[a]Adapted from Moskowitz and Goodman, 1985b.
[b]Values of 1.0 indicate no significant difference in binding levels between the control (C57) mice and the CXBK strain. Values of 0 imply no demonstrable mu_1 binding in the CXBK strain.

of mu_1 sites in many regions, including cortex (layers II, III, and V of the parietal cortex, layer I of the frontal cortex, and the pyramidal and plexiform layers of the pyriform cortex), limbic areas (interstitial nucleus of the stria terminalis, nucleus accumbens, and certain nuclei of the amygdala), and dorsal motor nucleus of the vagus. Of particular interest, however, were the low levels of mu_1 receptors in areas associated with antinociceptive actions such as the raphe nuclei, periaqueductal gray, and substantia gelatinosa of the spinal cord and trigeminal tract, consistent with pharmacological studies correlating mu_1 sites with analgesia (Pasternak and Wood, 1986).

Although individual regions can be examined for mu_1 sites using a grain-counting approach, it does not reveal a full distribution of the subtracted receptors. To overcome this limitation, we developed a computerized subtraction technique to generate an autoradiographic image of mu_1 receptors (Goodman and Pasternak, 1985). Conceptually, the procedure was essentially as outlined above. Instead of grain counting, sections in which mu_1 binding has been competed are subtracted from total binding pixel by pixel by the computer in essentially anatomically identical digitized autoradiograms, to yield a digitized image representing mu_1 binding sites (Fig. 1). This technique revealed a distribution of mu_1 sites in rat brain extremely similar to that in mice. Note the high levels of mu_1 receptors in the medial thalamus, periaqueductal gray, interpeduncular nucleus, and median raphe. This localization of mu_1 sites supports the association of mu_1 receptors with supraspinal analgesia.

5.3. Kappa Receptor Autoradiography

The distribution of kappa opioid receptors has proven difficult to evaluate and has received far less attention than mu or delta receptors. The lack of selectivity of most of the kappa [3H]ligands and the large species differences in levels of kappa binding sites have been problematic. Studies in rat brain using the standard radioligands [3H]ethylketazocine and [3H]bremazocine, which label mu and delta sites in addition to kappa receptors, were hampered by the small fraction of total specific binding corresponding to kappa receptors. In guinea pig brain, which contains far higher levels of kappa binding sites, their localization is unique.

The lack of selectivity of the kappa 3H-ligands required the elimination of mu and delta binding by including selective competitors, such as morphine and DADL, respectively, leaving only kappa sites labeled (Foote and Maurer, 1983; Chavkin et al., 1982;

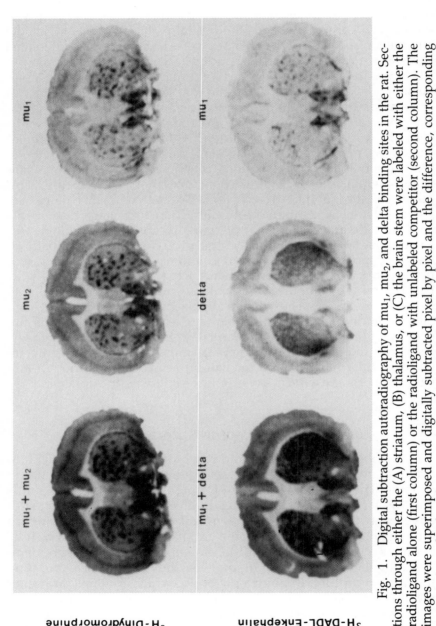

Fig. 1. Digital subtraction autoradiography of mu_1, mu_2, and delta binding sites in the rat. Sections through either the (A) striatum, (B) thalamus, or (C) the brain stem were labeled with either the radioligand alone (first column) or the radioligand with unlabeled competitor (second column). The images were superimposed and digitally subtracted pixel by pixel and the difference, corresponding to mu_1 sites, displayed as a separate image (third column) (from Goodman and Pasternak, 1985).

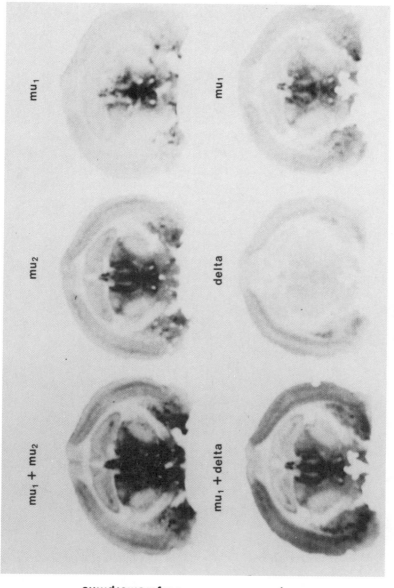

Fig. 1B.

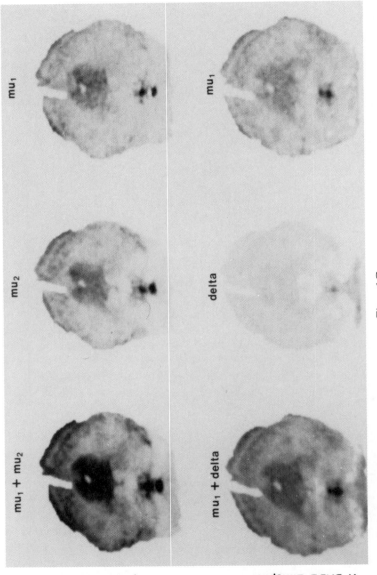

Fig. 1C.

Goodman and Snyder, 1982a,b). In the guinea pig, kappa receptors are concentrated in the deep layers (V and VI) of the cerebral cortex and in the pyriform cortex, caudate nucleus, and nucleus accumbens, as demonstrated in Fig. 2. [^{3}H]Bremazocine revealed similar neuroanatomical distributions in the guinea pig brain (Foote and Mauer, 1982, 1983). Although some binding of [^{3}H]bremazocine occurs in the dentate gyrus of the hippocampus and lateral habenula, the most dense labeling occurs in cortical layers V and VI. Further scrutinizing of the binding of [^{3}H]bremazocine revealed significant binding in the olfactory bulb and substantia nigra, as well as the deep layers of the cerebral cortex. Using guinea pig brain, Lewis et al. (1984) studied the binding of dynorphin A, a putative endogenous ligand for the kappa opioid receptor. The results support the localization of kappa opioid receptors to layers V and VI of the cerebral cortex. Significant species differences in the distribution of kappa opioid receptors exist. For example, kappa sites have been localized to the deep layer of the cerebral cortex in the guinea pig, but no such distribution is seen in the rat.

The suggestion that dynorphin A appears to be the endogenous kappa opioid (Lewis et al., 1982) located in the dorsal horn of the spinal cord and that kappa drugs such as ethylketazocine produce a spinal analgesia (Wood et al., 1981), led Slater and Patel (1983) to examine kappa opioid receptors in the rat spinal cord. They observed a concentration of kappa receptors in the substantia gelatinosa, consistent with a potential analgesic action of kappa sites.

In humans, [^{3}H]bremazocine labeled the deep cerebral cortical layers, especially layer VI, the molecular layers of the hippocampus and, the cerebellar cortex (Maurer et al., 1983). Others reported that [^{3}H]bremazocine and [^{3}H]naloxone binding sites are colocalized in rhesus monkey brain, as they are in rat brain (Lewis et al., 1982, 1983a,b). Interestingly, human brain (Maurer et al., 1983) and guinea pig brain (Foote and Maurer, 1982, 1983) do not contain such similar localizations of [^{3}H]bremazocine and [^{3}H]naloxone binding sites. In addition, [^{3}H]bremazocine strongly binds to the interpeduncular nucleus in the rhesus monkey brain, but not in the human brain (Maurer et al., 1983; Lewis et al., 1983a).

5.4. Epsilon Receptors

β-Endorphin's lack of binding selectivity has made autoradiographic studies of the distribution of the putative epsilon recep-

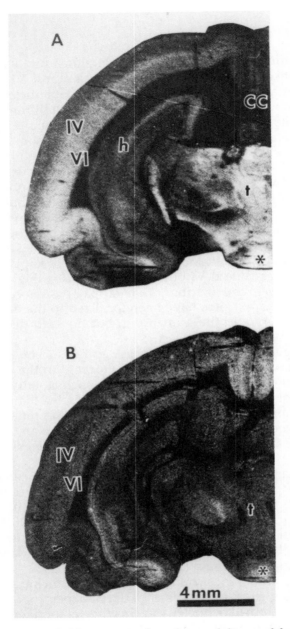

Fig. 2. Darkfield micrographs of mu, delta, and kappa binding sites in guinea pig brain. (A) Mu binding, labeled with [³H]dihydromorphine. Binding represents both mu₁ and mu₂ together. Note high densities in layers IV and VI of the cerebral cortex, the medial thalamus (t), and the interpeduncular nucleus (*). Moderate densities occur in layer V of the cerebral cortex and the molecular layer of the dentate gyrus. (B) Delta binding, measured by [³H]DADL in the presence of morphine. Note highest grain densities in layers V and VI of the cerebral cortex, the

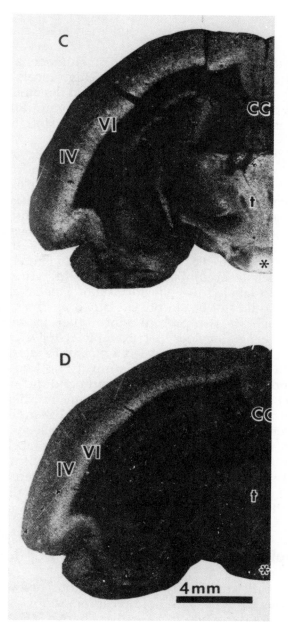

4mm

interpeduncular nucleus, and the ventral thalamus, with low densities in layer IV of the cortex and the molecular layer of the dentate gyrus. (C) [³H]Ethylketazocine binding, which is highest in layers V and VI of the cerebral cortex and in the same noncortical areas as [³H]dihydromorphine binding (*see* 2A). (D) Kappa binding, determined with [³H]ethylketazocine in the presence of morphine to compete mu binding. Note that the morphine eliminates noncortical labeling, without altering deep cortical labeling.

tors difficult (Schultz et al., 1979, 1981). Homogenate binding studies of different brain regions revealed high levels of binding in the striatum, hypothalamus, amygdala, and thalamus and very low levels of binding in the brain stem, midbrain, and cerebral cortex (Law et al., 1979; Johnson et al., 1982; Houghten et al., 1984).

Recently, we compared the autoradiographic distribution of [³H]β-endorphin with that of [³H]dihydromorphine and [³H]DADL in rat brain (Goodman et al., 1983). Close examination of the autoradiograms revealed differences consistent with β-endorphin-selective, or epsilon, binding sites within the brain (Fig. 3). At rostral levels, [³H]β-endorphin binding was similar to [³H]dihydromorphine, with significant labeling of the clusters and the subcallosal streak of the striatum, thalamus, hypothalamus, and nucleus accumbens. Unlike [³H]dihydromorphine, [³H]β-endorphin labeled the olfactory bulb. This labeling of the olfactory bulb could not be simply explained by cross binding to delta sites, which are also present, since other areas containing delta sites were not labeled. For example, [³H]DADL densely bound to the claustrum and revealed a medial-to-lateral gradient of increasing density within the striatum. [³H]β-Endorphin, on the other hand, did not label the claustrum and did not possess the same background density in the striatum. Furthermore, the small amount of cortical binding seen with [³H]β-endorphin was limited to layer IV in contrast to the delta binding seen in II/III and V. Finally, in the hippocampus [³H]β-endorphin labeled a thin, dense strip in the pyramidal cell layer, unlike the diffuse binding of the other two ligands. Although these results were quite suggestive, more studies are needed to definitively localize epsilon sites within the brain.

6. Opioid Receptors and Opioid Peptides

Correlating the distribution of the endogenous opioid peptides with the various subtypes of opioid receptors is obviously an important issue. As described in an earlier chapter, three different endogenous peptide systems have been identified and their precursors characterized: proopiomelanocortin (POMC), proenkephalin, and prodynorphin. POMC yields β-endorphin, ACTH, α-melanocyte stimulating hormone (α-MSH), and β-lipotropin. Proenkephalin contains six copies of [Met⁵]enkephalin and one of

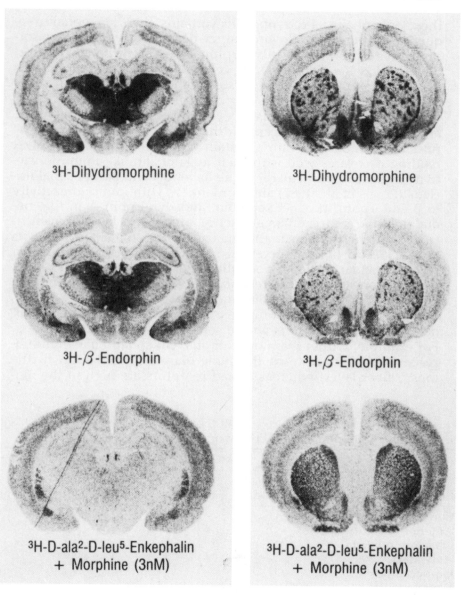

Fig. 3A and B.   [³H]β-Endorphin binding in rat brain. Sections through either the striatum (A) or the thalamus (B) were labeled with either [³H]dihydromorphine, [³H]β-endorphin, or [³H]DADL in the presence of morphine (from Goodman et al., 1983).

[Leu⁵]enkephalin. Prodynorphin contains [Leu⁵]enkephalin sequences within the following larger peptides: α- or β-neoendorphin, dynorphin A, and dynorphin B. A recent detailed report documented the distribution of cell bodies and fibers of neurons containing each of these precursors (Table 4; Khachaturian et al., 1985).

Opioid peptide systems innervate wide areas of the rat brain, and all of these areas, except for the globus pallidus and fastigial nucleus of the cerebellum, contain opioid receptors. [³H]Nalox binding correlates well with [Leu⁵]enkephalin-like immunoreactivity in the rat, particularly in the habenula and parabrachial nucleus (Lewis et al., 1982) and in monkeys with immunoreactivity to β-endorphin, [Lea⁵]enkephalin, and dynorphin A in the medial preoptic area, median eminence, arcuate nucleus, periventricular hypothalamic area, and nucleus of the solitary tract (Lewis et al., 1983a). In the interstitial nucleus of the stria terminalis, paraventricular nucleus, periaqueductal gray, and dorsal raphe, [³H]naloxone binding corresponded with β-endorphin and enkephalin, but not dynorphin immunoreactivity.

There is, however, a mismatch between opioid nerve terminals and opiate receptors within some of these anatomic regions. For example, within the hippocampus, enkephalin-like immunoreactivity is moderate in the molecular layer and high in the mossy fiber layer, whereas opioid receptors are high in the mo-

TABLE 4
Distribution of Opioid Precursors in Rat Brain and Pituitary[a]

Regions	POMC		Proenkephalin		Prodynorphin	
	Cell bodies	Fibers	Cell bodies	Fibers	Cell bodies	Fibers
Cerebral cortex			+	+	+	(+)
Anterior olfactory nucleus			+ +	+		
Olfactory tubercle			+ +	+	+	+
Amygdala		+	+ +	+	+	+
Hippocampus			+	+	(+)	+
Dentate gyrus			+	+	+	+
Nucleus accumbens		(+)	+	+		+
Corpus striatum			+	+	+	+
Nucleus diagonal band	+		+	+		(+)
Septal nuclei	+		+	+		
Globus pallidus			+ +			+ +
Ventral pallidum			+ +			+ +

(continued)

TABLE 4 (*continued*)
Distribution of Opioid Precursors in Rat Brain and Pituitary[a]

Regions	POMC Cell bodies	POMC Fibers	Proenkephalin Cell bodies	Proenkephalin Fibers	Prodynorphin Cell bodies	Prodynorphin Fibers
Bed n. stria terminalis		+ +	+	+	+	+
Thalamic n. (CM, AD, AM, AV, MG)				+ +		
Periventricular thalamus		+ +	+	+		(+)
Nucleus reuniens, thalamus		+	+	+		
Lateral geniculate			+	+		
Habenula				+		
Preoptic area		+	+	+		+
Hypothalamic nuclei	+ +*	+ +	+	+	+	+
Substantia nigra/pars compacta		+		+		
Substantia nigra/pars reticulata						+ +
Colliculi (sup. and inf.)		(+)	+	+		(+)
Periaqueductal gray		+ +	+ +	+	+	+
Interpeduncular nucleus			+	+		
Reticular formation			+	+		(+)
Parabrachial nucleus		+ +	+ +	+	+	+
Locus ceruleus				+		
Dorsal tegmental nucleus		(+)	+	+		
Trigeminal main sensory n.		(+)	+	+		
Facial nucleus				+		
Vestibular nucleus			+	+		(+)
Cochlear nucleus				+		
Raphe nuclei		+	+	+		+
Reticular gigantocellular n.		+	+	+		(+)
Paragigantocellular nucleus			+	+		(+)
N. tractus solitarius	+ +	+	+	+	+	+
Lateral reticular nucleus		+	+	+	+	+
Nucleus ambiguus		+		+		(+)
Dorsal motor n. of vagus		+		+		(+)
Fastigial n. of cerebellum			+	+		
Spinal trigeminal n.			+	+	+	+
Spinal cord dorsal gray			+	+	+	+
Pituitary						
Anterior lobe	+				+	
Intermediate lobe	+ +					
Posterior lobe				+		+ +

[a]Adapted from Khatchaturian et al., 1985.
[b]Symbols: (+), trace; +, medium; + +, dense; *, arcuate, medial, basal nucleus.

lecular layer and pyramidal cell layer and moderate in the mossy fiber layer (Stengaard-Pederson, 1983). Also, within the lateral geniculate body opioid receptors are restricted to the ventral band (Atweh and Kuhar, 1977b), whereas proenkephalin is present throughout the nucleus (Khatchaturian et al., 1985). Finally, opioid receptors are also found in layer IV of the cerebral cortex, whereas opioid peptide terminals occur only in superficial and deep layers.

Overall, the correspondence between receptors and peptides is quite good. There is no strong evidence, however, linking a particular subtype with a specific peptide on the basis of their anatomy. The distribution of prodynorphin overlaps extensively with that of proenkephalin, raising the possibility that specificity may involve the relative affinities of the peptides for the various binding subtypes, precursor processing and release, and not simply upon the location of terminals (Khatchaturian et al., 1985). At least two areas have been identified that contain opioid peptide terminals but no receptors, and several regions that contain receptors but no peptides. Kuhar (1985) has summarized this problem of "mismatch" and offered several possibilities: (1) these areas might be nonfunctional; (2) the receptors and/or peptides may be internal and/or undergoing transport; or (3) present techniques may not be sensitive enough to detect all receptors or peptides. Finally, the peptides may have a hormonal role that would not require a close match between terminals and receptors.

Species differences have been noted for the distribution of the peptides. For example, in the monkey, [Met^5]enkephalin-like immunoreactive fibers and terminals are dense in the substantia nigra compared to the rat, in which they are sparse (Haber and Elde, 1982). However, similarities are far more striking than differences.

7. Conclusion

In summary, much remains to be learned about the multiple subtypes of opioid receptors, but the vast amount of evidence obtained to date provides a compelling story of a neurotransmitter system important in a wide variety of central nervous system functions, including analgesia, sensory integration, autonomic functions, motor acts, and neuroendocrine and behavioral effects. The correlation of the regional distribution of the various subtypes of receptors with those brain regions mediating opioid actions, as obtained with autoradiography, is strong evidence for the relevance of these receptors. Ultrastructural studies and the development of more specific ligands are now needed to further understand opiate actions within the brain.

References

Abou-Khalil, B., Young, A. B., and Penney, J. B. (1984) Evidence for the presynaptic localization of opiate sites on striatal efferent fibers. *Brain Res.* **323**, 21–29.

Alexander, G. M., Schwarzman, R. J., Bell, R. D., Yu, J., and Renthal, A. (1981) Quantitative measurement of local cerebral metabolic rate for glucose utilizing tritiated 2-deoxyglucose. *Brain Res.* **223**, 59–67.

Atweh, S. F. and Kuhar, M. J. (1977a) Autoradiographic localization of opiate receptors in rat brain. I. Spinal cord and lower medulla. *Brain Res.* **124**, 53–67.

Atweh, S. F. and Kuhar, M. J. (1977b) Autoradiographic localization of opiate receptors in rat brain. II. The brain stem. *Brain Res.* **129**, 1–12.

Atweh, S. F. and Kuhar, M. J. (1977c) Autoradiographic localization of opiate receptors in rat brain. III. The telencephalon. *Brain Res.* **134**, 393–405.

Atweh, S. F. and Kuhar, M. J. (1983) Distribution and physiological significance of opioid receptors in the brain. *Br. Med. Bull.* **39**, 47–52.

Atweh, S. F., Murrin, L. C., and Kuhar, M. J. (1978) Presynaptic localization of opiate receptors in the vagal and accessory optic systems: An autoradiographic study. *Neuropharmacology* **17**, 65–71.

Chang, K. J. and Cuatrecasas, P. (1979) Multiple opiate receptors: Enkephalins and morphine bind to receptors of different specificity. *J. Biol. Chem.* **254**, 2610–2618.

Chang, K. J., Cooper, B. R., Hazum, E., and Cuatecasas, P. (1979) Multiple opiate receptors: Different regional distribution in the brain and differential binding of opiates and opioid peptides. *Mol. Pharmacol.* **16**, 91–104.

Chavkin, C., James, I. F., and Goldstein, A. (1982) Dynorphin is a specific endogenous ligand of the kappa opioid receptor. *Science* **215**, 413–415.

Clendenin, N. J., Petraitis, M., and Simon, E. J. (1976) Ontological development of opiate receptors in rodent brain. *Brain Res.* **118**, 157–160.

Coyle, J. T. and Pert, C. B. (1976) Ontogenetic development of ^{3}H-naloxone binding in rat brain. *Neuropharmacology* **15**, 555–560.

Csillik, B., Kiss, J., Knyihar-Csillike, E., and Lajtha, A. (1982) Effect of transganglionic degenerative atrophy on opiate receptors in the dorsal horn of the spinal cord. *J. Neurosci. Res.* **8**, 665–670.

Duka, T., Schubert, P., Wuster, M., Stoiber, R., and Herz, A. (1981a) A selective distribution pattern of different opiate receptors in certain areas of rat brain as revealed by in vitro autoradiography. *Neurosci. Lett.* **21**, 119–124.

Duka, T., Wuster, M., Schubert, P., Stoiber, R., and Herz, A. (1981b) Selective localization of different types of opiate receptors in hippocampus as revealed by in vitro autoradiography. *Brain Res.* **205,** 181–186.

Fields, H. L., Emson, P. C., Leigh, B. K., and Iversen, L. L. (1980) Multiple opiate receptor sites on primary afferent fibres. *Nature* **284,** 351–353.

Foote, R. W. and Maurer, R. (1982) Autoradiographic localization of opiate kappa receptors in guinea pig brain. *Eur. J. Pharmacol.* **85,** 99–103.

Foote, R. W. and Maurer, R. (1983) Kappa opiate binding sites in the substantia nigra and bulbus olfactorius of the guinea pig as shown by in vitro autoradiography. *Life Sci.* **33,** 243–246.

Gamse, R., Holzer, P., and Lembeck, F. (1979) Indirect evidence for presynaptic localization of opiate receptors on chemosensitive primary sensory neurones. *Arch. Pharmacol.* **308,** 281–285.

Garcin, F. and Coyle, J. T. (1976) Ontogenetic Development of ^{3}H-Naloxone Binding and Endogenous Morphine-Like Factor in Rat Brain, in *Opiates and Endogenous Opioid Peptides* (Kosterlitz, H. W., ed.) Elsevier/North Holland Biomedical Press, Amsterdam.

Gardner, E. L., Zukin, R. S., and Makman, M. H. (1980) Modulation of opiate receptor binding in striatum and amygdala by selective mesencephalic lesions. *Brain Res.* **194,** 232–239.

Goodman, R. R. and Snyder S. H. (1982a) Autoradiographic localization of kappa opiate receptors to deep layers of the cerebral cortex may explain unique sedative and analgesic effects. *Life Sci.* **31,** 1291–1294.

Goodman, R. R. and Snyder, S. H. (1982b) Kappa opiate receptors localized by autoradiography to deep layers of cerebral cortex: Relation to sedative effects. *Proc. Natl. Acad. Sci. USA* **79,** 5703–5707.

Goodman, R. R. and Pasternak, G. W. (1985) Visualization of mu$_1$ opiate receptors in rat brain using a computerized autoradiographic technique. *Proc. Natl. Acad. Sci. USA* **82,** 6667–6671.

Goodman, R. R., Adler, B. A. and Pasternak, G. W. (1985) Regional differences in mu$_1$ binding of ^{3}H-DADLE-enkephalin: Comparisons of thalamus and cortex. *Neurosci. Lett.* **59,** 155–158.

Goodman, R. R., Houghton, R. A., and Pasternak, G. W. (1983) Autoradiography of ^{3}H-β-endorphin binding in brain. *Brain Res.* **288,** 334–337.

Goodman, R. R., Snyder, S. H., Kuhar, M. J., and Young, III, W. S. (1980) Differentiation of delta and mu opiate receptor localizations by light microscopic autoradiography. *Proc. Natl. Acad. Sci. USA* **77,** 6239–6243.

Gulya K., Gehlert, D. R., Wamsley, J. K., Mosberg, H. I., Hruby, V. J., Duckles, S. P., and Yamamura, H. I. (1985) Autoradiographic localization of opioid receptors in the rat brain using a highly selective *bis*-penicillamine cyclic enkephalin analog. *Eur. J. Pharmacol.* **111,** 285–286.

Haber, S. and Elde, R. (1982) The distribution of enkephalin immunoreactive fibers and terminals in the monkey central nervous system: An immunohistochemical study. *Neuroscience* **5,** 1049–1095.

Hahn, E. F., Carroll-Buatti, M., and Pasternak, G. W. (1982) Irreversible opiate agonists and antagonists: The 14-hydroxydihydromorphinone azines. *J. Neurosci.* **2,** 572–576.

Hamel, E. and Beaudet, A. (1984) Electron microscopic autoradiographic localization of opioid receptors in rat neostriatum. *Nature* **312,** 155–157.

Herkenham, M. and Pert, C. B. (1980) In vitro autoradiography of opiate receptors in rat brain suggests loci of "opiatergic" pathways. *Proc. Natl. Acad. Sci. USA* **77**, 5532–5536.

Herkenham, M. and Sokoloff, L. (1984) Quantitative receptor autoradiography: Tissue defatting eliminates differential self-absorption of tritium radiation in gray and white matter of brain. *Brain Res.* **321**, 363–368.

Houghten, R. A., Johnson, N., and Pasternak, G. W. (1984) ^{3}H-Endorphin binding in rat brain. *J. Neurosci.* **4**, 2460–2465.

Jessell, T., Tsunoo, A., Kanazama, I., and Otsaka, M. (1979) Substance P: Depletion in the dorsal horn of rat spinal cord after section of the peripheral processes of primary sensory neurons. *Brain Res.* **168**, 247–259.

Johnson, N. and Pasternak, G. W. (1984) Binding of ^{3}H-naloxonazine to rat brain membranes. *J. Neurosci.* **26**, 477–483.

Johnson, N., Houghten, R., and Pasternak, G. W. (1982) Binding of ^{3}H-β-endorphin in rat brain. *Life Sci.* **31**, 1381–1384.

Kent, J. L., Pert, C. B., and Herkenham, M. (1982) Ontogeny of opiate receptors in rat forebrain: Visualization by in vitro autoradiography. *Dev. Brain Res.* **2**, 487–504.

Khachaturian, H., Lewis, M. E., Schater, M. K.-H., and Watson, S. J. (1985) Anatomy of the CNS opioid systems. *Trends Neurosci.* **8**, 111–119.

Kuhar, M. J. (1985) The mismatch problem in receptor mapping studies. *Trends Neurosci.* **5**, 109–191.

Kuhar, M. J. and Unnerstall, J. R. (1982) In vitro labeling receptor autoradiography: Loss of label during ethanol dehydration and preparative procedures. *Brain Res.* **244**, 178–181.

Kuhar, M. J. and Unnerstall, J. R. (1985) Quantitative receptor mapping by autoradiography: Some current technical problems. *Trends Neurosci.* **8**, 49–53.

Kuhar, M. J., Pert, C. B., and Snyder, S. H. (1973) Regional distribution of opiate receptor binding in monkey and human brain. *Nature* **245**, 447–450.

LaMotte, C. C., Snowman, A., Pert, C. B., and Snyder, S. H. (1978) Opiate receptor binding in rhesus monkey brain: Association with limbic structures. *Brain Res.* **155**, 374–379.

LaMotte, C., Pert, C. B., and Snyder, S. H. (1976) Opiate receptor binding in primate spinal cord: Distribution and changes after dorsal root section. *Brain Res.* **112**, 407–412.

Law, P. Y., Loh, H. H., and Li, C. H. (1979) Properties and localization of β-endorphin receptors in brain. *Proc. Natl. Acad. Sci. USA* **76**, 5455–5459.

Lewis, M. E., Khachaturian, H., and Watson, S. J. (1982) Visualization of opiate receptors and opioid peptides in sequential brain sections. *Life Sci.* **31**, 1347–1350.

Lewis, M. E., Khachaturian, H., and Watson, S. J. (1983a) Comparative distribution of opiate receptors and three opioid peptide neuronal systems in rhesus monkey central nervous system. *Life. Sci.* **33**, 239–242.

Lewis, M. E., Pert, A., Pert, C. B., and Herkenham, M. (1983b) Opiate receptor localization in rat cerebral cortex. *J. Comp. Neurol.* **216**, 339–358.

Lewis, M. E., Mishkin, M., Bragin, E., Brown, R. M., Pert, C. B., and Pert,

A. (1981) Opiate receptor gradients in monkey cerebral cortex: Correspondence with sensory processing hierarchies. *Science* **211,** 1166.

Lewis, M. E., Young, E. A., Houghten, R. A., Akil, H., and Watson, S. J. (1984) Binding of ^{3}H-dynorphin A to apparent kappa opioid receptors in deep layers of guinea pig cerebral cortex. *Eur. J. Pharmacol.* **98,** 149–150.

Lord, J. A. H., Waterfield, A. A., Hughes, J., and Kosterlitz, H. W. (1977) Endogenous opioid peptides: Multiple agonists and receptors. *Nature* **267,** 495–499.

Maurer, R., Cortez, R., Probst, A., and Palacios, J. M. (1983) Multiple opiate receptor in human brain: An autoradiographic investigation. *Life Sci.* **33,** 231–234.

Moskowitz, A. S., and Goodman, R. R. (1984) Light microscopic autoradiographic localization of mu and delta opioid binding sites in the mouse central nervous system. *J. Neurosci.* **4,** 1331–1342.

Moskowitz, A. S. and Goodman, R. R. (1985a) Autoradiographic distribution of mu_1 and mu_2 opioid binding in the mouse central nervous system. *Brain Res.* **360,** 117–129.

Moskowitz, A. S. and Goodman, R. R. (1985b) Autoradiographic analysis of mu_1 and mu_2 and delta opioid binding in the central nervous system of C57BL6BY and CXBK (opioid receptor-deficient) mice. *Brain Res.* **360,** 108–116.

Murrin, L. C., Coyle, J. T., and Kuhar, M. J. (1980) Striatal opiate receptors: Pre- and postsynaptic localization. *Life Sci.* **27,** 1175–1183.

Ninkovic, M., Hunt, S. P., and Gleave, R. W. (1982) Localization of opiate and histamine H1-receptors in the primate sensory ganglia and spinal cord. *Brain Res.* **241,** 197–206.

Ninkovic, M., Hunt, S. P., and Kelly, S. (1981) Effect of dorsal rhizotomy on the autoradiographic distribution of opiate and neurotensin receptors and neurotensin-like immunoreactivity within the rat spinal cord. *Brain Res.* **230,** 111–119.

Palacios, J. M., Niehoff, D. L., and Kuhar, M. J. (1981) Receptor autoradiography with tritium sensitive film: Potential for computerized dosimetry. *Neurosci. Lett.* **25,** 101–105.

Parenti, M., Tirone, F., Olgiati, V. R., and Groppetti, A. (1983) Presence of opiate receptors on striatal serotoninergic nerve terminals. *Brain Res.* **280,** 317–322.

Pasternak, G. W. and Wood, P. L. (1986) Multiple mu opiate receptors. *Life Sci.* **38,** 1889–1898.

Pasternak, G. W., Zhang, A-Z., and Tecott, L. (1980) Developmental differences between high and low affinity opiate binding sites: Their relationship to analgesia and respiratory depression. *Life Sci.* **27,** 1185–1190.

Pearson, J., Brandeis, L., Simon, E., and Hiller, J. (1980) Radioautography of binding of tritiated diprenorphine to opiate receptors in the rat. *Life Sci.* **26,** 1047–1052.

Penny, J. B., Frey, K., and Young, A. B. (1981) Quantitative autoradiography of neurotransmitter receptor using tritium sensitivefilm. *Eur. J. Pharmacol.* **72,** 421–422.

Pert, C. B., Kuhar, M. J., and Snyder, S. H. (1976) Autoradiographic l ocalization of opiate receptors in rat brain. *Proc. Natl. Acad. Sci. US A* **73,** 3729–3733.

Pert, C. B., Kuhar, M. J., and Snyder, S. H. (1975) Autoradiographic l ocalization of the opiate receptor in rat brain. *Life Sci.* **16,** 1849 –1854.

Pollard, M., Llorens, C., Schwartz, J. C., Gros, C., and Dray, F. (1978) Localization of opiate receptors and enkephalins in the rat striatum in relationship with the nigrostriatal dopaminergic system: Lesion studies. *Brain Res.* **151,** 392–398.

Pollard, M., Llorens, C., and Bonnet, J. J. (1977a) Opiate receptors on mesolimbic dopaminergic neurons. *Neurosci. Lett.* **7,** 295–299.

Pollard, M., Llorens-Cortes, C., and Schwartz, J. C. (1977b) Enkephalin receptors on dopaminergic neurones in rat striatum. *Nature* **268,** 745–747.

Quirion, R., Zajac, J. M., Morgat, J. L., and Roques, B. P. (1983) Autoradiographic distribution on mu and delta opiate receptors in rat brain using highly selective ligands. *Life Sci.* **33,** 227–230.

Rainbow, T. C., Bleisch, W. V., Biegon, A., and McEwen, B. S. (1982) Quantitative densitometry of neurotransmitter receptors. *J. Neurosci. Meth.* **5,** 127–138.

Recht, L. D., Kent, J., and Pasternak, G. W. (1985) Quantitative autoradiography of the development of mu opiate binding sites in rat brain. *Cell. Mol. Neurobiol.* **5,** 223–229.

Reisine, T. D., Nagy, J. I., Beaumont, K., Fibiger, H. C., and Yamamara, H. I. (1979) The localization of receptor binding sites in the substantia nigra and striatum of the rat. *Brain Res.* **177,** 241–252.

Roth, L. J., Diab, I. M., Natanabe, M., and Dinerstein, R. J. (1974) A correlative radioautographic fluorescent, and histochemical technique for cytopharmacology. *Mol. Pharmacol.* **10,** 986–998.

Schultz, R., Faaswe, E., Wuster, M., and Herz, A. (1979) Selective receptors for β-endorphin on the rat vas deferens. *Life Sci.* **24,** 843–850.

Schultz, R., Wuster, M., and Herz, A. (1981) Pharmacological characterization of the epsilon opiate receptor. *J. Pharmacol. Exp. Ther.* **216,** 604–609.

Slater, P. and Patel, S. (1983) Autoradiographic localization of opiate kappa receptors in rat spinal cord. *Eur. J. Pharmacol.* **92,** 159–160.

Stengaard-Pedersen, K. (1983) Comparative mapping of opioid receptors and enkephalin immunoreactive nerve terminals in the rat hippocampus. *Histochemistry* **79,** 311–333.

Unnerstall, J. R., Moliver, M. E., Kuhar, M. J., and Palacios, J. M. (1983) Ontogeny of opiate binding sites in the hippocampus, olfactory bulb and other regions of the rat forebrain by autoradiographic methods. *Dev. Brain Res.* **7,** 157–169.

Unnerstall, J. R., Neihoff, D. L., Kuhar, M. J., and Palacios, J. M. (1982) Quantitative receptor autoradiography using ^{3}H-Ultrafilm: Application to multiple benzodiazapine receptors. *J. Neurosci. Meth.* **6,** 59–73.

Wamsley, J. K. (1983) Opioid receptors: Autoradiography. *Pharmacol. Rev.* **35,** 69–83.

Wamsley, J. K., Zarbin, M. A., Young III, W. S., and Kuhar, M. J. (1982) Distribution of opiate receptors in the monkey brain: An autoradiographic study. *Neuroscience* **7,** 595–613.

Wise, S. P. and Herkenham, M. (1982) Opiate receptor distribution in the cerebral cortex of the rhesus monkey. *Science* **218,** 387–389.

Wolozin, B. L. and Pasternak, G. W. (1981) Classification of multiple morphine and enkephalin binding sites in the central nervous system. *Proc. Natl. Acad. Sci. USA* **78,** 6181–6185.

Wood, P. L., Rackham, A., and Richard, J. (1981) Spinal analgesia: Comparison of the mu agonist morphine and the kappa agonist ethylketocyclazocine. *Life Sci.* **28,** 219–2135.

Young III, W. S. and Kuhar, M. J. (1979) A new method for receptor autoradiography for 3H-opioid receptor labeling in mounted tissue sections. *Brain Res.* **179,** 255–270.

Zhang, A.-Z. and Pasternak, G. W. (1980) Mu and delta opiate receptors: Correlation with high and low affinity opiate binding sites. *Eur. J. Pharmacol.* **67,** 323–324.

Zhang, A.-Z. and Pasternak, G. W. (1981) Ontogeny of opioid pharmacology and receptors: High and low affinity site differences. *Eur. J. Pharmacol.* **73,** 29–40.

SECTION 4
MECHANISMS OF
RECEPTOR ACTION

Chapter 8

Opioid-Coupled Second Messenger Systems

Steven R. Childers

1. Introduction

Receptors are normally considered as composed of two separate parts: a specific ligand binding site and an effector component that causes a specific biological response subsequent to agonist binding. Historically, neurotransmitter receptors have been iden- tifed by both properties. For example, opioid receptors have been described by both specific radioligand binding assays (Pert and Snyder, 1973; Terenius, 1973; Simon et al., 1973) and bioassays measuring opioid inhibition of smooth muscle contraction in the guinea pig ileum and the mouse vas deferens (Kosterlitz and Waterfield, 1975). Connecting these two aspects of receptor func- tion is the second messenger system. For the purposes of this re- view, a second messenger system can be defined as the event(s) that occurs distal to ligand binding and initiates the sequence of events that lead to the biological response. For opiates, several biological responses have been measured, from inhibition of neu- rotransmitter release (Mudge et al., 1979), to modulation of pitui- tary hormone release (Grossman, 1983), to changes in cell firing rates (Duggan and North, 1983). All of these responses presuma- bly are associated with receptor-coupled second messenger sys- tems, but the nature of these systems has yet to be firmly estab- lished.

Most speculation regarding opioid-coupled second messenger systems has centered around several candidates. These include alterations in cyclic nucleotide metabolism (including inhibition of adenylate cyclase and increase in cyclic GMP levels), changes in protein phosphorylation, and opioid-mediated changes in calcium uptake and function in neurons. Moreover, since many electrophysiological experiments have provided direct evidence of opioid effects on membrane potentials, another second messenger system might be ion channels, with most current research focused on potassium and calcium channels (Duggan and North, 1983). Since electrophysiological actions of opioids will be considered elsewhere, this chapter will focus on the second messenger systems that have been determined by more biochemical procedures. The major focus of this review will be centered on opioid-inhibited adenylate cyclase, since the most attention and effort has been centered on this activity. Moreover, since this chapter deals directly with receptor-coupled second messenger systems, it will not review the physiological and in vivo experiments of opiates and cyclic nucleotides, which have been reviewed elsewhere (Wolleman, 1981).

With several second messenger system systems, especially the receptor-coupled adenylate cyclase system, direct interactions between receptors and second messenger systems do not occur. Instead, there are coupling, or membrane transduction, systems set up between receptors and second messengers. For example, receptor coupling to adenylate cyclase requires the presence of guanine nucleotide-binding proteins. Therefore, any description of second messenger systems will also involve a discussion of membrane transduction systems, and this chapter will review how these systems not only allow coupling of receptors with second messengers, but also allow for regulation of ligand binding to receptors. In order to understand the membrane transduction mechanisms involved with opioid receptors, it is first necessary to review the general field of receptor-coupled adenylate cyclase as it has been established in biochemical experiments with other neurotransmitter and hormone receptors.

2. Receptor-Coupled Adenylate Cyclase: The Ternary Complex Models

Most of the biochemical information known about coupling of receptors with adenylate cyclase comes from a series of experiments with β-adrenergic and glucagon receptors in specialized cell systems like adipocytes and S-49 lymphoma cells. These experiments have been exhaustively reviewed elsewhere (Rodbell, 1980; Gilman, 1984; Schramm and Selinger, 1984; Helmreich and Pfeuffer, 1985), and only the overall conclusions of these studies will be discussed here. In general, neurotransmitter and hormone receptors that are coupled to adenylate cyclase can be divided into two categories. The stimulatory class, such as β-adrenergic, glucagon, adenosine A_2, and dopamine D_1, act by stimulating the enzyme. The inhibitory class, which includes α_2-adrenergic, adenosine A_1, dopamine D_2, as well as opioids, inhibit adenylate cyclase activity, either directly by inhibition of basal activity, or indirectly by inhibition of receptor-stimulated activity. In general, stimulated adenylate cyclase activity has been better characterized than inhibited activity for both historical and technical reasons.

A major focus of research has been the mechanism of receptor-adenylate cyclase coupling. Although early speculation centered around the possibility that receptor-coupled adenylate cyclase might be part of a single macromolecular complex, results obtained since the mid1970s have made it clear that receptors and adenylate cyclase are separate proteins that are coupled by a third type of protein. An important early discovery was the key role played by guanine nucleotides in receptor-adenylate cyclase function. Receptor-mediated stimulation or inhibition of adenylate cyclase requires the presence of guanine nucleotides, especially GTP. The nucleotide triphosphate is an absolute requirement, since neither GDP nor GMP will support enzyme activation, although nonhydrolyzable analogs of GTP such as Gpp(NH)p will stimulate adenylate cyclase activity. In addition, guanine nucleotides regulate agonist binding to these receptors by increasing agonist dissociation rates and thus decreasing agonist affinity. A key feature of guanine nucleotide regulation of receptor binding is the universal finding that GTP decreases binding of agonists, but not antagonists. Presumably, this property means that the receptor exists in two different affinity states for agonists (depending upon the presence of guanine nucleotides), whereas antagonists bind with a single high affinity to both states (De Lean et al., 1980; Kent et al., 1980). The nucleotide specificity of the receptor regulation is somewhat different than that of adenylate cyclase coupling: although both effects require guanine (and not adenine) nucleotides, receptor regulation occurs with GDP as well as with GTP. These effects of GTP, both on coupling receptors with adenylate cyclase as well as regulating agonist binding to receptor sites, are unifying actions that occur with all adenylate cyclase-coupled receptors.

The effects of guanine nucleotides are mediated through specific GTP-binding proteins called either G-proteins or N-proteins depending on the style of nomenclature (Rodbell, 1980; Gilman, 1984). Stimulated adenylate cyclase is mediated by N_s, whereas inhibitory adenylate cyclase is mediated through N_i (Fig. 1). Each of these proteins are heterotrimers of subunit composition α_s, β, γ and α_i, β, γ. In other words, the beta and gamma subunits are identical in the two N-proteins, although the alpha subunit varies. The alpha subunits are best studied since they bind GTP and are the targets for ribosylation by cholera toxin and pertussis toxin (Northup et al., 1983b; Katada and Ui, 1982). Although α_s

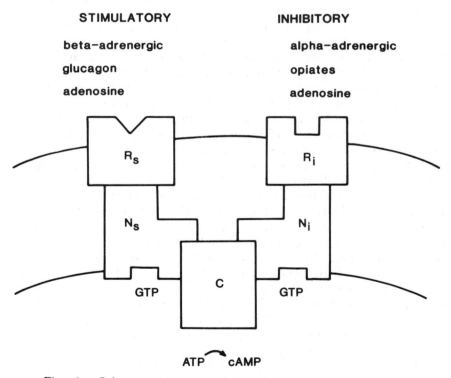

Fig. 1.   Schematic diagram of stimulatory and inhibitory receptors acting on the catalytic unit of adenylate cyclase through N_s and N_i proteins, respectively. Stimulatory receptors include β_1- and β_2-adrenergic, glucagon, and adenosine A_2, whereas inhibitory receptors include alpha$_2$-adrenergic, opioid, and adenosine A_1.

(molecular weight 42,000) and α_i (molecular weight 39,000) are different proteins, they exhibit considerable similarities. Both subunits possess GTPase activity and have considerable parallels in primary structure (Manning and Gilman, 1983). Bacterial toxins have proven to be valuable probes in the study of these subunits, since cholera toxin binds to α_s and pertussis toxin binds to α_i. In both cases, the toxin catalyzes ADP-ribosylation of the proteins (Northup et al., 1983b; Katada and Ui, 1982). In this reaction, in the presence of ATP, toxin catalyzes the transfer of an ADP moiety from NAD to the N-protein, with covalent reaction between the ribose portion of ADP and specific amino acid residues of the N-protein. This reaction produces essentially irreversible modification of N-protein function. Paradoxically, the functional consequences of toxin reactions with both N_s and N_i proteins lead to the same result: an increase in adenylate cyclase activity and resulting increase in intracellular cyclic AMP. In the case of α_s, cholera toxin-mediated ribosylation inactivates the GTPase associated with α_s that, as discussed below, normally inactivates adenylate cyclase (Northup et al., 1983b). Thus, cholera toxin is a potent irreversible stimulator of adenylate cyclase. In the case of α_i, pertussis toxin inactivates the inhibitory function of the subunit. Thus, pertussis toxin also causes stimulation of adenylate cyclase by removing the inhibitory component of the cycle (Katada and Ui, 1982).

Interestingly, other GTP-binding proteins also exhibit striking parallels to α_s and α_i. One is the alpha subunit of N_o, a GTP-binding protein isolated from brain and heart (Sternweis and Robishaw, 1984; Neer et al., 1984). The amino terminal sequence of the alpha subunit of N_o is highly homologous with corresponding subunits of N_s and N_i; the function of N_o is not yet clear, however. Recent studies have shown that α_o can be reconstituted with muscarinic cholinergic receptor solubilized from brain membranes to provide guanine nucleotide regulation of binding (Florio and Sternweis, 1985), and that α_o can be reconstituted with purified α_2-adrenergic receptors to provide α_2-stimulated GTPase activity (Cerione et al., 1986). The identity of the second messenger system associated with N_o function, however, is not yet known. Another similar protein is the alpha subunit of transducin in retinal rod outer segment membranes (Wheeler and Bitensky, 1977; Fung and Stryer, 1980). In this system, light-activated rhodopsin catalyses GTP-GDP exchange in transducin, which then activates cyclic GMP phosphodiesterase. Moreover, transducin can be ADP-ribosylated by both cholera toxin and pertussis toxin (Manning et al., 1984). The parallels between light-activated phosphodiesterase and receptor-stimulated adenylate cyclase are striking. Finally, recent studies have reported that an oncogene product, ras-21 protein, binds and hydrolyzes GTP (McGrath et al., 1984), and although the molecular weight of ras-21 is considerably smaller than that of the alpha subunits of the N-proteins (21,000 vs approximately 40,000), and although ras-21 cannot substitute for α_s or α_i in regulating adenylate cyclase (Helmreich and Pfeuffer, 1985), considerable structural homology exists between these classes of GTP-binding proteins.

The other two subunits of N_s and N_i, β and γ, are identical in the two N-proteins. The gamma subunit is small (molecular weight 8000) and its function in receptor–adenylate cyclase coupling is not yet known (Gilman, 1984; Helmreich and Pfeuffer, 1985). The beta subunit (molecular weight 35,000) apparently binds to the catalytic unit of adenylate cyclase to inactivate the enzyme (Northup et al., 1983a). Although most evidence suggests that β does not bind GTP (Northup et al., 1983a), recent studies with photo-affinity GTP probes have indicated that GTP binding to β does occur (Rasenick et al., 1984). These results suggest that our current understanding of the N-protein systems is far from complete.

The identification of several homologous members among a class of GTP-binding proteins has another implication for receptor-mediated second messenger systems. Receptors that are coupled to one N-protein or another may not necessarily be coupled to adenylate cyclase, but instead be coupled to other second messenger systems. An established example is the transducin system in the retinal rod outer segment, where the second messenger system is cyclic GMP phosphodieterase. In other cells, receptor-mediated changes in phosphoinositide turnover (Nishizuka, 1984) have been associated with N-protein coupling mechanisms. Recent results from Nakamura and Ui (1985) have shown attenuation of receptor-mediated stimulation of phospholipase A_2 and arachidonic acid release in mast cells by treatment with pertussis toxin. Moreover, in isolated membranes, guanine nucleotides stimulate phosphoinositide turnover (Cockcroft and Gomperts, 1985; Gonzales and Crews, 1985; Litosch et al., 1985), whereas in other systems, binding of agonists to receptors known to stimulate phosphoinositide turnover is regulated by guanine nucleotides (Evans et al., 1985). A third example is the receptor-coupled ion channel: a recent study has demonstrated that muscarinic cholinergic receptor-mediated potassium influx is regulated by guanine nucleotides (Pfaffinger et al., 1985). Therefore, identification of guanine nucleotide effects on receptor binding does not guarantee that the receptor system is coupled to adenylate cyclase.

Many experiments with purified N-proteins and genetic mutants of S-49 lymphoma cells have provided models for the actions of hormones and neurotransmitters in stimulating and inhibiting adenylate cyclase through N_s and N_i proteins. These models have been tested by experiments that reconstitute purified receptors, adenylate cyclase, and N-proteins into phospholipid vesicles (Cerione et al., 1984, 1986). Figure 2 illustrates our current understanding of these reactions and shows two different schemes. Panel A shows a model based upon the work of Gilman and others showing activation of adenylate cyclase by dissociation of N_s subunits and inhibition of adenylate cyclase by mass action principles. The stimulatory cycle is best understood. In this system, basal, or inactivated, adenylate cyclase is represented by the catalytic unit of adenylate cyclase (C) bound to $\beta\gamma$. Under these conditions, α_s is bound to GDP; in this state the subunits are bound together and adenylate cyclase is inhibited. Also, the receptor (R_s) is present as the high affinity binding state (R^*), bound to a $\alpha_s \beta\gamma$, whereas the ligand binding site is vacant. In the presence of the neurotransmitter or hormone (H_s), binding is facilitated because the receptor is present in the high-affinity state. The binding of the hormone causes displacement of GDP by GTP on α_s. GTP binding to α_s dissociates the N_s complex, thus dissociating $\beta\gamma$ from adenylate cyclase and producing the stimulated enzyme. The stimulation is terminated in two ways. First, GTP binding to α_s shifts the receptor from a high-affinity state into a low-affinity state, thus facilitating dissociation of the hormone from the receptor. Second, the GTPase activity in α_s hydrolyzes GTP into GDP, thus regenerating the GDP-bound form of α_s and causing reassociation of the N_s subunits. This reassociation returns the adenylate cyclase back to its inactive state and the receptor back to its high-affinity state. The crucial role of GTPase in terminating adenylate cyclase stimulation explains the actions of cholera toxin: by ribosylating α_s and inactivating GTPase activity in this subunit, the stimulation of adenylate cyclase is not terminated, and the result is persistent stimulation of adenylate cyclase.

The mechanism of receptor-mediated inhibition of adenylate cyclase is not as clear. There are many obvious parallels with the stimulatory cycle, but the precise series of reactions in the inhibi-

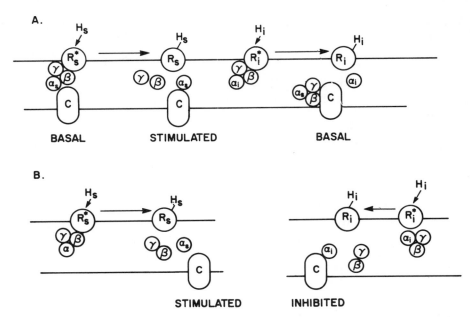

Fig. 2. Detailed models of N-protein subunit interactions during stimulation and inhibition of adenylate cyclase. (A) Dissociation model. In the inactivated state, the catalytic unit of adenylate cyclase (C) is bound to the α_s $\beta\gamma$ subunits of N_s, and α_s is bound to GDP. When a stimulatory hormone (H_s) binds to the high-affinity state of its receptor (R_s^*), it catalyzes the displacement of GDP by GTP on α_s, and dissociates the complex. Dissociation causes stimulation of C and changes the receptor to a low-affinity state (R_s). Binding of inhibitory hormone (H_i) to the high affinity form of its receptor (R_i^*) similarly dissociates N_i into its subunits α_i $\beta\gamma$, and free $\beta\gamma$ subunits react with free α_s to form inactivated (basal) enzyme. (B) Direct interaction model. Binding of either hormone to receptors causes dissociation of N-proteins, and interaction of α_s or α_i with C produces stimulation or inhibition, respectively.

tory cycle are still debated. Experiments by Gilman and colleagues (Manning and Gilman, 1983) suggest that a mechanism of subunit dissociation followed by mass action is responsible for adenylate cyclase inactivation. In this scheme (represented in Fig. 2 as the inhibitory portion of panel A), binding of the hormone to the receptor (in this case, H_i and R_i) promotes GTP binding to α_i and dissociation of the N_i subunits in a manner precisely analogous to the N_s cycle described above. In this case, however, dissociation of the N_s subunits produces an excess of free $\beta\gamma$. These subunits would then be free to associate with free α_s subunits that had been formed previously through the actions of the stimulatory hormones and receptors. The reaction of free α_s with the $\beta\gamma$ subunits liberated by the inhibitory cycle would tend, by simple mass action, to negate the actions of the stimulatory cycle and therefore cause inhibition of adenylate cyclase. This principle is described by the following reversible reaction:

$$\alpha_s\beta\gamma C \;\rightleftharpoons\; \alpha_s + \beta\gamma + C$$
$$\text{Inhibited} \qquad \text{Stimulated}$$

where an excess of free $\beta\gamma$ (formed from dissociation of N_i) would tend to push the reaction toward the left and result in inhibited adenylate cyclase.

Unfortunately, there are several drawbacks to this scheme of adenylate cyclase inhibition. First, it is not clear that the N-protein subunits are sufficiently mobile in the lipid milieu of cell membranes to allow mass action principles to dominate their actions. Second, there are several cases in which receptor-mediated inhibition of adenylate cyclase occurs in the absence of α_s proteins (Jakobs and Schultz, 1983; Childers and LaRiviere, 1984), a situation that clearly could not occur if α_s were necessary for the actions of N_i. An alternative possibility (shown by panel B in Fig. 2) is that α_i inhibits adenylate cyclase by direct interactions with the enzyme itself, but supporting evidence for this idea is lacking. Most of our models so far come from purifed proteins in artificial systems, and precise molecular interactions of these proteins in normal membranes may be quite different.

Another component of the receptor-mediated inhibitory cycle that has not yet been adequately explained is the role of sodium (Jakobs, 1979). For a number of inhibitory receptors, the addition of sodium produces a shift to low-affinity binding states, similar to the results seen in the presence of GTP. Moreover, sodium is required for receptor-mediated inhibition of adenylate cyclase, although its presence is irrelevant to the actions of the stimulatory receptors. The evidence that sodium actions on inhibitory receptors are related to N-proteins will be discussed later.

To summarize, there is a considerable body of data from different cell types to describe the properties of classical receptor-mediated inhibition of adenylate cyclase. Since opioid receptors also inhibit adenylate cyclase, we can use these data to predict several parameters that should also be true for the opioid receptor system if it works through similar mechanisms. These include:

1. Opioid agonist (but not antagonist) receptor binding should be decreased in the presence of guanine nucleotides.
2. Opioid agonist (but not antagonist) receptor binding should be decreased by sodium.
3. Inhibition of adenylate cyclase by opioid agonists should require the presence of GTP.
4. Inhibition of adenylate cyclase by opioid agonists should require the presence of sodium.
5. Inhibition of adenylate cyclase by opioid agonists should be attenuated by pertussis toxin; similar treatment might be expected to decrease formation of high-affinity agonist binding.
6. Opioid agonists should increase GTPase activity associated with N_i.

3. Actions of N-Proteins on Opioid Receptor Binding Sites

3.1. Effects of Guanine Nucleotides

The discovery that guanine nucleotides regulate binding of opioid receptor binding sites was the key finding that associated opioid receptors with traditional N-protein function. These early studies showed that guanine nucleotides decrease opioid agonist binding in both brain membranes (Blume, 1978a; Childers and Snyder, 1979, 1980a) and in NG108-15 cells (Blume, 1978b). In these preparations, effects are specific for guanine nucleotides, since adenine and other nucleotides have no effect. Among the guanine nucleotides, GTP, Gpp(NH)p (the nonhydrolyzable analog of GTP), and GDP are approximately equipotent, whereas GMP and guanosine are much less potent. Early results (Blume, 1978a,b) surprisingly showed that opioid antagonist as well as agonist binding was decreased by guanine nucleotides, but later experiments (Childers and Snyder, 1979, 1980a) showed that guanine nucleotides effectively discriminated between agonist and antagonist binding when assays were conducted in the presence of sodium. Therefore, guanine nucleotide regulation of opioid receptor binding parallels results from other receptor fields.

Other experiments have examined the receptor mechanisms of the guanine nucleotide effect. Kinetic experiments (Childers and Snyder, 1980a) have shown that guanine nucleotides increase both association and dissociation rates; since dissociation rates are increased more than association rates, the net result of GTP addition is a decrease in steady-state binding. Equilibrium saturation experiments have been more complicated, with results showing GTP-induced decrease in both affinity and numbers of binding sites. These apparent contradictions are easily resolved when the data are compared to results with other receptors. For example, with muscarinic cholinergic receptors, GTP eliminates agonist binding sites because the affinity of agonist binding has decreased to a point not detectable in receptor binding assays (Harden et al., 1983). The net result is a decrease in B_{max}, although the mechanism involves a decrease in affinity. The same interpretation can be made for opioid agonist sites, where the shape of the Rosenthal plots may depend upon the ability of the assay to detect the low affinity states produced by guanine nucleotides. In addition, when it is remembered that opioid receptor binding is complex anyway, with curvilinear Rosenthal plots in the absence of guanine nucleotides (Pasternak and Snyder, 1975a; Lord et al., 1977), it is not surprising that variable results can be seen.

The effects of divalent cations and guanine nucleotides have been explored in detail, not only because of the well-known effects of divalent cations (especially manganese) on opioid agonist binding (Pasternak et al., 1975a), but also because of the well-known requirement for magnesium for receptor stimulation and inhibition of adenylate cyclase (Schramm and Selinger, 1984). In most receptor systems, the addition of divalant cations attenuates the actions of guanine nucleotides on regulation of agonist binding (U'Prichard and Snyder, 1980), but this is not evident in the opioid receptor system. Although divalent cations inhibit the effect of GTP on opioid agonist binding, they do not affect the actions of the nonhydrolyzable analog Gpp(NH)p (Childers and Snyder, 1980a). This apparent paradox is explained by stimulation of membrane-bound phosphatases by divalent cations (Childers and Snyder, 1980b); by increasing hydrolysis of GTP, divalent cations would attenuate GTP but not Gpp(NH)p actions on receptor binding. Treatment of brain membranes with EDTA to chelate membrane-bound divalent cations does not affect opioid agonist binding itself, but does increase the ability of guanine nucleotides to inhibit agonist binding (Lambert and Childers, 1984), suggesting that membrane-bound divalent cations may play some role in regulating effects of guanine nucleotides on opioid receptor binding.

Identification of multiple opioid receptor subtypes (Lord et al., 1977; Chang and Cuatrecasas, 1979) has complicated the interpretation of guanine nucleotide effects on agonist binding. Early experiments on guanine nucleotide effects on opioid receptor binding clearly showed that effects of GTP varied with different labeled ligands. Pert and Taylor (1979) have described a classification of receptor subtypes based upon guanine nucleotide effects. In this system, type I receptors are regulated by GTP, and type II receptors are not. The implication was that the type II class might not be coupled to adenylate cyclase. Other workers have preferred to reclassify these receptors into more traditional subclasses, with mu receptors being type I and delta receptors being type II. However, whether these reclassifications are correct remains to be seen.

Several studies have indicated that delta receptors are less sensitive to guanine nucleotide regulation than mu receptors. Pfeiffer et al. (1982), Zajac and Roques (1985), and Chang et al. (1981) have shown that delta receptor binding sites are less sensitive to divalent cations, as well as guanine nucleotides. In these experiments, labeled agonist binding is decreased to a lower maximum inhibition level by GTP in the case of mu agonists compared to delta agonists, although the IC_{50} value for GTP is similar in both systems. These results illustrate the danger in extrapolating results from guanine nucleotide regulation of agonist binding into predictions about coupling of receptors with adenylate cyclase. Although delta receptors are less regulated by GTP, delta receptors in neuroblastoma $\times$ glioma NG108-15 cells are presumably coupled to adenylate cyclase (Blume et al., 1979). The lack of correlation between receptor binding regulation and receptor coupling with adenylate cyclase will be explored further in studies cited below.

A subject of some controversy has been the question of whether kappa opioid receptors are also regulated by guanine nucleotides. Several studies have shown that kappa agonist binding, as measured by [³H]ethylketocyclazocine (EKC) or [³H]bremazocine in the presence of unlabeled mu and delta ligands to block nonrelevant sites, is not regulated by GTP. Other studies (Mack et al., 1985), however, have demonstrated significant GTP regulation, although the effects of guanine nucleotides on [³H]EKC binding are even less evident than those previously reported on delta opioid receptor binding. It seems likely that this question will not be settled until kappa binding techniques are more carefully established between different laboratories.

Another opioid receptor subclass recently established is the high-affinity, or mu_1, class discovered by Pasternak and colleagues to be a common high-affinity site associated with all opiate ligand binding sites (Wolozin and Pasternak, 1981). Following treatment of membranes with naloxonazine, an opioid antagonist that binds irreversibly to mu_1 sites, Childers and Pasternak (1982) found that guanine nucleotide regulation of opioid agonist binding was not significantly affected, showing that removal of mu_1 sites retained a population of opioid receptors that were sensitive to GTP. More recent studies utilizing a new mu_1-selective binding assay indicate that these sites are very sensitive to both sodium ions and guanine nucleotides (Pasternak, personal communications). Indeed, of the various subtypes identified to date, the mu_1 sites appear to be most sensitive.

Long-term treatment of neuroblastoma cells with opioid antagonists, or chronic in vivo treatment of rats with naltrexone (Tempel et al., 1985), causes an increase, or up-regulation, of opioid receptors. An interesting question is whether these new receptor sites are also coupled to N-proteins. Tempel et al. (1985) found that the regulation of opioid agonist binding by guanine nucleotides was increased after chronic naltrexone treatment of rats, thus suggesting changes in receptor–N-protein interactions induced by up-regulation. No changes in guanine nucleotide regulation of binding were observed in neuroblastoma cells treated with naltrexone (Barg et al., 1984), however, and more recent experiments in rat brain failed to note any change in GTP regulation of binding nor in opioid-inhibited adenylate cyclase after chronic naltrexone treatment. Therefore, changes in receptor–N-protein interactions caused by receptor up-regulation remain an open question.

3.2. Sodium Regulation of Opioid Binding

The finding that sodium decreased opioid agonist binding without affecting antagonist binding was among the first discoveries of opioid receptor binding experiments (Pert et al., 1973; Simon et al., 1975). Interestingly, there are many parallels between the actions of sodium and those of guanine nucleotides, and there are several lines of evidence that both effects may be mediated through N-proteins. The similarities of sodium and GTP effects include:

1. Both sodium and GTP affect agonist and not antagonist binding, although the maximum agonist–antagonist differentiation of GTP effects are seen only in the presence of sodium (Childers and Snyder, 1980a).

2. Both affect kinetics of agonist binding by increasing agonist dissociation rates.

3. Effects of sodium and GTP on Rosenthal plots are equally confusing, with reports of both decrease in affinities and B_{max} values of labeled agonists (Pert and Snyder, 1974; Simon et al., 1975); these contradictions can be explained by the same reasoning as presented above for the effects of guanine nucleotides.

4. Effects of both are specific, with nucleotide effects specific for guanine nucleotides (especially GTP) and sodium effects mimicked somewhat by lithium, but not by potassium or rubidium.

5. Effects of both in several neurotransmitter systems are blocked by addition of divalent cations such as magnesium or manganese (U'Prichard and Snyder, 1980); although this blockade is apparent for sodium effects in the opioid receptor system (Pasternak et al., 1975a), it is not apparent for guanine nucleotide effects, as mentioned above.

6. The effects of both sodium and GTP are affected by reactions of sulfhydryl blocking reagents such as N-ethylmaleimide, (NEM) (Simon and Groth, 1975; Pasternak et al., 1975b; Larsen et al., 1981; Childers, 1984). Reagent effects are opposite for the two effects, however, decreasing regulation of binding by guanine nucleotides while increasing regulation of binding by sodium.

7. The effects of sodium and GTP are additive, at least for mu and delta sites (Childers and Snyder, 1980a), but probably not for kappa sites (Mack et al., 1985).

These results suggest that sodium and GTP may act at separate, though related, sites. The precise molecular relationship between sodium and GTP effects on opioid receptor binding has been explored in several ways. First, treatment of membranes or neuroblastoma cells with pertussis toxin to eliminate the function of N_i proteins has been used to examine the question of whether these effects are mediated by N-proteins. In experiments with neuroblastoma × glioma NG108-15 cells (Hsia et al., 1984), pertussis toxin decreased agonist binding, consistent with the idea that formation of high-affinity agonist binding sites requires interaction of receptors with N-proteins (De Lean et al., 1980; Kent et al., 1980). The binding that remained after toxin treatment was still regulated by both sodium and GTP, suggesting that the toxin had not eliminated all of the opioid receptor–N_i complexes in these cell membranes. In other experiments with NG108-15 cells, the action of pertussis toxin was more complex (Wuster et al.,

1984). Treatment of membranes with pertussis toxin had no effect on opioid agonist binding in the absence of sodium, but decreased agonist binding in the presence of sodium. Thus, pertussis toxin increased the effects of sodium on agonist binding. The effects of GTP were not affected by this treatment. These results suggest that inactivation of N_i by pertussis toxin did not disrupt interactions of N_i with receptors. Perhaps the interaction of receptors with N_i is very stable, since detergent solubilization of active opioid receptors from membranes yields preparations of soluble receptors that are still sensitive to guanine nucleotides (Koski et al., 1980). Unfortunately, experiments with pertussis toxin are complicated by the fact that this toxin not only reacts with N_i, but also with N_o (Sternweis and Robishaw, 1984). Moreover, because the ADP-ribosylation reactions of pertussis toxin are complex, requiring perhaps several soluble factors not yet characterized, it is conceivable that major differences in toxin effects may be more technical in nature rather than mechanistic. For example, even the effects of cholera toxin are complex on β-adrenergic receptors in frog erythrocytes (Stadel and Lefkowitz, 1981), a system much better characterized than the opioid receptor system.

Another useful probe in exploring the relationship between sodium and guanine nucleotide effects on opioid receptor binding has been specific sulfhydryl agents such as NEM. Work in other receptor fields has demonstrated the utility of agents like NEM in probing N-protein interactions with receptors. For example, in experiments with β-adrenergic receptors, NEM reduced high-affinity agonist binding only in the presence of guanine nucleotides (Vauquelin and Maguire, 1980); later experiments showed that NEM did not react with the beta receptor itself, but instead reacted with a crucial sulfhydryl group on the N_s protein that altered its ability to react with beta receptors (Heidenreich et al., 1982; Korner et al., 1982). Early opioid receptor binding experiments (Simon and Groth, 1975; Pasternak et al., 1975b) established the fact that incubation of brain membranes with NEM not only reduced opioid agonist binding, but also increased the regulation of agonist binding by sodium. Later experiments from Blume's group (Larsen et al., 1981) showed that in NG108-15 cells, treatment of membranes with NEM decreased the ability of GTP to regulate agonist binding. Moreover, a subclass of binding sites in the NG108-15 membranes was insensitive to NEM. In brain membranes, NEM also decreased guanine nucleotide regulation of binding, while simultaneously increasing sodium regulation (Childers and Jackson, 1984; Zukin et al., 1980). Taking advantage of these properties of NEM, other studies used selective protection experiments to explore the relationship of NEM effects on different sites within the opioid receptor complex. In these studies (Childers, 1984), the actions of NEM on GTP effects could be prevented by preincubating membranes with nonhydrolyzable analogs of GTP, whereas similar incubations did not prevent the NEM-induced increase in sodium regulation of binding. These results clearly show that although the sodium effect may be mediated through N-proteins (as the pertussis toxin experiments might tend to suggest), the sites for sodium and GTP regulation of binding are different. These results are summarized by the scheme in Fig. 3, which shows how occupation of different sites on the opioid receptor complex leads to conformational changes that affect the sensitivity of each site to NEM. The separate nature of sodium and GTP sites was confirmed by later studies (Lambert and Childers, 1984), which modified regulation of binding by guanine nucleotides by pretreatment of brain membranes at pH 4.5. In these experiments, low pH pretreatment increased the maximum effect of GTP, but did not change the effects of sodium on agonist binding.

Therefore, the current view of the topology of opioid receptors exhibits several parallels with other neurotransmitter receptor systems. The formation of high-affinity agonist binding sites presumably requires the interaction of opioid receptor binding sites with N_i proteins. The addition of GTP and/or sodium shifts the receptor into a low-affinity state, although whether this action occurs by dissociation of N_i away from the receptor has not yet been directly determined. The effect of sodium may be mediated by a site on N_i, but if so, the sodium site is physically distinct from the guanine nucleotide site. N_i probably also contains a specific divalent cation site, binding either magnesium or manganese to increase agonist binding affinities by antagonizing the actions of GTP and sodium; however, the physical relationship between the divalent cation site and the GTP and sodium site has not yet been determined.

4. Opioid-Inhibited Adenylate Cyclase

4.1. Studies in Cell Culture

Although initial studies on opioid inhibition of adenylate cyclase were conducted in brain membranes, most progress in this area

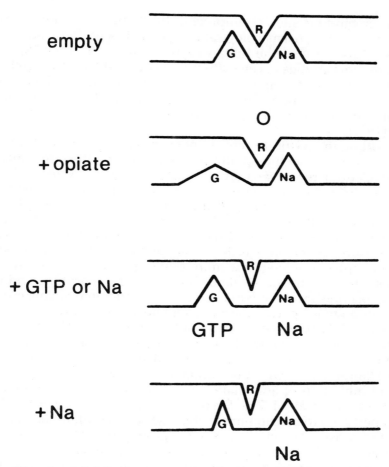

Fig. 3. Model of interactions between ligand binding sites and regulatory sites in the opioid receptor complex in brain membranes, summarizing effects of protecting ligands on N-ethylmaleimide (NEM) reactions. Binding of opiates to the receptor binding site (R) exposes SH groups at the GTP site, increasing sensitivity to NEM. Binding of GTP or sodium protects SH groups at the receptor binding site, decreasing sensitivity to NEM. Binding of sodium alone protects SH groups at both GTP and receptor binding sites (from Childers, 1984).

has been made in experiments with transformed cells. In these cells, usually neuroblastoma × glioma hybrids, opioid inhibition of adenylate cyclase activity is more pronounced than that of brain, presumably because of the biochemical simplicity of the transformed cells compared to brain. One strain, the NG108-15 cells, has been found to contain relatively high levels of opioid receptor binding sites (Hamprecht, 1977); further studies have shown that the pharmacological characteristics of these sites correspond to those of the delta subytpe (Chang et al., 1978). Although most studies in cell culture have utilized NG108-15 cells, a number of other transformed cell types also contain delta opioid receptors, including N4TG1, NiE-115, and N18TG2. Experiments on all these cell lines have been reviewed by Gilbert and Richelson (1983).

Although NG108-15 cells do not contain high levels of stimulatory receptors such as β-adrenergic receptors, they do contain prostaglandin receptors that stimulate adenylate cyclase (Hamprecht, 1977). Early experiments with NG108-15 cells showed that opioid agonists inhibited PGE_1-stimulated adenylate cyclase (Sharma et al., 1975a, b, 1977; Traber et al., 1975). This response is mediated by classical opioid receptors since inhibition is blocked by naloxone. Since these cells contain delta receptors, enkephalin and enkephalin analogs are more potent in inhibiting adenylace cyclase than are opiate alkaloids; nevertheless, morphine and related alkaloids inhibit adenylate cyclase at micromolar concentrations in a stereospecific manner. Opioid inhibition of adenylate cyclase in NG108-15 cells occurs not only for PGE-stimulated activity, but also for basal adenylate cyclase, as well as adenosine-stimulated and cholera toxin-stimulated adenylate cyclase (Propst and Hamprecht, 1981). Like other inhibitory receptor systems, opioid inhibition of adenylate cyclase requires both sodium and GTP (Blume et al., 1979). Finally, incubation of NG108-15 cells with pertussis toxin completely abolishes opioid inhibition of adenylate cyclase (Hsia et al., 1984), suggesting that N_i proteins (or, alternatively, N_0) are required for inhibitory activity.

Cell culture systems represent an excellent model system for examination of the relationship between receptor occupancy and efficacy of opioid inhibition of adenylate cyclase. In one study (Fantozzi et al., 1981), this relationship was explored by blocking receptor binding sites with the irreversible antagonist β-chlornaltrexamine. Interestingly, blockade of 95% of opiate receptor binding sites did not alter the inhibition of adenylate cyclase by opiate agonists, suggesting the presence of a large population of spare receptors in the NG108-15 cells. In detailed receptor binding studies by Law et al. (1985a), sodium and GTP produce three distinct agonist binding states of opiate receptors in NG108-15 cells whose agonist association rates are functions of receptor occupancy. These experiments directly demonstrated a decrease in opiate agonist affinity with respect to receptor occupancy during inhibition of adenylate cyclase by opioid agonists.

Since NG108-15 cells and the other cell types mentioned above contain only delta opioid receptors, an unresolved question in these studies is whether other opioid receptor subtypes may also be negatively coupled to adenylate cyclase. One approach to this question is to locate other transformed cell types containing different opioid receptor subtypes. Yu et al. (1986), by a systematic search through several cell lines, have located at least one type of human neuroblastoma cell line with both mu and delta receptor binding sites. Frey and Kebabian (1984) have identified mu opioid receptors in a pituitary tumor line designated 7315c. Interestingly, these receptors inhibit adenylate cyclase like the corresponding delta receptors in NG108-15 cells, except that in 7315c cells, morphine and related alkaloids are more potent than enkephalin analogs. These results suggest that mu receptors as well as delta receptors are negatively coupled to adenylate cyclase in transformed cells. An interesting variation of this theme occurs in the C-6 glioma cells, which contain high levels of β-adrenergic receptors, but, under normal conditions, no detectable opioid receptors. When C-6 cells are treated with desmethylimipramine for 24 h, however, β-adrenergic receptors are down-regulated and opiate receptor binding sites are detected (Tocque et al., 1984). Furthermore, as opioid receptor sites appear, opioid agonists inhibit cyclic AMP levels in intact cells. The pharmacological identity of these receptors has not yet been precisely determined, but preliminary results would suggest that they are not classical delta receptor sites (Tocque et al., 1984). Finally, there is presently some doubt as to whether the receptor coupled to adenylate cyclase in NG108-15 cells is indeed the classical delta site identified in binding studies. Costa et al. (1985) have demonstrated that several affinity states exist for agonist binding sites in NG108-15 cell membranes, and that the sites coupled to adenylate cyclase may not correspond to the delta sites identified in binding studies. Moreover, the studies from Blume's group cited earlier (Fantozzi et al., 1981) showed no effect on opioid-inhibited adenylate cyclase in NG108-15 cells after blockade of 95% of delta binding sites. The implications of these results will be discussed in more detail later in this review.

Interesting effects on adenylate cyclase occur when NG108-15 cells are chronically exposed to opioids. First, similar to other receptor systems, delta receptor down-regulation occurs, exhibited by a decrease in B_{max} of delta binding sites in NG108-15 cell membranes (Law et al., 1982). The down-regulation effect of chronic opioid exposure is explored in greater detail elsewhere in this volume. The second effect of chronic opioid exposure is a biphasic response of adenylate cyclase. Basal activity is first decreased by acute opiate agonist treatment because of direct inhibition of the enzyme by occupation of opiate receptors. During chronic exposure to opioids, however, cells show a gradual increase of adenylate cyclase activity close to normal (nontreated) levels. Moreover, when chronically treated NG108-15 cells are incubated with naloxone, a rebound effect occurs, in which a large (but transient) increase in adenylate cyclase is observed (Sharma et al., 1975a,b). These effects on basal adenylate cyclase have been used as a model system for tolerance and dependence, in which the slow increase from inhibited levels of adenylate cyclase activity represents the development of tolerance and the rebound actions of naloxone represent withdrawal (Sharma et al., 1975b). This conclusion has been questioned by more recent studies, however. First, adenylate cyclase in chronically treated cells can still be inhibited by opioid agonists, although response to some stimulatory agents like fluoride and guanine nucleotides is blunted. It is important to note that chronic treatment of NG108-15 cells by muscarinic or α-adrenergic agonists (both of which inhibit adenylate cyclase in these cells) produces exactly the same response as that seen by chronic exposure of cells to morphine (Gilbert and Richelson, 1983). Therefore, the gradual increase in adenylate cyclase during chronic treatment with inhibitory agonists is a general homeostatic principle of these cells. Moreover, other experiments (Griffin et al., 1983) have shown that the rebound effect of naloxone on chronically treated NG108-15 cells is either less than that reported by Sharma et al. (1975b) or not detectable at all (Wuster et al., 1983). More recent work from Greenspan and Musacchio (1984) has demonstrated, however, that some of the small rebound effects can be ascribed to slow dissociation of agonists from receptor binding sites. When etorphine-treated cells are washed before treatment with naloxone, a significant rebound effect is seen. A further description of tolerance and dependence effects on neuroblastoma cells is presented elsewhere in this volume.

4.2. Studies in Brain Membranes

Although more details about opioid-inhibited adenylate cyclase have been determined in cell culture, the original discovery of this activity was in mammalian brain membranes. In 1971, Chou et al. were the first to report inhibition of adenylate cyclase by opioids in brain membranes. Later, Collier and Roy (1974) reported that morphine inhibited PGE-stimulated adenylate cyclase in rat striatal membranes. Although several other papers appeared during this early period substantiating the role of opioid agonists in inhibiting brain adenylate cyclase (e.g., Minneman and Iversen, 1976; Tsang et al., 1978; Wilkening et al., 1976), and at least one paper appeared showing stimulation of adenylate cyclase by opioids (Puri et al., 1975), several groups were unable to reproduce these findings (Tell et al., 1975; Van Inwegen et al., 1975). As discussed above, the reasons for these discrepancies lay not only in the heterogeneities of brain membranes compared to cell culture, and in the disruption of coupling by homogenization procedures, but also in the lack of good biochemical information about the exact requirements for receptor-mediated changes in adenylate cyclase, especially GTP. As a result, most studies focused on neuroblastoma cells, on in vivo changes in cyclic nucleotide metabolism, or on brain slice experiments. In the latter type of experiment, several groups (Minneman and Iversen, 1976; Havemann and Kushinsky, 1978; Barchfeld et al., 1982) have described opioid inhibition of cyclic AMP levels in striatal slice preparations.

With the realization that guanine nucleotides were involved in receptor–adenylate cyclase coupling, later studies returned to brain membranes to obtain more reproducible results. Law et al. (1981) and Cooper et al. (1982) added GTP to their membrane preparations and thus were the first to accurately quantitate opioid inhibition of adenylate cyclase in these preparations. They showed that activity in brain, like in the cell culture experiments, is GTP-dependent, although some disagreement on sodium dependence of opioid inhibition has been seen. The pharmacological properties of opioid-inhibited adenylate cyclase in brain is similar to a delta receptor response, since opioid peptides are more potent than opioid alkaloids. This activity has remained difficult to quantitate, however, since the actual level of inhibition by opioid agonists is small, averaging around 20%.

Recognizing that opioid effects on adenylate cyclase activity are small even under ideal conditions, other studies have focused on techniques that selectively alter the function of N-proteins in brain membranes. In one such technique, brain membranes are preincubated in sodium acetate buffer at pH 4.5 before assay of receptors and adenylate cyclase at physiological pH (Childers et al., 1983). In low pH pretreated brain membranes, opioid receptor agonist binding in the absence of guanine nucleotides is not affected. Low pH pretreatment increases guanine nucleotide regulation of agonist binding, however, by increasing the maximal inhibition of agonist binding by GTP and Gpp(NH)p (Lambert and Childers, 1984). These results suggested that low pH pretreatment of brain membranes altered the interaction of N-proteins with receptors. Other experiments with adenylate cyclase (Childers and LaRiviere, 1984) showed that low pH pretreatment eliminates N_s-stimulated adenylate cyclase with no effect on basal enzyme activity or on activity stimulated by agents like forskolin and manganese, which act directly at the catalytic unit to stimulate adenylate cyclase (Table 1). Moreover, as N_s-stimulated adenylate cyclase is decreased by low pH pretreatment, inhibition of adenylate cyclase by opioid agonists is increased from a maximum effect of 10–15% in untreated membranes to 30–40% inhibition in treated membranes. These results suggested that there is an inverse correlation between N_s-stimulated and N_i-inhibited adenylate cyclase in brain membranes, and that significant opioid receptor-inhibited activity in brain membranes is masked when a large amount of N_s-stimulated activity is present.

Low pH treatment has also clearly showed differences in the properties of guanine nucleotide regulation of receptor binding and coupling of receptors with adenylate cyclase (Childers and LaRiviere, 1984). The effects of low pH pretreatment on adenylate

TABLE 1
Adenylate Cyclase Activity in Control (pH 7.4)
and pH 4.5 Pretreated Rat Striatal Membranes[a]

Agent	pH 7.4		pH 4.5	
	pmol/min/mg	% Basal	pmol/min/mg	% Basal
None	68 ± 7	100	72 ± 5	104
NaF (10 mM)	238 ± 15	350	74 ± 9	105
Gpp(NH)p (10 μM)	177 ± 16	260	95 ± 6	140
Forskolin	280 ± 30	411	291 ± 32	427
MnCl₂ (20 mM)	261 ± 31	380	284 ± 26	420
D-Ala enk (10 μM)	60 ± 6	90	47 ± 5	68
D-Ala enk + naloxone (0.5 μM)	65 ± 7	95	77 ± 8	109

[a]Low pH pretreatment of membranes has no effect on basal adenylate cyclase and no effect on stimulation by agents acting directly at the catalytic unit ($MnCl_2$ and forskolin), but eliminates stimulation by agents acting at N_s [Gpp(NH)p and NaF] and increases inhibition by opioid peptides.

cyclase are reversed by the addition of lipids such as phosphatidyl choline to treated membranes. These additions restore N_s-stimulated activity and reduce opioid-inhibited activity to levels of nontreated membranes. In the same membranes, however, addition of lipid has no effect on low pH pretreatment-induced increase in guanine nucleotide regulation of receptor binding. Therefore, these two actions of GTP are independent, and changes in one action of GTP may not affect the other.

The properties of opioid-inhibited adenylate cyclase in brain have now been examined in low pH pretreated membranes (Childers et al., 1986). Like all other receptor-inhibited activities, this reaction requires GTP. Unlike NG108-15 cells, sodium does not appear to be an absolute requirement for opioid inhibition, but the presence of 100 mM NaCl does provide maximal inhibited activity. Lineweaver-Burk plots (Fig. 4) show that opioid inhibition of adenylate cyclase is noncompetitive, decreasing V_{max} of the enzyme without affecting K_m of ATP. Regional distribution (Table 2) shows that opioid inhibition occurs primarily in only two brain regions, striatum and amygdala, with small inhibition in cortex and little or no inhibition in other regions. This distribution does not follow that of any known classical opioid receptor binding site. Moreover, the pharmacological profile of opioid-inhibited adenylate cyclase does not follow any known receptor binding site (Table 3). For example, the agonist profile resembles delta receptors, with enkephalin and enkephalin analogs more potent than mu agonists, but other opioid peptides such as β-endorphin and dynorphin are equipotent to enkephalin. Moreover, the antagonist profile does not match that of delta receptors, with mu antagonists such as naloxone and levallorphan blocking agonist inhibition at 50–100 nM concentrations, although the specific delta antagonist ICI 174864 does not block agonist inhibition at 10 μM concentration. To explore the relationship between classical opioid receptor binding sites and the identity of the receptor subtype(s) coupled to adenylate cyclase in brain, other experiments used specific blocking agents to inactivate the binding sites and determine effects on opioid-inhibited adenylate cyclase. One method used irreversible opiate antagonists and agonists such as β-flunaltrexamine, naloxonazine, and oxymorphine 4-nitrophenylhydrazone. In these experiments, the irreversible compounds blocked 75–95% of opioid receptor binding sites, depending on the ligand used. Even after blockade was established, however, opioid-inhibited adenylate cyclase was unaffected. Similar results were obtained with phospholipase A$_2$, an enzyme

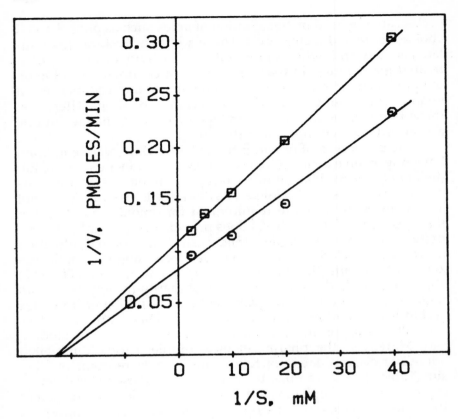

Fig. 4.   Lineweaver-Burk plot of adenylate cyclase activity in low pH pretreated striatal membranes, assayed in the absence (○) and presence (□) of 10μ*M* D-Ala enk (from Childers et al., 1986).

known to inhibit opioid receptor binding at low concentrations (Pasternak and Snyder, 1975b), but that does not decrease basal adenylate cyclase activity in brain membranes (Lad et al., 1979). In these experiments, decrease of opioid receptor binding sites by 93–100% still had no effect on opioid-inhibited adenylate cyclase (Table 4). These results are similar to those previously cited in NG108-15 cells, in which blockade of 95% of delta sites by β-chlornaltrexamine had no effect on opiate-inhibited adenylate cyclase (Fantozzi et al., 1981). In those studies, the conclusion was that there was a large population of spare receptors in the NG108-15 cells. That conclusion cannot be supported by these results in brain membranes, however, since the agonist dose-response

TABLE 2
Regional Distribution of Opioid-Inhibited Adenylate Cyclase
in Rat Brain Membranes

| Region | Basal activity, pmol/min/mg | Maximal % inhibition[a] | |
		+DSLET	+DAGO
Striatum	63.4	32	29
Amygdala	32.1	37	31
Thalamus	37.4	22	20
Sensomotor Cortex	13.8	15	11
Hypothalamus	53.4	10	11
Hippocampus	12.6	9	12
Frontal Cortex	10.7	5	0
Brain Stem	11.3	5	1
Cerebellum	34.4	4	1

[a]Assayed in the presence of 10 μM DSLET and 50 μM DAGO, together with 100 mM NaC1 and 50 μM GTP and crude rat brain membranes. Only striatum and amygdala show relatively high levels of inhibited activity.

TABLE 3
Agonist Specificity of Opioid-Inhibited Adenylate Cyclase
in Rat Striatal Membranes[a]

| Opioid | IC_{50}, μM | Maximal inhibition | |
		% Inhibition	conc., μM
Met-enk	0.8	33	10
Leu-enk	0.6	30	10
D-Ala enk-NH$_2$	0.8	32	10
DADL enk	0.7	32	10
DSLET	0.3	32	10
beta-end	0.8	40	10
N-Ac beta-end	—	11	50
Dyn (1-13)	0.7	30	10
Dyn A (1-17)	0.6	31	10
D-Ala Dyn A	0.6	40	10
Morphine	6	18	100
DAGO	10	24	50
Morphiceptin	10	15	50

[a]Enzyme activity assayed in low pH pretreated striatal membranes. Active agonists included delta receptor enkephalin analogs, dynorphin, and β-endorphin. Less active were mu receptor agonists; N-acetyl-β-endorphin was inactive.

TABLE 4
Effect of Phospholipase A_2 and Opioid Receptor Binding
and Opioid-Inhibited Adenylate Cyclase in Striatal Membranes[a]

Receptor binding				
	Control		Treated	
Ligand	Specific cpm	% Control	Specific cpm	% Control
[³H]DAGO	3166	100	91	3
[³H]DSLET	3169	100	12	0
[³H]EKC	1572	100	109	7

Adenylate cyclase		
	% Basal activity	
Additions	Control	Treated
None	100	118 (100)
D-Ala enk-NH₂	71	88 (74)
Naloxone + D-Ala enk-NH₂	97	117 (99)

[a]Striatal membranes were treated at pH 4.5, incubated with 0.5 μg/mL phospholipase A_2, and divided in half for receptor binding and adenylate cyclase assays. Despite the loss of 93–100% of high-affinity receptor sites, opioid-inhibited adenylate cyclase was unaffected by the enzyme treatment.

curves for opioid-inhibited adenylate cyclase are not altered by destruction of 75–100% of receptor binding sites. If spare receptors were the explanation, then destruction of such a large portion of binding sites would result in a right shift in the agonist dose–response curve. Therefore it seems possible that the opioid receptor coupled to adenylate cyclase in brain membranes does not correspond to any of the traditional receptor binding sites determined by binding studies and physiological experiments. This may not be too surprising since receptor binding experiments are conducted under conditions that would not allow for any significant coupling between receptors and adenylate cyclase. Moreover, as yet we have no information about the possible physiological role of opioid-inhibited adenylate cyclase in brain. It probably is not involved in analgesia mechanisms, since it is not found in regions that normally mediate pain information. Perhaps, since it is highest in striatum, it may be involved in extrapyramidal movement effects of opioids.

4.3. Opioid-Stimulated GTPase

One of the key features of the ternary complex model as discussed above is the role of GTP hydrolysis in receptor–adenylate cyclase coupling. For N_s systems, hydrolysis of GTP to GDP occurs on the alpha subunit of N_s, and this hydrolysis terminates the actions of N_s on adenylate cyclase (Cassel and Selinger, 1976). The role of GTP hydrolysis in N_i systems is not as clear, however. A major breakthrough in understanding this process was a study in NG108-15 cells by Koski and Klee (1981), who showed that opioid agonists stimulate GTPase activity in membranes from NG108-15 cells. This activity is receptor-mediated since naloxone blocks stimulation, and potencies of enkephalin and enkephalin analogs correlate with their affinities at delta receptors. It is important to place this receptor-stimulated GTPase in perspective with other GTP hydrolyzing enzymes. Since hydrolysis of GTP is clearly an important cellular activity, acting in reactions not related to neurotransmitter receptor actions, identification of the GTPase associated with opioid receptors must be differentiated from other nonspecific enzymes. In the case of NG108-15 cells, nonspecific GTPase activity is blocked by the addition of adenine nucleotides, and opioid-stimulated GTPase is specifically associated with low K_m form, with K_m for GTP less than $1\mu M$. The initial conclusion from these experiments was that the receptor-mediated GTPase represents a key intermediate in the coupling of opioid receptors with adenylate cyclase. The authors suggested that opioid-stimulated GTPase inhibits adenylate cyclase indirectly by decreasing intracellular levels of GTP that would be required for N_s stimulation. For several reasons, this interpretation is not generally accepted today. First, opioid inhibition of adenylate cyclase can occur in the absence of N_s stimulation (Childers and LaRiviere, 1984), whereas other inhibitory systems (e.g., somatostatin) exist in cells like the S-49 lymphoma cyc − cell, which has no functional N_s protein (Jakobs and Schultz, 1983). Furthermore, incubation of NG108-15 cells with opioid agonists has no effect on intracellular GTP levels (Musacchio and Schen, 1983). Therefore, N_i-associated GTPase does not function by inhibiting intracellular GTP concentrations necessary for N_s stimulation. An alternative model suggests that receptor-mediated GTPase is a function of N_i activity, just as GTPase is a similar function in N_s stimulation. In this model, GTPase would act to terminate actions of N_i as it does in the N_s system.

Although opioid-stimulated GTPase has now been identifed in several cell types (Gilbert and Richelson, 1983), other studies have attempted to identify this activiy in brain membranes. The problem of identification is even more difficult in brain membranes than in NG108-15 cells because brain contains an even greater proportion of nonspecific GTPase activities. Nevertheless, at least two studies (Barchfeld and Medzihradsky, 1984; Franklin and Ross, 1984) have identified opioid-stimulated GTPase in rat brain membranes. Like the activity in NG108-15 cells, receptor-stimulated GTPase in brain has a low (less than 1 μM) K_m for GTP. Although these results would suggest that GTPase is a required intermediate in adenylate cyclase inhibition, several cautions must be kept in mind. First, the regional distribution of opioid-stimulated GTPase in brain (Franklin and Ross, 1984) is much different than that of opioid-inhibited adenylate cyclase. Although GTPase occurs at equal levels in cortex, hippocampus, and striatum, adenylate cyclase has been observed primarily in striatum. Second, as mentioned previously, other second messenger systems besides adenylate cyclase may be coupled to receptors through N-proteins. Therefore, receptor-stimulated GTPase may be a reflection of all N-proteins coupled to opiate receptors, not just that portion that mediates adenylate cyclase inhibition.

5. Other Opioid Receptor-Coupled Second Messenger Systems

5.1. Cyclic GMP

Soon after the discovery that opioid agonists inhibit adenylate cyclase, other experiments showed that opioids increase levels of cyclic GMP in cells and brain slices. Minneman and Iversen (1976) showed that enkephalin increased intracellular cyclic GMP levels in slice preparations of rat striatum. Although these experiments showed that cyclic GMP stimulation is blocked by naloxone, detailed pharmacological studies were not completed in brain to determine the identity of the receptor causing cyclic GMP effects.

Work on opioid effects on cyclic GMP metabolism in cell culture was initially hampered by the controversy surrounding the work of Gullis, whose experiments showing opioid-induced increase in cyclic GMP levels in NG108-15 cells, were shown to be unreliable and were withdrawn (Gullis, 1977). Nevertheless, several later studies have shown opioid stimulatory effects on cyclic GMP levels in N4TG1 cells (Gwynn and Costa, 1983). Obviously, the molecular properties of the receptor-coupled guanylate cyclase are less well developed than those of adenylate cyclase, especially since guanylate cyclase is largely soluble, and direct coupling between receptors and guanylate cyclase has been difficult to establish. Therefore, such experiments are conducted with whole cells, using radioimmunoassays to determine levels of cyclic GMP. These studies have ruled out the possibility that opioids might increase cyclic GMP levels by inhibition of cyclic GMP phosphodiesterase, since phosphodiesterase inhibitors were used in several experiments. Moreover, in NG108-15 cells, stimulation of cyclic GMP levels appears to be mediated by a delta receptor response (Gwynn and Costa, 1983). Thus, occupation of delta receptors in NG108-15 cells may simultaneously increase cyclic GMP levels while decreasing levels of cyclic AMP.

5.2. Protein Phosphorylation

It is generally agreed that the immediate target of cyclic AMP actions in cells is cyclic AMP-dependent protein phosphorylation. Several neurotransmitters, whether they stimulate or inhibit adenylate cyclase, cause either increased or decreased phosphorylation of protein substrates in neuronal membranes (Nestler et al., 1984). Unfortunately, protein phosphorylation is a common reaction in cell membranes, and polyacrylamide gel electrophoresis has revealed more than 70 protein bands that are substrates for one form or another of phosphorylation reactions (Nestler et al., 1984). These reactions are generally classed as cyclic AMP-dependent, cyclic GMP-dependent, or calcium-dependent. Therefore, identifying and characterizing a single protein substrate that is coupled to opioid receptor reactions has not been straightforward. Nevertheless, several reports have identified opioid-induced changes in protein phosphorylation in brain membranes. For example, Ehrlich et al. (1978) showed that incubation of brain membranes with enkephalin inhibited phosphorylation of two proteins of molecular weight 47,000 and 10–20,000. In addition, β-endorphin increased phosphorylation of other membrane proteins in calcium-dependent reactions. These data suggested that β-endorphin caused changes in protein phosphorylation that would be evident during changes in calcium uptake. This suggestion has been supported by direct experiments showing opioid-induced changes in calcium uptake as discussed below.

Despite several positive experiments, the field of opioid-induced changes in protein phosphorylation is still in its early stages. There still has been no detailed characterization of the proteins affected by opioid receptors and no solid information about the identity of the second messenger system that couples opioid receptors with protein phosphorylation.

5.3. Effects of Opioids on Calcium Uptake

Although a review of current knowledge of effects of opiates on ion channels will be discussed elsewhere in this book, a large series of biochemical experiments has accumulated suggesting a role of calcium in opioid receptor function. These studies began with a series of in vivo experiments that examined the effect of opiate injections on brain calcium content. Initial experiments showing that calcium inhibits morphine analgesia (Harris et al., 1975) led to further studies (Ross and Cardenas, 1977; End et al., 1981) showing that opiate agonists reduce calcium content in brain.

These in vivo experiments have led to a series of biochemical studies to reveal the molecular basis for opioid effects on calcium levels. One focus of attention has been calmodulin. Nehmad et al. (1982) have demonstrated that opioids change the distribution of cytosolic and membrane-bound calmodulin in brain, and that chronic morphine treatment increases membrane levels of calmodulin. Although the significance of such changes is not known, these results suggest that opioid-mediated changes in calmodulin content and/or distribution would change activities of a variety of calcium-dependent enzymes, thus mediating cellular changes by opioids. Another potential site of opioid action is opioid peptide binding to calmodulin, seen especially with β-endorphin (Sellinger-Barnette and Weiss, 1982). Although the binding affinity of β-endorphin for calmodulin is not particularly high, there may be sufficient β-endorphin locally released from nerve endings to inactivate at least a portion of synaptic calmodulin. Nevertheless, these β-endorphin–calmodulin interactions are not true opioid-mediated phenomena, since they are not blocked by naloxone and the binding involves a nonopioid section of the primary sequence of β-endorphin (Giedroc and Puett, 1985).

Other experiments have focused on opioid effects on calcium uptake. As mentioned above, at least one study has demonstrated opioid-dependent changes in protein phosphorylation that require calcium (Ehrlich et al., 1978). Such studies may suggest that opioid receptors could change calcium uptake and thereby alter specific protein phosphorylation reactions. Biochemical experiments have demonstrated direct evidence for opioid-mediated changes in calcium uptake. Unfortunately, some of these studies contradict each other. For example, Guerrero-Munoz et al. (1979) showed that opioids inhibited ATP-depenent calcium uptake into synaptosomes, whereas Barr and Leslie

(1985) showed that opioids increased calcium uptake into synaptosomes from cortex and striatum. Part of the disagreement probably involves different regions and preparations, since the actions of opioids on calcium uptake appear to vary in different regions, and part of the problem lies in the question of voltage-dependent calcium uptake, in which effects would obviously vary depending upon the polarization state of the system studied. More informative studies have been obtained in electrophysiological experiments on neuroblastoma cells and cultured dorsal root ganglion cells (Werz and Macdonald, 1983); those experiments are reviewed elsewhere in this volume.

5.4. Opioid-Mediated Changes in Membrane Lipids

Besides cyclic nucleotides, another major second messenger system identified with different neurotransmitters in different cells is the receptor-mediated increase in phosphoinositide (PI) turnover, which ultimately leads to changes in calcium uptake (Nishizuka, 1984). As mentioned above, recent evidence suggests that receptors are coupled to PI turnover systems through N-proteins (Nakamura and Ui, 1985). Since most (if not all) opioid receptor subtypes are regulated by guanine nucleotides, and with the biochemical evidence cited above that opioids could change calcium uptake, it has been suggested that one potential opioid-coupled second messenger system is PI turnover. Unfortunately, in both brain slice preparations and neuroblastoma cells, no effect of opioids has yet been reported on PI turnover. Since this field is still in its infancy compared to the adenylate cyclase field, however, it may be premature to make any hard conclusions from these negative data.

Several studies have demonstrated the role of lipids and protein glyosylation in opioid receptor function. For example, incorporation of cerebroside sulfate increases the ability of enkephalin analogs to inhibit PGE-stimulated adenylate cyclase in N18TG2 cells, with no effect on receptor number or affinity (Law et al., 1983). Incubation of NG108-15 cells with tunicamysin, which inhibits protein glycosylation, decreases receptor binding, but does not affect the ability of etorphine to inhibit adenylate cyclase (Law et al., 1985b).

Other experiments have demonstrated effects of opioids on membrane lipid composition. The best characterized system is the opioid agonist-induced inhibition of ganglioside synthesis in neuroblastoma cells. In these systems, 24-hour incubation of cells with enkephalin analogs does not change phospholipid content, but produces a significant decrease in total ganglioside content that is blocked by naloxone. Moreover, the opioid-induced decrease in gangliosides is reversed by addition of cyclic AMP, suggesting that these effects of opioids may be mediated through inhibition of adenylate cyclase, presumably through inhibition of cyclic AMP-induced phosphorylation of glycosyltransferases. These effects may be limited to certain cell lines, however, since other cell lines that contain delta opioid receptors and opioid-inhibited adenylate cyclase do not appear to possess this action on gangliosides (Gilbert and Richelson, 1983).

6. Conclusions

Clearly, work to identify the biochemical reactions that take place after binding of opioid agonists to receptor sites has made some limited progress, but still lags behind most of the receptor research in this field. The best characterized system, opioid inhibition of adenylate cyclase, appears to work in similar ways to other neurotransmitter-inhibited adenylate cyclase systems, and conclusions from other systems may be extrapolated to this one. Many important questions remain about this and other second messenger systems, however:

1. What are the opioid receptor subtypes coupled to adenylate cyclase in brain and other nontransformed mammalian tissues? Although much important data have been obtained from transformed cells in culture systems, the act of cell transformation may cause important changes in receptor–adenylate cyclase coupling, producing coupled receptors that are not relevant to normal cells. Moreover, the continued use of nonphysiological conditions to assay high-affinity receptor binding sites, though they produce excellent binding assays with high-affinity binding of agonists and antagonists, may not provide the proper identification of receptor subtypes that exist under more physiological conditions.

2. What other second messenger systems are coupled to opioid receptors? In brain, only a small percentage of opioid receptor binding sites appear to be coupled to adenylate cyclase, and yet most (if not all) subtypes are regulated by guanine nucleotides. It is tempting to speculate that we have not yet identified all of the potential second messenger systems that cells utilize to couple to neurotransmitter receptors, and that opiate receptor-inhibited adenylate cyclase represents only a small percentage

of receptors that are coupled to other second messenger systems through N-proteins.

3. What happens after activation and/or inhibition of the opioid receptor-coupled second messenger system? As can be seen above, the available evidence for third messenger systems, such as protein phosphorylation or changes in calcium uptake, is meager and full of contradiction. A real challenge in this field is to identify those cellular components that are affected by opioid receptor-coupled second messenger systems and determine their role in determining the final biological response of opioids. To accomplish this goal, biochemists and electrophysiologists must work together to identify common components that act in their various systems.

References

Barchfeld, C. C., Maassen, Z., and Medzihradsky, F. (1982) Receptor-related interactions of opiates with PGE-induced adenylate cyclase in brain. *Life Sci.* **31,** 1661–1665.

Barchfeld, C. C. and Medzihradsky, F. (1984) Receptor-mediated stimulation of brain GTPase by opiates in normal and dependent rats. *Biochem. Biophys. Res. Commun.* **121,** 641–648.

Barg, J., Levy, R., and Simantov, R. (1984) Up-regulation of opiate receptors by opiate antagonists in neuroblastoma-glioma cell culture: The possibility of interaction with guanosine triphosphate-binding proteins. *Neurosci. Lett.* **50,** 133–137.

Barr, E. and Leslie, S. W. (1985) Opioid peptides increase calcium uptake by synaptosomes from brain regions. *Brain Res.* **329,** 280–284.

Blume, A. J. (1978a) Opiate binding to membrane preparations of neuroblastoma-glioma hybrid cells NG108-15: Effects of ions and nucleotides. *Life Sci.* **22,** 1843–1852.

Blume, A. J. (1978b) Interactions of ligands with opiate receptors of brain membranes: Regulation by ions and nucleotides. *Proc. Natl. Acad. Sci. USA* **75,** 1713–1717.

Blume, A. J., Lichtshtein, L., and Boone, G. (1979) Coupling of opiate receptors to adenylate cyclase: Requirement for sodium and GTP. *Proc. Natl. Acad. Sci. USA* **76,** 5626–5630.

Cassel, D. and Selinger, Z. (1976) Catecholamine-stimulated GTPase activity in turkey erythrocyte membranes. *Biochim. Biophys. Acta* **452,** 538–551.

Cerione, R. A., Codina, J., Benovic, J. L., Lefkowitz, R. J., Birnbaumer, L., and Caron, M. G. (1984) The mammalian beta-adrenergic receptor: Reconstitution of functional interactions between pure receptor and pure stimulatory guanine nucleotide binding protein of the adenylate cyclase system. *Biochemistry* **23,** 4519–4525.

Cerione, R. A., Regan, J. W., Nakata, H., Codina, J., Benovic, J. L., Geirschik, P., Somers, R. L., Spiegel, A. M., Birnbaumer, L., Lefkowitz, R. J., and Caron, M. G. (1986) Functional reconstitution of alpha(2)-adrenergic receptors with guanine nucleotide regulatory proteins in phospholipid vesicles. *J. Biol. Chem.* **261,** 3901–3909.

Chang, K. J. and Cuatrecasas, P. (1979) Multiple opiate receptors: Enkephalins and morphine bind to receptors of different specificity. *J. Biol. Chem.* **254,** 2610–2618.

Chang, K. J., Miller, R. J., and Cuatrecasas, P. (1978) Interaction of enkephalin with opiate receptors in intact cultured cells. *Mol. Pharmacol.* **14,** 961–970.

Chang, K. J., Hazum, E., Killian, A., and Cuatrecasas, P. (1981) Interactions of ligands with morphine and enkephalin receptors are differentially affected by guanine nucleotides. *Mol. Pharmacol.* **20,** 1–7.

Childers, S. R. (1984) Interaction of opiate receptor binding sites and guanine nucleotide regulatory sites: Selective protection from N-ethylmaleimide. *J. Pharmacol. Exp. Ther.* **230,** 684–691.

Childers, S. R. and Jackson, J. L. (1984) pH Selectivity of N-ethylmaleimide reactions with opiate receptor complexes in rat brain membranes. *J. Neurochem.* **43,** 1163–1170.

Childers, S. R. and LaRiviere, G. (1984) Modification of guanine nucleotide regulatory components in brain membranes. II. Relationship of guanosine-5′triphosphate effects on opiate receptor binding and coupling receptors with adenylate cyclase. *J. Neurosci.* **4,** 2764–2771.

Childers, S. R. and Pasternak, G. W. (1982) Naloxazone, a novel opiate antagonist: Irreversible blockade of rat brain opiate receptors in vitro. *Cell. Mol. Neurobiol.* **2,** 93–103.

Childers, S. R. and Snyder, S. H. (1979) Guanine nucleotides differentiate agonist and antagonist interactions with opiate receptors. *Life Sci.* **23,** 759–762.

Childers, S. R. and Snyder, S. H. (1980a) Differential regulation by guanine nucleotide of opiate agonist and antagonist receptor interactions. *J. Neurochem.* **34,** 583–593.

Childers, S. R. and Snyder, S. H. (1980b) Characterization of [^{3}H]-guanine nucleotide binding sites in brain membranes. *J. Neurochem.* **35,** 183–192.

Childers, S. R., Nijssen, P., Nadeau, P., Buckhannan, P., Li, P.-V., and Harris, J. (1986) Opiate-inhibited adenylate cyclase in mammalian brain membranes. *NIDA Monographs* **71,** 65–80.

Childers, S. R., Lambert, S. M., and LaRiviere, G. (1983) Selective alterations in guanine nucleotide regulation of opiate receptor binding and coupling with adenylate cyclase. *Life Sci.* **33,**(suppl. I), 215–218.

Chou, W. S., Ho, A. K. S., and Loh, H. H. (1971) Effect of acute and chronic morphine and norepinephrine on brain adenylate cyclase activity. *Proc. West. Pharmacol. Soc.* **14,** 42–46.

Cockcroft, S. and Gomperts, B. D. (1985) Role of guanine nucleotide binding protein in the activation of polyphosphinositide phosphodiesterase. *Nature* **314,** 534–536.

Collier, H. O. J. and Roy, A. C. (1974) Morphine-like drugs inhibit the stimulation by E prostaglandins of cyclic AMP formation by rat brain homogenates. *Nature* **248,** 24–27.

Cooper, D. M. F., Londos, C., Gill, D. L., and Rodbell, M. (1982) Opiate receptor-mediated inhibition of adenylate cyclase in rat striatal plasma membranes. *J. Neurochem.* **38,** 1164–1167.

Costa, T., Wuster, M., Gramsch, C., and Herz, A. (1985) Multiple states of opioid receptors may modulate adenylate cyclase in intact neuroblastoma × glioma hybrid cells. *Mol. Pharmacol.* **28,** 146–154.

De Lean, A., Stadel, J. M., and Lefkowitz, R. J. (1980) A ternary complex model explains the agonist-specific binding properties of the adenylate cyclase-coupled beta-adrenergic receptor. *J. Biol. Chem.* **255,** 1108–1111.

Duggan, A. W. and North, R. A. (1983) Electrophysiology of opioids. *Pharmacol. Rev.* **35,** 219–281.

Ehrlich, Y. H., Bonnet, K. A., Davis, L. G., and Brunngraber, E. G. (1978) Decreased phosphorylation of specific proteins in neostriatal membranes from rats after long-term narcotics exposure. *Life Sci.* **23,** 137–146.

End, D. W., Carchman, R. A., and Dewey, W. L. (1981) Interactions of narcotics with synaptosomal calcium transport. *Biochem. Pharmacol.* **30,** 674–676.

Evans, T., Martin, H. W., Hughes, A. R., and Harden, T. K. (1985) Guanine nucleotide-sensitive high affinity binding of carbachol to muscarinic cholinergic receptors of 1321nl astrocytoma cells is insensitive to pertussis toxin. *Mol. Pharmacol.* **27,** 32–37.

Fantozzi, R., Mullikin-Kirkpatrick, D., and Blume, A. J. (1981) Irreversible inactivation of the opiate receptors in neuroblastoma × glioma hybrid NG108-15 cells by chlornaltrexamine. *Mol. Pharmacol.* **20,** 8–15.

Florio, V. A. and Sternweis, P. C. (1985) Reconstitution of resolved muscarinic cholinergic receptors with purified GTP-binding proteins. *J. Biol. Chem.* **260,** 3477–3483.

Franklin, P. H. and Ross, W. (1984) Opiates stimulate low K_m GTPase in brain. *J. Neurochem.* **43,** 1132–1135.

Frey, A. and Kebabian, J. W. (1984) μ-Opiate receptor in 7315c tumor tissue mediates inhibition of immunoreactive prolactin release and adenylate cyclase activity. *Endocrinology* **115,** 1797–1804.

Fung, B. K.-K. and Stryer, L. (1980) Photolyzed rhodopsin catalyzes the exchange of GTP for bound GDP in retinal rod outer segments. *Proc. Natl. Acad. Sci. USA* **77,** 2500–2504.

Giedroc, D. P. and Puett, D. (1985) Binding of a synthetic beta-endorphin peptide to calmodulin. *Mol. Pharmacol.* **28,** 588–593.

Gilbert, J. A. and Richelson, E. (1983) Function of delta opioid receptors in cultured cells. *Mol. Cell. Biochem.* **55,** 83–91.

Gilman, A. G. (1984) G proteins and dual control of adenylate cyclase. *Cell* **36,** 577–579.

Gonzales, R. A. and Crews, F. T. (1985) Guanine nucleotides stimulate production of inositol triphosphate in rat cortical membranes. *Biochem. J.* **232,** 799–804.

Greenspan, D. L. and Mussachio, J. M. (1984) The effect of tolerance on opiate dependence as measured by the adenylate cyclase rebound response in the NG108-15 model system. *Neuropeptides* **5,** 41–44.

Griffin, M. T., Law, P. Y., and Loh, H. H. (1983) Modulation of adenylate cyclase by a cytosolic factor following chronic opiate exposure in neuroblastoma cells. *Life Sci.* **33,** (suppl. I), 365–368.

Grossman, A. (1983) Brain opiates and neuroendocrine function. *Clin. Endocrinol. Metab.* **12,** 725–746.

Guerrero-Munoz, F., Guerrero, M. L., and Way, E. L. (1979) Effect of beta-endorphin on calcium uptake in the brain. *Science* **206**, 89–91.

Gullis, R. J. (1977) Statement. *Nature* **265**, 764.

Gwynn, C. J. and Costa, E. (1983) Opioids regulate cyclic GMP formation in cloned neuroblastoma cells. *Proc. Natl. Acad. Sci USA* **79**, 690–694.

Hamprecht, B. (1977) Structural, electrophysiological, biochemical, and pharmacological properties of neuroblastoma × glioma cell hybrids in cell culture. *Int. Rev. Cytol.* **49**, 99—170.

Harden, T. K., Meeker, R. B., and Martin, H. W. (1983) Interaction of a radiolabeled agonist with cardiac muscarinic cholinergic receptors. *J. Pharmacol. Exp. Ther.* **227**, 570–577.

Harris, R. A., Loh, H. H., and Way, E. L. (1975) Effects of divalent cation chelators and an ionophore on morphine analgesia and tolerance. *J. Pharmacol. Exp. Ther.* **196**, 288–297.

Havemann, U. and Kushinsky, K. (1978) Interactions of opiates and prostaglandin E with regard to cyclic AMP in striatal tissue of rats *in vitro*. *Arch. Pharmacol.* **302**, 103–106.

Heidenreich, K. H., Weiland, G. A., and Molinoff, P. B. (1982) Effects of magnesium and N-ethylmaleimide on the binding of [^{3}H]-hydroxybenzylisoproterenol to beta-adrenergic receptors. *J. Biol. Chem.* **257**, 804–810.

Helmreich, E. J. M. and Pfeuffer, T. (1985) Regulation of signal transduction by beta-adrenergic hormone receptors. *Trends Pharmacol. Sci.* **6**, 438–443.

Hsia, J. A., Moss, J., Hewlett, E. L., and Vaughan, M. (1984) ADP-ribosylation of adenylate cyclase by pertussis toxin: Effects on inhibitory agonist binding. *J. Biol. Chem.* **259**, 1086–1090.

Jakobs, K. H. (1979) Inhibition of adenylate cyclase by hormones and neurotransmitters. *Mol. Cell. Endocrinol.* **16**, 147–156.

Jakobs, K. H. and Schultz, G. (1983) Occurrence of a homone-sensitive inhibitory component of the adenylate cyclase in S49 lymphoma cyc− variants. *Proc. Natl. Acad. Sci. USA* **80**, 3899–3905.

Katada, T. and Ui, M. (1982) Direct modification of the membrane adenylate cyclase system by islet-activating protein due to ADP-ribosylation of a membrane protein. *Proc. Natl. Acad. Sci. USA* **79**, 3129–3133.

Kent, R. S., De Lean, A., and Lefkowitz, R. J. (1980) A quantitative analysis of beta-adrenergic receptor interactions: Resolution of high and low affinity states of the receptor by computer modeling of ligand binding data. *Mol. Pharmacol.* **17**, 14–23.

Korner, M., Gilon, C., and Schramm, M. (1982) Locking of hormone in the beta-adrenergic receptor by attack on a sulfhydryl in an associated component. *J. Biol. Chem.* **257**, 3389–3397.

Koski, G. and Klee, W. A. (1981) Opiates inhibit adenylate cyclase by stimulating GTP hydrolysis. *Proc. Natl. Acad. Sci USA* **78**, 4185–4189.

Koski, G., Simonds, W. F., and Klee, W. A. (1980) Guanine nucleotides inhibit binding of agonists and antagonists to soluble opiate receptors. *J. Biol. Chem.* **256**, 1536–1538.

Kosterlitz, H. J. and Waterfield, A. A. (1975) In vitro models in the study of structure–activity relationships of narcotic analgesics. *Ann. Rev. Pharmacol. Toxicol.* **15**, 29–47.

Lad, P. M., Preston, M. S., Welton, A. F., Nielsen, T. B., and Rodbell, M. (1979) Effects of phospholipase A_2 and filipin on the activiation of adenylate cyclase. *Biochim. Biophys. Acta* **551**, 368–381.

Lambert, S. M. and Childers, S. R. (1984) Modification of guanine nucleotide regulatory components in brain membranes. I. Changes in guanosine-5'triphosphate regulation of opiate receptor binding sites. *J. Neurosci.* **4**, 2755–2763.

Larsen, N. E., Mullikin-Kirkpatrick, D., and Blume, A. J. (1981) Two different modifications of the neuroblastoma-glioma hybrid opiate receptors induced by N-ethylmaleimide. *Mol. Pharmacol.* **20**, 255–262.

Law, P. Y., Wu, J., Koehler, J. E., and Loh, H. H. (1981) Demonstration and characterization of opiate inhibition of the striatal adenylate cyclase. *J. Neurochem.* **36**, 1834–1846.

Law, P. Y., Hom, D. S., and Loh, H. H. (1982) Loss of opiate receptor activity in neuroblastoma × glioma NG108-15 hybrid cells after chronic opiate treatment: A multi-step process. *Mol. Pharmacol.* **22**, 1–4.

Law, P. Y., Griffin, M. T., Koehler, J. E., and Loh, H. H. (1983) Attenuation of enkephalin activity in neuroblastoma × glioma NG108-15 hybrid cells by phospholipases. *J. Neurochem.* **40**, 267–275.

Law, P. Y., Hom, D. S., and Loh, H. H. (1985a) Multiple affinity states of opiate receptors in neuroblastoma × glioma NG108-15 hybrid cells: Opiate agonist association rate is a function of receptor occupancy. *J. Biol. Chem.* **260**, 3561–3569.

Law, P. Y., Ungar, H. G., Hom, D. S., and Loh, H. H. (1985b) Effects of cycloheximide and tunicamycin on opiate receptor activities in neuroblastoma × glioma NG108-15 hybrid cells. *Biochem. Pharmacol.* **34**, 9–17.

Litosch, I., Lin, S.-H., and Fain, J. H. (1985) 5-Hydroxytryptamine stimulates inositol phosphate production in a cell-free system from blowfly salivary glands: Evidence for a role of GTP in coupling receptor activation to phosphoinositide breakdown. *J. Biol. Chem.* **260**, 5464–5471.

Lord, J. A. H., Waterfield, A. A., Hughes, J., and Kosterlitz, H. W. (1977) Endogenous opioid peptides: Multiple agonists and receptors. *Nature* **267**, 495–500.

Mack, K. J., Lee, M. F., and Wehenmeyer, J. A. (1985) Effects of guanine nucleotides and ions on kappa opioid binding. *Brain Res. Bull.* **14**, 301–306.

Manning, D. R. and Gilman, A. G. (1983) The regulatory components of adenylate cyclase and transducin: A family of structurally homologous guanine nucleotide binding proteins. *J. Biol. Chem.* **258**, 7059–7063.

Manning, D. R., Fraser, B. A., Kahn, R. A., and Gilman, A. G. (1984) ADP-ribosylation of transducin by islet-activating protein: Identification of asparagine as the site of ADP-ribosylation. *J. Biol. Chem.* **259**, 749–756.

McGrath, J. P., Capon, D. J., Goeddel, D. V., and Levinon, A. D. (1984) Comparative biochemical properties of normal and activated human *ras* p21 protein. *Nature* **310**, 644–649.

Minneman, K. P. and Iversen, L. L. (1976) Enkephalin and opiate narcotics increase cyclic GMP accumulation in slices of rat neostriatum. *Nature* **261**, 313–314.

Mudge, A. W., Leeman, S. E., and Fischbach, G. D. (1979) Enkephalin inhibits release of substance P from sensory neurons and decreases action potential duration. *Proc. Natl. Acad. Sci. USA* **76**, 526–530.

Musacchio, J. M. and Schen, C. (1983) Failure of opiates to increase the hydrolysis of GTP in neuroblastoma × glioma NG108-15 cells. *Life Sci.* **33**, 879–887.

Nakamura, T. and Ui, M. (1985) Simultaneous inhibitions of inositol-phospholipid breakdown, arachidonic acid release and histamine secretion in mast cells by islet activating protein, pertussis toxin: A possible involvement of the toxin-specific substrate in the calcium-mobilizing receptor-mediated biosignalling system. *J. Biol. Chem.* **260**, 3584–3593.

Neer, E. J., Lok, J. M., and Wolf, L. G. (1984) Purification and properties of the inhibitory guanine nucleotide regulatory unit of brain adenylate cyclase. *J. Biol. Chem.* **259**, 14222–14229.

Nehmad, R., Nadler, H., and Simantov, R. (1982) Effects of acute and chronic morphine treatment on calmodulin activity of rat brain. *Mol. Pharmacol.* **22**, 389–394.

Nestler, E. J., Walaas, S. I., and Greengard, P. (1984) Neuronal phosphoproteins: Physiological and clinical implications. *Science* **225**, 1357–1364.

Nishizuka, Y. (1984) Turnover of inositol phospholipids and signal transduction. *Science* **225**, 1365–1370.

Northup, J. K., Sternweis, P. C., and Gilman, A. G. (1983a) The subunits of the stimulatory regulatory component of adenylate cyclase: Resolution, activity, and properties of the 35,000-dalton (beta) subunit. *J. Biol. Chem.* **258**, 11361–11368.

Northup, J. K., Smigel, M. D., Sternweis, P. C., and Gilman, A. G. (1983b) The subunits of the stimulatory regulatory component of adenylate cyclase: Resolution of the activated 45,000-dalton (alpha) subunit. *J. Biol. Chem.* **258**, 11369–11376.

Pasternak, G. W. and Snyder, S. H. (1975a) Identification of novel high affinity opiate receptor binding in rat brain. *Nature* **253**, 563–565.

Pasternak, G. W. and Snyder, S. H. (1975b) Opiate receptor binding: Enzymatic treatments that discriminate between agonist and antagonist interactions. *Mol. Pharmacol.* **11**, 478–484.

Pasternak, G. W., Snowman, A. M., and Snyder, S. H. (1975a) Selective enhancement of [^{3}H]-opiate agonist binding by divalent cations. *Mol. Pharmacol.* **11**, 735–744.

Pasternak, G. W., Wilson, H. A., and Snyder, S. H. (1975b) Differential effects of protein-modifying reagents on receptor binding of opiate agonists and antagonists. *Mol. Pharmacol.* **11**, 340–351.

Pert, C. B., Pasternak, G. W., and Snyder, J. H. (1973) Opiate agonists and antagonists descriminated by receptor binding in brain. *Science* **182**, 1359–1361.

Pert, C. B. and Snyder, S. H. (1973) Opiate receptor: Demonstration in nervous tissue. *Science* **179**, 1011–1014.

Pert, C. B. and Snyder, S. H. (1974) Opiate receptor binding of agonists and antagonists affected differentially by sodium. *Mol. Pharmacol.* **10**, 868–879.

Pert, C. B. and Taylor, D. (1979) Type 1 and Type 2 Opiate Receptors: A Subclassification Scheme Based Upon GTP's Differential Effects on

Binding, in *Endogenous and Exogenous Opiate Agonists and Antagonists* (Way, E. L., ed.) Pergamon, New York.

Pfaffinger, P. J., Martin, J. M., Hunter, D., Nathanson, N. M., and Hille, B. (1985) GTP-binding proteins couple cardiac muscarinic receptors to a potassium channel. *Nature* **317,** 536–538.

Pfeiffer, A., Sadee, W., and Herz, A. (1982) Differential regulation of mu-, delta-, and kappa-opiate receptor subtypes by guanine nucleotides and metal ions. *J. Neurosci.* **2,** 912–917.

Propst, F. and Hamprecht, B. (1981) Opioids, noradrenaline and GTP analogs inhibit cholera toxin activated adenylate cyclase in neuroblastoma × glioma hybrid cells. *J. Neurochem.* **36,** 580–588.

Puri, S. K., Cochin, J., and Volicer, L. (1975) Effect of morphine sulfate on adenylate cyclase and phosphodiesterase activities in rat corpus striatum. *Life Sci.* **16,** 759–768.

Rasenick, M. M., Wheeler, G. L., Bitensky, M. W., Kosack, C. M., Malina, R. L., and Stein, P. J. (1984) Photoaffinity identification of colchinesolublized regulatory subunit from rat brain adenylate cyclase. *J. Neurochem.* **43,** 1447–1454.

Rodbell, M. (1980) The role of hormone receptors and GTP-regulatory proteins in membrane transduction. *Nature* **284,** 17–21.

Ross, D. H. and Cardenas, H. L. (1977) Nerve cell calcium as a messenger for opiate and endorphin actions. *Adv. Biochem. Psychopharm.* **20,** 301–336.

Schramm, M. and Selinger, Z. (1984) Message transmission: Receptor-controlled adenylate cyclase system. *Science* **225,** 1350–1356.

Sellinger-Barnette, M. and Weiss, B. (1982) Interaction of beta-endorphin and other opioid peptides with calmodulin. *Mol. Pharmacol.* **21,** 86–91.

Sharma, S. K., Niremberg, M., and Klee, W. (1975a) Morphine receptors as regulators of adenylate cyclase activity. *Proc. Natl. Acad. Sci. USA* **72,** 590–594.

Sharma, S. K., Klee, W. A., and Niremberg, M. (1975b) Dual regulation of adenylate cyclase accounts for narcotic dependence and tolerance. *Proc. Natl. Acad. Sci. USA* **72,** 3092–3096.

Sharma, S. K., Klee, W. A., and Niremberg, M. (1977) Opiate dependent modulation of adenylate cyclase activity. *Proc. Natl. Acad. Sci. USA* **74,** 3365–3369.

Simon, E. J. and Groth, H. (1975) Kinetics of opiate receptor inactivation by sulfhydryl reagents: Evidence for conformational change in the presence of sodium ions. *Proc. Natl. Acad. Sci. USA* **72,** 2404–2407.

Simon, E. J., Hiller, J. M., and Edelman, I. (1973) Stereospecific binding of the potent narcotic analgesic [^{3}H]-etorphine to rat brain homogenates. *Proc. Natl. Acad. Sci. USA* **70,** 1947–1949.

Simon, E. J., Hiller, J. M., Groth, J., and Edelman, I. (1975) Further properties of stereospecific opiate binding sites in rat brain: On the nature of the sodium effect. *J. Pharmacol. Exp. Ther.* **192,** 531–537.

Stadel, J. M. and Lefkowitz, R. J. (1981) Differential effects of cholera toxin on guanine nucleotide regulation of beta-adrenergic agonist high-affinity binding and adenylate cyclase activation in frog erythrocyte membranes. *J. Cyc. Nuc. Res.* **7,** 363–374.

Sternweis, P. C. and Robishaw, J. D. (1984) Isolation of two proteins with high affinity for guanine nucleotides from membranes of bovine brain. *J. Biol. Chem.* **259,** 13806–13813.

Tell, G. P., Pasternak, G. W., and Cuatrecasas, P. (1975) Brain and caudate nucleus adenylate cyclase: Effects of dopamine, GTP, E prostaglandins and morphine. *FEBS Lett.* **51,** 242–245.

Tempel, A., Gardner, E. L., and Zukin, R. S. (1985) Neurochemical and functional correlates of naltrexone-induced opiate receptor up-regulation. *J. Pharmacol. Exp. Ther.* **232,** 439–444.

Terenius, L. (1973) Characterisitcs of the 'receptor' for narcotic analgesics in synaptic plasma membrane fractions from rat brain. *Acta Pharmacol. Toxicol.* **33,** 377–384.

Tocque, B., Albouz, S., Boutry, J.-M., Le Saux, F., Hauw, J.-J., Bourdon, R., Baumann, N., and Zalc, B. (1984) Desipramine elicits the expression of opiate receptors and sulfogalactosylceramide synthesis in rat C-6 glioma cells. *J. Neurochem.* **42,** 1101–1106.

Traber, J., Fischer, K., Latzin, S., and Hamprecht, B. (1975) Morphine antagonizes action of prostaglandin in neuroblastoma × glioma hybrid cells. *Nature* **253,** 120–122.

Tsang, D., Tan, A. T., Henry, J. L., and Lal, S. (1978) Effect of opioid peptides on noradrenaline-stimulated cyclic AMP formation in homogenates of rat cerebral cortex and hypothalamus. *Brain Res.* **152,** 521–527.

U'Prichard, D. C. and Snyder, S. H. (1980) Interactions of divalent cations and guanine nucleotides at alpha(2)-adrenergic receptor binding sites in bovine brain membranes. *J. Neurochem.* **34,** 385–394.

Van Inwegen, R. G., Strada, S. J., and Robison, G. A. (1975) Effects of prostaglandins and morphine on brain adenylate cyclase. *Life Sci.* **16,** 1875–1876.

Vauquelin, G. and Maguire, M. E. (1980) Inactivation of beta-adrenergic receptors by N-ethylmaleimide in S49 lymphoma cells: Agonist induction of functional receptor heterogeneity. *Mol. Pharmacol.* **18,** 362–269.

Werz, M. A. and Macdonald, R. L. (1983) Opioid peptides with differential affinity for mu and delta receptors decrease sensory neuron calcium-dependent action potentials. *J. Pharmacol. Exp. Ther.* **227,** 394–401.

Wheeler, G. L. and Bitensky, M. W. (1977) A light-activated GTPase in vertebrate photoreceptors: Regulation of light-activated cyclic GMP phosphodiesterase. *Proc. Natl. Acad. Sci. USA* **74,** 4238–4242.

Wilkening, D., Mishra, R. K., and Makman, M. H. (1976) Effects of morphine on dopamine-stimulated adenylate cyclase and on cyclic GMP formation in primate brain amygdaloid nucleus. *Life Sci.* **19,** 1129–1138.

Wolleman, M. (1981) Endogenous opioids and cyclic AMP. *Prog. Neurobiol.* **16,** 145–154.

Wolozin, B. L. and Pasternak, G. W. (1981) Classification of multiple morphine and enkephalin binding sites in the central nervous system. *Proc. Natl. Acad. Sci. USA* **78,** 6181–6185.

Wuster, M., Costa, T., and Gramsch, C. (1983) Uncoupling of receptors is essential for opiate-induced desensitization (tolerance) in NG108-15 cells. *Life Sci.* **33,** (suppl. I), 341–344.

Wuster, M., Costa, T., Aktories, K., and Jakobs, K. H. (1984) Sodium regulation of opioid agonist binding is potentiated by pertussis toxin. *Biochem. Biophys. Res. Commun.* **123,** 1107–1115.

Yu, V. C., Richards, M. L., and Sadee, W. (1986) A human neuroblastoma cell line expresses mu and delta opioid receptor sites. *J. Biol. Chem.* **261,** 1065–1070.

Zajac, J.-M. and Roques, B. P. (1985) Differences in binding properties of mu and delta opioid receptor subtypes from rat brain: Kinetic analysis and effects of ions and guanine nucleotides. *J. Neurochem.* **44,** 1605–1614.

Zukin, R. S., Wallczak, S., and Makman, M. H. (1980) GTP modulation of opiate receptors in regions of rat brain and possible mechanism of GTP action. *Brain Res.* **186,** 238–244.

Chapter 9

Electrophysiology of Opiates and Opioid Peptides

Charles Chavkin

1. Overview

Electrophysiological methods have been used extensively to study the actions of opioids on cells in the nervous system. One of the principal motivations has been an interest in identifying the sites of opioid action and the pathways important for transmission of pain sensation (*see* Duggan and North, 1984; Basbaum and Fields, 1984, for recent reviews). The discovery of the endogenous opioids has created interest in the electrophysiological properties of these peptides as possible neurotransmitters. This has resulted in studies mapping the regional distribution of receptive cells and in studies comparing the effects of different endogenous opioids. Pharmacological characterization of multiple types of opioid receptors by behavioral and neurochemical assays gave impetus to the analysis of electrophysiological differences among receptor types. Recently this has led to important advances made by several groups identifying the receptor types involved in the cellular actions of opioids and the ionic conductances affected by opioid receptor activation.

Much has been learned already about the acute effects of opioids and synthetic opiates on neuronal physiology in the brain, spinal cord, and autonomic ganglia. The preponderant stereospecific action of opiate alkaloids or opioid peptides detected in most brain regions is depression of neuronal firing rate and reduction in transmitter release (Nicoll et al., 1977; Duggan and North, 1984; Henderson, 1983). There are certain regions, such as in the hippocampus and spinal cord, that respond to opioid application with a naloxone-sensitive increase in discharge rate and cellular excitability (Nicoll et al., 1977). Closer examination at these sites has revealed, however, that opioids are probably acting to inhibit presynaptic inputs of the excited cells (Zieglgansberger et al., 1979; Nicoll and Madison, 1984).

As has been discussed in several earlier chapters, there is considerable evidence to suggest the existence of multiple types of opioid receptors. Electrophysiological methods have provided some of this evidence and have been used to reveal important differences among the receptor types. This information has clearly provided substantiation for the concept of receptor heterogeneity.

Electrophysiological recording has also been a powerful technique to study the signal transduction mechanisms mediating drug responses (*see* North, 1986). In many cases, receptor activation initiates a sequence of biochemical events resulting in a change in concentration of a second messenger and/or a change in ion channel conductance. Electrophysiological methods are being used to study the role of particular second messenger systems and ionic species mediating the response to opioids. In this chapter, I will review the studies that describe the cellular effects of opioids in several different regions of the nervous system and review the data that link mu, delta, and kappa receptor types with specific transduction mechanisms. Results from several research groups support the concept that mu and delta receptors may be coupled to a potassium channel, whereas kappa receptors may be coupled to a calcium channel. The coupling between receptor and ion channel may be indirect, and it has been proposed that the mechanism regulating ion conductance change is via opioid inhibition of adenylate cyclase.

2. Receptor Identification

Cellular responses to applied opioids have been measured using both in vivo and in vitro recording techniques. Pharmacological analysis of these responses in vivo are complicated by problems associated with maintaining stable recordings and defining drug concentrations at sites of action. These difficulties can be largely circumvented by recording from brain slices, isolated tissue, or dispersed neuronal cultures. The development of these preparations has contributed to the rapid advancement of receptor characterization in the CNS. Precise definition of the receptor types involved in a drug response is obviously critical for understanding the cellular role of a specific opioid receptor. Since no one particular method is sufficient, several strategies of receptor identification are described below. These methods are evolving rapidly as new drugs are developed and as new receptor types are discovered.

Typically, receptor types are identified by the use of selective agonists. Although the receptor specificities of the available opioid agonists are not absolute, some inference can be made about the receptor types from the relative potencies of a series of selective agonists if differences in drug stability and penetration are considered. A large number of opioid active compounds have been synthesized and tested (see Goldstein and James, 1984a,b; Zukin and Zukin, 1981, for recent reviews). Some of the delta-selective agonists that have been used include [D-Ala^2,D-Leu^5]-enkephalin (DADLE), [D-Ser^2,L -Thr^6]-enkephalin (DSLET) (Fournie-Zaluski et al., 1981), [D-Pen^2,L-Pen^5]-enkephalin (DPLPE), and [D-Pen^2,D-Pen^5]-enkephalin (DPDPE) (Mosberg et al., 1983). The latter two compounds are cyclic enkephalin analogs with high selectivity for delta receptors: 1000–3000-fold higher agonist potency at delta than at mu or kappa receptors in a peripheral tissue bioassay (Mosberg et al., 1983). Mu receptor-selective agonists include normorphine, [D-Ala^2,MePhe^4,Gly^5]-enkephalin (DAGO), [D-Ala^2,MePhe^4,Met(O)^5]-met-enkephalin (FK 33-824) (Roemer et al., 1977), and (N-MePhe^3,D-Pro^4]-morphiceptin (PL017) (Chang et al., 1981). Kappa-selective agonists include ethylketocyclazocine, trans-($\pm$)-3,4-dichloro-N-methyl-N-[2-(1-pyrrolidinyl)cyclohexyl]-benzene-acetamide meth-ane sulfonate (U50488H), (5a,7a,8b)-($-$)-N-methyl-N-[7-(1-pyr-rolidinyl)-1-oxaspiro(4,5)-dec-8-yl] benzeneacetamide (U69593) (VonVoigtlander et al., 1983; Lahti et al., 1982), tifluadom (Romer et al., 1982), dynorphin A(1-17) (dyn-A), and dynorphin B (dyn-B) (Chavkin et al., 1982; Corbett et al., 1982; James et al., 1984).

The selectivities of these drugs have been defined using bioassay procedures as well as binding assays with generally good agreement between laboratories and procedures; assay conditions, however, including the ionic composition of the medium, temperature, and cofactor concentrations, are known to affect potency, receptor conformation, and agonist selectivity (Werling et al., 1985). It is extremely important to remember that none of the available agonists is absolutely specific. At sufficiently high concentration, each may occupy and activate other opioid receptor types (Lord et al., 1977; Chavkin et al., 1985a).

The second useful method of receptor identification relies on the selectivity of reversible antagonists. Naloxone has a 10-fold higher affinity for mu receptors than for either kappa or delta (Lord et al., 1977; Hutchinson et al., 1975; Chavkin et al., 1982). A new compound, ICI 174864 (N-bisallyl-Tyr-Aib-Aib-Phe-Leu; Aib = aminoisobutyrate), has greater than 200-fold higher potency at delta receptors than at either mu or kappa (Cotton et al., 1984). Kappa selective antagonists include 6beta, 6'beta [ethylenebis (oxyethyleneimino)] bis [17-(cyclopropylmethyl)-4,5alpha-epoxymorphinan-3,14-diol] (TENA) and binaltorphimine (BNI) synthesized by Portoghese and coworkers (Portoghese and Takemori, 1985; Portoghese et al., 1986). The relative sensitivity of an opioid agonist's action to these antagonists can be used to define the receptor type involved. The available antgonists lack absolute specificity, requiring that quantitative estimates of relative antagonist potency be made for definitive receptor identification.

Quantitative analysis of antagonist potency in bioassay preparations can be made using the method of Arunlakshana and Schild (Schild, 1947, 1949; Arunlakshana and Schild, 1959); the Schild equation $[K_i = (I)/(DR - 1)]$ allows for the estimation of the antagonist's apparent affinity. [K_i is the antagonist dissociation constant, DR is the dose ratio ($[A']/[A]$) of agonist concentrations in the absence $[A]$ and presence of antagonist $[A']$ necessary to achieve the same effect, and (I) is the concentration of antagonist used.] The method assumes that both agonist and antagonist drugs are at binding equilibrium (Kenakin, 1985); since agonist concentration need not be known with certainty, however, opioids can be applied by iontophoresis or micropressure pipet if application is reproducible. Receptor identification by antagonist-affinity determination can be more compelling than agonist potency measures, since the latter are strongly influenced by spare receptor concentration and differences in agonist efficacies (Chavkin and Goldstein, 1981b; Cox and Chavkin, 1983).

In addition to the reversible antagonists, the selective irreversible antagonists, beta-funaltrexamine (β-FNA) (*see* Takemori and Portoghese, 1985) or naloxazone (Pasternak et al., 1980; Hazum et al., 1981; Zhang et al., 1981; Hahn et al., 1982, 1985 can be used for opioid receptor identification. β-FNA is a derivative of the reversible opioid receptor antagonist naltrexone that has been shown to block specifically the effects of opioid agonists acting through the mu receptor (Portoghese et al., 1980; Takemori et al., 1981; Ward et al., 1982). The mu receptor selectivity of β-FNA has been challenged by several groups that report either no selectivity of the compound (Rothman et al., 1983, 1984; Corbett et al., 1985) or no effect of the ligand (McKnight et al., 1984). Our experience indicates that β-FNA is not a stable compound, and the potency and selectivity of β-FNA is dependent on its purity, storage conditions, and concentration used. In addition to irreversible mu antagonism, β-FNA also has reversible kappa agonist activity (Ward et al., 1981) and reversible delta antagonist activity (Mihara and North, 1986.) Naloxazone is selective for mu_1 sites (*see* chapter by Yossef Itzhak).

Selective receptor inactivation protocols have some theoretical advantages as methods of receptor identification. Under conditions in which only a single type of opioid receptor is present, the rank order of potencies of opioids in receptor assays will be particularly helpful in receptor identification. Certain tissues such as the rabbit ileum (Oka, 1980) normally express only a single type of opioid receptor; for most tissues that express multiple opioid receptor types, however, receptor homogeneity can be achieved by selective inactivation. In a typical experiment, the potencies of a series of agonists can be tested in a single preparation before and then again following treatment with the selective and irreversible antagonist. The receptor type affected is defined by the group of compounds whose potencies are reduced.

The third method of opioid receptor identification uses the principle of selective receptor protection (Chavkin and Goldstein, 1981b; Chavkin et al., 1982). Tissue containing opioid receptors can be treated with an irreversible opioid receptor antagonist, beta-chlornaltrexamine (β-CNA), a site-directed alkylating agent that will nonselectively inactivate mu, kappa, and delta receptors. In the presence of a reversible and receptor-selective ligand, one receptor type can be specifically protected from inactivation. This method has been applied successfully to the identification of receptor types in the guinea pig ileum myenteric plexus (Chavkin and Goldstein, 1981a; Chavkin et al., 1982), mouse vas deferens (Cox and Chavkin, 1983), and guinea pig brain membranes (James et al., 1982). Using this method, if the effects of two agonists are not protected by the same treatment, then they are likely to be acting through different opioid receptors. On the other hand, if both are protected by the same treatments, then it is possible (but not proven) that the two agonists are acting through the same receptor (Furchgott, 1966, 1972, 1978; Besse and Furchgott, 1976).

These techniques of receptor identification have been successfully used in several regions of the nervous system. The result is that a coherent image of the cellular effects of opioids is emerging as discussed below. The properties and tissue distribution of opioid receptor types are also becoming clearer. The goal of this chapter is to review the characteristics of the opioid receptors identified in the different regions of the nervous system.

3. Opioid Actions on Cells in Enteric Ganglia

The widespread therapeutic use of narcotics for the control of gastrointestinal activity has initiated an interest in the effects of opioids on that tissue. In addition, studies of the effects of opioids on the enteric ganglia in the guinea pig ileum longitudinal muscle have been particularly valuable in the characterization of differences between opioid receptor types (Lord et al., 1977; Chavkin et al., 1982; Ward et al., 1981, 1982; James and Goldstein, 1984). The guinea pig ileum longitudinal muscle contraction assay developed by Paton (1957) is a robust and quantitative measure of opioid activity. In this tissue, opioids were found to inhibit electrically stimulated contraction of the smooth muscle by reducing acetylcholine release at the neuromuscular junction (Cox and Weinstock, 1966). Opioid receptor types were identified using Schild analysis of antagonist potencies and receptor-selective irreversible antagonist paradigms. These methods were used to demonstrate that in the guinea pig ileum bioassay, mu and kappa, but not delta, receptors are normally involved in controlling the smooth muscle response (Hutchinson, et al., 1975; Lord et al., 1977; Chavkin et al., 1982; Ward et al., 1981, 1982). Typical delta selective agonists were found to activate mu-type receptors in this preparation.

Opioids were shown to inhibit acetylcholine release by acting on cholinergic neurons within the myenteric plexus, an autonomic ganglion embedded in the ileum longitudinal muscle (Paton, 1957; Cox and Weinstock, 1966). Intracellular recordings of myenteric neurons have distinguished two types of cells (Nishi and North, 1973; North, 1982). Both types respond to application of mu-selective opioids with a 3–7 mV hyperpolarization accompanied by a decrease in membrane resistance (Williams and North, 1979; Morita and North, 1982). An additional effect of morphine is to prolong the calcium-dependent hyperpolarization that normally follows a burst of action potentials in myenteric neurons (Tokimasa et al., 1981).

Several observations have demonstrated that the ionic basis of the hyperpolarization is an opioid-induced increase in potassium conductance. (1) The amplitude of the hyperpolarization depends on the external potassium concentration, and the reversal potential of the opioid activated current was found to be about − 100mV (a value close to the potassium equilibrium potential) (Morita and North, 1982; Tokimasa et al., 1981). (2) Potassium channel blockade by intracellular cesium injection blocks the mu receptor-mediated hyperpolarization (Cherubini and North, 1985). (3) Opioid-induced hyperpolarization persists in the absence of external calcium (Morita and North, 1982).

In addition to the membrane hyperpolarization, mu receptor activation depresses the cholinergic EPSPs generated by presynaptic stimulation (Cherubini and North, 1985). The reduction in EPSP amplitude recorded in the myenteric neuron is caused by the presynaptic inhibition of the release of acetylcholine (Nishi and North, 1973), since normorphine reduced the EPSP amplitude, but not the effect of iontophoretically applied acetylcholine (Cherubini and North, 1985). Pretreatment of the tissue with the irreversible mu-selective antagonist β-FNA blocks the effects of FK 33-824, morphine, and normorphine.

Kappa agonists (dynorphin A, tifluadom, and U50488H) also reversibly depress the EPSP measured in the myenteric neurons as do mu agonists. Kappa agonist effects are not mediated by the mu receptor, however, since the depression of the EPSP caused by kappa agonists is unaffected by β-FNA treatment (Cherubini and North, 1985). Additionally, low concentrations of barium (200–300 μM) added to the superfusion buffer blocked the effects of mu agonists, but did not alter the actions of kappa agonists

(Cherubini and North, 1985). Barium at low concentrations selectively reduces potassium conductances without significantly affecting membrane potential or action potential shape (Cherubini and North, 1985). Based on these observations, the authors proposed that mu agonists increase potassium conductance, whereas kappa agonists do not directly affect that conductance. Instead, intracellular recording of the myenteric neurons demonstrated that the kappa agonists, dynorphin A(1-17), tifluadom, and U50488H, reduce the calcium-dependent action potential duration (Cherubini and North, 1985). These results suggest that kappa receptors are present on myenteric neurons and are coupled to a calcium channel. Thus, the evidence suggests that kappa and mu receptors in this tissue are linked to different transduction mechanisms.

Intracellular recordings in the submucus plexus of the guinea pig ileum have shown that [Met^5]-enkephalin, [Leu^5]-enkephalin, DSLET, and DADLE hyperpolarize submucus plexus neurons (Surprenant and North, 1985; Mihara and North, 1986). On the same cells, normorphine, DAGO, FK 33-824, tifluadom, and dynorphin A were ineffective at concentrations of less than 2 μM. The receptor type activated by [Met^5]-enkephalin in the submucus plexus neurons was shown to be delta by the apparent dissociation constants of 50 nM for naloxone and 8 nM for ICI 174864 calculated by Schild analysis. The conductance change was very similar to that controlled by mu receptor activation in the myenteric plexus: hyperpolarization reversed at the potassium equilibrium potential and appeared to result from an outward potassium conductance. The potassium conductance increase caused by delta receptor activation also results in a decrease in calcium-mediated action potential in the submucus plexus neurons (Mihara and North, 1986).

4. Opioid Actions in Locus Ceruleus

Studies of intracellular effects of opioid receptor activation in other regions have given similar results. The principal cells of the rat locus ceruleus (a homogeneous group of catecholamine-containing neurons in the pons) respond to opioid application with a dose-dependent, naloxone-reversible membrane hyperpolarization and increase in membrane conductance (Pepper and

Henderson, 1980). Intracellular recordings of locus ceruleus neurons in rat brain slices have demonstrated that the membrane effects are caused by an increase in potassium conductance (Williams et al., 1982). The actions of opioids were mediated by mu, but not delta or kappa, receptors, as shown by the rank order of potency of a wide range of agonists, by the sensitivity of the opioid effect to β-FNA inactivation, and by the naloxone-apparent dissociation constants obtained (Williams and North, 1984).

Pharmacologic properties of the opioid-activated potassium conductance were characterized by adding various channel-blocking agents to the superfusion buffer and by intracellularly injecting antagonists through the recording pipet (North and Williams, 1985). Substitution of barium for calcium completely blocked the opioid-induced increase in potassium conductance. Intracellular injection of rubidium (RbC1) or cesium (CsC1) partially blocked the opioid induced increase in potassium current, presumably by blocking the efflux of potassium through the ionophore. Quinine (200 μM), shown to block specific potassium conductances in vertebrate and invertebrate neurons (Walden and Speckmann, 1981; Yoshida et al., 1986), also blocks the opioid-activated potassium conductance. The hyperpolarizing current induced by opioids is also sensitive to tetraethylammonium, but only at relatively high concentrations (25 mM), whereas 4-aminopyridine (0.1–1 mM) has no effect (North and Williams, 1985). These data indicate that mu receptor activation opens a type of potassium channel having properties different from the voltage-sensitive potassium conductance and from the muscarinic potassium conductance (Cole and Shinnick-Gallagher, 1984).

The properties of the mu receptor-linked potassium channel in the locus ceruleus closely resemble those described for the mu receptor in the myenteric and delta receptor in the submucus plexus of the guinea pig ileum. The opioid-induced change in conductance has a reversal potential at -110 mV, implicating potassium. Changes in external potassium concentration shift the reversal potential, as predicted by the Nernst equation (North and Williams, 1985). These data indicate that mu opioid receptors are linked to similar transduction mechanisms in different species and tissues.

Nonopioid agonists also activate similar potassium conductances. Aghajanian and coworkers have studied the relationship between the effects of opioids and clonidine, an alpha-2 adrenergic agonist, on locus ceruleus cells. Clonidine also hyperpolarized locus ceruleus neurons through an increase in potassium conductance (Aghajanian and VanderMaelen, 1982). Although opioids and alpha-2 adrenergic agonists act through different receptors, they probably activate the same population of ion channels (Andrade and Aghajanian, 1985). This finding may explain the ability of clonidine to attenuate opiate withdrawal (Aghajanian, 1978).

5. Opioid Actions in Dorsal Root Ganglia and Spinal Cultures

Jessel and Iversen (1977) first demonstrated that [D-Ala^{2}met^5]-enkephalin amide (DAEA) inhibits potassium-evoked release of substance P from slices of the rat trigeminal nucleus. Following on the observations made by Jessel and Iversen (1977), Mudge and coworkers (1979) used electrophysiological techniques to study opioid control of substance P release in chick dorsal root ganglion (DRG) cells in culture. DAEA was found to inhibit the release of substance P from chick DRG cells (Mudge et al., 1979). Intracellular recordings of chick DRG cells in culture demonstrated that the duration of the calcium-mediated action potential was reduced by DAEA without affecting the cell resting membrane potential or resting membrane conductance. Although quantitative dose–response curves were not obtained, the effects of DAEA were dose dependent; 10 μM had a large effect, 1.0 to 0.1 μM had smaller effects, and all of the effects were blocked by 1–50 μM naloxone. Based on these findings, Mudge et al. (1979) concluded that the opioid inhibition of the voltage-dependent calcium conductance could either be the result of a direct effect on the calcium channel or an indirect increase in a voltage-dependent potassium conductance. The authors argue for the former mechanism because the opioid effect was not blocked in the presence of barium at a concentration that should block the delayed, voltage-sensitive potassium conductance.

To further characterize the opioid receptors and the ionic transduction mechanisms involved, Werz and MacDonald (1983, 1984) have studied the electrophysiological effects of opioids applied to fetal mouse DRG cells in culture. In the mouse DRG cells, the calcium component of action potentials was enhanced by raising the calcium concentration from 1 to 5 mM and by including 5 mM tetraethylammonium in the recording culture medium to block sensitive potassium conductances. Action potentials were initiated by a brief depolarizing current injection through the recording electrode (300 μs), and as was seen in chick DRG cultures, opioids (e.g., morphiceptin and [Leu[5]]-enkephalin) reduced the duration of the calcium component of the action potential by approximately 20% (Werz and MacDonald, 1983).

Cells in the mouse DRG cultures varied greatly in their responsiveness to applied opioids. Some cells responded to Leu[5]-enkephalin, but not morphiceptin, and other cells were sensitive to both peptides. These authors have concluded that both mu and delta sites are present since both peptides are active, and that the differences in sensitivity are caused by an uneven distribution of receptor types (Werz and MacDonald, 1983). Since the peptides were applied by pressure pipet, however, the reported differences in agonist potency are difficult to evaluate. In support of their hypothesis, the presence of multiple receptor types is also suggested by the lower sensitivity of Leu[5]-enkephalin than morphiceptin to antagonism by naloxone. The 100-fold difference in naloxone sensitivity, however, is larger than the expected 10-fold difference in the affinity of naloxone for delta and mu sites (Lord et al., 1977).

Werz and MacDonald (1984, 1985) reported that kappa receptors are also present on dispersed mouse DRG cells in culture. Opioids such as dynorphin A(1-17), dynorphin A(1-8), dynorphin B, and alpha-neo-endorphin selectively reduced the voltage-sensitive calcium conductance, as did [Leu[5]]-enkephalin and morphiceptin (Werz and MacDonald, 1984, 1985). Intracellular recordings made using electrodes filled with cesium acetate (4M) can help to distinguish between potassium and calcium conductance changes. When all of the potassium conductances were blocked by filling the DRG cell with cesium, the effects of [Leu[5]]-enkephalin and morphiceptin were completely inhibited. This observation indicates that the reduction in calcium conductance caused by mu and delta receptors is produced indirectly by an increased potassium conductance. In contrast, cesium did not affect the reduction in calcium conductance caused by dynorphin A(1-17), dynorphin A(1-8), dynorphin B, and alpha-neo-endorphin. The authors therefore conclude that kappa receptors are directly coupled to a calcium ionophore in mouse DRG cells (Werz and MacDonald, 1984, 1985).

It is interesting to try to interpret the findings of Mudge et al. (1979) in light of the recent results of Werz and MacDonald. The identity, however, of the opioid receptor observed in chick DRG studied by Mudge et al. (1979) can not be ascertained because the concentration of DAEA used would not be receptor selective. Nevertheless, the barium-insensitive effects of opioids on calcium conductance observed by Mudge et al. (1979) suggest that it may have been kappa. Mu receptor effects were shown to be sensitive to barium or cesium (North and Williams, 1985; Werz and Mac-Donald, 1984).

6. Opioid Actions in the CA1 Region of the Hippocampus

Pharmacological effects of opioids in the rat hippocampus were first observed by Nicoll et al. (1977) and Hill et al. (1977) in iontophoretic surveys of the rat brain for regions sensitive to applied β-endorphin. The response to opioids in hippocampus differed from that seen in most other brain regions. Activation of the opioid receptors in this region has the unusual effect of increasing the firing rates of the neurons present (Nicoll et al., 1977; Zieglgansberger et al., 1979). In most other brain regions, the effect of applied opioid compounds is to decrease the neuronal firing rates (Henderson, 1983; Duggan and North, 1984).

Numerous groups have studied the effects of opioids in the CA1 region of the rat and guinea pig hippocampal slice (*see* Henderson, 1983; Duggan and North, 1984, for review). Electrical stimulation (in the stratum radiatum) of the Schaffer collateral neuronal fibers elicits a synchronous firing that can be measured by extracellularly recording the evoked response of the CA1 pyramidal cells. Under these conditions, opioids consistently increase the sensitivity of these cells to electrical stimulation. In other words, opioids decrease the stimulation intensity required to evoke a response without changing the maximal evoked response. Intracellular recording of CA1 pyramidal cells have shown that opioids do not change the intrinsic membrane properties (Dingledine, 1981; Siggins and Zieglgansberger, 1981).

The mechanism of the opioid effect on CA1 pyramidal cell excitability has been studied by several groups and is thought to be largely caused by an inhibition by opioids of an inhibitory GABA input to the CA1 pyramidal cells (e.g., excitation resulting from disinhibition), as proposed by Zieglgansberger et al. (1979). Extracellular recording of CA1 interneurons in vitro also showed that opioids directly reduce firing rates and excitability (Lee et al., 1980).

Additional support for this mechanism of opioid action in CA1 was obtained by Nicoll and Madison (1984) in a recent intracellular study of opioid effects on hippocampal inhibitory interneurons. Cells in the hippocampal slice were identified as interneurons by their tissue location, firing pattern, and morphology after dye filling (Schwartzkroin and Mathers, 1978). As predicted by the disinhibition hypothesis, DADLE and other opioids applied to the hippocampal slice were found to directly hyperpolarize interneurons by increasing their potassium conductance. The resulting reduction in firing rate and excitability of the interneurons would account for the reduction in GABA release and IPSP amplitude recorded in pyramidal cells.

Raggenbass et al. (1985) also studied the effects of opioids on non-pyramidal cells in the CA1 region of the rat hippocampus. DAGO, but not U50488H (1 μM), suppressed the firing of these cells. This action was post-synaptic, since elevated magnesium (6 mM) and reduced calcium (0.2 mM) in the medium did not block the effects of DAGO. The authors concluded that the mu receptor type was present, since the effect was shown to be produced by DAGO, but not U50488H, and was blocked by naloxone.

One of the earliest studies distinguishing mu and delta receptors in the rat hippocampus was done by French and Zieglgansberger (1982) using the technique of selective receptor tolerance. Hippocampal slices taken from rats exposed for 7 d to subcutaneous morphine pellets were insensitive to the excitatory action of normorphine measured using extracellular field potential recording. Separate delta receptors were inferred by the lack of cross tolerance to [Met[5]]-enkephalin. Earlier reports had concluded from relative agonist potencies that mu, but not kappa, receptors were present (Gahwiler and Maurer, 1981).

We have determined the relative potencies of several opioids by comparing the concentration necessary to increase the CA1 pyramidal cell response to orthodromic stimulation (Chavkin et al., 1985a). The rank order of potency found was DADLE > normorphine > dynorphin A = dynorphin B = [Leu[5]]-enkephalin > U504488H ethylketocyclazocine. The kappa-selective opiates, U50488H and ethylketocyclazocine, each required concentrations greater than 10–50 μM. The low potency of ethylketocyclazocine had been reported earlier by Valentino and Dingledine (1982) and also by Brookes and Bradley (1984). Although this measure of potency does not differentiate the contributions of drug stability, penetration to the receptor, and receptor affinity, the relatively low potencies of kappa-selective opioids suggest that these compounds were acting through opioid receptors other than kappa to change CA1 cell excitability.

To further define the receptor types that mediate opioid action in the CA1 region of the hippocampus, we adapted a selective receptor inactivation paradigm (Chavkin et al., 1985a). Pretreatment of the hippocampal slice with 1.0 μM β-FNA for 15 min was the minimal treatment condition we found necessary for consistent blockade of the effects of the mu-selective agonist, normorphine. β-FNA-treated slices were insensitive to the effects of normorphine (10 μM) and PL017 (10 μM). Moreover, following β-FNA, the effects of both 10 μM dynorphin A and 10 μM dynorphin B were almost completely blocked. In contrast, the response to DADLE (1.0 μM) or DSLET (1.0 μM) were not changed significantly by β-FNA treatment. β-FNA is unlikely to have blocked the normorphine or dynorphin effects by a nonspecific (toxic) action, since evoked responses could still be elicited at pretreatment stimulation intensities, and since DADLE, [Leu^5]-enkephalin, and DSLET could still enhance the cellular response to electrical stimulation.

In contrast to the selectivity of β-FNA antagonism, 1 μM naloxone blocked the effects of each agonist tested. Schild analysis of the naloxone-induced shift in agonist does–response curves confirms that normorphine, PL017, and dynorphin A(1-17) are highly sensitive to naloxone antagonism (apparent dissociation constants were between 1 and 5 nM) (Neumaier and Chavkin, 1986a,b). In contrast, the naloxone sensitivity of DSLET was significantly lower (15–30 nM) (Neumaier and Chavkin, 1986a,b). These results support the conclusion that the CA1 region of the rat hippocampus contains mu and delta receptors, but not kappa, and that at high concentrations, the dynorphin opioids can activate mu receptors.

There is some disagreement among the published reports on the effects of dynorphin A(1-17) in the CA1 region. These differences can best be attributed to differences in technique and cell sampling. We consistently see low-potency excitatory actions of dynorphin A in the rat hippocampal slice preparation (Chavkin et al., 1985a; Neumaier and Chavkin, 1986a,b). Others report dynorphin A(1-17) is excitatory at low concentrations (0.1 nM), but inhibitory at higher concentrations (Vidal et al., 1984). The inhibitory effects were not reversed by naloxone. Naloxone-insensitive inhibition of extracellularly recorded single-unit firing rate was observed following in vivo iontophoretic application of dynorphin A(1-17) (Walker et al., 1982; Henriksen et al., 1982; Moises and Walker, 1985). Des-tyr-dynorphin A(2-17), a dynorphin analog lacking opioid receptor affinity (Chavkin and Goldstein, 1981a), had similar inhibitory action (Walker et al., 1982). Thus, at low to moderate concentrations (0.1 nM–1 µM), dynorphin A(1-17) can activate mu receptors; whereas at higher concentrations, nonspecific and naloxone-insensitive depression of pyramidal cell activity is observed.

In summary, the CA1 region seems to contain mu and delta receptors on nonpyramidal cells. These cells respond to opioids by increasing potassium conductance. The resulting hyperpolarization reduces GABA release in the region, thus causing an increase in excitability measured in CA1 pyramidal cells. The reduction in inhibition of the pyramidal cell has several effects: somatic EPSP amplitudes become larger and dendritic IPSP amplitudes become reduced (Siggins and Zieglgansberger, 1981; Dingledine, 1981; Henderson, 1983).

7. Opioid Actions in the CA3 Region of the Hippocampus

Interest in the actions of opioids in the CA3 region of the hippocampus was greatly stimulated by the immunocytochemical localization of proenkephalin- and prodynorphin-derived opioids in the dentate gyrus and mossy fiber pathway of the rat hippocampus (Gall et al., 1981; Gall, 1984; McGinty et al., 1983). In addition, using specific radioimmunoassays and high-pressure liquid chromatography techniques, all five prodynorphin-derived peptides were detected in high concentrations and are present in hippocampal extracts in their opioid active molecular forms (Chavkin et al., 1983, 1985b).

Using specific radioimmunoassays, additional evidence supporting the hypothesis that these endogenous opioids are neurotransmitters in this region has been obtained. Calcium-dependent release of dynorphin A(1-17), dynorphin A(1-8), dynorphin B, α-neo-endorphin, β-neo-endorphin, and [Leu^5]-enkephalin after in vitro depolarization of hippocampal tissue was detected (Chavkin et al., 1983, 1985b). Since the five known prodynorphin-derived opioid peptides are each potent opioid agonists having relatively high preference for the kappa type of opioid receptor, it has been suggested that the dynorphins are the natural endogenous ligands for the kappa receptor (Wuster et al., 1981; Chavkin et al., 1982; James et al., 1984). Our hypothesis is that the products of prodynorphin processing may be released at sites in the nervous system to act on postsynaptic kappa receptors.

In the CA3 region, [Leu^5]-enkephalin and DADLE consistently increase the excitability of the pyramidal cells as recorded both in vivo (Henriksen et al., 1982; Moises and Walker, 1985) and in vitro (Masukawa and Prince, 1982; Gruol et al., 1983). In contrast, the effects of dynorphin A(1-17) on CA3 pyramidal cell excitability are neither robust nor consistent (Gruol et al., 1983; Chavkin and Bloom, 1986; Iwama et al., 1986). Using extracellular field-potential recording methods, we have compared the effects of dynorphin A(1-17) and [Leu^5]-enkephalin on CA1 and CA3 pyramidal cell excitability (Gruol et al., 1983). [Leu^5]-enkephalin consistently enhanced the pyramidal cell responses. Dynorphin A(1-17) added to the superfusion buffer was found to have mixed effects: on different slices, dynorphin A(1-17) either increased or decreased the response evoked by mossy fiber stimulation. Both of the dynorphin A(1-17) effects were blocked by naloxone. Iwama and coworkers (1986) report similarly mixed effects observed in guinea pig hippocampal slices. In the latter study, the depressions produced by dynorphin A(1-17) were also produced by U50488H and bremazocine at very high concentrations (100 µM) and were not reversed by naloxone (100 µM). Iwama et al. (1986) suggest that the inhibitory action may be mediated by kappa receptors; however, based on the low potency of kappa agonists and the insensitivity of the effect to naloxone antagonism, this depression is not likely to be mediated by an opioid receptor.

Henriksen and coworkers (1982) have studied the effects of iontophoretic and micropneumatic application of the dynorphins on hippocampal pyramidal cell firing rates in vivo. In halothane-anesthetized rats, a majority (77%) of the identified CA3 pyramidal cells tested were excited by application of dynorphin A(1-17), dynorphin A(1-8), alpha-neo-endorphin, or dynorphin B. The spontaneous firing rates of only 10% of the CA3 cells were inhibited. The dynorphin effects are believed to be mediated by an opioid receptor since the nonopioid analog, des-tyr-dynorphin A(2-17), was found to be inactive, and the excitatory effects reported could be blocked by naloxone applied either systemically or iontophoretically. Similarly, Bradley and Brookes (1984) found all CA1 and CA3 neurons that responded to iontophoretically applied dynorphin A(1-13) in vivo were inhibited in a naloxone-reversible manner.

In contrast, these findings were not confirmed by Walker and coworkers (1982), who have reported that in the CA3 region, dynorphin A(1-17) had only naloxone-insensitive inhibitory effects. In their hands, des-tyr-dynorphin also reduced the CA3 spontaneous firing rates, and the observed inhibitions were again not naloxone reversible. The basis for this controversy has not yet been resolved. The discrepancy may be related to differences in anesthesia, recording technique, or cell sampling bias.

To further investigate the actions of dynorphin A(1-17) in the CA3 region, we have also recorded intracellularly from hippocampal pyramidal cells (Gruol et al., 1983). All CA3 hippocampal neurons studied displayed spontaneous activity consisting of synaptic potentials, single action potentials, and bursts of spike discharges followed by after-hyperpolarizations. Exogenously applied dynorphin A(1-17) produced variable effects on the spontaneous activity, although individual cells displayed consistent responses. The component of spontaneous activity most affected was the burst discharges, which are thought to be generated by intrinsic mechanisms. Clear membrane potential changes were produced by dynorphin in many CA3 neurons, but these changes did not necessarily correlate with the changes in spontaneous activity. Neither synaptic potentials evoked by orthodromic activation nor resting input resistance were significantly altered by dynorphin A(1-17). In contrast, [Leu^5]-enkephalin reduced IPSPs with no change in membrane potential or input resistance in CA3, in accord with previous studies in CA1 (Masukawa and Prince, 1982). After-hyperpolarizations were occasionally altered in CA3 neurons, but most cells showed no change in after-hyperpolarization amplitude.

We have observed that the predominant effect of dynorphin B(1-13) in vitro is a dose-dependent depolarization (Chavkin and Schwartzkroin, unpublished observations). Dynorphin B was applied in the region of the proximal dendrites near the recording electrode by a micropipet filled with 100 μM dynorphin B(1-13) dissolved in HEPES-buffered saline (pH 7.4). Brief pulses (40 psi, 20–100 ms duration) applied to the peptide-containing pipet consistently elicited a moderately long-duration (0.1–10 s) depolarizing response of 5–20 mV. Naloxone completely blocked the dynorphin B-induced depolarizations. No consistent effect of dynorphin B was seen on the other components of the spontaneous or synaptically activated responses, including IPSPs evoked by mossy fiber stimulation or the after-hyperpolarization following intrinsic bursts. The basis for the difference between our results with dynorphin B in the guinea pig hippocampal slice and the results observed earlier is unclear, but may be related to differences in the tissue preparation or method of peptide application.

Based on the typical inhibitory actions of opioids seen in other regions studied, we would expect that dynorphin has presynaptic disinhibitory effects in CA3; but neither the receptor types present nor the ionic basis for the opioid actions in the CA3 region have yet been established.

8. Opioid Actions in Dentate Region of the Hippocampus

Previous studies (Chavkin et al., 1983, 1985b) have provided strong anatomical and neurochemical evidence suggesting that the proenkephalin- and prodynorphin-derived opioids are present and can be released within the rat hippocampus. The site of action within the hippocampus is not yet known, however. As discussed earlier, intracellular and extracellular recordings, as well as behavioral data, indicate that opioids have effects on the dentate granule cells (Haas and Ryall, 1980; Tielen et al., 1981; Linseman and Corrigall, 1982; Collier and Routtenberg, 1984; Christian et al., 1985). Opioid binding sites are present in this region, as demonstrated by autoradiography (Foote and Maurer, 1982; Zamir et al., 1985). Since precise anatomical localization of the opioid synapses is not yet available, we do not know which processes of the dentate granule cells release opioid peptides.

Dentate granule cells can be orthodromically activated by stimulation of the perforant path. Extracellular recording in the stratum granulosum following perforant path stimulation measures an evoked response that is proportional to the intensity of the stimulus. The evoked response was shown to be orthodromic by its complete absence after 10 mM $MgCl_2$ was added to the superfusion buffer (Neumaier and Chavkin, 1986b). This evoked response has been shown to be sensitive to opioids (Tielen et al., 1981; Neumaier and Chavkin, 1986b). Using rat and guinea pig hippocampal slices, Tielen et al. (1981) found that [D-ala^2]-met-enkephalin added to the superfusion buffer depressed the evoked response at peptide concentrations between 0.3 and 1 μM.

The effects of [D-ala^2]-met-enkephalin were blocked by naloxone (0.1–1 μ*M*), but not by bicuculline.

Normorphine applied either by micropipet to the granule cell layer near the recording pipet or by addition to the superfusion buffer caused a dose-dependent increase in the amplitude of the after-potential (Neumaier and Chavkin, 1986a,b). The effect is reversed 1–5 min after drug application by micropipet, and is also completely blocked by the addition of 50 n*M* naloxone to the superfusion buffer.

The normorphine-induced increase in sensitivity to electrical stimulation can be quantitated by measuring the amplitude of the after-potential recorded in the dentate. Dose-response curves can be used to measure agonist potency, and Schild analysis can be used to measure the apparent binding affinity of an antagonist. Based on the results of the normorphine sensitivity to different concentrations of naloxone, Schild analysis yielded an apparent dissociation constant of 2.3 ± 0.8 n*M* ($n = 5$). This value is very close to the apparent affinity for naloxone to the mu opioid receptor (Lord et al., 1977) and is consistent with normorphine acting through the mu receptor in the dentate region of the rat hippocampus.

Using the same extracellular recording paradigm described above, the effects of dynorphin A(1-17) have been measured following application by micropipet. Dynorphin A(1-17) also caused the appearance of an after-potential recorded in the dentate cell layer (Neumaier and Chavkin, 1986a,b). The dynorphin effect was reversed by naloxone, but required a 10-fold higher concentration (500 n*M*) than that required to antagonize the actions of normorphine. The lower sensitivity of dynorphin A(1-17) effects to naloxone in the dentate region suggests that these effects are mediated by kappa receptors (Neumaier and Chavkin, 1986a,b). The similarity of the opioid effects in the dentate region to those seen in the CA1 region suggests that a common disinhibitory mechanism and a common synaptic arrangement may be involved.

9. Role of Adenylate Cyclase in the Electrophysiological Actions of Opioids

Andrade and Aghajanian (1985) found that both opioids and alpha-2 adrenergic agonists activate the same pool of potassium channels in locus ceruleus cells. The linkage between the two receptors and the potassium channels may not be direct, however, since the maximal potassium conductance increase caused by one type of agonist could not be increased by the simultaneous application of the other. This finding suggests that there may be a common second messenger system linking both the mu opioid receptor and alpha-2 adrenergic receptor to the potassium channel in locus ceruleus cells.

Similarly, in guinea pig ileum submucus plexus, norepinephrine and somatostatin acting through separate receptors also elicit the same increase in potassium conductance as delta-selective opioid agonists (Mihara and North, 1986). When maximal concentrations of each were applied simultaneously under voltage clamp conditions, the effects were not additive. These results indicate that the same population of potassium channels is affected and that the receptors are indirectly coupled to the ionophore.

The mechanism of coupling between each of the opioid receptors and their respective channels is not yet known. Several groups have presented strong evidence, however, that delta opioid receptors (in NG108-15 neuroblastoma-glioma cells) control adenylate cyclase activity via an interaction with the GTP binding protein, N_i. Delta-selective opioids were found to inhibit adenylate cyclase and decrease production of cyclicAMP, and pertussis toxin pretreatment of the cells blocked the action of opioids (Sharma et al., 1975, 1977; Law et al., 1985; Wuster et al., 1985). In a related study, Abood et al. (1985) demonstrated that the opioid inhibition of adenylate cyclase in rat striatal membranes could also be blocked by pretreatment of the membranes with pertussis toxin. Pertussis toxin will uncouple receptors linked to adenylate cyclase through the N_i or N_o membrane protein (Ui, 1984). These results suggest that the regulation of potassium conductance by opioid receptors may normally be by controlling adenylate cyclase activity.

Electrophysiological evidence for a linkage between an opioid receptor and adenylate cyclase is beginning to accumulate. Andrade and Aghajanian (1985) have found that cyclicAMP analogs, 8-bromo-cyclicAMP and dibutyrl cyclicAMP, reverse the effects of opioids and clonidine on locus ceruleus cells without altering the basal conductance of the cells. Furthermore, pertussis toxin pretreatment blocks the outward potassium currents evoked by opioids and alpha-2 adrenergic agonists measured in locus ceruleus brain slices (Aghajanian and Wang, 1986). These observations have led Aghajanian and coworkers to propose that the mu receptor indirectly opens potassium channels in the locus ceruleus by first inhibiting the production of cyclicAMP.

Crain et al. (1986) measured the effects of cyclicAMP levels on the response to opioids in mouse spinal cord–dorsal root ganglion explants. Electrical stimulation of the afferent fibers in the organ culture evokes an extracellularly detectable response in the spinal explant. Opioids act in a naloxone-reversible, dose-dependent manner to depress the amplitude of the response. Activation of the adenylate cyclase by forskolin (10–50 μM) blocked the effects of morphine and DADLE. Dibutyryl cyclicAMP and dioctanoyl cyclicAMP also reduced the sensitivity of the response to opioids. Although the receptor type involved has not been identified, the observations are consistent with the hypothesis that an opioid receptor in the preparation may act by reducing intracellular cyclicAMP concentration.

In conflict with the proposed involvement of cyclicAMP, North and Williams (1985) have found that activation of the adenylate cyclase by forskolin treatment (1 μM) of locus ceruleus slices had no effect on the membrane hyperpolarization or outward current induced by [Met[5]]-enkephalin. In addition, North and Vitek (1980) found in the mouse vas deferens smooth muscle bioassay that depression of norepinephrine release by opioids was not affected by dibutyryl cyclic AMP or phosphodiesterase inhibitors. Karras and North (1979) also found that opioid receptor-mediated responses recorded in myenteric neurons were not blocked by dibutyryl cyclicAMP.

The suggested link between opioid receptors and adenylate cyclase was also examined in the guinea pig ileum longitudinal muscle myenteric plexus. Several groups have studied the effects of pertussis toxin treatment on the opioid sensitivity of the guinea pig ileum with conflicting results. Lux and Schulz (1985, 1986) injected guinea pigs with pertussis toxin (20 or 60 μg/kg) 3 or 6 d prior to testing the actions of opioids. Neither normorphine nor ethylketocyclazocine potency was affected. Identical results were obtained using the mouse vas deferens bioassay (Lux and Schulz, 1986). Collier et al. (1983), using a crude preparation of pertussis toxin, also found that normorphine potency in the guinea pig ileum assay was not changed. In contrast, similar pertussis toxin treatment (60 μg/kg for 6 d) by Lujan and coworkers (1984) dramatically reduced the sensitivity of the tissue to morphine. The basis for this discrepancy is not yet evident, but will need to be resolved before a conclusion about the involvement of adenylate cyclase and cyclicAMP in opioid action can be reached.

Interpretation of studies showing that dibutyryl cyclicAMP affects opioid action is complicated by the wide range of effects this compound has on the cell physiology. In addition, interpretation of the pertussis toxin experiments is confounded by the ability of the toxin to uncouple other transduction systems as well as adenylate cyclase (Ui, 1984; Pfaffinger et al., 1985). Cardiac muscarinic receptor control of potassium conductance is known not to be mediated by cyclicAMP, yet muscarinic activation of potassium channels is blocked by pertussis toxin treatment (Pfaffinger et al., 1985). Thus, although the proposal is attractive and consistent with data from these and other systems, the hypothesis that mu or delta receptors normally control potassium conductance indirectly through inhibition of adenylate cyclase activity in other cells is not yet fully substantiated. Single-channel measurement of potassium channel activation by opioids using patch clamp recording will be necessary to resolve this question. The mechanism of kappa receptor control of calcium conductance is similarly uncertain.

10. Summary

There is strong evidence to suggest that mu-selective opioids open a specific type of potassium channel. The molecular aspects of this channel have only been partly defined. The opioid-activated potassium conductance change is linear over a wide range of membrane voltages, and is therefore distinguishable from the potassium conductance regulated by muscarinic agonists (North and Williams, 1985). The pharmacological characteristics of the opioid-sensitive conductance also help to define its properties: it is sensitive to inhibition by barium (North and Williams, 1983; Cherubini and North, 1985), high concentration of tetraethylammonium, and quinine present in the tissue bathing medium (North and Williams, 1985; Cherubini and North, 1985). Intracellular application of cesium also blocks the opioid-induced potassium conductance (North and Williams, 1983).

The effect of mu receptor activation is similar to the actions of alpha-2 adrenergic agonists and GABA-B agonists (Cherubini et al., 1985). Thus mu receptor activation opens a type of potassium channel having characteristic properties different from the voltage-sensitive potassium conductance and different from the muscarinic potassium conductance (Cole and Shinnick-Gallagher, 1984), but similar to other ligand gated ion channels.

Based on studies of the submucus plexus and of DRG cultures, the properties of the delta receptor-activated potassium channel are indistinguishable from the mu receptor channel. The similarity in mechanism may reflect a close evolutionary relationship between the mu and delta receptors and suggests that there may be other common features. In contrast, kappa receptors have been shown to control calcium conductance. It is interesting that the net effect on cell excitability is the same regardless of which mechanism is used. The consequence of the increased potassium conductance is the reduction in excitability of the postsynaptic cell and a decrease in the transmitter release at the nerve terminal. The kappa receptor-mediated inhibition of calcium conductance will similarly reduce cell excitability by reduction of the calcium component of the action potential and may directly reduce transmitter release if kappa receptors are also located at the nerve terminals. Additional work is required to define the cellular distribution of the receptors. In the future, one can be optimistic that single-channel recording of each of the receptor types will answer the questions about possible second messenger linkages between the receptor and the ion channel.

Acknowledgment

The work done in the author's laboratory was supported by NIH grant NS23483 and a PMA research starter grant.

References

Abood, M. E., Law, P. Y., and Loh, H. H. (1985) Pertussis toxin treatment modifies opiate action in the rat brain striatum. *Biochem. Biophys. Res. Comm.* **127,** 477–483.

Aghajanian, G. K. (1978) Tolerance of locus coeruleus neurones to morphine and suppression of withdrawal response by clonidine. *Nature* **276,** 186–188.

Aghajanian, G. K. and VanderMaelen, C. P. (1982) Alpha 2-adrenoceptor-mediated hyperpolarization of locus coeruleus neurons: Intracellular studies in vivo. *Science* **215,** 1394–1396.

Aghajanian, G. K. and Wang, Y.-Y. (1986) Pertussis toxin blocks the outward currents evoked by opiate and alpha2-agonists in locus coeruleus neurons. *Brain Res.* **371,** 390–394.

Andrade, R. and Aghajanian, G. K. (1985) Opiate- and alpha2-adrenocep-tor-induced hyperpolarizations of locus coeruleus neurons in brain slices: Reversal by cyclic adenosine 3':5'-monophosphate analogues. *J. Neurosci.* **5**, 2359–2364.

Arunlakshana, O. and Schild, H. O. (1959) Some quantitative uses of drug antagonists. *Br. J. Pharmacol.* **14**, 48–58.

Basbaum, A. I. and Fields, H. L. (1984) Endogenous pain control systems: Brainstem spinal pathways and endorphin circuitry. *Ann. Rev. Neurosci.* **7**, 309–338.

Besse, J. C. and Furchgott, R. F. (1976) Dissociation constants and relative efficacies of agonists acting on alpha adrenergic receptors in rabbit aorta. *J. Pharmacol. Exp. Ther.* **197**, 66–78.

Bradley, P. B. and Brookes, A. (1984) A microiontophoretic study of the actions of mu-, delta-, and kappa-opiate receptor agonists in the rat brain. *Br. J. Pharmacol.* **83**, 763–772.

Brookes, A. and Bradley, P. B. (1984) The effects of kappa opioid agonists in the rat hippocampal slice. *Neuropeptides* **5**, 261–264.

Chang, K., Killian, A., Hazum, E., Cuatrecasas, P., and Chang, J. (1981) Morphiceptin (NH_4-Tyr-Pro-Phe-Pro-$CONH_2$): A potent and specific agonist for morphine (mu) receptors. *Science* **212**, 75–77.

Chavkin, C. and Bloom, F. (1986) Opiate antagonists do not alter neuronal responses to stimulation of opioid-containing pathways in rat hippocampus. *Neuropeptides* **7**, 19–22.

Chavkin, C. and Goldstein, A. (1981a) Specific receptor for the opioid peptide dynorphin: Structure–activity relationships. *Proc. Natl. Acad. Sci. USA* **78**, 6543–6547.

Chavkin, C. and Goldstein, A. (1981b) Demonstration of a specific dynorphin receptor in guinea pig ileum myenteric plexus. *Nature* **291**, 591–593.

Chavkin, C., Henriksen, S. J., Siggins, G. R., and Bloom, F. E. (1985a) Selective inactivation of opioid receptors in rat hippocampus demonstrates that dynorphin-A and -B may act on mu-receptors in the CA1 region. *Brain Res.* **331**, 366–370.

Chavkin, C., Shoemaker, W. J., McGinty, J. F., Bayon, A., and Bloom, F. E. (1985b) Characterization of the prodynorphin and proenkephalin neuropeptide systems in rat hippocampus. *J. Neurosci.* **5**, 808–816.

Chavkin, C., Bakhit, C., Weber, E., and Bloom, F. E. (1983) Relative contents and concomitant release of prodynorphin/neoendorphin-derived peptides in rat hippocampus. *Proc. Natl. Acad. Sci. USA* **80**, 7669–7673.

Chavkin, C., James, I. F., and Goldstein, A. (1982) Dynorphin is a specific endogenous ligand of the kappa opioid receptor. *Science* **215**, 413–415.

Cherubini, E. and North, R. A. (1985) Mu and kappa opioids inhibit transmitter release by different mechanisms. *Proc. Natl. Acad. Sci. USA* **82**, 1860–1863.

Cherubini, E., Morita, K., and North, R. A. (1985) Opioid inhibition of synaptic transmission in the guinea-pig myenteric plexus. *Br. J. Pharmacol.* **85**, 805–817.

Christian, E. P., West, M. O., and Deadwyler, S. A. (1985) Opiates and opioid peptides modify sensory evoked potentials and synaptic excitability in the rat dentate gyrus. *Neuropharmacology* **24**, 607–615.

Cole, A. E. and Shinnick-Gallagher, P. (1984) Muscarinic inhibitory transmission in mammalian sympathetic ganglia mediated by increased potassium conductance. *Nature* **307**, 270–271.

Collier, T. J. and Routtenberg, A. (1984) Selective impairment of declarative memory following stimulation of dentate gyrus granule cells: A naloxone-sensitive effect. *Brain Res.* **310,** 384–387.

Collier, H. O. J., Plant, N. T., and Tucker, J. F. (1983) Pertussis vaccine inhibits the chronic but not acute action of normorphine on the myenteric plexus of guinea-pig ileum. *Eur. J. Pharmacol.* **91,** 325–326.

Corbett, A. D., Kosterlitz, H. W., McKnight, A. T., Paterson, S. J., and Robson, L. E. (1985) Pre-incubation of guinea-pig myenteric plexus with beta- funaltrexamine: Discrepancy between binding assays and bioassays. *Br. J. Pharmacol.* **85,** 665–673.

Corbett, A. D., Paterson, S. J., Mcknight, A. T., Magnan, J., and Kosterlitz, H. W. (1982) Dynorphin(1-8) and dynorphin(1-9) are ligands for the kappa- subtype of opiate receptor. *Nature* **299,** 79–81.

Cotton, R., Giles, M. G., Miller, L., Shaw, J. S., and Timms, D. (1984) ICI 174864: A highly selective antagonist for the opioid delta-receptor. *Eur. J. Pharmacol.* **97,** 331–332.

Cox, B. M. and Chavkin, C. (1983) Comparison of dynorphin-selective kappa receptors in mouse vas deferens and guinea pig ileum. *Mol. Pharmacol.* **23,** 36–43.

Cox, B. M. and Weinstock, M. (1966) The effect of analgesic drugs on the release of acetylcholine from electrically stimulated guinea-pig ileum. *Br. J. Pharmacol.* **27,** 81–92.

Crain, S. M., Crain, B., and Peterson, E. R. (1986) Cyclic AMP or forskolin rapidly attenuates the depressant effects of opioids on sensory-evoked dorsal-horn responses in mouse spinal cord-ganglion explants. *Brain Res.* **370,** 61–72.

Dingledine, R. (1981) Possible mechanisms of enkephalin action on hippocampal CA1 pyramidal neurons. *J. Neurosci.* **1,** 1022–1035.

Duggan, A. W. and North, R. A. (1984) Electrophysiology of opioids. *Pharmacol. Rev.* **35,** 219–281.

Foote, R. W. and Maurer, R. (1982) Autoradiographic localization of opiate kappa-receptors in the guinea-pig brain. *Eur. J. Pharmacol.* **85,** 99–103.

Fournie-Zaluski, M., Gacel, G., Maigret, B., Premilat, S., and Roques, B. P. (1981) Structural requirements for specific recognition of mu or delta opiate receptors. *Mol. Pharmacol.* **20,** 484–491.

French, E. D. and Zieglgansberger, W. (1982) The excitatory response of in vitro hippocampal pyramidal cells to normorphine and methionine-enkephalin may be mediated by different receptor populations. *Exp. Brain Res.* **48,** 238–244.

Furchgott, R. F. (1966) The use of beta-haloalkylamines in the differentiation of receptors and in the determination dissociation constants of receptor-agonist complexes. *Adv. Brain Res.* **3,** 21–55.

Furchgott, R. F. (1972) The Classification of Adrenoceptors (Adrenergic Receptors). An Evaluation from the Standpoint of Receptor Theory, *Catecholamines* (Blaschko, H. and Muscholl, E., eds.) Springer-Verlag, Berlin.

Furchgott, R. F. (1978) Pharmacological characterization of receptors: Its relation to radioligand-binding studies. *Fed. Proc.* **37,** 115–120.

Gahwiler, B. H. and Maurer, R. (1981) Involvement of mu-receptors in the opioid-induced generation of bursting discharges in hippocampal pyramidal cells. *Reg. Peptides* **2,** 91–96.

Gall, C. (1984) Ontogeny of dynorphin-like immunoreactivity in the hippocampal formation of the rat. *Brain Res.* **307**, 327–331.

Gall, C., Brecha, N., Karten, H. J., and Chang, K. (1981) Localization of enkephalin-like immunoreactivity to identified axonal and neuronal populations of the rat hippocampus. *J. Comp. Neurol.* **198**, 335–350.

Goldstein, A. and James, I. F. (1984a) Multiple opioid receptors: Criteria for identification and classification. *Trends Pharmacol. Sci.* **5**, 503–505.

Goldstein, A. and James, I. F. (1984b) Site-directed alkylation of multiple opioid receptors. II. Pharmacological selectivity. *Mol. Pharmacol.* **25**, 343–348.

Gruol, D. L., Chavkin, C., Valentino, R. J., and Siggins, G. R. (1983) Dynorphin-A alters the excitability of pyramidal neurons of the rat hippocampus in vitro. *Life Sci.* **33**, 533–536.

Haas, H. L. and Ryall, R. W. (1980) Is excitation by enkephalins of hippocampal neurons in the rat due to presynaptic facilitation or to disinhibition? *J. Physiol.* **308**, 315–330.

Hahn, E. F., Itzhak, Y., Nishimura, S., Johnson, N., and Pasternak, G. W. (1985) Irreversible opiate agonists and antagonists. III. Phenylhydrazone derivatives of naloxone and oxymorphone. *J. Pharmacol. Exp. Ther.* **235**, 846–850.

Hahn, E. F., Carroll-Buatti, M., and Pasternak, G. W. (1982) Irreversible opiate agonists and antagonists: The 14-hydroxydihydromorphinone azines. *J. Neurosci.* **2**, 572–576.

Hazum, E., Chang, K., Cuatrecasas, P., and Pasternak, G. W. (1981) Naloxazone irreversibly inhibits the high affinity binding of [125I]D-ala2-D-leu5-enkephalin. *Life Sci.* **28**, 2973–2979.

Henderson, G. (1983) Electrophysiological analysis of opioid action in the central nervous system *Br. Med. Bull.* **39**, 59–64.

Henriksen, S. J., Chouvet, G., and Bloom, F. E. (1982) In vivo cellular responses to electrophoretically applied dynorphin in the rat hippocampus. *Life Sci.* **31**, 1785–1788.

Hill, R., Mitchell, J., and Pepper, C. (1977) The excitation and depression of hippocampal neurons by iontophoretically applied enkephalins. *J. Physiol.* **272**, 50–51p.

Hutchinson, M., Kosterlitz, H. W., Leslie, F. M., and Waterfield, A. A. (1975) Assessment in the guinea-pig ileum and mouse vas deferens of benzomorphans which have strong antinociceptive activity but do not substitute for morphine in the dependent monkey. *Brit. J. Pharmacol.* **55**, 541–546.

Iwama, T., Ishihara, K., Satoh, M., and Takagi, H. (1986) Different effects of dynorphin A on in vitro guinea pig hippocampal CA3 pyramidal cells with various degrees of paired- pulse facilitation. *Neurosci. Lett.* **63**, 190–194.

James, I. F. and Goldstein, A. (1984) Site-directed alkylation of multiple opioid receptors I. Binding selectivity. *Mol. Pharmacol.* **25**, 337–342.

James, I. F., Chavkin, C., and Goldstein, A. (1982) Preparation of brain membranes containing a single type of opioid receptor highly selective for dynorphin. *Proc. Natl. Acad. Sci. USA* **79**, 7570–7574.

James, I. F., Fischli, W. and Goldstein, A. (1984) Opioid receptor selectivity of dynorphin gene products. *J. Pharmacol. Exp. Ther.* **228**, 88–93.

Jessell, T. M. and Iversen, L. L. (1977) Opiate analgesics inhibit substance P release from rat trigeminal nucleus. *Nature* **268**, 549–551.

Karras, P. J. and North, R. A. (1979) Inhibition of neuronal firing by opiates: Evidence against the involvement of cyclic nucleotides. *Br. J. Pharmacol.* **65**, 647–652.

Kenakin, T. P. (1985) Schild regressions as indicators of non-equilibrium steady-states and heterogeneous receptor populations. *Trends Pharmacol. Sci.* **6**, 68–71.

Lahti, R. A., VonVoigtlander, P. F., and Barsuhn, C. (1982) Properties of a selective kappa agonist, U-50,488H. *Life Sci.* **31**, 2257–2260.

Law, P., Wu, J., Koehler, J., and Loh, H. (1981) Demonstration and characterization of opiate inhibition of the striatal adenylate cyclase. *J. Neurochem.* **36**, 1834–1846.

Law, P., Louie, A. K., and Loh, H. H. (1985) Effect of pertussis toxin treatment on the down-regulation of opiate receptors in neuroblastoma glioma NG108–15 hybrid cells. *J. Biol. Chem.* **260**, 14818–14823.

Lee, H. K., Dunwiddie T., and Hoffer, B. (1980) Electrophysiological interactions of enkephalins with neuronal circuitry in the rat hippocampus. II. Effects on interneuron excitability. *Brain Res.* **184**, 331–342.

Linseman, M. A. and Corrigall, W. A. (1982) Effects of morphine on CA1 versus dentate hippocampal field potentials following systemic administration in freely-moving rats. *Neuropharmacology* **21**, 361–366.

Lord, J. A. H., Waterfield, A. A., Hughes, J., and Kosterlitz, H. W. (1977) Endogenous opioid peptides: Multiple agonists and receptors. *Nature* **267**, 495–499.

Lujan, M., Lopez, E., Ramirez, R., Aguilar, H., Martinez-Olmedo, M. A., and Garcia-Sainz, J. A. (1984) Pertussis toxin blocks the action of morphine, norepinephrine and clonidine on isolated guinea-pig ileum. *Eur. J. Pharmacol.* **100**, 377–380.

Lux, B. and Schulz, R. (1985) Opioid dependence prevents the action of pertussis toxin in the guinea-pig myenteric plexus. *Naunyn Schmeidebergs Arch. Pharmacol.* **330**, 184–186.

Lux, B. and Schulz, R. (1986) Effect of cholera toxin and pertussis toxin on opioid tolerance and dependence in the guinea-pig myenteric plexus. *J. Pharmacol. Exp. Ther.* **237**, 995–1000.

Masukawa, L. M. and Prince, D. A. (1982) Enkephalin inhibition of inhibitory input to CA1 and CA3 pyramidal neurons in the hippocampus. *Brain Res.* **249**, 271–280.

McGinty, J. F., Henriksen, S. J., Goldstein, A., Terenius, L., and Bloom, F. E. (1983) Dynorphin is contained within hippocampal mossy fibers: Immunochemical alterations after kainic acid administration and colchicine-induced neurotoxicity. *Proc. Natl. Acad. Sci. USA* **80**, 589–593.

McKnight, A., Paterson, S., Corbett, A., and Kosterlitz, H. (1984) Acute and persistent effects of beta-funaltrexamine on the binding and agonist potencies of opioids in the myenteric plexus of the guinea-pig ileum. *Neuropeptides* **5**, 169–172.

Mihara, S. and North, R. A. (1986) Opioids increase potassium conductance in submucous neurons of guinea-pig caecum by activating delta-receptors. *Br. J. Pharmacol.* **88**, 315–322.

Moises, H. C. and Walker, J. M. (1985) Electrophysiological effects of dynorphin peptides on hippocampal pyramidal cells in rat. *Eur. J. Pharmacol.* **108,** 85–98.

Morita, K. and North, R. A. (1982) Opiate activation of potassium conductance in myenteric neurons: Inhibition by calcium ion. *Brain Res.* **242,** 145–150.

Mosberg, H. I., Hurst, R., Hruby, V. J., Gee, Kelvin, Yamamura, H. I., Galligan, J. J., and Burks, T. F. (1983) Bis-penicillamine enkephalins possess highly improved specificity toward delta opioid receptors. *Proc. Natl. Acad. Sci. USA* **80,** 5871–5874.

Mudge, A. W., Leeman, S. E., and Fischbach, G. D. (1979) Enkephalin inhibits release of substance P from sensory neurons in culture and decreases action potential duration. *Proc. Natl. Acad. Sci. USA* **76,** 526–530.

Neumaier, J. and Chavkin, C. (1986a) Opioid receptor activity in the dentate gyrus of the rat hippocampus. *NIDA Res. Monogr.,* in press.

Neumaier, J. and Chavkin, C. (1986b) Multiple opioid receptor types in the rat hippocampus. *Soc. Neurosci. Abst.* **12,** (2), 1013.

Nicoll, R. and Madison, D. (1984) The action of enkephalin on interneurons in the hippocampus. *Soc. Neurosci. Abst.* **10** (1), 660.

Nicoll, R. A., Siggins, G. R., Ling, N., Bloom, F. E., and Guillemin, R. (1977) Neuronal actions of endorphins and enkephalins among brain regions: A comparative microiontophoretic study. *Proc. Natl. Acad. Sci. USA* **74,** 2584–2588.

Nishi, S. and North, R. A. (1973) Intracellular recording from the myenteric plexus of the guinea-pig ileum. *J. Physiology* **231,** 471–490.

North, R. A. (1986) Opioid receptor types and membrane ion channels. *Trends Neurosci.* **9,** 114–117.

North, R. (1982) Electrophysiology of the enteric nervous system. *Neuroscience* **7,** 315–326.

North, R. A. and Vitek, L. V. (1980) A study of the role of cyclic adenosine 3′,5′-monophosphate in the depression by opiates and opioid peptides of excitatory junction potentials in the mouse vas deferens. *Br. J. Pharmacol.* **71,** 307–313.

North, R. A. and Williams, J. R. (1985) On the potassium conductance increased by opioids in rat locus coeruleus neurons. *J. Physiology* **364,** 265–280.

North, R. A. and Williams, J. T. (1983) Opiate activation of potassium conductance inhibits calcium action potentials in rat locus coeruleus neurons. *Br. J. Pharmacol.* **80,** 225–228.

Oka, T. (1980) Enkephalin receptor in the rabbit ileum. *Br. J. Pharmacol.* **68,** 193–195.

Pasternak, G. W., Childers, S. R., and Snyder, S. H. (1980) Naloxazone, a long-acting opiate antagonist: Effects on analgesia in intact animals and on opiate receptor binding in vitro. *J. Pharmacol. Exp. Ther.* **214,** 455–462.

Paton, W. D. M. (1957) The action of morphine and related substances on contraction and on acetylcholine output of coaxially stimulated guinea-pig ileum. *Br. J. Pharmacol.* **12,** 119–127.

Pepper, C. M. and Henderson, G. (1980) Opiates and opioid peptides hyperpolarize locus coeruleus neurons in vitro. *Science* **209,** 394–396.

Pfaffinger, P., Martin, J., Hunter, D. D., Nathanson, N., and Hille, B. (1985) GTP-binding proteins couple cardiac muscarinic receptors to a K channel. *Nature* **317**, 536–538.

Portoghese, P. S. and Takemori, A. (1985) TENA, a selective kappa opioid receptor antagonist. *Life Sci.* **36**, 801–805.

Portoghese, P. S., Larson, D. L., Sayre, L. M., Fries, D. S., and Takemori, A. E. (1980) A novel opioid receptor site directed alkylating agent with irreversible narcotic antagonistic and reversible agonistic activities. *J. Medicinal Chem.* **23**, 233–234.

Portoghese, P. S., Lipowski, A. W., and Takemori, A. E. (1986) Binaltorphimine: A highly selective, kappa opioid receptor antagonist. *Abst. Int. Narcotics Res. Conf.* 0–74.

Raggenbass, M., Wuarin, J. P., Gahwiler, B. H., and Dreifuss, J. J. (1985) Opposing effects of oxytocin and of a mu-receptor agonistic opioid peptide on the same class of non-pyramidal neurons in rat hippocampus. *Brain Res.* **344**, 392–396.

Roemer, D., Buescher, H., Hill, R. C., Pless, J., Bauer, W., Cardinaux, F., Closse, A., Hauser, D., and Huguenin, R. (1977) A synthetic enkephalin analogue with prolonged parenteral and oral analgesic activity. *Nature* **268**, 547–549.

Romer, D., Buscher, H. H., Hill, R. C., Maurer, R., Petcher, T. J., Zeugner, H., Benson, W., Finner, E., Milkowski, W., and Thies, P. W. (1982) An opioid benzodiazepine. *Nature* **298**, 759–760.

Rothman, R. B., Bowen, W. D., Schumacher, U. K., and Pert, C. B. (1983) Effect of beta-FNA on opiate receptor binding: Preliminary evidence for two types of mu receptors. *Eur. J. Pharmacol.* **95**, 147–148.

Rothman, R. B., Schumacher, U. K., and Pert, C. B. (1984) Effect of beta-FNA on opiate delta receptor binding. *J. Neurochem.* **43**, 1197–1200.

Schild, H. O. (1947) The use of drug antagonists for the identification and classification of drugs. *Br. J. Pharmacol.* **2**, 251–258.

Schild, H. (1949) pAx and competitive drug antagonism. *Br. J. Pharmacol.* **4**, 277–280.

Schwartzkroin, P. A. and Mathers, L. H. (1978) Physiological and morphological identification of a nonpyramidal hippocampal cell type. *Brain Res.* **157**, 1–10.

Sharma, S. K., Klee, W. A., and Nirenberg, M. (1977) Opiate-dependent modulation of adenylate cyclase. *Proc. Natl. Acad. Sci. USA* **74**, 3365–3369.

Sharma, S. K., Nirenberg, M., and Klee, W. A. (1975) Morphine receptors as regulators of adenylate cyclase activity. *Proc. Natl. Acad. Sci. USA* **72**, 590–594.

Siggins, G. R. and Zieglgansberger, W. (1981) Morphine and opioid peptides reduce inhibitory synaptic potentials in hippocampal pyramidal cells in vitro without alteration of membrane potential. *Proc. Natl. Acad. Sci. USA* **78**, 5235–5239.

Surprenant, A. and North, R. (1985) mu-Opioid receptors and alpha2-adrenoceptors coexist on myenteric but not submucous neurons. *Neuroscience* **16**, 425–430.

Takemori, A. E. and Portoghese, P. S. (1985) Affinity labels for opioid receptors. *Ann. Rev. Pharmacol. Toxicol.* **25**, 193–223.

Takemori, A. E., Larson, D. L., and Portoghese, P. S. (1981) The irreversible narcotic antagonistic and reversible agonistic properties of the fumaramate methyl ester derivative of naltrexone. *Eur. J. Pharmacol.* **70,** 445–451.

Tielen, A. M., Lopes Da Silva, F. H., Mollevanger, W. J., and DeJong, F. H. (1981) Differential effects of enkephalin within hippocampal areas. *Exp. Brain Res.* **44,** 343–346.

Tokimasa, T., Morita, K., and North, A. (1981) Opiates and clonidine prolong calcium-dependent after- hyperpolarizations. *Nature* **294,** 162–163.

Ui, M. (1984) Islet-activating protein, pertussis toxin: A probe for functions of the inhibitory guanine nucleotide regulatory component of adenylate cyclase. *Trends Pharmacol. Sci.* **5,** 277–279.

Valentino, R. J. and Dingledine, R. (1982) Pharmacological characterization of opioid effects in the rat hippocampal slice. *J. Pharmacol. Exp. Ther.* **223,** 502–509.

Vidal, C., Maier, R., and Zieglgansberger, W. (1984) Effects of dynorphin A (1-17), dynorphin A (1-13) and D-ala2- D-leu5-enkephalin on the excitability of pyramidal cells in CA1 and CA2 of the rat hippocampus in vitro. *Neuropeptides,* **5,** 237–240.

VonVoigtlander, P. F., Lahti, R. A., and Ludens, J. H. (1983) U-50,488: A selective and structurally novel non-mu (kappa) opioid agonist. *J. Pharmacol. Exp. Ther.* **224,** 7–12.

Walden, J. and Speckmann, E.-J. (1981) Effects of quinine on membrane potential and membrane currents in identified neurons of helix pomatia. *Neurosci. Lett.* **27,** 139–143.

Walker, J. M., Moises, H. C., Coy, D. H., Baldrighi, G., and Akil, H. (1982) Nonopiate effects of dynorphin and des-tyr-dynorphin. *Science* **218,** 1136–1138.

Ward, S. J., Portoghese, P. S., and Takemori, A. E. (1981) Pharmacological characterization in vivo of the novel opiate, beta-funaltrexamine. *J. Pharmacol. Exp. Ther.* **220,** 494–498.

Ward, S. J., Portoghese, P. S., and Takemori, A. E. (1982) Pharmacological profiles of beta-funaltrexamine (beta-FNA) and beta-chlornaltrexamine (beta-CNA) on the mouse vas deferens preparation. *Eur. J. Pharmacol.* **80,** 377–384.

Werling, L. L., Zarr, G. D., Brown, S. R., and Cox, B. M. (1985) Opioid binding to rat and guinea-pig neural membranes in the presence of physiological cations at 37°C. *J. Pharmacol. Exp. Ther.* **233,** 722–728.

Werz, M. A. and MacDonald, R. L. (1985) Dynorphin and neoendorphin peptides decrease dorsal root ganglion neuron calcium-dependent action potential duration. *J. Pharmacol. Exp. Ther.* **234,** 49–56.

Werz, M. A. and MacDonald, R. L. (1984) Dynorphin reduces calcium-dependent action potential duration by decreasing voltage-dependent calcium conductance. *Neurosci. Lett.* **46,** 185–190.

Werz, M. A. and MacDonald, R. L. (1983) Opioid peptides with differential affinity for mu and delta receptors decrease sensory neuron calcium-dependent action potentials. *J. Pharmacol. Exp. Ther.* **227,** 394–402.

Williams, J. T. and North, R. A. (1984) Opiate-receptor interactions on single locus coeruleus neurons. *Mol. Pharmacol.* **26,** 489–497.

Williams, J. T. and North, R. A. (1979) Effects of endorphins on single myenteric neurons. *Brain Res.* **165,** 57–65.

Williams, J. T., Egan, T. M., and North, R. A. (1982) Enkephalin opens potassium channels on mammalian central neurons. *Nature* **299,** 74–77.

Wuster, M., Rubini, P., and Schulz, R. (1981) The preference of putative pro-enkephalins for different types of opiate receptors. *Life Sci.* **29,** 1219–1227.

Wuster, M., Schulz, R., and Herz, A. (1985) Opioid tolerance and dependence: Re-evaluating the unitary hypothesis. *Trends Pharmacol. Sci.* **6,** 64–67.

Yoshida, S., Fujimura, K., and Matsuda, T. (1986) Effects of quinidine and quinine on the excitability of pyramidal neurons in guinea-pig hippocampal slices. *Pflugers Arch.* **406,** 544–546.

Zamir, N., Quirion, R., and Segal, M. (1985) Ontogeny and regional distribution of proenkephalin- and prodynorphin-derived peptides and opioid receptors in rat hippocampus. *Neuroscience* **15,** 1025–1034.

Zhang, A., Chang, J., and Pasternak, G. W. (1981) The actions of naloxazone on the binding and analgesic properties of morphiceptin (NH2Tyr-Pro-Phe-Pro-CONH2), a selective mu-receptor ligand. *Life Sci.* **28,** 2829–2836.

Zieglgansberger, W., French, E. D., Siggins, G. R., and Bloom, F. E. (1979) Opioid peptides may excite hippocampal pyramidal neurons by inhibiting adjacent inhibitory interneurons. *Science,* **205,** 415–417.

Zukin, R. S. and Zukin, S. R. (1981) Multiple opiate receptors: Emerging concepts. *Life Sci.* **29,** 2681–2690.

SECTION 5
PHARMACOLOGICAL
CORRELATION OF
BINDING SITES WITH FUNCTION

Chapter 10

Central Actions of Opiates and Opioid Peptides
In Vivo Evidence for Opioid Receptor Multiplicity

Paul L. Wood and Smriti Iyengar

1. Introduction

The in vivo study of opiates and opioid peptides is complicated by the multiple receptor affinities of the drugs presently available (Wood et al., 1981b; Wood, 1982a; Wood, 1983a). This property of the majority of compounds available for study demands that both extensive dose–response studies and naloxone reversibility be performed. If possible, stereospecificity for both the agonist actions and the reversal by an antagonist should be examined (Wood et al., 1984b). A further complication is also evident; namely, species differences that appear to be dependent upon species differences in the proportion of mu, delta, and kappa receptors in a brain area (Gillan and Kosterlitz, 1982; Wood, 1983a,b; Frischknecht et al., 1983) and in the proportion of presynaptic to postsynaptic opioid receptors on a given neuronal population (Wood and Richard, 1982). Multiple receptor types on the same neuron may be a further complication; however, the problems of receptor dualism via separate neuronal populations have been clearly demonstrated (Wood et al., 1983a). In this example, the Ag/Ant butorphanol, which possesses a bell-shaped dose–response curve with regard to increases in striatal dopamine metabolites, has an initial agonist action directly on dopamine neurons that is subsequently antagonized by another receptor action at a neuronal population caudal to the substantia nigra (Wood et al., 1983a).

With these constraints in mind, the following central actions of opiates and opioid peptides are reviewed.

2. Analgesia

Opiates and the opioid peptides have the unique ability to selectively relieve the subjective component of pain without affecting primary sensory modalities, such as touch, vibration, vision, and hearing, making them the preferred clinical class of drug for severe pain. Opiates, however, produce their actions through modulation of a wide variety of neurotransmitter systems, including acetylcholine, dopamine, and serotonin. Studies of the interactions of opioids with these transmitters are discussed later in this chapter.

Opioids can modulate pain sensation at several levels of the CNS, but most experimental work has focused on the spinal cord, specifically, laminae I and II, nucleus raphé magnus and the periaqueductal gray (PAG). The physiology of this system has been extensively studied (Basbaum, 1984). In addition to multiple anatomical sites within the CNS, opiates and opioid peptides can mediate analgesia through multiple opioid receptor types. The concept of these multiple opioid receptor populations was first reviewed by Martin (1967), and is covered elsewhere in this volume. Discussion of the receptor subtypes mediating analgesia is complicated, requiring consideration of the level of the CNS affected and the receptor selectivity of the drugs employed, which is dependent upon the dose of drug.

2.1. Mu and Delta Agonists

With morphine and codeine as standards, it is not surprising that pharmacologists first associated analgesia with mu receptors (Martin, 1967). Even today, most investigators agree that mu receptor activation yields the most consistent and efficacious analgesia. Mu analgesia is mediated predominantly supraspinally, with the PAG being a key site of action (Yaksh and Rudy, 1978). Microinjection into the PAG of small quantities of morphine (1–5 μg) elicits profound analgesia, whereas intrathecal morphine in the rat is much weaker in analgesic tests (Wood et al., 1981a). Intrathecal delta agonists are potent analgesics both in animals (Yaksh, 1985) and in humans (Moulin et al., 1984). Intraventricular administration of delta agonists, however, is not as efficacious in eliciting analgesia (Wood, 1982a), and via this route, the more delta-specific peptides are relatively weak analgesics (Ronai et al., 1981). β-Endorphin, like mu agonists, is a more potent analgesic via the intraventricular route (Tseng et al., 1983).

Recently, it has been proposed that mu_1 sites mediate the morphine analgesia (Pasternak and Wood, 1986; Pasternak, 1981). Naloxazone and naloxonazine, two long-acting, mu_1-selective antagonists, dramatically decrease morphine analgesia in both rats and mice (Table 1; Pasternak et al., 1980a,b; Zhang and Pasternak, 1981a). Additional studies have revealed that mu_1 blockade also attenuates the analgesic actions of a series of other opiates, consistent with their affinity for the mu_1 binding site (Ling et al., 1983). The correlation between mu_1 receptors and sensitivity toward morphine analgesia seen in the naloxazone studies is also found among strains of mice (Moskowitz and Goodman, 1985a,b) and in developmental studies (Zhang and Pasternak, 1981b; Pasternak et al., 1980c).

The importance of the PAG in alleviating pain rests upon the strong, naloxone-reversible analgesia elicited by either the microinjection of morphine or many enkephalins or by electrical stimulation, which presumably releases endogenous opioid peptides (Reynolds, 1969; Mayer and Liebeskind, 1974; Akil et al., 1974). Recent work now suggests that mu_1 receptors mediate opioid analgesia in the PAG, nucleus raphe magnus, locus

TABLE 1
Effects of Mu_1 Blockade In Vivo on Opioid Analgesia[a]

Drug	Analgesic ED_{50}, mg/kg		
	Control	Mu_1 Blockade	Shift
Morphine (sc)	6.1	70	11-fold
Ketocyclazocine (sc)	7.4	55	7-fold
EKC (sc)	0.06	0.27	5-fold
Metkephamid (sc)	29	71	2-fold
DADLE (ivt)	1.1 μg	3.9 μg	3-fold

[a]Data from Ling et al., (1983) and Pasternak (1981). Abbreviations: sc, subcutaneous; ivt, intraventricular.

ceruleus, and nucleus reticularis gigantocellularis (Bodnar, Williams, and Pasternak, personal communication). Microinjection of morphine directly into these regions elicits a strong antinociceptive response that is antagonized by naloxonazine. Both [D-Ser^2-Leu^5]enkephalin-Thr^6 (DSLET) and [D-Pen^2-D-Pen^5]enkephalin (DPDPE) are potent delta ligands, but only DSLET has significant activity at mu_1 receptors (Clark et al., 1986; Itzhak and Pasternak, 1987). Microinjections of DSLET, but not DPDPE, into these regions produces analgesia that is antagonized by naloxonazine. Thus, supraspinal mechanisms of opioid analgesia involve the mu_1 subtype of mu receptors.

2.2. Kappa Agonists

Kappa receptor agonists are potent analgesics in a large number of experimental pain paradigms; writhing, tailflick (Table 2), Randall and Selitto hyperesthesia, tail clip, and hot plate and shock titration (Romer and Hill, 1981; Wood et al., 1982a; Upton et al.,

TABLE 2
Analgesic Actions of Opioid Receptor Agonists
in the Rat Tail Flick Assay[a]

Receptor	Drug	ED$_{50}$, mg/kg
Mu	Morphine	2.0
	Methadone	0.8
	Etorphine	0.002
	Phenazocine	0.5
	Buprenorphine	0.06
	Metkephamid	0.2
	FK 33.824	0.4
Delta	DADLE	5.0 μg, ivt
Kappa	EKC	2.0
	Mr2034	0.5
	Tifluadom	2.0
	U50488H	8.0
Ag/Ant	Butorphanol	0.6
	Nalbuphine	4.0
	Pentazocine	40.0
	Cyclazocine	IA
	Nalorphine	IA

[a]Data are comparative since they are all from one laboratory (Wood et al., 1980; Wood, 1984b). Abbreviations: IA, inactive; ivt, intraventricular.

1983; Wood, 1984b; Piercey et al., 1982a,b). The actions of kappa agonists are unique in that they are only analgesic in areas of primary afferent input; the trigeminal N (Skingle and Tyers, 1980) and the spinal cord (Wood et al., 1981a). The spinal actions of kappa agonists are potent, as has been demonstrated in spinal animals (Wood et al., 1981a) and by intrathecal injections of both kappa opiates (Wood et al., 1981a; Piercey et al., 1982a,b) and kappa opioid peptides (Piercey et al., 1982b; Han and Xie, 1982). In spinal animals, kappa opiates are the only analgesics that have demonstrated no loss of analgesic activity as assessed by the tail flick test (Wood et al., 1981a). These potent actions are presumably mediated by the numerous kappa receptors that have been quantitated in the dorsal spinal cord of the rat, guinea pig, and humans (Kelly et al., 1982; Gouarderes et al., 1982; Czlonkowski et al., 1983).

At more rostral local injection sites in the CNS, kappa agonists are inactive. Clearly, intraventricular kappa opiates (Wood et al., 1981a) and kappa opioid peptides (Hollt et al., 1982) are inactive as analgesics. Similarly, local injections of kappa agonists into the periaqueductal grey (PAG) do not elicit analgesia, whereas mu agonists are potent analgesics after local injections into this region (Wood et al., 1981a).

The antagonist properties of kappa receptor agonists are also clearly evident in analgesic dose ranges such that all kappa agonists examined to date (Wood, 1984a) block the actions of mu and delta agonists on DA neurons and delta agonists on ACh neurons. Similarly, at analgesic doses, the kappa agonist bremazocine blocks the constipation induced by both morphine and DADLE (Petrillo et al., 1984). These data clearly explain the multiple receptor affinities observed with kappa agonists using in vitro receptor binding assays (Wood, 1982a). These in vitro receptor affinities probably include kappa agonism, delta antagonism, and mu_2 antagonism in vivo (Wood, 1983a; 1984a).

2.3. Agonist/Antagonist Analgesics

The analgesia induced by the agonist/antagonist agents is probably the least understood of all forms of opiate analgesia at the present time. These drugs are characterized by ceilings to their analgesic efficacy as monitored both in the clinic and basic laboratory (Wood, 1984b).

At the spinal level, these agents, unlike mu and kappa agonists, are inactive in analgesic tests (Table 3) as has been described with both intrathecal injections (Yaksh and Rudy, 1978; Russell

TABLE 3
Analgesic Profiles of Mu, Kappa, and Ag/Ant Agents[a]

Analgesic test	Mu agonist	Kappa agonist	Ag/Ant
	Active analgesic, yes or no		
Tail flick			
Parenteral	Yes	Yes	Yes
PAG	Yes	No	No
Intrathecal	Yes	Yes	No
Spinal animals	No	Yes	No
Potency ranking			
Tail flick > hot plate	Yes	Yes	No
Tail clip > tail immersion	No	Yes	?

[a]Data from Wood (1984a) and Upton et al. (1983).

and Yaksh, 1982; Schmauss et al., 1983) and parental administration in spinal animals (Satoh et al., 1979; Inukai and Takagi, 1979). In fact, the only activity that has been observed at the spinal level is a mu antagonist action that is critically dependent upon the correct dose ratio for morphine and the agonist/antagonist agent (Russell and Yaksh, 1982; Shimada et al., 1984). At the level of the PAG, the agonist/antagonist agents are also inactive as analgesics (Yaksh and Rudy, 1978). These data are suggestive of an undefined site of action for the agonist/antagonist analgesics; a suggestion supported by the different pA_2 values of naloxone for reversing agonist/antagonist vs. mu-dependent analgesia (Smits and Takemori, 1970).

The one exception to these generalizations appears to be butorphanol, which is a potent analgesic after injection into the PAG, with cross tolerance to morphine, suggesting a mu_1 agonist action of this drug (Wood et al., 1983a).

3. Behavioral/Autonomic Actions

3.1. Respiratory Depression

Classical mu opiates and opioid peptides consistently depress respiration in all species that have been tested. These actions appear to involve both decreased responsiveness of CNS centers to CO_2 and a decrease in the CNS respiratory frequency controller (Eckenhoff and Oech, 1960; Borison, 1977). In animal experiments, decreases in the peak discharge frequency, but not the basal frequency of cell firing, have been monitored in the tractus solitarius, N ambigus and N parabrachialis after iontophoretic application of either morphine or enkephalins (Denavit-Saubie et al., 1978). These actions on bulbar and pontine respiratory centers are naloxone-reversible, with low doses reversing the depressant actions of both morphine and β-endorphin and higher doses reversing the actions of Leu- and Met-enkephalin (McQueen, 1983). These data would support separate mu and delta inputs to the respiratory centers and might indicate that the actions of β-endorphin (Moss and Friedman, 1978) are mu receptor-mediated. Determination of the pA_2 values for naloxone reversal of mu- and delta-dependent respiratory depression also supports a role for separate mu and delta sites regulating respiration (Pazos and Florez, 1983). In addition, some tonic enkephalinergic input is suggested since naloxone alone can increase the inspiratory rate and enhance the sensitivity of these centers to CO_2 (Lawson et al., 1979; Beubler, 1980; McQueen and Ribeiro, 1980).

Clearly, mu (Green, 1959) and delta (McQueen, 1983) agonists depress respiration. In the case of the partial mu agonist, buprenorphine, a ceiling in the respiratory actions, as assessed by pCO_2 measurements, has been reported (50% of morphine effect; Cowan et al., 1977). Similarly with the agonist/antagonist analgesics, a ceiling in the respiratory depression has been observed both in the lab and clinic with pentazocine, nalbuphine, and butorphanol (Eckenhoff and Oech, 1960; Bellville and Forrest, 1968; Heel et al., 1978; Romagnoli and Keats, 1980; Gal et al., 1982). These actions are, however, paralleled by ceilings in the analgesic actions of these drugs. Analysis of the pA_2 values for naloxone reversal of the respiratory depression induced by morphine, levallorphan, and pentazocine clearly indicated that these agents act at a common receptor (McGilliard and Takemori, 1978) to induce respiratory depression. These data would suggest that the respiratory depressant actions of agonist/antagonist agents is mu receptor-mediated, with the ceiling in activity being dependent upon a lesser intrinsic activity for these analgesics at the mu receptor. This is supported by the antagonism of morphine-dependent respiratory depression by Ag/Ant analgesics if administered in a critical dose ratio range (Eckenhoff and Oech, 1960; Martin, 1967).

Further studies of the mu receptor mediating respiratory depression have suggested that a mu isoreceptor site is involved. Initially, the mu agonist meptazinol was found not to depress respiration in the analgesic dose range (Goode et al., 1979; Spiegel and Pasternak, 1984). Subsequently, the mu_1 antagonist, naloxonazine, was found not to alter the actions of morphine in increasing pCO_2, suggesting a mu_2 receptor action of morphine and dissociating the receptor mechanisms responsible for analgesia and respiratory depression (Ling et al., 1983, 1985). Consistent with this receptor classification, kappa agonists (e.g., EKC, Mr2034), which possess mu_2 antagonist properties (Wood, 1984a), will block the respiratory depressant actions of morphine (Wood et al., 1982a). The kappa agonists alone elicit minimal respiratory depressant actions.

3.2. Catalepsy

Mu agonists (Tseng et al., 1979; Ling and Pasternak, 1982), delta agonists (Tseng et al., 1979), and β-endorphin (Tseng et al., 1979; Bloom et al., 1978) all elicit catalepsy in the rat. Since the actions of morphine in the rat can be reversed by naloxonazine (Ling and Pasternak, 1982), catalepsy appears to be mu_1-mediated. This suggestion is supported by the observations that there is a high correlation between the sites of action of etorphine analgesia (i.e., mu_1) and catalepsy (Thorn and Levitt, 1980). The catalepsy induced by the delta agonist, [D-Ala^2-D-Leu^5]enkephalin, is unique in that in contrast to morphine and β-endorphin, the catalepsy is present without muscular rigidity (Tseng et al., 1979).

Although the kappa opiates do not induce catalepsy in the rat, the kappa opioid peptide, dynorphin (1-13) does induce catalepsy that is independent of the mu receptor, as demonstrated in tolerance experiments (Herman and Goldstein, 1981).

In contrast to the catalepsy observed in the rat, these agents all produce motor excitement in the mouse (Katz et al., 1978; Wood, 1982a), except for the kappa agonists (Tepper and Woods, 1978). The observed motor activation after mu and delta agonists in the mouse appears to involve dopaminergic pathways and to be mu_2 receptor-mediated (Wood and Richard, 1982; Wood, 1984a). Locomotor activation can also be induced in the rat by local injections of β-endorphin (Stinus et al., 1980), Met-enkephalin (Broekkamp et al., 1979), and morphine (Joyce and Iverson, 1979) into the ventral tegmental area.

In the cat, morphine and β-endorphin produce psychomotor excitation (Megans and Cools, 1982; Beleslin et al., 1982). Septal epsilon receptors appear to be the final common point of action for eliciting this syndrome (Megans and Cools, 1982).

Local injections of opiates and opioid peptides into the pars reticulata of the rat substantia nigra have suggested that although mu agonists induce ipsilateral turning behavior, both delta and kappa agonists induce contralateral rotation (Jacquet, 1982; Herrera-Marschitz et al., 1984). In rats with unilateral nigral lesions, both mu agonists and Ag/Ant analgesics induce ipsilateral turning behavior (Iwamoto et al., 1976).

3.3. Substance P-Induced Scratching

Intracisternal or intrathecal injections of substance P induce a spinally mediated reciprocal scratching of the hindlimbs in the mouse (Share and Rackham, 1981; Rackham et al., 1981). This behavior is potently antagonized by delta (Hylden and Wilcox, 1983), mu, and kappa agonists and by some agonist/antagonist analgesics (Wood et al., 1982a). Agonist/antagonist agents with a Na^+ ratio of greater than five in the $[^3H]$naloxone binding assay appear to be effective in blocking this response (Table 4). This may be reflective of the greater kappa agonist affinities of these agonist/antagonist or the greater mu antagonist actions of the

TABLE 4
Actions of Mu, Kappa, and Ag/Ant Agents in Analgesic Tests
and Substance P-Induced Scratching in the Mouse[a]

Drug	Hot plate	Tail flick	Substance-P scratching	Sodium ratio $[^3H]$naloxone binding
		ED_{50}, mg/kg, ip		
MU				
Morphine	5.0	2.4	10.1	30.0
Levorphanol	0.5	0.2	1.4	10.0
Dihydromorphine	5.0	3.0	5.4	47.0
Kappa				
EKC	7.8	1.2	0.65	7.5
Bremazocine	>4.0	0.5	1.0	1.3
Mr2034	1.0	0.19	0.6	16.9
Ag/Ant				
Butorphanol	0.1	0.6	3.5	5.1
Pentazocine	31.0	40.0	21.0	12.0
Nalbuphine	2.0	5.0	10.0	6.2
Levallorphan	16.0	>64	>64	3.0
Nalorphine	48.0	>128	>64	2.1
Cyclazocine	3.0	>16	>64	2.1

[a]Data from Wood et al. (1982a).

agonist/antagonist with a low Na$^+$ ratio (Wood, 1982a). Indeed, opiate antagonists potentiate the substance P-induced behavior, suggestive of an endogenous opioid tone in the spinal dorsal horn (Share and Rackham, 1981).

These data would suggest that at the spinal level, the neurons receiving a substance P input from the dorsal root also possess both mu and kappa receptors that can negatively modulate this excitatory peptidergic input.

3.4. Feeding

Opiates have also been implicated in the control of feeding behaviors (reviewed by Morley et al., 1983). Pure antagonists such as naloxone suppress deprivation-induced (Brown and Holtzman, 1979; Cooper, 1980) or glycolytic (Lowy et al., 1980) feeding. Naloxone and naltrexone are also active in the "cafeteria diet" model, which utilizes highly palatable diets (Apfelbaum and Mandenoff, 1981; Mandenoff et al., 1982; Cooper et al., 1985a,b). In view of the ability of antagonists to reduce food intake, reports of increased feeding following opiate agonists were not unexpected. However, all opioid receptor subtypes appear to be involved: mu (Jalowiec et al., 1981; Sanger and McCarthy, 1980); kappa (Morley et al., 1983); delta (Jackson and Sewall, 1985; McLean and Hoeber, 1983; Tepperman and Hirst, 1983); and epsilon (Grandison and Guidotti, 1977b). Thus the actions of opiates and opioid peptides on feeding are complex, involving both anatomical and receptor differences.

Another approach to the issue of receptor subtypes involved in feeding has been to use naloxonazine to selectively block mu_1 sites (Simone et al., 1985). In these experiments, naloxonazine antagonized both free feeding and deprivation-induced feeding in a long-acting manner, implying a mu_1 mechanism in these feeding mechanisms, but had no effect on glucoprivic feeding.

4. Neuroendocrinology

It has long been known that opiates like morphine can alter endocrine secretion. Subsequent to the discovery of endogenous opiates, the study of the ability of enkephalins and endorphins to modify endocrine secretion has led to an interest in in vivo actions of opiates and opioid peptides on neuroendocrine regulation and has been extensively reviewed by Pfeiffer and Herz (1984) and

Millian and Herz (1985). Multiplicity of both opioid receptor types and opioid peptides has further complicated the study of opiate effects on hormone release.

4.1. Corticosterone-ACTH

In rats, mice, and dogs, opiates stimulate the hypothalamic-pituitary-adrenal (HPA) axis (George and Way, 1959; Lotti et al., 1969; Gibson et al., 1979; Levin et al., 1981; Buckingham, 1982), whereas in humans, they inhibit this axis (Grossman et al., 1982a). The action of morphine has been most studied on this axis and appears to be centrally mediated: (1) it develops tolerance; (2) it is abolished by hypophysectomy, dexamethasone, or lesions of the median eminence; (3) it is reproduced by central administration; and (4) in vitro it does not affect the release of ACTH from pituitaries, but stimulates the release of CRF from hypothalami (Kokka and George, 1974; Levin et al., 1981; Harasz et al., 1981; Buckingham, 1982; de Souza and Van Loon, 1982; Buckingham and Cooper, 1984). The in vivo rise in corticosterone in response to morphine is accompanied by a rise in ACTH and changes in hypothalamic levels of CRF. Similarly, injections of β-endorphin into the brain also cause a stimulation of the HPA axis. Buckingham and Cooper (1984) have also shown that Leu- and Met-enkephalin can elicit the release of CRF from isolated hypothalami in vitro.

Other opiate drugs having an affinity for the kappa opioid receptor have been shown to stimulate this axis by various workers: U50488H (Lahti and Collins, 1982), EKC (Eisenberg, 1982; Pechnick et al., 1985a,b,c), bremazocine (Fuller and Leander, 1984), and MRZ 2549 (Pfeiffer and Pfeiffer, 1984), and the agonist/antagonist, cyclazocine (Lahti and Collins, 1982), and SKF 10,047 (Pechnick et al., 1985a; Eisenberg, 1985), a sigma drug with multiple receptor affinities.

The most thorough investigation of various opiate drugs has been reported by Iyengar et al. (1986) (Table 5). This study demonstrated that although morphine caused potent, dose-dependent increases in both corticosterone and ACTH, both DADLE, the delta agonist, and various kappa drugs were more potent in releasing corticosterone. The key characteristics of these kappa actions were: (1) stereospecific increases in plasma corticosterone and corresponding changes in ACTH; (2) stereospecific reversal by opiate antagonists; (3) dose dependency with a rank order of potency similar to that observed in the rabbit vas deferens (which

TABLE 5
Effect of Opiate Drugs on Plasma Corticosterone in the Rat[a]

Drug	Receptor	Effect	Reversibility	
			Naloxone	WIN 44441-3
Morphine	Mu	S	Y	Y
Etorphine	Mu	S	—	Y
DADLE	Delta	S	Y	N
U50488H	Kappa	S	Y	N
Mr2034	Kappa	S	Y	N
1-EKC	Kappa	S	Y	Y
d-EKC	Sigma	NE	—	—
Tifluadom	Kappa	S	Y	Y
(−)-Bremazocine	Kappa	S	—	—
(+)-Bremazocine	Kappa	NE	—	—
d,l-Cyclazocine	Ag/Ant	S	—	Y
d-Cyclazocine	Sigma	NE	—	—
Butorphanol	Ag/Ant	S	—	Y
Naloxone	Mu, delta, kappa	I		
l-WIN 44441	Mu, delta, kappa	I		
d-WIN 44441		NE		

[a]Abbreviations: S, stimulatory; I, inhibitory; NE, no effect; Y, yes; N, no.

is a kappa specific tissue); (4) potent effects at doses far below those needed to elicit analgesia; (5) inactivity in hypophysectomized animals; (6) normal release of ACTH in adrenalectomized animals; (7) tolerance in subchronic studies, but no cross tolerance with mu agonists; and (8) kappa agonist action of the agonist/antagonist opiates and no sigma receptor role in these actions. These data suggest a potent kappa regulation of the HPA axis. In further antagonist studies it was found that although naloxone reversed the actions of all the kappa drugs, the long-acting antagonist WIN 44441-3 reversed the actions of tifluadom and 1-EKC, but not those of Mr2034 and U50488H, even at doses of 5 mg/kg, a dose that is effective in blocking the mu agonists in this system. These data are suggestive of the presence of kappa isoreceptor populations being involved in the stimulation of the HPA axis.

The antagonists naloxone and WIN 44441-3 by themselves inhibited the HPA axis, suggesting a role of endogenous opioid peptides. In further studies with intracerebroventricular (icv) administration of endogenous peptides (Iyengar et al., 1987), it was found that dynorphin (1-13), Met-enkephalin-Arg-Phe (MEAP), β-endorphin, and DADLE potently released corticosterone in a dose-dependent, naloxone-reversible manner (Table 6). β-Endorphin was the most potent and efficacious. However, dynorphin (1-13) also elicited profound increases in corticosterone, in keeping with the observations seen with kappa agonist drugs. Several in vitro binding studies have revealed (Attali et al., 1982; Audiger et al., 1982; Pilapil and Wood, 1983) a kappa site possessing high affinity for MEAP and β-endorphin. MEAP also caused potent increases in corticosterone; together with the differences in WIN 44441-3 antagonism among kappa drugs, these data indicate the involvement of two kappa receptor subtypes in stimulation of the HPA axis. To test this hypothesis further (Table 7), these four peptides were injected icv into animals made tolerant to either morphine or the kappa agonist U50488H. The effects of DADLE,

TABLE 6
Effect of Opioid Peptides on Rat Plasma Corticosterone

	Dose, μg icv	Plasma corticosterone, % of control
β-Endorphin	0.5	940[a]
	5	1400[a]
	20	2000[a]
	5 + Nal (5)	270[a]
DADLE	0.5	150[a]
	2	300[a]
	10	600[a]
	2 + Nal (2)	99
Dynorphin (1-13)	1	146[a]
	5	813[a]
	10	1300[a]
	10 + Nal (5)	120
MEAP	5	175[a]
	25	750[a]
	50	675[a]
	50 + Nal (5)	280[a]

[a]$p < 0.05$ compared to control, 60 min, $n = 7$–10. Nal, naloxone given twice (-6, $+30$ min). MEAP injected with enzyme inhibitors captopril (869 μg) and bestatin (50 μg).

TABLE 7
Effect of Opioid Peptides on Plasma Corticosterone in Morphine-Tolerant
and U50488H-Tolerant Rats

| Drug, µg, icv | Corticosterone, % of control | |
	Morphine-tolerant rats	U50488H-tolerant rats
Morphine (16 mg/kg,ip)	135	700[a]
U50488H (8 mg/kg,ip)	1350[a]	220[a]
DADLE (10)	680[a]	525[a]
β-Endorphine (5)	600[a]	925[a]
Dynorphin (1–13) (10)	880[a]	25
MEAP (50)	755[a]	149

[a]$p < 0.05$ compared to naive control, 60 min, $n = 8$–10. Tolerance induced by injecting successively every 12 h, 10, 15, 23, 34, 51, 77 mg/kg morphine or U50488H (ip) and
treated acutely with opiates or peptides on day 4.

dynorphin, and MEAP were not inhibited in the morphine-tolerant animal, whereas those of β-endorphin were only partially inhibited. In the U50488H-tolerant animals, the response of DADLE
was not inhibited and the response of β-endorphin was partially
inhibited, whereas those of dynorphin and MEAP were completely inhibited. These data clearly indicated that the actions of
both dynorphin and MEAP were mediated by kappa receptors. It
must be noted that U50488H is believed to bind to both isoreceptor populations (Su, 1985). These data also indicate that the actions of DADLE and β-endorphin occur at a site distinct from
morphine and the U50488H site. These studies demonstrate further that the HPA axis is independently stimulated by multiple
opioid receptors.

It should be noted here that although we observed an inhibitory influence of two opiate antagonists on the HPA axis, some
workers have reported a stimulatory effect of high doses of naloxone (Levin et al., 1981; Jezova et al., 1982; Eisenberg, 1984; Pechnick et al., 1985b). Buckingham (1982), however, did not observe
changes in the release of CRF-like activity in isolated hypothalami
with naloxone, whereas Lahti and Collins (1982), Fuller and Leander (1985), and Pechnick et al. (1985b) were able to show naloxone
reversibility of the effects of U50488H, bremazocine, and EKC on
corticosterone release. In humans, both naloxone (Volavka et al.,
1979a; Morley et al., 1980; Naber et al., 1981; Judd et al., 1981,
1985; Cohen et al., 1985) and naltrexone (Volavka et al., 1979b)
increase ACTH and corticosterone release.

4.2. Thyroid-Stimulating Hormone (TSH)

Opiates are known to inhibit TSH secretion in the rat (Bruni et al., 1977; Sharp et al., 1981). This decrease seems to be at the level of the hypothalamus; microinjections into the mediobasal hypothalamus and hypothalamic lesioning studies support this hypothesis (Lomax and George, 1966; Lomax et al., 1970). Moreover opiates have been shown to inhibit potassium-evoked TRH release from superfused hypothalami in vitro. Both morphine and dynorphin are unable to inhibit TRH-stimulated TSH release, whereas antagonists are unable to stimulate this response (Morley et al., 1980; Delitala et al., 1981; Sharp et al., 1981; Mitsuma and Nogimori, 1983a,b). Further, morphine blocks the cold-induced rise in TSH, which is centrally mediated (Sharp et al., 1981). Opioids do not decrease TSH secretion from anterior pituitary either in the presence or absence of TRH (Judd and Hedge, 1982). The role of opiates in humans is controversial. Naloxone was reported to have no effect on basal TSH release in humans by Morley et al. (1980), Delitala et al. (1981), and Rolandi et al. (1982), whereas Grossman et al. (1981) found a decrease in TSH. Both Morley et al. (1980) and Grossman et al. (1982b), however, found naloxone not to have any effect on TSH in primary hypothyroid patients.

Our own studies have confirmed the inhibitory effect of various opiates in the rat (Iyengar and Wood, 1985) (Table 8). Besides morphine, several kappa opiate agonists, U50488H, Mr2034, U69593, and bremazocine caused very potent inhibition of TSH secretion that was naloxone-reversible and dose-dependent. Two other kappa agonists, tifluadom and 1-EKC, also caused inhibition, but their effects were more pronounced at higher doses. The effects of U50488H and Mr2034 were not reversible by WIN 44441-3, whereas those of tifluadom and 1-EKC were. These results are similar to our observations regarding the antagonism of kappa modulation of corticosterone release and again point to the presence of kappa receptor subtypes.

Both agonist/antagonist opiates tested, cyclazocine and butorphanol, were not potent inhibitors of TSH. It may be noted that Pechnick et al. (1985c) saw an inhibition of TSH at low doses with the partial mu agonist buprenorphine, but an antagonist action at higher doses.

Of the peptides tested (manuscript in preparation), DADLE and β-endorphin caused significant dose-dependent inhibition of TSH release when given centrally. Dynorphin (1-13) also inhibited TSH release, but the effect was most pronounced only at the

TABLE 8
Summary of Opiate Drug Actions on Plasma TSH[a]

Drug	Receptor	Effect	Reversibility	
			Naloxone	WIN
Morphine	Mu	I	Y	Y
DADLE	Delta	I	Y	Y*
U69593	Kappa	I	—	—
U50488H	Kappa	I	Y	N
Mr2034	Kappa	I	Y	N
Tifluadom	Kappa	I	Y	Y
l-EKC	Kappa	I +	Y	—
d-EKC	Sigma	NE	—	—
(−)-Bremazocine	Kappa	I	—	—
(+)-Bremazocine		NE	—	—
d,l-Cyclazocine	Ag/Ant	NE	—	—
d-Cyclazocine	Sigma	NE	—	—
Butorphanol	Ag/Ant	NE	—	—
Naloxone	Mu, delta, kappa	NE	—	—
l-WIN 44441	Mu, delta, kappa	NE	—	
d-WIN 44441		NE		

[a]Abbreviations: I, inhibitory; NE, no effect; Y, yes; N, no; —, not tested; *, partial; +, at highest dose only.

highest dose tested, unlike the effect of the other kappa agonists. Mitsuma and Nogimori (1983a) have previously shown inhibition of TSH release by dynorphin (1-13) when given intravenously. MEAP had no effect on the release of this hormone (Table 9). In subchronic tolerance studies, the effects of both morphine and U50488H demonstrated tolerance, but not cross-tolerance, to each other. The effect of β-endorphin, in both morphine- and U50488H-tolerant rats, was still evident, indicating a site of action that was independent of these two drugs. The actions of DADLE were partially decreased in morphine-tolerant animals, whereas full activity was seen in the U50488H-tolerant rats (Table 10). Surprisingly, dynorphin was active in both morphine and U50488H-tolerant animals. Thus, the role of kappa opioids in TSH release seems to be more complicated than in corticosterone release. This study also revealed that the effects of both morphine and U50488H were not present in hypophysectomized rats and were attenuated in thyroidectomized rats, thus making it more difficult to pinpoint the loci of action of opiates on TSH release. It seems clear from these studies, however, that the release of TSH is also under multiple opioid receptor regulation.

TABLE 9
Effect of Opioid Peptides on Rat Plasma TSH

	Dose, μg, icv	TSH, % of control
DADLE	0.5	61
	2	53[a]
	10	40[a]
	2 + Nal (5)	110
β-Endorphin	0.5	115
	5	37[a]
	20	37[a]
	5 + Nal (5)	120
Dynorphin (1-13)	1	85
	5	80
	10	55[a]
	10 + Nal (5)	97
MEAP	5	90
	25	75
	50	104

[a]$p < 0.05$ compared to control, 60 min, $n = 7$–10. Nal, naloxone given twice (-6, $+30$ min); MEAP injected with captopril (869 μg) and bestatin (50 μg).

4.3. Prolactin

Opioids have also been implicated in the regulation of prolactin (PRL) release in the rat. Opiate agonists stimulate PRL release, whereas opiate antagonists reduce basal release and block stimulus-induced secretion of this hormone (Bruni et al., 1977; Shaar et al., 1977; Rivier et al., 1977; Grandison and Guidotti, 1977a; Du-

TABLE 10
Effect of Opioid Peptides on Plasma TSH in Morphine-Tolerant
and U50488H-Tolerant Rats

	TSH, % of control	
Drug, μg, icv	Morphine-tolerant rats	U50488H-tolerant rats
Morphine (16 mg/kg)	61	33[a]
U50488H (8 mg/kg)	56	21[a]
DADLE (10)	51[a]	29[a]
β-Endorphin (5)	38[a]	39[a]
Dynorphin (1-13) (10)	42[a]	55[a]

[a]$p < 0.05$ compared to control, 60 min, $n = 8$–10. Tolerance paradigm same as in Table 7.

pont et al., 1979; Meites et al., 1979; VanVugt et al., 1979). This stimulation seems to be centrally mediated: (1) The basal release of PRL from lactotrophs in vitro is not stimulated by opioids (Rivier et al., 1977; Shaar et al., 1977; Brown et al., 1978) and (2) opiate actions on prolactin release appear to be via inhibition of tuberoinfundibular dopaminergic neurons (Gudelsky and Porter, 1979; Deyo et al., 1979; Alper et al., 1980; Okajima et al., 1980; Haskins et al., 1981; Gudelsky et al., 1983; Arita and Porter, 1984). There is also evidence that opioid modulation of serotonergic mechanisms may be involved (Spampinato et al., 1979; Koenig et al., 1979; Callahan et al., 1985). Injections of morphine into the dorsal raphe also elevate serum levels of PRL (Johnson, 1982).

Lactation can be initiated by daily injection of morphine (Meites, 1966); morphine does not increase PRL during lactation, however (Rabii et al., 1984; Callahan et al., 1985). Naloxone inhibits the suckling-induced rise in PRL in rats (Ferland et al., 1980). Naloxone also blocks the proestrous surge of PRL (Ieiri et al., 1980) and attenuates estrogen-induced rise in PRL. It is therefore possible that estrogen may modulate opioid function in the female rat.

Stress-induced increases in serum prolactin also appear to involve opioid mechanisms (VanVugt et al., 1978; Rossier et al., 1980). Naloxone inhibits stress-induced rises in PRL caused by heat, ether, immobilization, and foot-shock in rats (Deyo and Miller, 1982; Ferland et al., 1980; Grandison and Guidotti, 1977; Meites et al., 1979).

In monkeys, naloxone also decreases serum PRL levels (Gold et al., 1978). In cynomolgus monkeys, administration of the enkephalin analogue FK 33-824 (a mu peptide) into the medial basal hypothalamus increased prolactin release (Belchetz, 1981). In humans, opiates including morphine, methadone, β-endorphin, and the synthetic enkephalin analog FK 33-824 cause potent increases in prolactin (Tolis et al., 1975; Stubbs et al., 1978; Von Graffenried et al., 1978; Foley et al., 1979; Del Pozo et al., 1980; Rolandi et al., 1985). Several workers have shown, however, that naloxone does not affect the basal release of PRL in humans (Volavka et al., 1980; Morley et al., 1980; Grossman et al., 1981; Naber et al., 1981; Janowsky et al., 1979; Cohen et al., 1985). The elevated levels of PRL occurring in patients with prolactinomas are also not affected by naloxone (Blankstein et al., 1979; Tolis et al., 1982). Interestingly, Judd et al. (1982) have shown a blunted PRL response to methadone in a subpopulation of depressed patients.

Naloxone has been shown to attenuate increases in PRL in humans after surgery, and in some instances insulin-hypoglycemia or exercise induced increases in PRL (Morley et al., 1980; Spiler and Molitch, 1980; Grossman et al., 1981; Serri et al., 1981; Pontiroli et al., 1982; Morreti et al., 1983). Martin et al. (1979) did not find naloxone to affect sleep-related patterns in PRL levels, but Ferland et al. (1980) found that naloxone blocked nocturnal rises in PRL in postmenopausal women.

The actions of morphine on prolactin release have been shown to occur at the mu_1 opioid isoreceptor site (Spiegel et al., 1982) in the rat. Besides morphine, other mu agonists like methadone and meperidine elevate plasma prolactin (Lien et al., 1979). Studies with endogenous peptides and their analogs and opiates having affinities to multiple opioid receptors, however, have clearly shown that more than one receptor may be involved in the regulation of prolactin release. Met-enkephalin and the synthetic analog FK 33-824 have been shown to increase PRL in the rat (Bruni et al., 1977; Romer and Hill, 1981; Meites et al., 1979; Brown et al., 1978). It may be pointed out that, in humans, the latter peptide showed physiological changes different from that of morphine, and unlike morphine the prolactin increase was not blocked by nalorphine (Foley et al., 1979).

Of drugs having kappa receptor affinity, Krulich et al. (1986a) have shown that both U50488H and bremazocine can elicit increases in prolactin. Pechnick et al. (1985a) observed elevations of PRL with EKC only at the lowest doses and no effect at higher doses, and a similar biphasic effect with the partial mu agonist buprenorphine (Pechnick et al., 1985c). Brown et al. (1978), however, found no changes with either buprenorphine or the agonist/antagonist cyclazocine. Lien et al. (1979) also found two other agonist/antagonists, pentazocine and meptazinol, to have no effect, whereas levallorphan, nalorphine, and ciramadol lowered PRL and suppressed morphine-induced increases in PRL. Krulich et al. (1986b) have also shown a suppression of morphine-induced PRL increases by the kappa agonist bremazocine, but not by U50488H. SKF 10,047, the sigma agonist with other opioid affinities, inhibited the release of PRL (Pechnick et al., 1985a).

Of the endogenous peptides, besides β-endorphin and enkephalin, Kato et al. (1981) and VanVugt et al. (1981) have shown stimulation of PRL by dynorphin (1-13). We were unable to show any stimulation with MEAP. In cross-tolerance studies, however (same paradigm as in Table 10), we found that the effect of 10 μg dynorphin (icv) was not blocked in morphine-tolerant rats, although it was blocked in U50488H-tolerant rats. Interestingly, the effect of β-endorphin (5 μg, icv) was not blocked in either the morphine-tolerant or the U50488H-tolerant rat (Iyengar et al., 1987), thus indicating actions at a unique site, distinct from mu and kappa opioid receptors. It was recently shown by Callahan et al. (1985, personal communication) that lactating female rats did not respond to morphine by increasing PRL, whereas both DADLE and β-endorphin, could elicit large increases in PRL when given centrally. In the same animals, morphine caused an increase in growth hormone (GH), clearly indicating that the drug was bioavailable. In our studies, β-endorphin did cause the most significant increases in plasma prolactin (17.5-fold at 0.5 μg dose) in the male rat. Whether the stimulation of PRL release is under a unique "epsilon" receptor modulation remains to be investigated. Foley et al. (1979) noted that in humans the hormonal effects of β-endorphin occurred at doses lower than those needed to produce analgesia, and that when both hormonal and analgesic effects were observed together, the hormonal response preceded the analgesic and behavioral responses. At this point, it is once again clear that the release of PRL is quite complex and involves more than one opioid receptor.

4.4. Growth Hormone (GH)

Morphine and opioid peptides are known to have a stimulatory response on GH release (Kokka et al., 1973; Martin et al., 1975). This in vivo action is thought to be elicited in the hypothalamus (Kokka and George, 1974; Martin et al., 1975; Shaar et al., 1977; Rivier et al., 1977; Dupont et al., 1977; Chihara et al., 1978; Grandison et al., 1980). Opioids were found to inhibit potassium-stimulated release of somatostatin from isolated rat hypothalami in vitro (Drouva et al., 1981), but not basal release of somatostatin in a similar preparation. Immunoneutralization with antisera to somatostatin also did not block GH responses to opiates (Dupont et al., 1977; Chihara et al., 1978). β-Endorphin administered icv failed to alter levels of somatostatin in portal plasma even though it increased GH (Abe et al., 1981). It thus seems likely that opioid actions probably occur through a GH-releasing factor (Guillemin et al., 1982). In rats an alpha-adrenergic mechanism has been implicated in the opioid effects on GH (Koenig et al., 1980; Katakami et al., 1981), as has GABA (Koenig et al., 1980; Eriksson et al., 1981; Terry et al., 1982). In dogs (Casaneuva et al., 1981) and humans (Penalva et al., 1983; Delitala et al., 1983), cholinergic and histaminergic mechanisms have also been implicated.

Although in rat both morphine and β-endorphin cause an increase in GH, in humans both opiates, when given iv, do not cause any changes in GH (Tolis et al., 1975; Foley et al., 1979). Similarly, baboons given an enkephalin analog, D-Ala²-Nor⁵-enkephalinamide, administered iv, did not show any increase in GH. β-Endorphin administered icv, however, decreased GH in humans (Foley et al., 1979). Belchetz (1981) also suggested that injections of the enkephalin analog DAMME at sites lateral, anterior, and dorsal to the mediobasal hypothalamus (a site that elicited PRL increases) caused GH increases in the cynomolgus monkeys. In other human studies, patients with affective disorders demonstrated a blunted GH response to methadone (Judd et al., 1982). Von GraffenFried et al. (1978) and Allolio et al. (1982) found a dose-dependent increase in plasma GH levels with the enkephalin analog FK 33-824 in humans. Naloxone does not affect basal GH release in humans (Morley et al., 1980; Volavka et al., 1980), nor does it affect nocturnal GH releases (Martin et al., 1979).

In rats, morphine (Bruni et al., 1977; Lien et al., 1979; Pechnick et al., 1985a; Krulich et al., 1986a), enkephalin (Bruni et al., 1977), β-endorphin (Dupont et al., 1977; Chihara et al., 1978), and dynorphin (1-13) (Kato et al., 1981) have all been shown to stimulate GH release, though the latter effect was not as robust. Lien et al. (1979) also reported that methadone and meperidine can elevate GH. Spiegel et al. (1982), however, demonstrated that the effect of morphine on GH release was through a mu₂ and/or delta opioid receptor, rather than a mu₁ receptor, unlike that of PRL release. Further, Koenig et al. (1984) indicated that this effect could be blocked by the selective delta antagonist ICI 154129, but not by naloxonazine or β-FNA, both mu receptor blockers. In lactating females, Callahan et al. (1985) found that morphine as well, as DADLE and β-endorphin, could cause GH increases, but the β-endorphin effect was not as profound as with PRL. Also, morphine was unable to stimulate PRL in this model. Pechnick et al. (1985a,c) found both EKC and buprenorphine to cause dose-dependent elevations in GH. Lien et al. (1979) found levallorphan, nalorphine, pentazocine, meptazanol, and ciramadol, all Ag/Ants, to elevate GH. In contrast, bremazocine and U50488H, kappa agonists, inhibited basal GH release (Krulich et al., 1986a) and clonidine-induced GH release (Krulich et al., 1986b).

Many of these actions were studied together with PRL release, and interestingly, the two hormones appear to be regulated very differently. The effects of various opiates on the two hormones are summarized in Table 11. Although this anterior pituitary hormone seems to be under multiple opioid receptor control, it is interesting that the actions of various ligands are not necessarily in the same di-

TABLE 11
Published Effects of Opiates on PRL and GH Release[a]

Opiate	Type	Species	PRL	GH
Morphine (iv, icv)	Mu	Rat	S	S
+ Naloxonazine	Mu$_1$	Rat	I (mu$_1$)	S
+ β-FNA	Mu	Rat	I	S
+ ICI 154129	Delta	Rat		I
Morphine (iv)	Mu	Human	S	NE
β-Endorphin (iv)	Ep, mu, delta	Human	S	NE
β-Endorphin (icv)	Ep, mu, delta	Human	S	I
β-Endorphin (iv, icv)	Ep, mu, delta	Rat	S	S
Methadone	Mu	Rat	S	S
Meperidine	Mu	Rat	S	S
Morphine (lact. female)	Mu	Rat	NE	S
Methadone (lact. female)	Mu	Rat	NE	S
β-Endorphin (lact. female)	Mu, delta, ep	Rat	S	S
DADLE (lact. female)	Delta	Rat	S	S
Met-enkephalin	Delta	Rat	S	S
FK 33-824	Delta	Rat	S	S
DAMME	Delta	Rat	S	S
DAMME (central)	Delta	Monkey	S (MBH)	S (OS)
Dynorphin	Kappa	Rat	S	S
U50488H	Kappa	Rat	S	I
Bremazocine	Kappa	Rat	S	I
EKC	Kappa, Ag/Ant	Rat	Biphasic	S
Buprenorphine	Ag/Ant	Rat	Biphasic	S
Cyclazocine	Kappa, Ag/Ant	Rat	NE	—
Levallorphan	Ag/Ant	Rat	I	S
Nalorphine	Ag/Ant	Rat	I	S
Ciramadol	Ag/Ant	Rat	I	S
Pentazocine	Ag/Ant	Rat	NE	S
Meptazinol	Ag/Ant	Rat	NE	S
NANMT	Sigma	Rat	I	NE
Naloxone	Mu, delta, kappa	Rat	I	I
Naloxone	Mu, delta, kappa	Human	NE	NE

[a]Abbreviations: S, stimulatory; I, inhibitory; NE, no effect; —, not tested; MBH, medial basal hypothalamus; OS, other sites; d, delta; ep, epsilon; lact., lactating.

rection, and here one may find a clearer example of how multiple opioid receptors can differentially regulate neuroendocrine function.

4.5. Luteinizing Hormone (LH)

Opiate agonists inhibit LH release (Cicero et al., 1976; Bruni et al., 1977). The ability of opiates to inhibit ovulation has been known since the early studies of Barraclough and Sawyer (1955). Naloxone causes a rise in LH (Bruni et al., 1977; Cicero et al., 1976). LHRH antagonists block naloxone-induced rises in portal plasma LH levels (Ching, 1983). The actions of opioids on LH seem to be mediated by DA, serotonin, and norepinephrine (NE) (Van Loon and deSouza, 1978; Kordon et al., 1979; Kalra, 1981; Kalra and Simpkins, 1981; Drouva et al., 1981; Rotsztejn et al., 1982; Johnson, 1982; Moore and Johnston, 1982), although their precise roles under physiological conditions remain unresolved (Millian and Herz, 1985).

Opiates are unable to inhibit LH secretion from anterior pituitaries in vitro (Cicero et al., 1976; Bhanot and Wilkinson, 1983), whereas DA- and potassium-induced release of LHRH from hypothalami in vitro could be inhibited by opiates (Rotsztejn et al., 1978; Drouva et al., 1981). It is thus clear that opiate actions on LH release are mediated centrally. Further experiments seem to confirm this. Kalra (1981) observed increases of LH by implantation of minute amounts of naloxone into discrete areas of the hypothalamus, especially into the median-eminence-arcuate nucleus and the medial-preoptic area. It may be noted that these were areas where Iyengar and Rabii (1984a,b) observed age-related changes and sex differences in [^{3}H]naloxone binding. Several studies have shown that age, sex, and the steroid environment are important for opiate effects on LH release. Naloxone greatly enhances LH release in prepubertal female rats, but not in prepubertal male rats (Blank et al., 1979; Ieiri et al., 1979; Schulz et al., 1982). Direct introduction of antisera to β-endorphin and dynorphin into the medial-basal hypothalamus in prepubertal female rats also elevated plasma LH levels (Schulz et al., 1981). Forman et al. (1983) also showed antiserum of β-endorphin to elevate LH in male rats. Chronic exposure to morphine prenatally during a critical period in development caused increases in [^{3}H]naloxone binding in several hypothalamic regions important to LH release in female offspring, but not in males (Iyengar and Rabii, 1984a).

Opioid suppression of LH in gonadectomized, immature fe-

males again parallels changes in feedback suppression by steroids. In adult female rats, β-endorphin content in discrete hypothalamic nuclei varies with the estrous cycle (Barden et al., 1981;
Knuth et al., 1983). Naloxone also potentiates the duration and
magnitude of the proestrous-related surge of LH and increases
the number of ova shed (Ieiri et al., 1980; Koves et al., 1981;
Marton et al., 1981; Gabriel et al., 1983).

In humans and monkeys, naloxone is most effective in the
luteal phase, but ineffective in the early follicular stage, in stimulating LH release (Quigley and Yen, 1980; Browning et al., 1981;
Blankstein et al., 1979). Endogenous opioids appear to play a role
in modulating the pattern of LH release in the human female
(Ropert et al., 1981). Naloxone can also restore pulsatile LH release in secondary ammenorrhea (Blankstein et al., 1979). Opiate
agonists decrease LH in human males (Mirin et al., 1976; Stubbs
et al., 1978), and antagonists increase LH (Mirin et al., 1976;
Mendelson et al., 1979; Morley et al., 1980).

In addition to morphine, β-endorphin, and naloxone, the
kappa agonists bremazocine and EKC also reduced LH in rats
(Marko and Romer, 1983; Pechnick et al., 1985a), whereas WIN
44441-3 elevated LH (Pechnick et al., 1985b). The partial mu agonist buprenorphine did not change LH (Pechnick et al., 1985c).
EKC was also equipotent with morphine in suppressing LH in immature females (Schulz et al., 1982). This is in keeping with the
observations of Schulz et al. (1981) that dynorphin antisera elevate serum LH in immature females. Thus there seems to be multiple opioid regulation of LH, but more studies are needed to evaluate the complex circuitry.

In summary, it can be seen that opiates affect secretion of
several hormones from the anterior pituitary in various species,
including humans, and this seems to be an important in vivo
function of these peptides. These actions, as we have seen, are
central and involve endogenous opioids acting at several opioid
receptor subtypes. Moreover, the modulation of each hormone is
different from the others and thus presents an opportunity to
evaluate in vivo actions and multiple receptor affinities of endogenous opioids and opiate drugs.

5. Neurochemistry

5.1. Acetylcholine (ACh)

Several cholinergic systems are regulated by opioid receptors (Table 12). Morphine depresses acetylcholine (ACh) turnover in the

TABLE 12
Summary of Opioid and Opiate Actions on ACh Turnover
in the Rat Cortex and Hippocampus

Drug	Action	ACh Turnover	
		Hippocampus	Neocortex
Morphine	Mu	Decrease	Decrease
Buprenorphine	Partial mu	Decrease[a]	Decrease[a]
DADLE	Delta	Decrease	Decrease
β-Endorphin	Epsilon	Decrease	Decrease
Mr2034	Kappa	No effect	No effect
Pentazocine	Ag/Ant	No effect	Decrease
Naloxone	Ant	No effect	No effect

[a]Reversal of effect at high doses.

parietal and occipital cortices, hippocampus, and N accumbens. It has no such effect in the frontal cortex, striatum, amygdala, substantia nigra, dorsal raphe, septum, or N interpeduncularis (Cheney et al., 1974; Costa et al., 1975; Zsilla et al., 1976, 1977; Schmidt and Buxbaum, 1978; Wood and Stotland, 1980). Thus only specific pathways possess an inhibitory enkephalinergic regulation. The septal-hippocampal and N basalis-cortical cholinergic pathways have mu, delta, and epsilon modulation, but lack a kappa receptor regulation (Moroni et al., 1977, 1978; Wood et al., 1979; Wood and Stotland, 1980; Wood and Rackham, 1981; Wood et al., 1984c). This regulation is at the level of the cholinergic cell bodies in the septal-hippocampal pathway (Wood et al., 1984a,c), whereas the N basalis appears to receive a regulatory afferent, which itself is under opioid control at a more caudal site (Wood et al., 1984c). The location of these receptors remains to be defined, however. Several studies have shown inactivity of opioids at the level of cholinergic nerve endings in the neocortex (Szerb, 1974; Jhamandas et al., 1971, 1975; Wood et al., 1984b,c) and indicate inhibitory opioid synapses outside the cortex or substantia innominata (Wood et al., 1984b,c).

Mu- and delta-induced ACh turnover changes appear to involve distinct receptor populations. Delta agonists demonstrate a greater resistance to reversal by naloxone and exhibit full agonist activity in morphine-tolerant rats (Wood et al., 1979, 1984c). Studies (Zsilla et al., 1977) of mu agonist actions on hippocampal acetylcholine turnover demonstrated significant correlations between the ED_{50} for analgesia and decreases in acetylcholine turnover. Subsequent studies with kappa agonists further suggested a mu_1 opioid receptor regulation of these neurons (Wood et al.,

1984c). In these studies, kappa agonists alone did not alter ACh turnover, although reversing the actions of delta, but not mu, agonists in a stereospecific and dose-dependent manner. These studies support the hypothesis (Wood et al., 1984c) that cholinergic neurons innervating the cortex and hippocampus possess delta and mu_1 opioid receptor regulation.

Partial mu agonists like buprenorphine act as classical mu agonists to depress ACh turnover in both pathways. At higher dose levels, however, these actions reverse (Wood and Rackham, 1981). On the other hand agonist/antagonist agents like pentazocine, cyclazocine, and butorphanol have no action on hippocampal ACh turnover, but depress neocortical ACh turnover (Wood and Stotland, 1980). This naloxone-reversible receptor action, which is clearly not kappa- or delta opioid-mediated, remains to be elucidated. β-Endorphin, an epsilon opioid receptor agonist, depresses both pathways. Studies of hippocampal ACh turnover after intraseptal injections of β-endorphin have suggested a site of endorphin receptor action at the cholinergic cell bodies in the septal region (Moroni et al., 1977).

5.2. Dopamine (DA)

5.2.1. Nigrostriatal Pathway

Opioids affect dopaminergic neurotransmission in several regions of the brain (Wood, 1983b). Mu agonist analgesics are potent stimulants of dopamine synthesis in the striatum of both rat (Ahtee and Kaariainen, 1973; Gauchy et al., 1973; Costa et al., 1975; Wood et al., 1980) and mouse (Smith et al., 1972; Loh et al., 1973; Wood et al., 1980, 1983b; Wood and Richard, 1982). Opioid receptors in this system are located at multiple sites in the rat: (1) the dopaminergic nerve endings in the striatum (Pollard et al., 1977, 1978; Trabucchi et al., 1978; Gardner et al., 1980; Murrin et al., 1980); (2) the cell bodies of the substantia nigra (Llorens-Cortes et al., 1979); (3) afferent nerve endings to the substantia nigra (Llorens-Cortes et al., 1979; Gale et al., 1979); and (4) enkephalinergic nerve terminals have also been visualized in close proximity to nigral dendrites and afferents (Johnson et al., 1980).

In both the rat and the mouse, the nigrostriatal dopaminergic pathway has been shown to be regulated by mu and delta opioid receptor populations (Biggio et al., 1978; Wood et al., 1980; Wood and Richard, 1982), in both the striatum and substantia nigra of the rat, but in only the substantia nigra of the mouse. In the case of mu receptor actions, these are reversed by the kappa agonists, which have been shown to be mu_2 selective antagonists (Wood et al., 1980, 1982b, 1983a; Wood, 1984a). In addition, the actions of morphine are not reversed by the mu_1 antagonist naloxonazine (Wood and Pasternak, 1983), suggesting that the nigrostriatal pathway is modulated by both delta and mu_2 opioid receptors, and kappa opiate agonists function only as mu_2 and delta antagonists in this system, possessing no agonist actions of their own (Wood, 1983a, 1984a). The actions of agonist/antagonist analgesics on this system were unique in that bell-shaped dose-response curves were obtained (Wood, 1983a; Wood et al., 1982a, 1983a,b). Throughout this bell-shaped curve, these agents act as mu_2 and delta antagonists and demonstrate a lack of cross-tolerance between mu, delta, and agonist/antagonist drugs. The receptor involved therefore remains to be defined. β-Endorphin also increases dopamine metabolism in the rat striatum, presumably via a mu receptor action (Wood et al., 1980).

Although mu and delta receptor activation produces increases in nerve ending DA metabolism, no increase in DA release, as measured by 3-methoxytyramine (3-MT) levels, was seen in the rat (Wood, 1983b). In contrast, DA release was increased in the mouse (Wood et al., 1980; Wood and Richard, 1982). Using local injections and hemitransections, these studies demonstrated that only the rat possesses presynaptic opioid control of dopaminergic nerve endings in the striatum. This finding supported direct binding studies in the two species (Pollard et al., 1977; Trabucchi et al., 1978; Murrin et al., 1980). Increased DA metabolism after morphine was also observed in the hamster and gerbil, but increased release was seen only in the hamster, and no opiate action could be detected on ascending dopaminergic pathways in the pigeon (Wood, 1983b).

Nigrostriatal dopaminergic neurons also possess a phasic enkephalinergic input, as shown in studies with the enkephalinase-inhibitor thiorphan (Wood, 1982b). Inhibition of this enzyme resulted in elevated striatal DOPAC and HVA in a dose-dependent manner and was reversed by low doses of naloxone. The effect of various opiate classes on nigrostriatal DA metabolism is summarized in Table 13.

5.2.2. Mesocortical DA Metabolism

Electrophysiological studies (Palmer and Hoffer, 1980; Williams and Zieglgansberger, 1981) of the actions of enkephalins in the

TABLE 13
Multiple Opiate Effects on Nigrostriatal DA Metabolism

Opiate class	Striatal action[a]	Reversal[a]
Mu (mu$_2$)	Increase DA met.	Nal, WIN, K ag.
Delta	Increase DA met.	Nal, WIN, K ag.
Epsilon	Increase DA met.	Nal
Kappa	Inactive, reverses mu$_2$ and delta	—
Agonist/antagonist	Bell-shaped DR	Nal, WIN
Enkephalinase inhibitor	Increase DA met.	Nal

[a]Abbreviations: met., metabolism; Nal, naloxone; WIN, WIN 44441-3; K ag, kappa agonists; DR, dose–response.

frontal cortex of the rat have suggested that opioid actions in this brain region involve postsynaptic interactions with the dopaminergic innervation and do not involve an action on transmitter release. Our studies on DA metabolism in four cortical regions (cingulate, pyriform, prefrontal, and entorrhinal cortices, Table 14) revealed that morphine increased DOPAC and HVA in the first three regions, but not in the entorrhinal cortex. Previous studies with parenteral morphine have reported increases in HVA in the frontal cortex (Westerink and Korf, 1976). Local injections of morphine (Joyce and Iverson, 1979) and enkephalin (Broekkamp et al., 1979) into the ventral tegmental area (VTA) stimulate these mesocortical dopamine neurons. These data suggest that our observations on cortical DA metabolism may be dependent on actions within the VTA. Both kappa agonists and the agonist/antagonist butorphanol had no effect on DA metabolism in any of these cortical regions (Iyengar et al., manuscript in preparation).

TABLE 14
Effect of Morphine (16 mg/kg, sc)
on Cortical DA Metabolism in the Rat

Region	% of control	
	DOPAC	HVA
Cingulate cortex	150[a]	165[a]
Prefrontal cortex	170[a]	220[a]
Pyriform cortex	185[a]	190[a]
Entorrhinal cortex	95	100

[a]$p < 0.05$, SEM < 10%, 60 min. All actions were naloxone-reversible (2 mg/kg, ip).

5.2.3. Mesolimbic DA Metabolism

Small increases in septal DOPAC and HVA were observed after high (16 mg/kg) doses of morphine (Wood, 1983b). Collu et al. (1980) also described small increases in septal DOPAC after high doses of the enkephalin analog D-Ala^2-Leu^5-enkephalinamide. The actions of other opiate drugs have not been studied in this region. Trulson and Arasteh (1985) noted from in vitro studies, using mouse brain slices, that morphine produced a dose-dependent, naloxone-reversible increase in DA release from the DA-containing neurons in the VTA, whereas Mathews and German (1984) reported electrophysiological evidence for excitation of rat ventral tegmental area DA neurons by morphine.

Morphine caused potent increases in DA metabolism in the N accumbens (Wood, 1983b) (Table 15). We also have observed dose-dependent, naloxone-reversible increases in N accumbens dopamine metabolism with β-endorphin (Table 15). Although the effects of kappa agonists were not tested in this region, the agonist/antagonist butorphanol caused dose-dependent increases in DOPAC and HVA that were partially reversed by naloxone (Table 15). Thus this action of butorphanol was different from the bell-shaped dose–response curve seen in the striatum.

It is clear from these studies that mesolimbic and nigrostriatal dopaminergic neurons have multiple opioid inputs (Table 16). In this region, although both morphine and DADLE cause potent,

TABLE 15
Effect of Some Opiates on DA Metabolism
in the N Accumbens

Drug		DOPAC	HVA	DA
		% of control		
Morphine (mg/kg, sc)[a]	2	155[b]	170[b]	100
	16	219[b]	263[b]	92
β-Endorphin (μg, icv)	5	170[b]	170[b]	125
	20	160[b]	155[b]	115
N (5) +	5	106	116	83
Butorphanol (mg/kg)	8	120	125	107
	24	150[b]	145[b]	110
	64	145[b]	155[b]	115
N (5) +	24	120	125	113

[a] Wood, 1983b.
[b] $p < 0.05$, 60 min, SEM < 10%.

TABLE 16
Effect of Opiates on DA Metabolism
in the Olfactory Tubercle (60 min)

Drug, mg/kg, ip		Receptor type	DOPAC	HVA	DA
			% of control		
Morphine		Mu			
	4		170[a]	170	110
	16		185[a]	185	115
W (2) +	16		130	125	100
N (2) +	16		120	115	90
DADLE (μg, icv)		Delta			
	2		130[a]	140[a]	106
	10		165[a]	190[a]	97
W (5) +	2		125	130[a]	101
N (5) +	10		113	119	101
β-Endorphin (μg, icv)		Mu, delta, epsilon			
	5		134[a]	151[a]	98
	20		150[a]	155[a]	110
N (5) +	5		120	124	95
Butorphanol		Ag/Ant, kappa			
	2		83	90	130
	8		85	90	119
	24		82	85	117
U50488H		Kappa			
	2		125	125	119
	16		150[a]	130[a]	100
W (5) +	16		145[a]		105
N (5) +	16		97	107	110
Mr2034		Kappa			
	2		135[a]	125[a]	95
	4		150[a]	140[a]	114
W (5) +	4		135[a]	130[a]	110
N (5) +	4		110	110	109
1-EKC		Kappa			
	2		115	115	95
	16		120	115	90
Tifluadom		Kappa			
	2		100	115	100
	16		105	120	101

[a] $p < 0.05$, W, WIN 44441-3 (-10 min); N, naloxone (-6, $+10$ min).

dose-dependent increases in dopamine metabolism that are naloxone-reversible, they are differentially reversed by WIN 44441-3, indicating independent modulation of the two receptors. Although the action of morphine is reversed by low doses of the latter antagonist, that of DADLE is not. Another interesting observation is that two kappa agonists, Mr2034 and U50488H, cause significant naloxone-reversible increases in DA metabolism, indicating an agonist action for these kappa drugs, unlike in the nigrostriatal dopaminergic pathway. These actions are not reversed, however, by the long-acting opiate antagonist WIN 44441-3. More surprising, two other kappa agonists, 1-EKC and tifluadom, have no action on DA metabolism. This is the first neurochemical evidence for the presence of potential kappa opioid isoreceptors (Table 16). The agonist/antagonist butorphanol has no action on DA metabolism in the olfactory tubercle. Two endogenous opioid peptides, MEAP and dynorphin, also had no effect (unpublished observations), whereas β-endorphin caused dose-dependent, naloxone-reversible increases in dopamine metabolism (Table 16).

5.3. Serotonin

Unlike the effect of opiates on dopamine metabolism, which have been extensively studied, the effect of opiates on the neurochemistry of serotonin (5-HT) have not been as thoroughly documented. There have been reports of the effect of morphine on several brain regions (Snelgar and Vogt, 1980). Johnson and Moore (1983) demonstrated that morphine caused naloxone-reversible increases in 5-HT metabolism in the rat striatum, arcuate nucleus, medial preoptic area, and suprachiasmatic nucleus. Cervo et al. (1983) implicated forebrain 5-HT in naloxone-precipitated jumping in morphine-dependent rats, whereas Kruszewska and Langwinski (1983) implicated central 5-HT in the morphine-abstinence syndrome. Spampinato et al. (1985) found systemic morphine to increase 5-HIAA in the striatum, nucleus accumbens, and cortex, although it had no effect on hippocampus. Similar changes were found when morphine was injected in the dorsal raphe, whereas only N accumbens showed increased metabolism when morphine was injected into the medial raphe. The effect of dorsal raphe injections was blocked by PCPA, a serotonin synthesis inhibitor, suggesting that morphine increases forebrain 5-HT metabolism through activation of 5-HT cells in the nucleus raphe

TABLE 17
Mu$_1$ and Mu$_2$ Isoreceptor Classification Scheme[a]

Mu$_1$ action	Mu$_2$ and/or delta action
Supraspinal analgesia	Growth hormone release
Catalepsy	Respiratory depression
Cortical ACh neurons	Striatal DA neurons
Prolactin release	Spinal analgesia (also kappa)
Feeding (free and	Guinea pig ileum (also kappa)
deprivation-induced)	Bradycardia
	Reversal of endotoxic shock
	Physical dependence signs

[a]Data from Pasternak and Wood, 1986.

dorsalis. Broderick (1985a,b) also reported increased serotonin release in response to morphine from N accumbens and striatum.

Although morphine was found to elevate spinal dorsal horn 5-HIAA in a dose-dependent and naloxone-reversible manner, other mu, delta, and kappa opioid receptor agonists did not alter 5-HIAA levels (Wood, 1985). These studies indicate that 5-HT pathways are not essential for opiate analgesia.

6. Overview

It is now clear that there are both multiple opioid receptors and multiple endogenous opioid ligands. It is, therefore, essential that in the study of potential opioid regulation of any new physiological system, the key limitations observed in previous studies be considered in both the study design and evaluation.

These key areas include: (1) species differences in the proportion of mu, delta, and kappa receptor populations; (2) the role of mu isoreceptors (Table 17); (3) the role of presynaptic vs neuronal receptors; (4) the role of receptor dualism with agents possessing multiple receptor affinities; and (5) the possible complications of an endogenous opioid tone.

With these limitations in mind, the design of better studies is possible and will aid in the clearer definition of the opioid control and modulation of CNS circuitry.

References

Abe, H., Kato, Y., Chihara, K., Iwasaki, Y., and Imura, H. (1981) Effects of drugs infused into a rat hypophysial portal vessel on prolactin and growth hormone release. *Proc. Soc. Exp. Biol. Med.* **165,** 248–252.

Ahtee, L. and Kaariainen, I. (1973) The effect of narcotic analgesics on homovanillic acid content of rat nucleus caudatus. *Eur. J. Pharmacol.* **22,** 206–208.

Akil, H., Mayer, D. J., and Liebeskind, J. C. (1974) Antagonism of stimulation-produced analgesia by naloxone, a narcotic antagonist. *Science* **191,** 961–962.

Allolio, B., Winkelman, W., Hipp, F. X., Kaulen, D., and Mies, R. (1982) Effects of a met-enkephalin analogue on ACTH, growth hormone and prolactin in patients with ACTH hypersecretion. *J. Clin. Endocrinol. Metab.* **55,** 1–7.

Alper, R. H., Demerest, K. T., and Moore, K. E. (1980) Morphine differentially alters synthesis and turnover of dopamine in central neuronal systems. *J. Neural Trans.* **48,** 157–165.

Apfelbaum, M. and Mandenoff, A. (1981) Naltrexone suppresses hyperphagia induced in the rat by a highly palatable diet. *Pharmacol. Biochem. Behav.* **15,** 89–91.

Arita, J. and Porter, J. C. (1984) Relationship between dopamine release into hypophyseal portal blood and prolactin release after morphine treatment in rats. *Neuroendocrinology* **38,** 62–67.

Attali, B., Gouarderes, C., Mazarguil, H., Audigier, Y., and Cros, J. (1982) Evidence for multiple kappa binding sites by use of opioid peptides in the guinea-pig lumbo-sacral spinal cord. *Neuropeptides* **3,** 53–64.

Audiger, Y., Attali, B., Mazarguil, H., and Cros, J. (1982) Characterization of ^{3}H-etorphine binding in the guinea-pig striatum after blockade of mu and delta sites. *Life Sci.* **31,** 1287–1290.

Barden, N., Merand, Y., Rouleau, D., Garon, M., and Dupont, A. (1981) Changes in the β-endorphin content of discrete hypothalamic nuclei during the estrous cycle of the rat. *Brain Res.* **80,** 291–301.

Barraclough, C. A. and Sawyer, C. H. (1955) Inhibition of the release of pituitary ovulatory hormone in the rat by morphine. *Endocrinology* **57,** 329–337.

Basbaum, A. I. (1984) Anatomical Substrates of Pain and Pain Modulation and Their Relationship to Analgesic Drug Action, in *Analgesics: Neurochemical, Behavioral, and Clinical Perspectives* (Kuhar, M. J. and Pasternak, G. W., eds.) Raven, New York.

Belchetz, P. E. (1981) Functional and anatomical segregation of hypothalamic opiate receptors involved in prolactin and growth hormone secretion in cynomolgus monkeys. *Life Sci.* **28,** 2961–2971.

Beleslin, D. B., Samarddzic, R., and Krstic, S. K. (1982) Beta-endorphin-induced psychomotor excitation in the cat. *Physiol. Behav.* **28,** 195–197.

Bellville, J. W. and Forrest, W. H. (1968) Respiratory and subjective effects of *d*- and *l*-pentazocine. *Clin. Pharmacol. Ther.* **9,** 142–151.

Beubler, E. (1980) Naloxone increases carbon dioxide stimulated respiration in the rabbit. *Naunyn Schmiedebergs Arch. Pharmacol.* **311,** 199–203.

Bhanot, R. and Wilkinson, M. (1983) Opioidergic control of gonadotropin secretion during the puberty in the rat. *Endocrinology* **113,** 596–603.

Biggio, G., Casu, M., Corda, M. G., DiBello, C., and Gessa, G. L. (1978) Stimulation of dopamine synthesis in caudate nucleus by intrastriatal enkephalins and antagonism by naloxone. *Science* **200,** 552–554.

Blank, M. S., Panerai, A. E., and Friesan, H. G. (1979) Opioid peptides modulate luteinizing hormone secretion during sexual maturation. *Science* **203,** 1129–1131.

Blankstein, J., Reyes, F., Winter, J., and Faiman, C. (1979) Failure of naloxone to alter growth hormone and prolactin levels in acromegalic and in hyperprolactinaemic patients. *Clin. Endocrinol.* **11,** 475–479.

Bloom, F. E., Rossier, J., Battenberg, E. L. F., Bayon, A., French, E., Henriksen, S. J., Siggins, G. R., Segal, D., Browne, R., Ling, N., and Guillemin, R. (1978) Beta endorphin: Cellular localization, electrophysiological and behavioral effects. *Adv. Biochem. Psychopharmacol.* **18,** 89–109.

Borison, H. L. (1977) Central nervous respiratory depressants—narcotic analgesics. *Pharmacol. Ther.* **3,** 227–237.

Broderick, P. A. (1985a) In vivo electrochemical studies of rat striatal dopamine and serotonin release after morphine. *Life Sci.* **36,** 2269–2275.

Broderick, P. A. (1985b) Opiate regulation of mesolimbic serotonin release: In vivo semiderivative electrochemical analyses. *Neuropeptides* **5,** 587–590.

Broekkamp, C. L. E., Phillips, A. G., and Cools, A. R. (1979) Stimulant effects of enkephalin microinjection into the dopaminergic A10 area. *Nature* **278,** 560–562.

Brown, D. R. and Holtzman, S. F. (1979) Suppression of deprivation-induced food and water intake in rats and mice by naloxone. *Pharmacol. Biochem. Behav.* **11,** 567–573.

Brown, B., Dettmar, P. W., Dobson, P. R., Lynn, A. G., Metcalf, G., and Morgan, B. A. (1978) Opiate analgesics: The effect of agonist–antagonist character on prolactin secretion. *J. Pharm. Pharmacol.* **30,** 644–645.

Browning, A. J. F., Butt, W. R., and London, D. R. (1981) The interaction of female sex-steroids and endogenous opioids on the inhibition of pituitary gonadotropin release. *Acta Endocr.* **243,** (suppl.): 191.

Bruni, J. F., VanVugt, D., Marshall, S., and Meitis, J. (1977) Effects of naloxone, morphine and methionine enkephalin on serum prolactin, luteinizing hormone, follicle stimulating hormone, thyroid stimulating hormone and growth hormone. *Life Sci.* **21,** 461–466.

Buckingham, J. C. (1982) Secretion of corticotrophin and its hypothalamic releasing factor in response to morphine and opioid peptides. *Neuroendocrinology* **35,** 111–116.

Buckingham, J. C. and Cooper, T. A. (1984) Differences in hypothalamo-pituitary-adrenocortical activity in the rat after acute and prolonged treatment with morphine. *Neuroendocrinology* **38,** 411–417.

Callahan, P., Janik, J., Grandison, L., and Rabii, J. (1985) Alterations in the sensitivity of the prolactin regulatory mechanism to opiates during lactation. *Soc. Neurosci.* **11,** 1199.

Casaneuva, F., Betti, R., Cocchi, D., Chieli, T., Mantegazza, P., and Mueller, E. E. (1981) Proof for histaminergic but not for adrenergic involvement in the growth hormone releasing effect of an enkephalin analog in the dog. *Endocrinology* **108,** 157–163.

Cervo, L., Romandini, S., and Samanin, R. (1983) Evidence that 5HT in naloxone precipitated jumping in morphine dependent rats. *Br. J. Pharmacol.* **79,** 993–996.

Cheney, D. L., Trabucchi, M., Racagni, G., Wang, C., and Costa, E. (1974) Effects of acute and chronic morphine on regional rat brain acetylcholine turnover rate. *Life Sci.* **15,** 1977–1990.

Chihara, K., Arimura, A., Coy, D. H., and Schally, A. V. (1978) Studies on the interaction of endorphins, substance P, and endogenous somatostatin in growth hormone and prolactin release in rats. *Endocrinology* **102,** 281–290.

Ching, M. (1983) Morphine suppresses the proestrous surge of GnRH in pituitary portal plasma of rats. *Endocrinology* **112,** 2209–2211.

Cicero, T. J., Meyer, E. R., Bell, R. D., and Koch, G. A. (1976) Effects of morphine and methadone on serum testosterone and luteinizing hormone levels and on the secondary sex organs of the male rat. *Endocrinology* **98,** 367–372.

Clark, J. A., Itzhak, Y., Hruby, V. J., Yamamura, H. I., and Pasternak, G. W. (1986) [D-Pen^2,D-Pen^5]Enkephalin (DPDPE): a delta-selective enkephalin with low affinity for mu$_1$ opiate sites. *Eur. J. Phamacol.* **128.** 303–304.

Cohen, M. R., Cohen, R. M., Pickar, D., Kreger, D., McLellan, C., and Murphy, D. (1985) Hormonal effects of high dose naloxone in humans. *Neuropeptides* **6,** 373–380.

Collu, R., Stefanini, E., Vernaleone, F., Marchisio, A. M., Devoto, P., and Argiolas, A. (1980) Biochemical characterization of the dopaminergic innervation of the rat septum. *Life Sci.* **26,** 1665–1673.

Cooper, S. J. (1980) Naloxone: Effects on food and water consumption in the non-deprived and deprived rat. *Psychopharmacology* **71,** 1–6.

Cooper, S. J., Barber, D. J., and Barbour-McMullen, J. (1985a) Selective attenuation of sweetened milk consumption by opiate receptor antagonists in male and female rats of the Roman strains. *Neuropeptides* **5,** 349–352.

Cooper, S. J., Jackson, A., Morgan, R., and Carter, R. (1985b) Evidence for opiate receptor involvement in the consumption of a high palatability diet in nondeprived rats. *Neuropeptides* **5,** 345–348.

Costa, E., Cheney, D. L., Racagni, G., and Zsilla, G (1975) An analysis at the synaptic level of the morphine action in striatum and N. accumbens, dopamine and acetylcholine interaction. *Life Sci.* **17,** 1–8.

Cowan, A., Doxey, J. C., and Harry, E. J. R. (1977) The animal pharmacology of buprenorphine, an oripavine analgesic agent. *Br. J. Pharmacol.* **60,** 547–554.

Czlonkowski, A., Costa, T., Przewlocki, R., Pasi, A., and Herz, A. (1983) Opiate receptor binding sites in human spinal cord. *Brain Res.* **267,** 392–396.

Delitala, G., Grossman, A., and Besser, G. M. (1983) The participation of hypothalamic dopamine in morphine induced prolactin release in man. *Clin. Endocrinol.* **19,** 437–444.

Del Pozo, E., von Graffenried, B., Brownell, J., Derrer, F., and Marbach, P. (1980) Endocrine effect of a methionine enkephalin derivative (FK 33–824) in man. *Hormone Res.* **13,** 90–97.

Denavit-Saubie, M., Champagnat, J., and Zieglgansberger, W. (1978) Effects of opiates and methionine enkephalin on pontine and bulbar respiratory neurons of the cat. *Brain Res.* **155,** 55–67.

de Souza, E. B. and Van Loon, G. R. (1982) D-Ala-Met-Enkephalinamide, a potent opioid peptide, alters pituitary-adrenocortical secretion in rats. *Endocrinology* **111,** 1483–1490.

Deyo, S. N. and Miller, R. J. (1982) The role of endogenous opioids in the stress and estrogen induced activation of PRL release. *Life Sci.* **31,** 2171–2175.

Deyo, S. N., Swift, R. M., and Miller, R. J. (1979) Morphine and endorphins modulate dopamine turnover in rat median eminence. *Proc. Natl. Acad. Sci. USA* **76,** 3006–3339.

Drouva, S. V., Epelbaum, J., Tapia-Arancibia, L., Laplante, E., and Kordon, C. (1981) Opiate receptors modulate LHRH and SRIF release from mediobasal hypothalamic neurons. *Neuroendocrinology* **32,** 163–167.

Dupont, A., Cusan, L., Garon, M., Labrie, F., and Li, C. H. (1977) Beta-endorphin stimulation of growth hormone release in vitro. *Proc. Natl. Acad. Sci. USA* **74,** 358–359.

Dupont, A., Cusan, L., Ferland, L., Lemay, A., and Labrie, F. (1979) Evidence for a Role for Endorphins in the Control of Prolactin Secretion, in *Central Nervous System Effects of Hypothalamic Hormones and Other Peptides* (Collu, R., Barbeau, A., Ducharine, J. R., and Rockefort, J. G., eds.) Raven, New York.

Eckenhoff, J. E. and Oech, S. R. (1960) The effects of narcotics and antagonists upon respiration and circulation in man. A review. *Clin. Pharmacol. Ther.* **1,** 483–524.

Eisenberg, R. M. (1982) Effects of ethylketocyclazocine and N-allylnormetazocine on plasma corticosterone. *Pharmacologist* **24,** 125.

Eisenberg, R. M. (1984) Effects of naltrexone on plasma corticosterone in opiate-naive rats: A central action. *Life Sci.* **34,** 1185–1191.

Eisenberg, R. M. (1985) Plasma corticosterone changes in response to central or peripheral administration of kappa and sigma opiate agonists. *J. Pharm. Exp. Ther.* **233,** 863–869.

Ericksson, E., Eden, S., and Modigh, K. (1981) Importance of norepinephrine-induced rat growth hormone secretion. *Neuroendocrinology* **33,** 91–96.

Ferland, L., Labrie, F., Cusan, L., DuPont, A., Lepine, J., Bedulie, M., Denizeau, F., and Lemay, A. (1980) Role of the Tuberoinfundibular Dopaminergic System in the Control of Prolactin Secretion, in *The Endocrine Functions of the Brain* (Motto, M., ed.) Raven, New York.

Foley, K. M., Kourides, I. A., Inturrisi, C. E., Kaiko, R. F., Zaroulis, C. G., Posner, J. B., Houde, R. W., and Li, C. H. (1979) β-Endorphin: Analgesic and hormonal effects in humans. *Proc. Natl. Acad. Sci. USA* **76,** 5377–5381.

Forman, L. J., Sonntag, W. E., and Meitis, J. (1983) Elevation of plasma LH in response to systemic injection of β-endorphin antiserum in adult male rats. *Proc. Soc. Exp. Biol. Med.* **173,** 14–16.

Frischknecht, H. -R., Siegfried, B., Riggio, G., and Waser, P. G. (1983) Inhibition of morphine-induced analgesia and locomotor activity in strains of mice: A comparison of long-acting opiate antagonists. *Pharmacol. Biochem. Behav.* **19,** 939–944.

Fuller, R. W. and Leander, J. D. (1985) Elevation of serum corticosterone in rats by bremazocine, a κ-opioid agonist. *J. Pharm. Pharmacol.* **36,** 345–346.

Gabriel, S. M., Simpkins, J. W., and Kalra, S. P. (1983) Modulation of endogenous opioid influence on LH secretion by progesterone and estrogen. *Endocrinology* **113,** 199.

Gal, T. J., DiFazio, C. A., and Moscicki, J. (1982) Analgesic and respiratory depressant activity of nalbuphine: A comparison with morphine. *Anesthesiology* **57,** 367–374.

Gale, K., Moroni, F., Kumakura, K., and Guidotti, A. (1979) Opiate receptors in substantia-nigra and ventral tegmental area demonstrated by combined histofluorescence-immunochemistry *Neuropharmacology* **18,** 427–430.

Gardner, E. L., Zukin, R. S., and Makman, M. H. (1980) Modulation of opiate receptor binding in striatum and amygdala by selective mesencephalic lesions. *Brain Res.* **194,** 232–239.

Gauchy, C., Agid, Y., Glowinski, J., and Cheramy, A. (1973) Acute effects of morphine on dopamine synthesis and release and tyrosine metabolism in the rat striatum. *Eur. J. Pharmacol.* **22,** 311–319.

George, R. and Way, E. L. (1959) Studies on the mechanism of pituitary-adrenal activation by morphine. *Br. J. Pharmacol. Chemother.* **10,** 260–264.

Gibson, A., Ginsburg, M., Hall, M., and Hart, S. L. (1979) The effects of opiate receptor agonists on the stress induced secretion of corticosterone in mice. *Br. J. Pharmacol.* **65,** 139–146.

Gillan, M. G. and Kosterlitz, H. W. (1982) Spectrum of the mu-, delta- and kappa-binding sites in homogenates of rat brain. *Br. J. Pharmacol.* **77,** 461–469.

Gold, M. S., Redmond, D. E., Jr., and Donabedian, R. K. (1978) Increase in serum prolactin by exogenous and endogenous opiates: Evidence for antidopamine and antipsychotic effects. *Am. J. Psychiatry* **135,** 1415.

Goode, P. G., Rhodes, K. F., and Waterfall, J. F. (1979) The analgesic and respiratory effects of meptazinol, morphine and pentazocine in the rat. *J. Pharm. Pharmacol.* **31,** 793–795.

Gouarderes, C., Audigier, Y., and Cros, J. (1982) Benzomorphan binding sites in rat lumbo-sacral spinal cord. *Eur. J. Pharmacol.* **78,** 483–486.

Grandison, L. and Guidotti, A. (1977a) Evidence for regulation of prolactin release by endogenous opiates. *Nature* **270,** 357–359.

Grandison, L. and Guidotti, A. (1977b) Stimulation of food intake by muscimol and beta-endorphin. *Neuropharmacology* **16,** 533–536.

Grandison, L., Fratta, W., and Guidotti, A. (1980) Localization and characterization of opiate receptors regulating pituitary secretion. *Life Sci.* **26,** 1633–1642.

Green, A. F. (1959) Comparative effects of analgesics on pain threshold, respiratory frequency and gastrointestinal propulsion. *Br. J. Pharmacol.* **14,** 26–34.

Grossman, A., Stubbs, W. A., Gaillard, R. C., Delitala, G., Rees, L. H., and Besser, G. M. (1981) Studies on the opiate control of PRL, GH and TSH. *Clin. Endocrinol.* **14,** 381–386.

Grossman, A., Gaillard, R. C., McCartney, P., Rees, L. H., and Besser, G. M. (1982a) Opiate modulation of the pituitary adrenal axis: Effect of stress and circadian rhythm. *Clin. Endocrinol.* **17,** 279–286.

Grossman, A., West, S., Williams, J., Evans, J., Rees, L. H., and Besser, G.

M. (1982b) The role of opiate peptides in the puerperium and TSH in primary hypothyroidism. *Clin. Endocrinol.* **16**, 317–320.

Gudelsky, G. A. and Porter, J. C. (1979) Morphine and opioid peptides induced inhibition of the release of dopamine from tuberoinfundibular neurons. *Life Sci.* **25**, 1697–1702.

Gudelsky, G. A., Siminovic, M., Passaro, E., and Meltzer, H. Y. (1983) The inhibitory effect of morphine on rat prolactin secretion: Role of tuberoinfundibular dopaminergic neurons. *Endocrinology* **112** (suppl.), 165.

Guillemin, R., Brazeau, P., Boehlen, P., Esch, F., Ling, N., and Wehrenberg, W. B. (1982) Growth hormone releasing factor from a human pancreatic tumor that caused acromegaly. *Science* **218**, 585–587.

Han, J. -S. and Xie, C. -W. (1982) Dynorphin: Potent analgesic effect in spinal cord of the rat. *Life Sci.* **31**, 1781–1784.

Harasz, J. L., Bloom, A. S., Wang, R. I. H., and Tseng, L. -P. (1981) Effect of intraventricular β-endorphin and morphine on hypothalamo-pituitary-adrenal activity and the release of pituitary β-endorphin. *Neuroendocrinology* **33**, 170–175.

Haskins, J. T., Gudelsky, G. A., Moss, R. L., and Porter, J. C. (1981) Iontophoresis of morphine into the arcuate nucleus: Effects on dopamine concentrations in the hypophyseal portal plasma and serum prolactin concentrations. *Endocrinology* **108**, 767–771.

Heel, R. C., Brogden, R. N., Speight, T. M., and Avery, G. S. (1978) Butorphanol: A review of its pharmacological properties and therapeutic efficacy. *Drugs* **16**, 473–505.

Herman, B. H. and Goldstein, A. (1981) Cataleptic effects of dynorphin-(1-13) in rats made tolerant to a mu opiate receptor agonist. *Neuropeptides* **2**, 13–22.

Herrera-Marschitz, M., Hokfelt, T., Ungerstedt, U., Terenius, L., and Goldstein, M. (1984) Effect of intranigral injections of dynorphin, dynorph in fragments and alpha-neoendorphin on rotational behavior in the rat. *Eur. J. Pharmacol.* **102**, 213–227.

Hollt, V., Tulunay, F. C., Woo, S. K., Loh, H. L., and Herz, A. (1982) Opioid peptides derived from pro-enkephalin A but not from pro-enkephalin B are substantial analgesics after administration into brain of mice. *Eur. J. Pharmacol.* **85**, 355–356.

Hylden, J. L. K. and Wilcox, G. L. (1983) Intrathecal opioids block a spinal action of substance P in mice: Functional importance of both mu and delta receptors. *Eur. J. Pharmacol.* **86**, 95–98.

Ieiri, T., Chen, H. T., and Meitis, J. (1979) Effects of morphine and naloxone on LH and PRL in prepubertal male and female rats. *Neuroendocrinology* **29**, 288–293.

Ieiri, T., Chen, H. T., Campbell, G. A., and Meitis, J. (1980) Effects of naloxone and morphine on the proestrous surge of prolactin and gonadotropins in the rat. *Endocrinology* **106**, 1568–1570.

Inukai, T. and Takagi, H. (1979) Site of anti-nociceptive action of a new benzomorphan derivative ID-1229. *Arch. Int. Pharmacodyn.* **242**, 262–272.

Itzhak, Y. and Pasternak, G. W. (1987) Interaction of [D-Ser^2,Leu^5]Enkephalin-Thr^6 (DSLET), a relatively selective delta ligand, with mu$_1$ opioid binding sites. *Life Sci.* **40**, 307–311.

Iwamoto, E. T., Loh, H. H., and Way, E. L. (1976) Circling behavior after narcotic drugs and during naloxone-precipitated abstinence in rats with unilateral nigral lesion. *J. Pharmacol. Exp. Ther.* **197,** 503–516.

Iyengar, S. and Rabii, J. (1984a) Sex differences in opiate receptor binding as determined by quantitative autoradiography in several areas of the rat brain. *Soc. Neurosci.* **10,** 582.

Iyengar, S. and Rabii, J. (1984b) The influence of prenatal exposure to morphine on postnatal opiate receptor density in the rat brain. Excerpta Medica, Int. Congress Series 652, p. 745.

Iyengar, S. and Wood, P. L. (1985) Kappa opiate modulation of thyroid stimulating hormone (TSH) release in the rat. *Soc. Neurosci.* **11,** 908.

Iyengar, S., Kim, H., and Wood, P. L. (1986) Kappa opiate agonists modulate the hypothalamo-pituitary-adrenocortical axis in the rat. *J. Pharmacol. Exp. Ther.* **238,** 429–436.

Iyengar, S., Kim, H. S., and Wood, P. L. (1987) Mu, delta, kappa and epsilon opioid receptor modulation of the hypothalamic-pituitary-adrenocortical (HPA) axis: Sub-chronic tolerance studies of endogenous opioid peptides. *Brain Res.* (submitted).

Jackson, H. C. and Sewell, R. D. E. (1985) Are delta-opioid receptors involved in the regulation of food and water intake? *Neuropharmacology* **24,** 885–888.

Jacquet, Y. (1982) Met-enkephalin: Potent contraversive rotation after microinjection in rat substantia nigra. *Brain Res.* **264,** 340–343.

Jaloweic, J. E., Panksepp, J., Zolovick, A. J., Najam, N., and Herman, B. (1981) Opioid modulation of ingestive behavior. *Pharmacol. Biochem. Behav.* **15,** 477–484.

Janowsky, D., Judd, L., Huey, L., Roitman, N., and Parker, D. (1979) Naloxone effects on serum growth hormone and prolactin in man. *Psychopharmacology* **65,** 95–97.

Jezova, D., Vigas, M., and Jurcovicova, J. (1982) ACTH and corticosterone response to naloxone and morphine in normal, hypophysectomized and dexamethasone treated rats. *Life Sci.* **31,** 307–314.

Jhamandas, K., Phyllis, J. W., and Pinsky, C. (1971) Effect of narcotic analgesics and antagonists on the in vivo release of acetylcholine from the cerebral cortex of the rat. *Br. J. Pharmacol.* **43,** 53–66.

Jhamandas, K., Hron, V., and Sutak, M. (1975) Comparative effects of opiate agonists methadone, levorphanol and their isomers on the release of cortical ACh in vivo and in vitro. *Can. J. Pharmacol. Physiol.* **50,** 5762.

Johnson, J. H. (1982) Release of prolactin in response to microinjection of morphine into mesencephalic dorsal raphe nucleus. *Neuroendocrinology* **37,** 248–257.

Johnson, R. P., Sar, M., and Stumpf, W. E. (1980) A topographic localization of enkephalin on the dopamine neurons of the rat substantia-nigra and ventral tegmental area demonstrated by combined histofluorescence-immunochemistry. *Brain Res.* **194,** 566–571.

Johnston, C. A. and Moore, K. E. (1983) The effect of morphine on 5-hydroxy-tryptamine synthesis and metabolism in the striatum and several discrete hypothalamic regions of the rat brain. *J. Neural. Transm.* **57,** 65–73.

Joyce, E. M. and Iverson, S. D. (1979) The effect of morphine applied locally to mesencephalic dopamine cell bodies on spontaneous motor activity in the rat. *Neurosci. Lett.* **14**, 207–212.

Judd, A. M. and Hedge, G. A. (1982) The roles of opioid peptides in controlling thyroid stimulating hormone release. *Life Sci.* **31**, 2529–2536.

Judd, L. L., Parker, D. C., Janowsky, D. S., Segal, D., Risen, S., and Huey, L. (1982) The effect of methadone on the behavioral and neuroendocrine responses of manic patients. *Psychiat. Res.* **7**, 163.

Judd, L. L., Janowsky, D. S., and Segal, D. S. (1981) Effects of naloxone HCl on cortisol levels in patients with affective disorders and normal controls. *Psychiat. Res.* **4**, 277.

Judd, L. L., Risch, S. C., Segal, D. S., Janowsky, D. S., and Huey, L. Y. (1985) Behavioral and neuroendocrine effects of opioid receptor agonists in psychopathalogic states. *Psychiat. Clin. N. Am.* **6**, 393–402.

Kalra, S. P. (1981) Neural loci involved in naloxone-induced luteinizing hormone release: Effects of a norepinephrine synthesis inhibitor. *Endocrinology* **109**, 1805–1810.

Kalra, S. P. and Simpkins, J. W. (1981) Evidence for noradrenergic mediation of opioid effects on luteinizing hormone secretion. *Endocrinology* **109**, 776–781.

Katakami, H., Kato, Y., Matsushita, N., Hiroto, S., Shimatsu, A., and Imura, H. (1981) Involvement of α-adrenergic mechanisms in growth hormone release induced by opioid peptides in rats. *Neuroendocrinology* **33**, 129–135.

Kato, Y., Matsushita, N., Katakami, A., Shimatsu, A., and Imura, H. (1981) Stimulation by dynorphin of prolactin and growth hormone secretion in the rat. *Eur. J. Pharmacol.* **73**, 353–355.

Katz, R. J., Carroll, B. J., and Baldrighi, G. (1978) Behavioral activation by enkephalins in mice. *Pharmacol. Biochem. Behav.* **8**, 493–496.

Kelly, P. D., Rance, M. J., and Traynor, J. R. (1982) Properties of opiate binding in the rat spinal cord. *Neuropeptides* **2**, 319–324.

Knuth, V. A., Sikand, G. S., Casamera, G. S., Havlicek, V., and Friesen, H. G. (1983) *Life Sci.* **33** (suppl. 1), 1443–1450.

Koenig, J., Mayfield, M. A., McCann, S. M., and Krulich, L. (1979) Stimulation of PRL by morphine: Role of central serotoninergic system. *Life Sci.* **25**, 853–864.

Koenig, J., Mayfield, M. A., Coppings, R. J., McCann, S. M., and Krulich, L. (1980) Role of central nervous system neurotransmitters in mediating the effects of morphine on growth hormone and prolactin secretion in the rat. *Brain Res.* **197**, 453–468.

Koenig, J. I., Mayfield, M. A., McCann, S. M., and Krulich, L. (1984) Differential role of the opioid m and d receptors in the activation of prolactin (PRL) and growth hormone (GH) secretion by morphine in the male rat. *Life Sci.* **34**, 1829–1837.

Kokka, N. and George, R. (1974) Effects of Narcotic Analgesics, Anesthetics and Hypothalamic Lesions on Growth Hormone and Adrenocorticotropic Hormone Secretion in Rats, in *Narcotics and the Hypothalamus* (Zimmerman, E. and George, R., eds.) Raven, New York.

Kokka, N., Garcia, J. F., and Elliot, J. W. (1973) Effects of acute and chronic administration of narcotics on growth hormone and ACTH secretion in rats. *Prog. Brain Res.* **39**, 347–360.

Kordon, C., Enjalbert, A., Epelbaum, J., and Rotsztejn, W. (1979) Neurotransmitter Interactions with Adrenohypophyseal Regulation, in *Brain Peptides: A New Endocrinology* (Gotto, A. M., Peck, E. J., and Boyd, A. E., eds.) Elsevier, Amsterdam.

Koves, K., Masrton, J., Molnar, J., and Halasz, B. (1981) (D-met², Pro⁵)-enkephalinamide-induced blockade of ovulation and its reversal by naloxone in the rat. *Neuroendocrinology* **32**, 82–86.

Krulich, L., Koenig, J. I., Conway, S., McCann, S., and Mayfield, M. A. (1986a) Opioid κ receptors and the secretion of prolactin and growth hormone (GH) in the rat. I. Effects of opioid κ receptor agonists brema-zocine and U-50488 on secretion of PRL and GH: Comparison with mor-phine. *Neuroendocrinology* **42**, 75–81.

Krulich, L., Koenig, J. I., Conway, S., McCann, S. M., and Mayfield, M. A. (1986b) Opioid κ receptors and the secretion of prolactin (PRL) and growth hormone (GH) in the rat. II. GH and PRL release-inhibiting ef-fects of the opioid κ receptor agonists bremazocine and U-50488. *Neuro-endocrinology* **42**, 82–87.

Kruszewska, A. and Langwinski, R. (1983) The role of central serotoninergic neurotransmission in the morphine abstinence syndrome in rats. *Drug Alcohol Depend.* **12**, 273–278.

Lahti, R. A. and Collins, R. J. (1982) Opiate effects on plasma corticoste-roids: Relationship to dysphoria and reinforcement. *Pharmacol. Biochem. Behav.* **17**, 107–109.

Lawson, E. E., Waldrop, T. G., and Eldridge, F. L. (1979) Naloxone en-hances respiratory output in cats. *J. Appl. Physiol.* **47**, 1105–1111.

Levin, E. R., Sharp, B., Meyer, N. V., and Carlson, H. E. (1981) Morphine and naloxone: Effects on β-endorphin immunoreactivity in canine plasma and secretions from rat pituitaries. *Endocrinology* **109**, 146–151.

Lien, E. L., Morrison, A., and Dvonch, Wm. (1979) The effects of partial opiate agonists on plasma prolactin and growth hormone levels in the rat. *Life Sci.* **25**, 1709–1716.

Ling, G. S. F. and Pasternak, G. W. (1982) Morphine catalepsy in the rat: Involvement of mu-1 (high affinity) opioid binding sites. *Neurosci. Lett.* **32**, 193–196.

Ling, G. S. F., Spiegel, K., Nishimura, S. L., and Pasternak, G. W. (1983) Dissociation of morphine's analgesic and respiratory depressant ac-tions. *Eur. J. Pharmacol.* **86**, 487–488.

Ling, G. S. F., Spiegel, K., Lockhart, S. H., and Pasternak, G. W. (1985) Separation of opioid analgesia from respiratory depression: Evidence for different receptor mechanisms. *J. Pharmacol Exp. Ther.* **232**, 149–155.

Llorens-Cortes, C., Pollard, H., and Schwartz, J. C. (1979) Localization of opiate receptors in substantia-nigra evidence by lesion studies. *Neuro-sci. Lett.* **12**, 165–170.

Loh, H. H., Hitzemann, R. J., and Way, E. L. (1973) Effect of acute mor-phine administration on the metabolism of brain catecholamines. *Life Sci.* **12**, 33–41.

Lomax, P. and George, R. (1966) Thyroid activity following administration of morphine in rats with hypothalamic lesions. *Brain Res.* **2**, 316.

Lomax, P., Kokka, N., and George, R. (1970) Thyroid activity following intracerebral injection of morphine in the rat. *Neuroendocrinology* **6**, 146–151.

Lotti, V. J., Kokka, N., and George, R. (1969) Pituitary-adrenal activation following intrahypothalamic microinjection of morphine. *Neuroendocrinology* **4**, 326–332.

Lowy, M. T., Maickel, R. P., and Yim, G. K. W. (1980) Naloxone reduction of stress-related feeding. *Life Sci.* **26**, 2113–2118.

Mandenoff, A., Fumeron, F., Apfelbaum, M., and Margules, D. L. (1982) Endogenous opiates and energy balance. *Science* **215**, 1536–1537.

Marko, M. and Romer, D. (1983) Inhibitory effect of a new opioid agonist on reproductive endocrine activity in rats of both sexes. *Life Sci.* **33**, 233–234.

Martin, W. R. (1967) Opioid antagonists. *Pharmacol. Rev.* **19**, 463–521.

Martin, J. B., Audet, J., and Saunders, A. (1975) Effects of somatostatin and hypothalamic ventromedial lesions on GH release induced by morphine. *Endocrinology* **96**, 839–846.

Martin, J. B., Tolis, G., Wood, I., and Guyda, H. (1979) Failure of naloxone to influence physiological growth hormone and prolactin secretion. *Brain Res.* **168**, 210–215.

Marton, J., Molaer, J., Koues, K., and Halasz, B. (1981) Naloxone reversal of the pentobarbital-induced blockade of ovulation in the rat. *Life Sci.* **28**, 737–743.

Mathews, R. T. and German, D. C. (1984) Electrophysiological evidence for excitation of rat ventral tegmental area dopamine neurons by morphine. *Neuroscience* **11**, 617–625.

Mayer, D. J. and Liebeskind, J. C. (1974) Pain reduction by focal electrical stimulation of the brain: An anatomical approach. *Brain Res.* **68**, 73–93.

McGilliard, K. L. and Takemori, A. E. (1978) Antagonism by naloxone of narcotic-induced respiratory depression and analgesia. *J. Pharmacol. Exp. Ther.* **207**, 494–503.

McLean, S. and Hoebel, B. G. (1983) Feeding induced by opiates injected into the paraventricular hypothalamus. *Peptides* **4**, 287–292.

McQueen, D. S. (1983) Opioid peptide interactions with respiratory and circulatory systems. *Br. Med. Bull.* **39**, 77–82.

McQueen, D. S. and Ribeiro, J. A. (1980) Inhibitory actions of methionine-enkephalin and morphine on the cat carotid chemoreceptors. *Br. J. Pharmacol.* **71**, 297–305.

Megens, A. A. P. H. and Cools, A. R. (1982) Intraseptally injected opiate agents: Effects on morphine-induced behavior of cats. *Pharmacol. Biochem. Behav.* **17**, 297–304.

Meites, J. (1966) Control of Mammary Growth and Lactation, in *Neuroendocrinology* (Martini, L. and Ganong, W. F., eds.) Academic, New York.

Meites, J., Bruni, J. F., VanVugt, D. A., and Smith, A. F. (1979) Relation of endogenous opioid peptides and morphine to neuroendocrine functions. *Life Sci.* **24**, 1325–1336.

Mendelson, J., Ellingboe, J., Keuhnle, J., and Mello, N. (1979) Effects of naltrexone on mood and neuroendocrine function in normal adult males. *Psychoneuroendocrinology* **3**, 231–236.

Millian, M. J. and Herz, A. (1985) The endocrinology of the opioids. *Int. Rev. Neurobiol.* **26**, 1–83.

Mirin, S. M., Mendelson, J. H., Ellinboe, J., and Meyer, R. E. (1976) Acute effects of heroin and naltrexone on testosterone and gonadotropin secretion: A pilot study. *Psychoneuroendocrinology* **1**, 359–369.

Mitsuma, T. and Nogimori, T. (1983a) Dynorphin (1-13) effects on thyroid-releasing hormone and thyrotropin secretion in rats. *Acta Endocrinologica* **103**, 359–364.

Mitsuma, T. and Nogimori, T. (1983b) Effects of leucine-enkephalin on hypothalamic-pituitary-thyroid axis in the rat. *Life Sci.* **32**, 241–248.

Moore, K. E. and Johnston, C. A. (1982) Median Eminence: Aminergic Control Mechanisms, in *Neuroendocrine Perspectives* (E. E. Mueller and R. M. McLeod, eds.) vol. 1, Elsevier, Amsterdam.

Morley, J. E., Baranetzky, G., Wingert, T. D., Carlson, H. E., Weitzman, R., Chang, R. J., and Varner, A. A. (1980) Endocrine effects of naloxone induced opiate receptor blockade. *J. Clin. Endo. Metab.* **50**, 251–257.

Morley, J. E., Levine, A. S., Grace, M., and Kniep, J. (1983) Opioid modulation of appetite. *Neurosci. Biobehav. Rev.* **7**, 281–305.

Moroni, F., Cheney, D. L., and Costa, E. (1977) Inhibition of acetylcholine turnover in rat hippocampus by intraseptal injections of beta-endorphin and morphine. *Naunyn Schmiedebergs Arch. Pharmacol.* **299**, 149–153.

Moroni, F., Cheney, D. L., and Costa, E. (1978) The turnover rate of acetylcholine in brain nuclei of rats injected intraventricularly and intraseptally with alpha and beta-endorphin. *Neuropharmacology* **17**, 191–196.

Morreti, C., Fabbri, A., Gnessi, L., Cappa, M., Calzolari, A., Grossman, A., and Besser, M. (1983) Naloxone inhibits exercise induced release of PRL and GH in athletes. *Clin. Endocrinol.* **18**, 135–138.

Moskowitz, A. S. and Goodman, R. R. (1985a) Autoradiographic distribution of mu_1 and mu_2 opioid binding in the mouse central nervous system. *Brain Res.* **360**, 117–129.

Moskowitz, A. S. and Goodman, R. R. (1985b) Autoradiographic analysis of mu_1 and mu_2 and delta opioid binding in the central nervous system of C57BL6BY and CXBK (opioid receptor-deficient) mice. *Brain Res.* **360**, 108–116.

Moss, I. R. and Friedman, E. (1978) Beta-endorphin: Effects on respiratory regulation. *Life Sci.* **23**, 1271–1276.

Moulin, D. E., Max, M., Kaiko, R. F., Inturrisi, C. E., Maggard, J., and Foley, K. (1984) The analgesic efficacy of intrathecal (IT) D-Ala-D-Leu-enkephalin (DADL) in cancer patients with chronic pain. *Pain* (suppl.) **2**, 511.

Murrin, L. C., Coyle, J. T., and Kuhar, M. J. (1980) Striatal opiate receptors: Pre- and postsynaptic localization. *Life Sci.* **27**, 1175–1183.

Naber, D., Pickar, D., Davis, G., Cohen, R. M., Jimerson, D. C., Elchisak, M. A., Defraites, E. G., Kalin, N. H., Risch, S. C., and Buchsbaum, M. S. (1981) Naloxone effects on beta-endorphin, cortisol, prolactin, growth hormone, HVA and MHPG in plasma of normal volunteers. *Psychopharmacology* **74**, 125–128.

Okajima, T., Motomatsu, T., Kato, K., and Ibayashi, H. (1980) The stimulatory effect of beta-endorphin on the plasma prolactin levels was diminished in the rats treated with 6-hydroxydopamine. *Life Sci.* **26**, 699–705.

Palmer, M. R. and Hoffer, B. J. (1980) Catecholamine modulation of enkephalin-induced electrophysiological responses in cerebral cortex. *J. Pharmacol. Exp. Ther.* **213**, 205–215.

Pasternak, G. W. (1981) Opiate, enkephalin and endorphin analgesia: Relations to a single subpopulation of opiate receptors. *Neurology* **31,** 1311–1315.

Pasternak, G. W. and Wood, P. L. (1986) Minireview: Multiple mu opiate receptors. *Life Sci.* **38,** 1889–1898.

Pasternak, G. W., Childers, S. R., and Snyder, S. H. (1980a) Opiate analgesia: Evidence for mediation by a subpopulation of opiate receptors. *Science* **208,** 514–515.

Pasternak, G. W., Childers, S. R., and Snyder, S. H. (1980b) Naloxazone, a long-acting opiate antagonist: Effects on analgesia in intact animals and on opiate receptor binding in vitro. *J. Pharmacol. Exp. Ther.* **214,** 455–462.

Pasternak, G. W., Zhang, A.-Z., and Tecott, L. (1980c) Developmental differences between high and low affinity opiate binding sites: Their relationship to analgesia and respiratory depression. *Life Sci.* **27,** 1185–1190.

Pazos, A. and Florez, J. (1983) Interaction of naloxone with mu- and delta-opioid agonists on the respiration of rats. *Eur. J. Pharmacol.* **87,** 309–314.

Pechnick, R., George, R., and Poland, R. E. (1985a) Identification of multiple opiate receptors through neuroendocrine responses. 1. Effects of agonists. *J. Pharmacol. Exp. Ther.* **232,** 163–169.

Pechnick, R., George, R., and Poland, R. E. (1985b) Identification of multiple opiate receptors through neuroendocrine responses. II. Antagonism of mu, kappa and sigma agonists by naloxone and WIN 44441-3. *J. Pharmacol. Exp. Ther.* **232,** 170–179.

Pechnick, R., George, R., and Poland, R. E. (1985c) The effects of the acute administration of buprenorphine hydrochloride on the release of anterior pituitary hormones in the rat: Evidence for the involvement of multiple opiate receptors. *Life Sci.* **37,** 1861–1868.

Penalva, A., Villaneuva, L., Casaneuva, F., Cavagnini, F., Gomez-pan, A., and Mueller, E. E. (1983) Cholinergic and histaminergic involvement in the growth hormone releasing effect of an enkephalin analog FK-33824 in man. *Psychopharmacology* **80,** 120–124.

Petrillo, P., Gambino, M. C., and Tavani, A. (1984) Bremazocine induces antinociception, but prevents opioid-induced constipation and catatonia in rats and precipitates withdrawal in morphine-dependent rats. *Life Sci.* **35,** 917–927.

Pfeiffer, A. and Herz, A. (1984) Endocrine actions of opioids. *Horm. Metabol. Res.* **16,** 386–397.

Pfeiffer, A. and Pfeiffer, D. G. (1984) Central mu- and kappa-opiate receptors may mediate the opiate-induced release of GH and ACTH in rats. *Acta Endocrinol.* **105** (suppl. 264), 40–41.

Piercey, M. F., Lahti, R. A., Schroeder, L. A., Einsphar, F. J., and Barsuhn, C. (1982a) U-50488H, a pure kappa receptor agonist with spinal analgesic loci in the mouse. *Life Sci.* **31,** 1197–1200.

Piercey, M. F., Varner, K., and Schroeder, L. A. (1982b) Analgesic activity of intraspinally administered dynorphin and ethylketocyclazocine. *Eur. J. Pharmacol.* **80,** 283–284.

Pilapil, and Wood, P. L. (1983) [^{3}H]-SKF 10047 binding to rat brain membranes: Evidence for kappa isoreceptors. *Life Sci.* **33,** 263–265.

Pollard, H., Llorens, C., and Schwartz, J. C. (1977) Enkephalin receptors on dopaminergic neurons in rat striatum. *Nature* (Lond.) **268**, 745–747.

Pollard, H., Llorens, C., Schwartz, J. C., Gros, C., and Dray, F. (1978) Localization of opiate receptors and enkephalins in the rat striatum in relationship with the nigrostriatal dopaminergic system: Lesion studies. *Brain Res.* **151**, 392–398.

Pontiroli, A. E., Baio, G., Stella, L., Crescenti, A., and Girardi, A. M. (1982) Effects of naloxone on prolactin, luteinizing hormone and cortisol responses to surgical stress in humans. *J. Clin. Endocrinol. Metab.* **55**, 378–380.

Quigley, M. E. and Yen, S. S. (1980) The role of endogenous opiates on LH secretion during the menstrual cycle. *J. Clin. Endocrinol. Metab.* **52**, 179–181.

Rabii, J., Safier, P., and Grandison, L. (1984) The effect of morphine on basal release of prolactin in lactating rats. *Soc. Neurosci.* **10**, 1110.

Rackham, A., Therriault, M., and Wood, P. L. (1981) Substance P: Evidence for spinal mediation of some behavioral effects. *Neuropharmacology* **20**, 753–755.

Reynolds, D. V. (1969) Surgery in the rat during electrical analgesia induced by focal brain stimulation. *Science* **164**, 444–445.

Rivier, C., Vale, W., Ling, N., Brown, M., and Guillemin, R. (1977) Stimulation in vivo of the secretion of prolactin and growth hormone by β-endorphin. *Endocrinology* **100**, 238–241.

Rolandi, E., Marabini, A., Magnani, G., Sannia, A., and Barreca, T. (1982) Influence of low dose naloxone on pituitary secretion in man. *Eur. J. Clin. Pharmacol.* **22**, 213–216.

Rolandi, E., Perria, C., Franceschini, R., Siani, C., Messina, V., Francaviglia, N., and Barreca, T. (1985) Variations of prolactin content in human cerebrospinal fluid after metoclopramide and morphine. *Life Sci.* **36**, 901–905.

Romagnoli, A. and Keats, A. S. (1980) Ceiling effect for respiratory depression by nalbuphine. *Clin. Pharmacol. Ther.* **27**, 478–485.

Romer, D. and Hill, R. C. (1981) Preclinical development of analgesics. *Triangle* **20**, 49–53.

Ronai, A. Z., Berzetei, I. P., Szekeley, J. I., Miglecz, E., Kurgyis, J., and Bajusz, S. (1981) Enkephalin-like character and analgesia. *Eur. J. Pharmacol.* **69**, 263–271.

Ropert, J., Quigley, M. E., and Yen, S. S. C. (1981) Endogenous opiates modulate pulsatile luteinizing hormone release in humans. *J. Clin. Endocrinol. Metab.* **52**, 583–585.

Rossier, J., French, E., Rivier, C., Shibasaki, T., and Guillemin, R. (1980) Stress-induced release of PRL: Blockade by dexamethasone and naloxone may indicate beta-endorphin mediation. *Proc. Natl. Acad. Sci. USA* **77**, 666–669.

Rotsztejn, W. H., Drouva, S. V., Pattou, E., and Kordon, C. (1978) Met-enkephalin inhibits in vitro dopamine induced LH-RH release from mediobasal hypothalamus of male rats. *Nature* **274**, 281–282.

Rotsztejn, W., Drouva, S. V., Pollard, K., Sokoloff, P., Pattou, E., and Kordon, C. (1982) Further evidence for the existence of opiate binding sites on neurosecretory LHRH mediobasal hypothalamic terminals. *Eur. J. Pharmacol.* **80,** 139–141.

Russell, B. and Yaksh, T. L. (1982) Antagonism by phenoxybenzamine and pentazocine of the antinociceptive effects of morphine in the spinal cord. *Neuropharmacology* **20,** 575–579.

Sanger, D. J. and McCarthy, P. S. (1980) Differential effects of morphine on food and water intake in food deprived and freely-feeding rats. *Psychopharmacology* **72,** 103–106.

Satoh, M., Kawairi, S., Yamamoto, M., Foong, F. -W., and Masuda, C. (1979) Analgesic action of cyclazocine: Blocking nociceptive responses induced by intra-arterial bradykinin injection and tooth pulp stimulation. *Arch. Int. Pharmacodyn.* **241,** 300–306.

Schmauss, C., Doherty, C., and Yaksh, T. L. (1983) The analgesic effects of an intrathecally administered partial opiate agonist, nalbuphine hydrochloride. *Eur. J. Pharmacol.* **86,** 1–7.

Schmidt, D. E. and Buxbaum, D. M. (1978) Effect of acute morphine administration on regional acetylcholine turnover in the rat. *Brain Res.* **147,** 194–200.

Schulz, R., Wilhelm, A., Pirke, K. M., Gramsch, C., and Herz, A. (1981) Beta-endorphin and dynorphin control serum luteinizing hormone level in immature-female arts. *Nature* **294,** 757–759.

Schulz, R., Wilhelm, A., Pirke, K., and Herz, A. (1982) Regulation of luteinizing hormone secretion in prepubertal male and female rats. *Life Sci.* **31,** 2167–2170.

Serri, O., Rasio, E., and Somma, M. (1981) Effects of naloxone on insulin induced release of pituitary hormones. *J. Clin. Endocrinol. Metab.* **53,** 206–208.

Shaar, C. J., Frederickson, R. C. A., Dininger, N. B., and Jackson, L. (1977) Enkephalin analogues and naloxone modulate the release of growth hormone and prolactin-evidence for regulation by an endogenous opioid peptide. *Life Sci.* **21,** 853–860.

Share, N. N. and Rackham, A. (1981) Intracerebral substance P in mice: Behavioral effects and narcotic agents. *Brain Res.* **211,** 379–386.

Sharp, B., Morley, J. C., Carlson, S. E., Gordon, J. B., Melmed, S., and Hershman, J. M. (1981) The role of opiates and endogenous opioid peptides in the regulation of rat TSH secretion. *Brain Res.* **219,** 335–344.

Shimada, A., Iizuka, H., and Yanagita, T. (1984) Agonist–antagonist interactions of pentazocine with morphine studied in mice. *Pharmacol. Biochem. Behav.* **20,** 531–535.

Simone, D. A., Bodnar, R. J., Goldman, E. J., and Pasternak, G. W. (1985) Involvement of opioid receptor subtypes in rat feeding behavior. *Life Sci.* **36,** 829–833.

Skingle, M. and Tyers, M. B. (1980) Further studies on opiate receptors that mediate antinociception: Tooth pulp stimulation in the dog. *Br. J. Pharmacol.* **70,** 323–327.

Smith, C. B., Sheldon, M. T., Bednarczyk, J. H., and Villar-real, J. E. (1972) Morphine-induced increases in the incorporation of 14C-tyrosine into 14C-dopamine and 14C-norepinephrine in the mouse brain: Antagonism by naloxone and tolerance. *J. Pharmacol. Exp. Ther.* **180,** 547–557.

Snelgar, R. S. and Vogt, M. (1980) Mapping, in the rat central nervous system, of morphine-induced changes in turnover of 5-hydroxytryptamine. *J. Physiol.* **314,** 395–410.

Spampinato, S., Locatelli, V., Cocchi, L., Vinventini, L., Bajusz, S., Ferri, S., and Mueller, E. (1979) Involvement of brain serotonin in the prolactin releasing effect of opioid peptides. *Endocrinology* **105,** 163–170.

Spampinato, S., Esposito, E., Romandini, S., and Samanin, R. (1985) Changes of serotonin and dopamine metabolism in various forebrain areas of rats injected with morphine either systemically or in the raphe nuclei dorsalis and medianus. *Brain Res.* **328,** 89–95.

Spiegel, K. and Pasternak, G. W. (1984) Meptazinol: A novel mu-1 selective opioid analgesic. *J. Pharmacol. Exp. Ther.* **228,** 414–418.

Spiegel, K., Kourides, I. A., and Pasternak, G. W. (1982) Different receptors mediate morphine-induced prolactin and growth hormone release. *Life Sci.* **31,** 2177–2180.

Spiler, I. J. and Molitch, M. E. (1980) Lack of modulation of pituitary hormone stress response by neural pathways involving opiate receptors. *J. Clin. Endocrinol. Metab.* **50,** 516–520.

Stinus, L., Koob, G. F., Ling, N., Bloom, F. E., and LeMoal, M. (1980) Locomotor activation induced by infusion of endorphins into the ventral tegmental area: Evidence for opiate-dopamine interactions. *Proc. Natl. Acad. Sci USA* **77,** 2323–2327.

Stubbs, W. A., Jones, A., Edwards, C. R. W., Delitala, G., Jeffcoate, W. J., Ratter, S. J., Besser, G. M., Bloom, S. R., and Aberti, K. G. M. M. (1978) Hormonal and metabolic responses to an enkephalin analogue in normal man. *Lancet* **2,** 1225–1227.

Su, T. -P. (1985) Further demonstration of kappa opioid binding sites in the brain: Evidence for heterogeneity. *J. Pharmacol. Exp. Ther.* **232,** 144–148.

Szerb, J. (1974) Lack of effect of morphine in reducing the release of labelled acetylcholine from brain slices stimulated electrically. *Eur. J. Pharmacol.* **29,** 192–194.

Tepper, P. and Woods, J. H. (1978) Changes in locomotor activity and naloxone-induced jumping in mice produced by WIN 35, 197-2 (ethylketazocine) and morphine. *Psychopharmacology* **58,** 125–129.

Tepperman, F. S. and Hirst, M. (1983) Effect of intrahypothalamic injection of [D-ala^2,D-leu^5]enkephal in on feeding and temperature in the rat. *Eur. J. Pharmacol.* **96,** 243–249.

Terry, C. L., Crowley, W. R., and Johnson, M. D. (1982) Regulation of episodic growth hormone secretion by central epinephrine system. *J. Clin. Invest.* **69,** 104–112.

Thorn, B. E. and Levitt, R. A. (1980) Etorphine induction of analgesia and catatonia in the rat: Systemic or intracranial injection. *Neuropharmacol.* **19,** 203–207.

Tolis, G., Hickey, J., and Guyda, H. (1975) Effects of morphine on serum growth hormone, cortisol, prolactin and thyroid-stimulating hormone in man. *J. Clin. Endocrinol. Metab.* **41,** 797–800.

Tolis, G., Jukier, L., Wiesen, M., and Krieger, D. T. (1982) Effect of naloxone on pituitary hypersecretory syndromes. *J. Clin. Endocrinol. Metab.* **54**, 780–784.

Trabucchi, M., Poli, A., Tonon, G. C., and Spano, P. F. (1978) Interaction Among Enkephalinergic and Dopaminergic Systems in Striatum and Limbic Forebrain, in *Catecholamines: Basic and Clinical Frontiers* (Usdin, E., Kopin, I. J., and Barchas, J., eds.) Pergamon, New York.

Trulson, M. E. and Arasteh, K. (1985) Morphine increases the activity of midbrain dopamine neurons in vitro. *Eur. J. Pharmacol.* **114**, 105–109.

Tseng, L. -F., Ostwald, T. J., Loh, H. H., and Li, C. H. (1979) Behavioral activities of opioid peptides and morphine sulfate in golden hamsters and rats. *Psychopharmacology,* **64**, 215–218.

Tseng, L. -F., Cheng, S. S., and Fujimoto, J. M. (1983) Inhibition of tail-flick and shaking responses by intrathecal and intraventricular D-Ala²-D-Leu⁵-enkephal and be ta-endorphin in anesthetized rats. *J. Pharmacol. Exp. Ther.* **224**, 51–54.

Upton, N., Gonzalez, J. P., and Sewell, R. D. E. (1983) Characterization of a kappa agonist-like antinoiceptive action of tifluadom. *Neuropharmacology* **22**, 1241–1242.

Van Loon, G. R. and deSouza, E. B. (1978) Effects of β-endorphin on brain serotonin metabolism. *Life Sci.* **23**, 971–978.

VanVugt, D. A., Bruni, J. F., and Meitis, J. (1978) Naloxone inhibition of stress-induced increase in PRL secretion. *Life Sci.* **22**, 85–90.

VanVugt, D. A., Bruni, J. F., Sylvester, P. W., Chen, H. T., Ieiri, T., and Meitis, J. (1979) Interaction between opiates and hypothalamic dopamine on prolactin release. *Life Sci.* **24**, 2361–2368.

VanVugt, D. A., Sylvester, P. W., Aylsworth, C. F., and Meitis, J. (1981) Comparison of acute effects of dynorphin and β-endorphin on prolactin release in the rat. *Endocrinology* **108**, 2017–2018.

Volavka, J., Cho, D., and Mallaya, A. (1979a) Naloxone increases ACTH and cortisol levels in man. *N. Engl. J. Med.* **300**, 1056.

Volavka, J., Mallya, A., Bauman, J., Pevnick, J., Cho, D., Reker, D., James, B., and Dornbush, R. (1979b) Hormonal and other effects of naltrexone in normal men. *Adv. Exp. Med. Biol.* **116**, 291–305.

Volavka, J., Bauman, J., Pevnick, J., Reker, D., James, B., and Cho, D. (1980) Short-term hormonal effects of naloxone in man. *Psychoneuroendocrinology* **5**, 225–234.

Von GraffenFried, B., Del Pozo, E., Roubicek, J., Krebs, E., Poldinger, W., Burmeister, P., and Kerp, L. (1978) Effects of the synthetic analogue FK 33-824 in man. *Nature* **729**, 730.

Westerink, B. H. C. and Korf, J. (1976) Comparison of effects of drugs on dopamine metabolism in the substantia nigra and the corpus striatum of rat brain. *Eur. J. Pharmacol.* **40**, 131–136.

Williams, J. T. and Zieglgansberger, W. (1981) Neurons in the frontal cortex of the rat carry multiple opiate receptors. *Brain Res.* **226**, 304–308.

Wood, P. L. (1982a) Multiple opiate receptors: Support for unique mu, delta, and kappa sites. *Neuropharmacology* **21**, 487–497.

Wood, P. L. (1982b) Phasic enkephalinergic modulation of nigrostriatal dopamine metabolism: Potentiation with enkephalinase inhibitors. *Eur. J. Pharmacol.* **82**, 119–120.

Wood, P. L. (1983a) Opioid receptor affinities of kappa agonists, agonist/ antagonists and antagonists in vitro and in vivo. *Prog. Neuropsychopharmacol. Biol. Psychiat.* **7**, 657–662.

Wood, P. L. (1983b) Opioid regulation of CNS dopaminergic pathways: A review of methodology, receptor types, regional variations and species differences. *Peptides* **4**, 595–601.

Wood, P. L. (1984a) Kappa agonist analgesics: Evidence for mu-2 and delta opioid receptor antagonism. *Drug Dev. Res.* **4**, 429–435.

Wood, P. L. (1984b) Animal Models in Analgesic Testing, in *Analgesics: Neurochemical, Behavioral and Clinical Perspectives* (M. Kuhar and G. Pasternak, eds.) Raven, New York.

Wood, P. L. (1985) In vivo evaluation of mu, delta and kappa opioid receptor agonists on spinal 5-HT metabolism in the rat. *Neuropeptides* **5**, 319–322.

Wood, P. L. and Pasternak, G. W. (1983) Specific mu-2 opioid isoreceptor regulation of nigrostriatal neurons: In vivo evidence with naloxonazine. *Neurosci. Lett.* **37**, 291–293.

Wood, P. L. and Rackham, A. (1981) Actions of kappa, sigma and partial mu narcotic receptor agonists on rat brain acetylcholine turnover. *Neurosci. Lett.* **23**, 75–80.

Wood, P. L. and Richard, J. W. (1982) Morphine and nigrostriatal function in the rat and mouse: Role of nigral and striatal opiate receptors. *Neuropharmacology* **21**, 1305–1310.

Wood, P. L. and Stotland, L. M. (1980) Actions of enkephalin, mu and partial agonist analgesics on acetylcholine turnover in rat brain. *Neuropharmacology* **19**, 975–982.

Wood, P. L., McQuade, P. S., and Nair, N. P. V. (1984a) GABAergic and opioid regulation of the substantia innominata-cortical cholinergic pathway in the rat. *Prog. Neuropsychopharmacol. Biol. Psychiat.* **8**, 789–792.

Wood, P. L., Pilapil, C., Thakur, M., and Richard, J. W. (1984b) WIN 44,441: A stereospecific and long-acting narcotic antagonist. *Pharmaceut. Res.* **1**, 46–48.

Wood, P. L., Stotland, L. M., and Rackham, A. (1984c) Opiate Receptor Regulation of Acetylcholine Metabolism: Role of Mu, Delta, Kappa and Sigma Narcotic Receptors, in *Dynamics of Neurotransmitter Function* (Hanin, I., ed.) Raven, New York.

Wood, P. L., McQuade, P., Richard, J. W., and Thakur, M. (1983a) Agonist/ antagonist analgesics and nigrostriatal dopamine metabolism in the rat: Evidence for receptor dualism. *Life Sci.* **33**, 759–762.

Wood, P. L., Sanschagrin, D., Richard, J. W., and Thakur, M., (1983b) Multiple opiate receptor affinities of kappa and agonist/antagonist analgesics: In vivo assessment. *J. Pharmacol. Exp. Ther.* **226**, 545–550.

Wood, P. L., Hudgin, R. L., and Rackham, A. (1982a) Neuropharmacology of Kappa and Agonist/Antagonist Analgesics, in *Quo Vadis? Analgesia and Enkephalinases* Groupe Sanofi, Montpellier.

Wood, P. L., Richard, J. W., and Thakur, M. (1982b) Mu opiate isoreceptors: Differentiation with kappa agonists. *Life Sci.* **31**, 2313–2317.

Wood, P. L., Rackham, A., and Richard, J. (1981a) Spinal analgesia: Comparison of the mu agonist morphine and the kappa agonist ethylketazocine. *Life Sci.* **28**, 2119–2125.

Wood, P. L., Charleson, S. E., Lane, D., and Hudgin, R. L. (1981b) Multiple opiate receptors: Differential binding of mu, kappa and delta agonists. *Neuropharmacology* **20**, 1215–1220.

Wood, P. L., Stotland, M., Richard, J. W., and Rackham, A. (1980) Actions of mu, kappa, sigma, delta and agonist/antagonist opiates on striatal dopaminergic function. *J. Pharmacol. Exp. Ther.* **215**, 697–703.

Wood, P. L., Cheney, D. L., and Costa, E. (1979) An investigation of whether septal gamma-aminobutyrate-containing interneurons are involved in the reduction of the turnover rate of acetylcholine elicited by substance P and β-endorphin in the hippocampus. *Neuroscience* **4**, 1479–1484.

Yaksh, T. L. (1985) The physiology and pharmacology of spinal opiates. *Ann. Rev. Pharmacol. Toxicol.* **25**, 433–462.

Yaksh, T. L. and Rudy, T. A. (1978) Narcotic analgesics: CNS sites and mechanisms of action as revealed by intracerebral injection techniques. *Pain* **4**, 299–359.

Zhang, A. -Z. and Pasternak, G. W. (1981a) Opiates and enkephalins: A common binding site mediates their analgesic actions in rats. *Life Sci.* **29**, 843–857.

Zhang, A. -Z. and Pasternak, G. W. (1981b) Ontogeny of opioid pharmacology and receptors: High and low affinity site differences. *Eur. J. Pharmacol.* **73**, 29–40.

Zsilla, G., Cheney, D. L., Racagni, G., and Costa, E. (1976) Correlation between analgesia and the decrease of acetylcholine turnover rate in cortex and hippocampus elicited by morphine, meperidine, viminol R2 and azidomorphine. *J. Pharmacol. Exp. Ther.* **199**, 662–668.

Zsilla, G., Racagni, G., Cheney, D. L., and Costa, E. (1977) Constant rate infusion of deuterated phosphorylcholine to measure the effects of morphine on acetylcholine turnover rate in specific nuclei of rat brain. *Neuropharmacology* **16**, 25–31.

Chapter 11

Peripheral Actions Mediated by Opioid Receptors

Brian M. Cox

1. Introduction

The earliest references to the use of extracts of opium for therapeutic purposes refer not to their use in pain relief, but to their
effectiveness in relieving the symptoms of diarrhea and dysentery
(Jaffe and Martin, 1985), and this remains a very useful attribute
of opiate drugs. As we shall see later, at least part of this effect
can be attributed to local actions of the drug in the gastrointestinal
tract. For several reasons, there is again increasing interest in the
actions of opioids on peripheral tissues. There are potential therapeutic benefits to be obtained from a better understanding of
some of these actions, and analysis of opioid actions on peripheral systems may contribute to an understanding of the modes of
actions of opioids both in peripheral tissues and in the central
nervous system.

It is not always clear what actions of a drug should be described as "opioid." In this chapter, actions of drugs or peptides
will be considered in the light of two functional criteria. First, the
effect should be much more readily produced by one isomer, usually the $(-)$-isomer of an enantiomeric pair of opiates, than the
other. The stereoselectivity of opioid actions was noted by Beckett
and Casy (1954) more than 30 yr ago, and continues to be a widely
regarded criterion. Recently $(+)$-morphine has been synthesized

and is available for comparison with ($-$)-morphine (Jaquet et al., 1977), in addition to the frequently used enantiomeric pairs, levorphanol, dextrorphan, and ($-$)- and ($+$)-methadone. Second, the actions of drugs and peptides that are antagonized by naloxone at reasonably low concentrations (less than 5–10 μM) or by reasonably low doses of naloxone in intact animals (less than 10–20 mg/kg) will be defined as "opioid," unless other evidence strongly suggests that opioid receptors are not implicated in the effect. Stereoselectivity is also a feature of opioid antagonist action. The recent availability of ($+$)-naloxone (Iijima et al., 1978) makes a comparison of the antagonistic effects of the two naloxone isomers a useful secondary criterion for characterization of a drug effect. Actions of drugs or peptides that are not prevented or reversed by ($-$)-naloxone administration will be considered to arise from some different mechanism in which opioid receptors are not implicated. It will be apparent immediately that this functional definition implies that naloxone antagonizes actions of opioids not only at mu receptors, but also at delta, kappa, and other types of opioid receptors. There is good evidence that naloxone can antagonize agonist actions at delta and kappa receptors in in vitro preparations (*see* section 2), although it is possible that in intact animals some actions mediated through delta or kappa receptors may be difficult to antagonize by quite high doses of naloxone. Actions of opioids at epsilon receptors (Schulz et al., 1979a) appear to be sensitive to naloxone antagonism, but the ability of naloxone to antagonize actions of drugs at sigma receptors is uncertain (compare Martin et al., 1976 and Brady et al., 1982). This aspect of naloxone pharmacology probably needs further clarification. At present, however, there is little information available on the distribution and function of sigma receptors in peripheral tissues.

The methods available for the discrimination of the types of receptors mediating the actions of opioids in peripheral tissues also require some comment. The apparent presence in the central nervous system of several types of opioid binding sites has received much support from radiolabeled ligand binding studies, which have demonstrated the heterogeneous nature of binding sites for opioid drugs and peptides in membrane preparations derived from brain homogenates (*see* chapter by Yossef Itzhak). However, attempts to measure radiolabeled opioid binding in peripheral tissues have often been less successful, with the exception of studies conducted in guinea pig ileum. There are several reasons for this. In some tissues, it is possible that studies with a radiolabeled ligand with receptor-type selectivity appropriate to the receptor type present have not yet been attempted. In other cases, the receptors probably are present only in the neural elements of the tissue, which comprise a very small fraction of the total tissue mass. Specific binding then becomes a very small fraction of the total binding of the labeled ligand in such tissues, and is too unreliable to permit meaningful analysis. These problems may be overcome in the future by the application of quantitative autoradiographic techniques to peripheral opioid receptors.

Conclusions about the receptors mediating opioid effects may also be drawn from an analysis of the opioid action. There are several methods that can be used to characterize receptors on the basis of the effects they induce. Classically, measurement of the effectiveness of an antagonist in shifting the agonist dose–response curve to the right along the concentration axis, allowing the computation of the apparent equilibrium dissociation constant of the antagonist for the receptor, has been an effective method for characterizing receptors. Kosterlitz and coworkers (Kosterlitz and Watt, 1968; Lord et al., 1977) have shown that quantitation of naloxone antagonism of opioid actions in peripheral tissues can be used to discriminate effects produced by different types of opioid receptors. Naloxone has higher affinity at mu-type receptors than at delta and kappa receptors, however, and it is not suitable for discriminating between delta and kappa receptors. Naloxone may also have similar affinities at mu and epsilon receptors (compare Lord et al., 1977 and Schulz et al., 1979a). Eventually, it seems likely that pure, potent antagonists with unique selectivity for delta or kappa receptors will become available. Some progress toward that goal has been achieved with the synthesis of ICI 174864, a synthetic analog of enkephalin with fairly good selectivity for delta receptors (Cotton et al., 1984).

Other approaches are also needed. The occurrence of opioid receptor heterogeneity was predicated on the basis of experiments in which the relative potencies of a series of agonists in inducing a spectrum of pharmacological effects were compared (Martin et al., 1976), and comparison of agonist potencies remains a useful initial method for providing preliminary characterization of the receptor types mediating a particular effect. As ligands with almost complete specificity for one receptor type become available, this method will continue to be useful. Most stable opioids presently available, however, have some ability to react with more than one type of opioid receptor type; a purely qualitative analysis of their actions is therefore inadequate to discriminate receptors mediating their effects. Estimation of agonist affinity from a consideration of the effects mediated by the agonist is also fraught with difficulty. Theoretical aspects of the analysis of agonist actions are the subject of a recent review (Black and Leff, 1983). Differences in the intrinsic efficacy of agonists and in the magnitude of receptor reserves (or in the number of "spare" receptors) in different tissues make comparisons of estimates of agonist potency (ED_{50}, A_{50}) relatively uninformative. Furchgott (1978), however, has described a procedure, based on the comparison of agonist dose–response curves before and after occlusion of a fraction of the receptors with an irreversible antagonist, which allows for the estimation of agonist affinity at the receptors mediating the observed effect. With the development of irreversible antagonists for opioid receptors (e.g., β-CNA, β-FNA: Portoghese et al., 1979; naloxonazine: Hahn et al., 1982), this method is applicable to opioid receptors. At this time, it has been applied in a few studies of actions of opioids, mainly in peripheral tissues in vitro (Porreca and Burks, 1983). It is noteworthy that the estimates of agonist affinity determined from such functional studies yield affinity estimates that are severalfold lower than the affinities of opioids for receptors estimated from radiolabeled ligand binding studies. It is generally assumed that this discrepancy results from the absence in washed membrane preparations of critical ions and nucleotides, factors that normally regulate agonists binding and probably also mediate coupling of the receptors to effector systems within the cell (Blume et al., 1979). Further study is needed to confirm that this is the basis for the apparent anomaly.

In the sections that follow, the actions of opioids on various peripheral tissues will be described, and information that is available regarding the nature of the receptors mediating these effects will be reviewed. Where information is available, the distribution of endogenous opioids in peripheral tissues will also be briefly considered, since it is probable that opioid drugs and peptides will exert some effects at sites at which endogenous opioids are secreted (except where the secreted endogenous opioids serve an endocrine function on some distant structure).

2. Opioid Actions Related to the Enteric Nervous System

2.1. Endogenous Opioids in the Gastrointestinal Tract

Immunocytochemical studies have demonstrated the presence of numerous neurons containing enkephalin-like and dynorphin-like peptides in most regions of the gastrointestinal tract. Bioassays of intestinal extracts confirm the presence of enkephalin peptides in intestinal extracts (Hughes et al., 1977). In all mammalian species studied, neurons in the myenteric plexus staining with anti-enkephalin antisera have been found. The relative number of these enkephalin-containing cells appears to vary both with regard to location along the gastrointestinal tract from esophagus to colon and among species (Elde et al., 1976; Linnoila et al., 1978; Jessen et al., 1980; Schultzberg et al., 1980; Uddman et al., 1980). In general, fibers from the enkephalin-containing cells run from and between myenteric plexus ganglia and distribute extensively through the circular and longitudinal muscle layers. Some fibers also innervate the submucus plexus and the mucosa, but enkephalin cell bodies are rare or absent in the submucus plexus. Antisera to enkephalins and other peptides derived from proenkephalin A, including [Met⁵]enkephalyl-Arg-Phe and [Met⁵]enkephalyl-Arg-Gly-Leu, also stain gastrointestinal endocrine cells, including enterochromaffin cells and some of the gastrin-containing cells of the stomach antral mucosa in dog, pig, and man (Polak et al., 1977; Alumets et al., 1978; Jonsson, 1985).

There is indirect evidence suggesting that release of enkephalin from guinea pig intestine occurs in response to electrical stimulation. The concentration of enkephalin in an isolated segment of ileum is reported to fall after repeated electrical stimulation (Corbett et al., 1980). It is assumed that the decline in tissue concentration of enkephalin resulted from stimulated release (and subsequent degradation) of enkephalin from myenteric plexus neurons. Other investigators have noted that at a stimulation frequency of 10 Hz there was an initial wave of contractions followed by a transient inhibition of motility when the stimulus was turned off. Since the inhibition was antagonized by naloxone, it was assumed that endogenous opioid had been released in response to repeated stimuli or contractions (Puig et al., 1977). It has also been suggested that endogenous opioids might participate in the declining effectiveness of sustained increases in intraluminal pressure in inducing peristaltic contractions, since opioids depress peristaltic activity (see below) and naloxone apparently reduces the "fatigue" that occurs during prolonged exposure to pressure stimulation (van Neuten et al., 1976).

Dynorphin immunoreactivity has also been shown to occur in myenteric plexus neurons (Watson et al., 1981; Vincent et al., 1984), and dynorphin A has been extracted, purified, and sequenced from porcine duodenum (Tachibana et al., 1982). Dynorphin-containing cells are found less frequently than enkephalin-containing cells in myenteric plexus, and there are fewer dynorphin-containing fibers. Their distribution is generally similar to enkephalin-containing fibers, with networks of fibers running into circular and longitudinal muscle layers. Dynorphin immunoreactivity has been shown to be released into perfusates of guinea pig ileum segments during peristalsis (Kromer et al., 1981; Donnerer et al., 1984).

Since both dynorphin A and enkephalins have been found in the gastrointestinal tract, it may be assumed that all opioid peptides derived from proenkephalin and prodynorphin are present in the tract and may be released in response to appropriate physiological stimuli, to act on gastrointestinal opioid receptors. In contrast, β-endorphin and related peptides derived from proopiomelanocortin have not been reported to be intrinsic to the gastrointestinal tract. β-Endorphin circulating in blood might conceivably exert effects on opioid receptors in the gastrointestinal tract. However, reported concentrations of β-endorphin in plasma, even after severe stimuli provoking maximum secretion of β-endorphin, do not appear to be high enough to occupy a significant fraction of opioid receptors in the gut (Cox and Baizman, 1982). The possibility that opioids secreted from adrenal medulla act on gastrointestinal opioid receptors cannot be evaluated at present, since the concentrations of adrenal opioid peptides in arterial blood are not known.

2.2. Effects of Opioids on Gastrointestinal Motility

Opioids can exert several different actions on gastrointestinal motility, and the effect that is most apparent depends both on the species and the method of investigation. In intact animals, the overall result of these actions is a decline in propulsive activity, resulting in a delay in the passage of gastrointestinal contents. After systemic administration, opioids can act at both central and peripheral sites to alter gastrointestinal function (Schulz et al., 1979b; Manara and Bianchetti, 1985). In this section, discussion will be limited to consideration of studies in which opioids have been applied locally to tissues of the gastrointestinal tract.

2.2.1. Opioid Stimulation of Gastrointestinal Muscle

Many early studies (summarized by Vaughan Williams, 1954) demonstrated that morphine induced an increase in "tone" in the gastrointestinal tract of rabbit, dog, and man. These observations appeared in conflict with the overall effect of reduced propulsion of gut contents, resulting in constipation. However, Vaughan Williams was able to show that the increase in "tone" was associated with increased segmenting activity and a resulting decline in aboral transport of fluid (Vaughan Williams, 1954). Work of gastrointestinal muscle was increased, but propulsion reduced. This effect of morphine on gastrointestinal motility appears to predominate in most mammalian species. The mechanism by which morphine increases gastrointestinal contractions has been investigated in a series of studies by Burks and coworkers. Pretreatment of dogs with reserpine to deplete intestinal stores of serotonin, or treatment of isolated ileal segments with serotonin antagonists such as cyproheptadine or cinanserin, reduced or prevented the stimulant action of morphine. The stimulation was also prevented by tetrodotoxin. These results suggest that morphine induced the release of serotonin from neurons (Burks, 1973). Since serotonin is a powerful stimulant of gut musculature, it is probable that serotonin release is a major factor in the morphine stimulant effect. The effects of both morphine and serotonin were antagonized by tetrodotoxin and atropine. Burks (1973) has therefore suggested that released serotonin may increase contractions through a stimulation of excitatory cholinergic neurons.

There is some evidence indicating that opioids may have a particular role in the functions of sphincter muscles throughout the gastrointestinal tract. In cats, stimulation of the vagus nerve induced a contraction of the pyloric sphincter that was antagonized by naloxone (Edin et al., 1980). Intraarterial injections of morphine and enkephalins also induced pyloric contraction. The tone in the lower esophageal sphincter of the opossum has also been reported to be sensitive to modulation by opioids: in this tissue, both contractile and relaxant actions were observed with different opioids (Rattan and Goyal, 1983).

The nature of the opioid receptors that mediate the contractile actions of morphine and other opioids has not been determined with certainty. Similar effects on dog intestine are produced by opioid peptides, including [Met^5]- and [Leu^5]enkephalin, [D-Ala^2-Met^5]enkephalin-NH$_2$, β-endorphin, α-endorphin, γ-endorphin, morphiceptin, and dynorphin A (1-13) (Burks et al., 1982; Davis et al., 1983). The actions of all these peptides were antagonized by naloxone, but quantitative estimates of naloxone potencies against each agent are not available. The effectiveness of mu-selective agonists like morphine and morphiceptin and kappa-selective agonists like dynorphin A (1-13) suggests that more than one opioid receptor type may be capable of mediating contractile actions on gastrointestinal muscle. Opioid induced contractions of rat ileum have also been reported (Nijkamp and van Ree, 1980; Huidobro-Toro and Way, 1981). In this tissue, estimates of the naloxone equilibrium constants in antagonizing contractions induced by normorphine, enkephalins, and β-endorphin have been made (Shaw, 1979). A naloxone K_e (apparent equilibrium dissociation constant) of about 4 nM against normorphine contrasts with K_e values of between 20 and 30 nM against the peptide opioids. These results indicate that mu receptors mediate the actions of normorphine, whereas delta receptors probably mediate the effects of enkephalins and β-endorphin in this tissue. In sheep, intravenous administration of mu- and kappa-selective agonists induced an increase in duodenal motility, which could be prevented by a quaternized derivative of naloxone or by methyl atropine administration (Ruckebusch et al., 1984), suggesting the presence of mu and kappa receptors mediating increased contractions in this species.

There is some indication that the stimulant actions of some opioids may not be entirely attributable to neuronally mediated release of a stimulant agent. In dog intestine, the stimulant actions of [Met^5]enkephalin were largely resistant to tetrodotoxin, in contrast to the actions of other opioids (Burks et al., 1982). Similarly, some of the stimulant actions of opioids in rat rectum were not antagonized by tetrodotoxin (Nijkamp and van Ree, 1980). Thus, it is possible that some opioids can either directly stimulate smooth muscle cells or release a stimulatory agent to contract muscle cells through an action that does not require activation of neuronal sodium channels. The direct contraction of gastric and intestinal circular muscle cells by opioids has been reported (Bitar and Makhlouf, 1982, 1985). In these studies, cells of guinea pig stomach or guinea pig and human intestine were isolated by enzymatic tissue dispersion and sieving. Changes in muscle cell length induced by applied agents were observed and quantified optically. Contractions of circular but not longitudinal muscle cells were induced by submicromolar concentrations of dynorphin A (1-13), [Met^5]enkephalin, [Met^5]enkephalyl-Arg-Phe, β-neo-endorphin, morphine, and [Leu^5]enkephalin (in order of decreasing potency). Although antagonist affinity estimates are not available, comparisons of the sensitivities of each opioid to antagonism by naloxone, and the benzomorphan antagonist Mr2266, which has relatively more antagonist effect at kappa receptors, suggest that at least mu and kappa receptors are capable of mediating this action (Bitar and Mahklouf, 1985). The possible involvement of other types of opioid receptor cannot be ruled out. These results provide fairly strong evidence that opioids can directly stimulate gut circular muscle cells. Electron microscopic evidence of the absence of neuronal terminals adhering to the dispersed muscle cells is not available, however, and experiments testing the sensitivity of this stimulant action to tetrodotoxin have not been reported. It is important to establish these points, since at most sites opioids appear to alter the activity of muscle, endocrine, or other secretory cells, indirectly through modification of neuronal activity. Whatever mechanism is involved, the presence of a network of opioid peptide-containing nerve fibers in gastrointestinal circular muscle layers is well established (see section 2.1). Thus, opioid stimulation of circular muscle fibers may play an important physiological role in the control of gastrointestinal function.

2.2.2. Inhibitory Actions of Opioids on Gastrointestinal Muscle

It has long been known that opioids inhibit the peristaltic reflex (Trendelenburg, 1917). It was also shown that this effect was produced only by the analgesically active isomer of enantiomeric pairs of opioids (Schaumann et al., 1952) and was antagonized by the opiate partial agonist, nalorphine (Green, 1959). Thus, there were many early indications that the inhibitory effects of opioids on the gastrointestinal tract were mediated by receptor mechanisms with some important similarities to the mechanisms underlying opiate analgesia.

The guinea pig ileum has been an extremely convenient tissue for the study of opioid inhibitory properties. This seems to be largely attributable to the lack of rhythmic "spontaneous" contractions in isolated segments of ileum from guinea pig. In other species, such rhythmic activity masks possible inhibitory actions of opioids and makes reliable quantitation almost impossible. In the guinea pig, however, the lack of inherent tone makes it possible to induce quantitatively consistent contractions by chemical, mechanical, or electrical stimulation. Contractions induced by nicotine, serotonin, and barium were shown to be inhibited by morphine, whereas responses to directly acting agents like acetylcholine and histamine were not (Kosterlitz and Robinson, 1958). Paton (1957) reported that electrical stimulation of isolated guinea pig ileum segments produced contractions that could be inhibited by morphine, and showed that the opiates acted by inhibiting the release of acetylcholine from nerve terminals. Subsequently, opiate inhibition of acetylcholine release was shown to be stereospecific, and potencies of opiates were shown to be correlated with their analgesic potencies (Cox and Weinstock, 1966). Nalorphine inhibited contractions in this tissue with a potency equivalent to that of morphine. Lower concentrations were shown to antagonize the effects of morphine, however (Cox and Weinstock, 1966). It is now known that these complex actions of nalorphine can be explained by its antagonistic activity at mu receptors through which morphine acted, and its agonist activity at kappa receptors.

Later, the pure antagonist, naloxone, became available. The importance of naloxone as an antagonist for use in the characterization of opioid receptors was recognized by Kosterlitz and Watt (1968). They introduced a method by which the apparent equilibrium dissociation constant (K_e) for naloxone antagonism of opioid inhibition of electrically stimulated contractions of guinea pig ileum could be measured. Their single-dose method was applicable to partial opioid agonists and led to the recognition that there were differences in the manner in which various synthetic opiates activated opioid receptors in guinea pig ileum. In studies with naloxone, however, which has negligible agonist activity, it is preferable to examine the effects of several concentrations of naloxone in shifting the agonist dose–response curve in order to estimate the antagonist K_e, using the procedure originally described by Schild (1949). Kappa agonists (Hutchison et al., 1975) and delta agonists (Lord et al., 1977) were shown to be less sensitive to antagonism by naloxone than agonist acting through mu receptors.

Opioid receptors in guinea pig ileum can also be examined by measurement of radiolabeled ligand binding (Terenius, 1973; Creese and Snyder, 1975). In general, binding sites in this tissue have similar properties to binding sites in brain. Antagonist affinity estimates based on inhibition of opioid agonist activity in smooth muscle are closely comparable to estimates of affinity determined by direct estimates of radiolabeled naloxone binding to brain or ileum homogenates (Table 1). Sodium and guanine nucleotides reduce agonist affinity at guinea pig ileum receptors, as in the central nervous system (Creese and Snyder, 1975; Zukin and Gintzler, 1980). With receptor-type selective labeled agonists, the presence of mu, kappa, and delta opioid binding sites in homogenates of guinea pig ileum longitudinal muscle (with associated myenteric plexus) has been demonstrated (Leslie et al., 1980). In view of the high potencies of mu and kappa agonists in guinea pig ileum, the presence of receptors of these types is not surprising. The observation of delta-type binding sites was unexpected, since estimates of antagonist potencies suggest that even agonists with potency at delta receptors in other tissues usually inhibit electrically induced contractions of guinea pig ileum by activating mu receptors (Lord et al., 1977; Chavkin and Goldstein, 1981). This suggests that delta receptors are present, but not usually functional in guinea pig ileum myenteric plexus and longitudinal muscle. It is possible that the delta receptors are located on neurons passing from the myenteric plexus to the mucosa, since it has been shown that mucosal secretion is inhibited by opioids acting on delta receptors (Kachur and Miller, 1982). It is also possible that some or all of the cholinergic neurons regulating longitudinal muscle contraction have a relatively low concentration of delta receptors. In preparations rendered selectively tolerant to mu agonists, some inhibition of electrically stimulated contractions through delta receptors has been reported (Gintzler and Scalisi, 1982). It is noteworthy that lower specific binding of opioids is apparent in homogenates of rabbit and rat longitudinal muscle–myenteric plexus, and the few binding sites observed have the properties of delta receptors (Leslie et al., 1980). Oka (1980) has reported that enkephalins, but not mu selective agonists like morphine, inhibit electrically evoked contractions of rabbit ileum longitudinal muscle. Naloxone antagonized this action, with a K_e of 43 nM, suggesting mediation by a delta receptor.

Further insights into the receptors mediating opioids effects on guinea pig ileum have come from experiments with irreversible antagonists. Pretreatment of the tissue with naloxonazine, which irreversibly blocks mu_1 receptors, did not block the actions of mu agonists on isolated guinea pig ileum (Gintzler and Pasternak, 1983). It is presumed, therefore, that the receptors through which morphine and many opioid peptides inhibit ace-

TABLE 1
Opioid Receptors in the Gastrointestinal Tract

Location/species	Function	Antagonist	K_e, nM[a] Agonist[c]	Receptor type	Comments	Reference
Lower esophageal sphincter, opussum	Contraction	Naloxone	nd[b]	Delta (?)	DADLE active, meperidine inactive	Rattan and Goyal, 1983
Lower esophageal sphincter, opussum	Inhibition	Naloxone	nd[b]	Mu, kappa (?)	Ketocyclazocine, meperidine active	Rattan and Goyal, 1983
Stomach circular muscle, guinea pig	Contraction	Naloxone	nd[b]	Mu, kappa (?)	Normorphine, dynorphin active	Bitar and Makhlouf, 1982
Duodenum, sheep	Increased motility	N-Methylnaloxone naloxone	nd[b]	Mu, kappa (?)	Morphine, U50488H active	Ruckebusch et al., 1984
Intestine, dog	Contraction	Naloxone	nd[b]	Mu, delta, kappa, (epsilon) (?)	Morphiceptin, enkephalins, dynorphin A, β-endorphin active	Burks et al., 1982
Ileum, guinea pig	Inhibition of binding	Naloxone	2, [³H]DHM	Mu	—	Leslie et al., 1980
Illeum, guinea pig	Inhibition of binding		nd[b]	Delta	High affinity [³H]DADLE binding, DAGO low affinity	Leslie et al., 1980

Tissue	Response	Antagonist	K_e, Agonist	Receptor	Comments	Reference
Ileum, guinea pig	Hyperpolarization, myenteric plexus neurons	Naloxone	2, Normorphine	Mu	—	Morita and North, 1982
Ileum, guinea pig	Inhibition of contraction	Naloxone	2–4, Normorphine	Mu_2	—	Lord et al., 1977; Chavkin and Goldstein, 1981; Gintzler Pasternak, 1983
	Inhibition of contraction	Naloxone	15–30, EKC, dyn A	Kappa	—	Lord et al., 1977; Chavkin and Goldstein, 1981
	Inhibition of contraction	Naloxone	nd^b	Delta	DADLE active in mu tolerant tissues	Gintzler and Scalisi, 1982
Ileum, rabbit	Inhibition of contraction	Naloxone	43, Met^5-enkephalin	Delta	Morphine inactive	Oka, 1980
Ileum, guinea pig	Inhibition of Cl^- secretion	Naloxone	60–100, Enkephalins	Delta	Morphine, EKC, very low potency	Kachur and Miller, 1982
	Inhibition of Cl^- secretion	ICI 154129	750 DADLE	Delta		Vinayek et al., 1983
Rectum, rat	Contraction	Naloxone	4, Normorphine	Mu	—	Shaw, 1979
	Contraction	Naloxone	20–30, Enkephalins	Delta	—	Shaw, 1979

[a]K_e, apparent equilibrium dissociation constant.
[b]nd, not determined.
[c]Abbreviations: DHM, dihydromorphine; DADLE, [D-Ala[2]-D-Leu[5]]enkephalin; DAGO, Tyr-D-Ala-Gly-N(Me)Phe-Gly-ol; EKC, ethylketo-cyclazocine.

tylcholine release in this tissue are of the mu_2 type. The mu receptor antagonist, β-funaltrexamine (β-FNA), also antagonized the actions of mu-selective agonists, but did not significantly antagonize kappa-selective agonists such as ethylketocyclazocine and dynorphin A (1-13) (Huidobro-Toro et al., 1982). The less receptor-type selective irreversible antagonist, β-chlornaltrexamine (β-CNA), antagonizes the actions of mu-, delta-, and kappa-selective agonists in isolated guinea pig ileum preparations (Chavkin and Goldstein, 1981). However, by using high concentrations of agonists with known receptor selectivity to protect specific receptors from inactivation by β-CNA, it was possible to demonstrate that the mu agonist, normorphine, and the kappa agonist, dynorphin A (1-13), were acting on different receptor populations to inhibit contractions of the guinea pig ileum preparation (Chavkin and Goldstein, 1981). In these studies, it was also shown that [Leu[5]]enkephalin, a peptide with preferential activity at delta receptors in other tissues, acts through mu receptors in guinea pig ileum. Studies with β-CNA have also demonstrated that there is a large "reserve" of mu and kappa receptors in this tissue. Pretreatment with low concentrations of β-CNA produced a parallel shift to the right in the dose–response curves for normorphine or dynorphin A (Chavkin and Goldstein, 1984). Only at higher concentrations of β-CNA was the maximum response to these agonists reduced. The magnitude of the parallel shift in dose–response curves suggests that there was a spare receptor fraction of about 90%, for both mu and kappa receptors.

Irreversible antagonists have also been used in the determination of agonist dissociation constants for opioids at receptors in isolated guinea pig ileum preparations, using the method described by Furchgott (1978). A normorphine dissociation constant of 1.5 μM has been reported by both Porreca and Burks (1983) and Chavkin and Goldstein (1984). The dynorphin A (1-13) dissociation constant, determined by the same procedure, is 10 nM (Chavkin and Goldstein, 1984). The IC_{50} values for both normorphine and dynorphin A (1-13) were about one-twentieth of the estimated dissociation constants. After induction of tolerance to mu agonists through the implantation of morphine pellets, the spare receptor fraction for normorphine was significantly reduced, without any significant change in the apparent affinity for normorphine (Porreca and Burks, 1983; Chavkin and Goldstein, 1984). This result might indicate that tolerance to morphine is associated with a reduction in the number of mu receptors. Measurements of radiolabeled ligand binding, however, both in morphine-tolerant guinea pig ileum (Cox and Padhya, 1977) and in brain membrane preparations from morphine tolerant animals (Klee and Streaty, 1974; Dum et al., 1979), indicate that the number of opioid binding sites is not changed by prior chronic treatment with morphine. It therefore seems probable that the coupling between opioid mu receptors and tissue effector systems is impaired in morphine tolerance. Thus, the fraction of receptors needed to be occupied for induction of a given effect is increased and the receptor reserve reduced.

The mechanisms by which opioids inhibit the release of acetylcholine from guinea pig myenteric neurons has been studied in some detail at an electrophysiological level. Opioids that are mu selective have been reported to induce a naloxone-reversible hyperpolarization of many myenteric plexus neurons. This effect was attributed to an opening of potassium channels (Morita and North, 1982). Hyperpolarization was not observed with kappa selective agonists (Cherubini and North, 1985), however. Both mu and kappa agonists reduced excitatory postsynaptic potentials (EPSP) in myenteric plexus neurons. The reduction in EPSP amplitude induced by morphine was inhibited by low concentrations of barium, confirming that this effect also resulted from an opening of potassium channels, but the reduction in EPSP amplitude induced by dynorphin was not depressed by the same concentration of barium. Measurement of calcium conductance indicated that kappa agonists induced a direct reduction of calcium influx, an effect not observed with normorphine or other mu agonists (Cherubini and North, 1985). It is therefore clear that mu and kappa agonists reduce transmitter release in the guinea pig myenteric plexus by modulating different ionic conductances. The reported ability of dynorphin A (1-13) to restore the potency of morphine in guinea pig ileum preparations rendered tolerant to morphine (Rezvani and Way, 1984), may be explained by the different mechanisms by which these agents inhibit acetylcholine release. The mu receptor–potassium channel system displays tolerance to morphine, but the sensitivity of the kappa receptor–calcium channel system is little changed by morphine pretreatment (Schulz et al., 1981). Synergism between these two different mechanisms for reduction of calcium influx during depolarization might not be very obvious in normal tissues, where there is a very large receptor reserve in both systems. When the receptor reserve for mu regulation of potassium channels is reduced in morphine tolerant tissues (perhaps by influencing coupling between receptor and channel), however, synergism between the two systems may have a more significant effect on the opioid regulation of local intracellular calcium concentrations. Synergism would not be anticipated with ethylketocyclazocine, since this compound is reported to be an antagonist at mu receptors (Martin et al., 1976).

The mechanism by which opioid receptors regulate ion channels in myenteric plexus neurons is not known. Attempts to implicate an inhibition of the action of adenylate cyclase in the actions of opioids in myenteric plexus have generally failed to provide strong evidence in support of this hypothesis (Sawynok and Jhamandas, 1979). Guanine nucleotide binding proteins may have a significant role in the actions of mu agonists, however. As noted earlier, agonist binding at mu sites in guinea pig ileum homogenates is inhibited by guanine nucleotides (Zukin and Gintzler, 1980). Recent studies have also indicated that pertussis toxin, a toxin that selectively ADP-ribosylates nonstimulatory guanine nucleotide binding proteins (Kurose et al., 1983), can inhibit the actions of mu agonists in guinea pig ileum (Lujan et al., 1984; Tucker, 1984). The toxin can also inhibit the development of tolerance and dependence on normorphine if given to the guinea pig prior to the initiation of chronic opioid treatment (Tucker, 1984). The action of the toxin is reduced, however, if administration is delayed more than 12 h after the start of opioid treatment (Lux and Schulz, 1985). These results clearly implicate guanine nucleotide binding proteins in both the acute and chronic actions of mu agonists, although the mechanisms remain to be elucidated. These studies do not, however, provide specific support for a role for inhibition of adenylate cyclase in mu agonist action, since there is increasing evidence that guanine nucleotide binding proteins may participate in the coupling of receptors to other effectors systems in addition to adenylate cyclase. The recent report of a potassium channel in cardiac membranes that is coupled to muscarinic receptors through a guanine nucleotide binding protein raises the possibility that mu agonists may open potassium channels by a similar GTP-regulated mechanism (Pfaffinger et al., 1985). At this time, there is no evidence suggesting that kappa agonists regulate calcium conductance through an inhibition of adenylate cyclase.

2.3. Effects of Opioids on Gastrointestinal Secretion

Opioids may potentiate or reduce gastrointestinal secretions. These actions have generally been assumed to be exerted locally in the gastrointestinal tract, although in many in vivo studies the site of action of opioids on gastrointestinal secretion has not been determined. As in the case of motility effects of opioids, the effects of opioids on secretion may vary among different gastrointestinal structures and among species. There are contradictory reports concerning the effects of opioids on gastric and pancreatic secretions (for references, *see* the recent review by Schick and Schusdziarra, 1985).

Studies of opioid effects on isolated segments or sheets of intestinal tissue have provided evidence of a local antisecretory effect of opioids. Strips of intestinal mucosa from which the muscle layers have been removed are mounted in Ussing chambers between two buffer compartments into which drugs can be introduced. Drugs can be applied on either side, allowing drug effects on the serosal or mucosal surfaces to be studied (Kachur et al., 1980; Dobbins et al., 1980; McKay et al., 1981; Kachur and Miller, 1982). Secretion is associated with a net transport of chloride ions into the chamber on the mucosal side. Changes in ion transport across the mucosa are monitored by measuring the potential difference and short circuit current (I_{sc}). In rabbit ileum preparations, Dobbins et al. (1980) found that enkephalins applied to the serosal surface reduced the potential difference and I_{sc}. Kachur and Miller (1982), using guinea pig intestinal mucosa, examined the opioid receptor mediating this effect in more detail. The most potent agonist was [D-Ala^2,D-Leu^5]enkephalin (DADLE), a potent delta and mu agonist. Other mu agonists with lower activity at delta receptors (e.g., morphine and fentanyl), and kappa agonists (ethylketocyclazocine and dynorphin A (1-13)), were less potent or completely ineffective. These results suggest the likely involvement of delta receptors. Naloxone antagonized the enkephalin effect with K_e of 60–100 nM. This low naloxone potency is consistent with delta receptor involvement, although the K_e estimate is higher than has been observed at other delta receptors (Table 1). A peptide opioid antagonist, ICI 154129, with some selectivity (although low potency) for delta receptors (Shaw et al., 1982), antagonizes enkephalin inhibition of ion transport in guinea pig intestinal mucosa with a K_e of 750 nM (Vinayek et al., 1983). The very low potency of morphine has been confirmed by McKay et al. (1981), using rabbit ileum mucosa. It is noteworthy that McKay et al. found that the maximum reduction of the potential difference across the mucosa induced by morphine was substantially less than that observed with enkephalins (Dobbins et al., 1980; Kachur and Miller, 1982). This suggests that morphine does not have full efficacy in inhibiting ion transport in intestinal mucosa. Similarly, morphine does not have full efficacy in inhibiting adenylate cyclase through delta receptors in NG108-15 cells (Law et al., 1983). Thus, morphine may behave as a partial agonist at delta receptors in several systems.

The mechanism by which delta agonists reduce chloride secretion in ileal mucosa is not entirely understood. It is possible that they act directly on enterocytes. The presence of [Leu^5]enkephalin binding sites in enterocytes isolated from guinea pig ileum has been reported (Lopez-Ruiz et al., 1985). In these cells, enkephalins were observed to stimulate adenylate cyclase activity. These binding sites do not have the properties normally associated with delta (or other opioid) receptors, however. The [Leu^5]enkephalin affinity was in the micromolar range, and some D-Ala^2-substituted enkephalins had much lower affinities. The very low affinity might be attributed to measurement in intact cells, where guanine nucleotides might lower affinity of agonists substantially, relative to affinities measured in membrane suspensions. In other intact cells with delta receptors, however, enkephalin affinities two or three orders of magnitude higher than in enterocytes have been noted (Chang et al., 1978). Unfortunately, the enkephalin analogs used by Lopez-Ruiz et al. (1985) are different from those used by Kachur and Miller (1982) to inhibit chloride secretion, and are not well suited to discriminate between opioid receptors. On the basis of the evidence currently available, however, it seems unlikely that the low-affinity enkephalin binding sites are responsible for enkephalin inhibition of chloride secretion. Other workers have failed to find evidence of high-affinity enkephalin binding sites in rabbit ileal enterocytes (Binder et al., 1984).

There is some indirect evidence suggesting that the opioid inhibition of chloride secretion is neurally mediated. Binder and colleagues (Dobbins et al., 1980; Binder et al., 1984) observed that the enkephalin effect was inhibited by tetrodotoxin, an inhibitor of sodium channels in neurons but not in other tissues. Thus, enkephalins may indirectly affect chloride secretion, either by inhibiting excitatory neurons or stimulating inhibitory neurons. Further support for an action of enkephalins on the neural control of secretion is provided by electrophysiological studies on neurons of the submucus plexus in guinea pig cecum. Mihara and North (1986) have demonstrated that enkephalins (but not morphine) induce hyperpolarization of some submucus plexus neurons by opening potassium channels. The receptor mediating this effect had delta receptor characteristics, since the K_e values for both naloxone and the delta selective antagonist ICI 174864 were about 20 nM. The enkephalin inhibition of chloride secretion in rabbit ileum was not inhibited by phentolamine, haloperidol, or 6-hydroxydopamine treatment (Dobbins et al., 1980). Enkephalins were still active in the presence of muscarinic receptor agonists and were not antagonized by atropine. Collectively, these results suggest that the delta receptor-mediated local inhibition of chloride secretion in ileum is mediated by hyperpolarization of nonadrenergic, noncholinergic submucus plexus neurons.

2.4. Actions of Antidiarrheal Agents

All of the actions described above probably contribute to the antidiarrheal actions of opiates. There is likely to be a synergistic interaction between the reduction in motility and antisecretory effects of opiates. The reduction in propulsion of gastrointestinal contents allows longer time for fluid reabsorption. A reduction in fluid secretion also contributes to the production of dry, compacted feces (Powell, 1981). It is possible that both central and local actions of opioids contribute to these effects. The relative contributions of each component of opioid action on the gastrointestinal tract will vary among opioids, however, depending on both their ability to penetrate the central nervous system, and thus induce centrally mediated effects on motility and secretion, and their selectivities for the receptor types regulating gut function in the periphery. Since there are considerable species differences in the location and functions of different types of opioid receptors, especially in peripheral tissues, some opioid antidiarrheal agents will be more effective in some species than others. The etiology of diarrhea is also variable, and thus it is likely that the effectiveness of opioids in alleviating pathological diarrhea will be at least partly dependent on the nature of the causative agent.

Morphine is, of course, the oldest of the opioid antidiarrheal drugs. The actions of morphine are primarily exerted at mu receptors (e.g., see Lord et al., 1977). Morphine acts mainly by its effects on gastrointestinal motility; it has little effect on gastrointestinal secretion in guinea pig (Kachur et al., 1980), but has been reported to reduce prostaglandin-stimulated fluid secretion after systemic administration in rat (Coupar, 1978). The relative contributions of central and peripheral actions of systemically administered morphine on gastrointestinal propulsion have been assessed by Manara and colleagues (Manara and Bianchetti, 1985). After treatment of rats with quaternary opiate antagonists (Tavani et al., 1979; Ferretti et al., 1981), morphine and FK 33-824 were much less effective in reducing intestinal transit. Measurement of local tissue levels at various times after drug administration revealed a much better correlation between the reduction of gastrointestinal transit and the level of morphine in the gut than the level of morphine in brain (Bianchi et al., 1983). Fiocchi et al. (1982) have reported that reduction of propulsive movements in the small intestine is more important than delayed gastric emptying in the reduction of gastrointestinal transit by morphine in the rat.

Although morphine usually provides useful symptomatic relief of diarrhea, its actions in the central nervous system and its addictive liability limit its therapeutic value. Drugs with actions limited to the gastrointestinal tract are often more useful. Two such opioid agents have now become established as effective and useful antidiarrheal agents. Loperamide and diphenoxylate are mu-selective opioid agonists that do not penetrate the central nervous system in significant concentration (Awouters et al., 1983). Much of their effectiveness probably lies in their ability to reduce gastrointestinal propulsion. Recent studies have suggested, however, that they may also reduce gastrointestinal secretion through a nonopioid mechanism. Miller et al. (1985) have demonstrated a noncompetitive antagonism by loperamide of the substance P-stimulated influx of calcium into isolated enterocytes. This effect was not blocked by naloxone. Thus, a combination of opioid effects on gastrointestinal motility and nonopioid effects on secretion may contribute to the actions of these antidiarrheal agents. The demonstration by Miller and coworkers (Kachur and Miller, 1982) that gastrointestinal secretions can be reduced by activation of delta opioid receptors suggests that drugs with delta agonist activity might usefully complement the currently available antidiarrheal agents. Because of the many potential causes of diarrhea, treatment is likely to be facilitated by the availability of agents reducing gastrointestinal transit and secretion by different mechanisms.

3. Opioid Actions Related to the Sympathetic Nervous System

In this section, peripheral actions of opioids on the function of the sympathetic nervous system and tissues receiving major sympathetic innervation will be considered. Discussion of opioid actions on sympathetic regulation of cardiac function will be considered in section 4, however, where the sensitivity to opioids of both sympathetic and parasympathetic innervation of the heart will be reviewed. Likewise, the actions of opioids on the sympathetic innervation of vas deferens will be considered in section 5, in relation to opioid actions in the reproductive tract.

3.1. Endogenous Opioids and the Sympathetic Nervous System

Early biochemical studies by Hughes et al. (1977) demonstrated the presence of enkephalin-like biological activity in sympathetic nerve trunks, and immunocytochemical studies revealed the presence of enkephalins in adrenal medulla (Schultzberg et al., 1978). Subsequently, adrenal medullary tissue has been used as a major source of enkephalin precursors (Lewis et al., 1980) and of proenkephalin mRNA (Noda et al., 1982; Gubler et al., 1982, Comb et al., 1982). Enkephalins and the larger molecular weight peptides are released from adrenal medulla together with catecholamine in response to potassium perfusion of the gland or stimulation of the splanchnic nerve (Viveros et al., 1979; Chaminade et al., 1984).

The presence of enkephalin-like material in sympathetic ganglia has been demonstrated and, as in adrenal gland, has been shown to consist of both the pentapeptide enkephalins and higher molecular weight enkephalin containing peptides (Di Giulio et al., 1978). The immunocytochemical localization of enkephalin peptides in sympathetic ganglia of guinea pig, rat, and human, has also been described (Schultzberg et al., 1979; Hervonen et al., 1981). β-Endorphin does not appear to be present in the sympathetic nervous system. The levels of peptides derived from prodynorphin are very low in rat adrenal gland, but higher levels may be present in other species. There is a a small number of dynorphin-containing neurons in the peripheral sympathetic nervous system of the guinea pig, but with the exception of the celiac–superior mesenteric ganglion complex, dynorphin-immunoreactive fibers and neurons are absent from rat sympathetic ganglia (Vincent et al., 1984).

3.2. Actions of Opioids on Transmission at Sympathetic Ganglia

The ability of morphine to inhibit contractions of the cat nictitating membrane elicited by stimulation of the cervical sympathetic nerve was one of the earliest peripheral actions of morphine to be studied (Trendelenburg, 1957; Cairnie et al., 1961). Most of this effect appears to be related to an action on the postganglionic sympathetic nerve terminals, which will be discussed below (section 3.5). Trendelenburg (1957) demonstrated, however, that very low doses of morphine (5–20 μg, iv) antagonized the contractions of the nictitating membrane induced by intraarterial administration of histamine, pilocarpine, or serotonin, to the superior cervical ganglion. These very low doses of morphine had no effect on the response of the end-organ to postganglionic stimulation, and thus appeared to be a direct action of the opiate drug on the superior cervical ganglion. Stimulation of the ganglion by local administration of nicotine or potassium was not affected by these low doses of morphine. Thus, morphine did not directly affect the primary cholinergic transmission path in the ganglion, but was able to inhibit potential modulators of ganglionic transmission.

More recent electrophysiological studies by Otsuka and coworkers (Konishi et al., 1979, 1981) have confirmed that opioids can exert a presynaptic modulatory role on cholinergic transmission in sympathetic ganglia. In guinea pig celiac-superior mesenteric and inferior mesenteric ganglia incubated in vitro, [Met[5]]- and [Leu[5]]enkephalin, at concentrations from 0.5 to 20 μM, depressed the postsynaptic epsp. Metabolically stable analogs of enkephalin were substantially more potent than the natural enkephalins, and none of the opioids inhibited the postsynaptic response to acetylcholine (Konishi et al., 1979). The possibility that inhibition of acetylcholine release from presynaptic fibers might be inhibited by endogenous enkephalin released from presynaptic neurons has been tested. The effects of a conditioning volley of stimuli on the postsynaptic epsps induced by a subsequent test stimulus was determined (Konishi et al., 1981). After an 8-s, 50-Hz stimulus, the epsp response to a subsequent test stimulus was reduced by about 50%. This effect was antagonized by naloxone, 1–3 μM. Thus, a potential role for physiologically released opioids in sympathetic ganglia appears probable. The nature of the opioid receptors mediating this effect remains unclear. Since both morphine and enkephalins appear to be capable of modulating ganglionic transmission (albeit, in different ganglia, in different species), possible roles for both mu and delta receptors must be considered.

3.3. Actions of Opioids in Adrenal Gland

Specific binding sites for opioids have been demonstrated in homogenates of bovine adrenal gland. Chavkin et. al. (1979) first reported high-affinity naloxone binding, with characteristics similar to naloxone binding sites in the central nervous system. Subsequently, these binding sites have been characterized further. Leslie et al. (1980) reported that sites with properties similar to those of both mu and delta receptors could be identified. With the availability of receptor-type selective ligands, more complete analyses have been possible. Using several radiolabeled ligands and nonlinear curve fitting procedures for data analysis. Castanas et al. (1984) have proposed the presence of five independent opioid binding sites with differing agonist selectivities in bovine adrenal medulla. In addition to mu and delta sites, it is proposed that two of the binding sites are subtypes of kappa receptors. The final site was identified as a benzomorphan binding site. Lemaire et al. (1981), examining inhibition of etorphine binding, have claimed a very high potency for dynorphin (IC_{50}, 0.4 nM), thus also suggesting that kappa sites are probably present, Saiani and Guidotti (1982), however, also using etorphine as the radiolabeled ligand, found dynorphin to be a relatively weak inhibitor (IC_{50}, 500 nM). Both groups found β-endorphin to have fairly high potency (IC_{50}, 10–12 nM). The reasons for these discrepancies in estimates of dynorphin potency are unclear, unless they are related to differences in the method of adrenal medullary membrane preparation (Saiani and Guidotti, 1982). Saiani and Guidotti (1982) have also reported that the number of etorphine binding sites is more than twice the sum of binding sites with high affinity for dihydromorphine, ethyketocyclazocine, SKF 10,047, and DADLE. Thus, most of the binding sites labeled by etorphine in these studies do not have the properties of conventional mu, delta, kappa, or sigma receptors. It is not clear if these etorphine binding sites should be characterized as epsilon sites with high selective affinity for β-endorphin. At this time, it would seem reasonable to conclude that mu, delta, and kappa receptors are present in bovine adrenal medulla, although further studies will be needed to determine the nature of the additional etorphine binding sites.

There is also uncertainty regarding the functional role of opioid binding sites in adrenal gland. It has been reported that opioids inhibit the release of catecholamines from primary cultures of bovine adrenal chromaffin cells (Kumakara et al., 1980; Saiani and Guidotti, 1982). A noteworthy feature of these studies is the high concentration of opioid required to produce significant inhibition of acetylcholine stimulated catecholamine release. The IC_{50} for etorphine, the most potent opioid tested, was found to be 100 nM. Antagonism of etorphine by naloxone and diprenorphine was demonstrated. The mu-selective synthetic peptide FK 33-824 was 2.5-fold less potent that etorphine, whereas the IC_{50} values for morphine and DADLE were higher than 50 μM. The relative agonist potencies noted in this system are not similar to those observed in other in vitro opioid bioassays and do not suggest mediation of the inhibition of catecholamine release by mu, delta, or kappa receptors. Lemaire et al. (1981) also examined the potencies of opioids in inhibiting stimulated catecholamine release from bovine adrenal medullary cells. He, like Saiani and Guidotti, found that the antagonism of acetylcholine stimulation was noncompetitive; the maximum release induced by acetylcholine was reduced by the opioids, with no change in the concentrations of acetylcholine required to elicit release. Lemaire et al. also showed that inhibition was restricted to acetylcholine- and nicotine-stimulated release, whereas release induced by potassium or calcium ionophores was unaffected. In this study, the IC_{50} for all opioids was in excess in 1 μM, and dextrophan was of equal potency to levorphanol. Di-iodo derivatives of dynorphin and β-endorphin had equal or higher potency than the parent compounds, although di-iodination was shown to dramatically reduce their potencies in displacing radiolabeled etorphine binding and in the guinea pig ileum opioid bioassay. Furthermore, Lemaire et al. (1981) found that the effect of opioids was not antagonized by naloxone. Thus, in this study, it appears that the inhibitory effects of the high concentrations of opioids were not mediated by opioid receptors. The differences between the results of Saiani and Guidotti (1982) and Lemaire et al. (1981) may be partly explained by differences in the procedures used to disperse the adrenal medullary cells. Lemaire et al. used cells 24 h after incubation with a fairly high concentration of collagenase, whereas Saiani and Guidotti allowed the cells to grow in culture dishes for 2–3 d before use, during which time they became attached to the dishes. It is possible that some cell surface receptors are lost, or at least uncoupled from effector systems, during the cell dispersion, requiring a recovery period of longer than 24 h before opioid effects can be observed.

Thus, the functions of opioids in adrenal medulla remain unclear at this time. Specific opioid binding sites are present, but no effects on adrenal medullary function that can be clearly attributed to these sites have been demonstrated. In addition to possible local actions, it is quite likely that opioids secreted by adrenal medulla act in an endocrine manner at distant sites. The higher molecular weight forms of enkephalins would be particularly suited to this role, since they are more stable than the pentapeptide enkephalins in blood and may possess significant affinity for kappa, as well as mu and delta, receptors. Possible target tissues include all peripheral structures carrying opioid receptors, including the heart and blood vessels, the gastrointestinal tract, the posterior lobe of pituitary, the reproductive tract, and the immune system.

3.4. Actions of Opioids on Blood Vessels

The ability of enkephalins to depress vasoconstrictor responses to sympathetic nerve stimulation in the rabbit isolated ear artery was first noted by Knoll (1976). Subsequently, other groups have confirmed this effect (Ronai et al., 1982; Illes et al., 1983, 1985a). The locus of action has been shown to be at the presynaptic nerve terminal, since the responses to injected norepinephrine are not modified. In this tissue, alkaloids like morphine are less effective than peptide opioids. Illes et al. (1985a) have shown that the potencies of a series of peptides in inhibiting [^{3}H]norepinephrine release parallel their ability to inhibit the vasoconstrictor response to sympathetic nerve stimulation. [Met^5]enkephalin and DADLE were the most potent peptides, with IC_{50} values of 20–30 nM. Other agonists with good affinity at delta receptors were also effective. Peptides derived from prodynorphin with good kappa receptor activity were effective, but less potent than the enkephalins. β-Endorphin had very low potency, a surprising observation since this peptide is thought to have reasonable affinity and efficacy at delta receptors. The effects of the peptides were antagonized by addition of 100 nM naloxone to the perfusate. This concentration of naloxone did not by itself affect the response to sympathetic nerve stimulation. Illes et al. (1985a) have concluded that delta and kappa receptors present on sympathetic nerve endings in this tissue can exert a regulatory role on sympathetic vasoconstrictor responses. Since naloxone, in low concentrations, did not directly affect the response to sympathetic nerve stimulation, no evidence is presently available to suggest that opioids are coreleased during sympathetic stimulation to exert an immediate feedback of norepinephrine secretion.

Opioid effects on the sympathetic regulation of other blood vessels have been proposed. Sun and Zhang (1985) have reported that dynorphin A (1-13) inhibited the response of dog mesenteric artery to electrical stimulation, the effect being antagonized by naloxone. Enkephalins were almost without effect on this tissue. Illes et al. (1985b) have observed that [Met^5]enkephalin inhibited the response of rabbit mesenteric artery to electrical stimulation in a naloxone reversible manner. A more detailed study has been conducted in a branch of the rabbit ileocolic artery. Comparison of relative agonist potencies and of the abilities of naloxone and the delta-selective peptide antagonist, ICI 154129, to reverse the effects of agonists, suggested that, as in the rabbit ear artery, both delta and mu receptors are present on sympathetic terminals in this artery (von Kugelgen et al., 1985). An early study (Hanko and Hardebo, 1978) has also demonstrated that enkephalins and morphine induce dilatation of feline pial arteries contracted by infusion of prostaglandin. The nature of the receptors mediating this effect is not clear, although the effectiveness of [Leu^5]enkephalin, the low potency of morphine, and the relatively low sensitivity to antagonism by naloxone suggest the possible involvement of delta receptors. The location of these receptors was not determined in this study. It is possible that the prostaglandin-induced increase in vascular tone was fully or partially dependent on stimulation of sympathetic nerve terminals, but a direct action on the arterial smooth muscle has not been excluded.

Enkephalins can exert nonopioid effects on blood vessels. Pulmonary vasoconstriction induced by [Leu^5]enkephalin is not reversed by naloxone or diprenorphine, and other enkephalins, including [Met^5]enkephalin and DADLE, do not induce the same vasoconstrictor effect (Crooks et al., 1984). Thus, a nonopioid mechanism is assumed to be responsible for this effect.

3.5. Actions of Opioids on Cat Nictitating Membrane

Trendelenburg (1957) demonstrated that morphine inhibited the contractions of the nictitating membrane, the third eyelid in the cat, to stimulation of the postganglionic cervical sympathetic nerve trunk, but had no effect on the response of the tissue to injections of norepinephrine. Trendelenburg concluded that morphine was inhibiting the stimulated release of norepinephrine from the postganglionic neuron. These studies were extended by Cairnie et al. (1961), who showed that cocaine antagonized the action of morphine, presumably by inhibiting reuptake of released norepinephrine. The nature of the opioid receptors mediating the inhibition has not been determined. The potency of morphine suggests a probable role for mu receptors. The effects of opioid antagonists do not appear to have been examined. It should be noted that not all sympathetically innervated smooth muscle is sensitive to regulation by morphine; Cairnie et al. (1961) tested the ability of morphine to inhibit the response of the cat spleen and heart to sympathetic nerve stimulation, but found no effect.

4. Actions of Opioids on the Heart

4.1. Endogenous Opioids and Opioid Binding in the Heart

Endogenous opioids have been reported to be present in guinea pig and rat heart (Hughes et al., 1977; Spampinato and Goldstein, 1983; Lang et al., 1983). In a recent study, acid extracts from guinea pig heart were fractionated by high performance liquid chromatography and assayed for opioid activity by the mouse vas deferens bioassay (Weihe et al., 1985). Activities corresponding in elution positions to the enkephalins, C-terminally extended enkephalin peptides, and the opioid peptides derived from prodynorphin were all found in the extracts. In general, levels of the peptides were slightly higher in the atria than in the ventricles. Proenkephalin mRNA has also been found in rat heart (Howells et al., 1985). There are two remarkable features of this study. First, the heart was found to contain larger amounts of enkephalin mRNA than any other tissue. Second, 95% of the mRNA was found in the ventricles, which contain very low concentrations of enkephalin, relative to both atria and to other tissues like brain (Weihe et al., 1985). The cellular location of the mRNA and opioid peptides within the atria and ventricles is not known at present, although Weihe et al. (1985) suggest, without direct evidence, that the peptides are localized in the sympathetic and parasympathetic innervation of the heart. Since myocytes in the atria of mammalian heart contain many peptide storage granules (Jamieson and Palade, 1964), and high concentrations of peptides such as atrial natriuretic peptide (Currie et al., 1983), a possible localization of the opioids in muscle of the heart cannot be excluded.

High-affinity saturable opioid binding has also been reported in homogenates of heart (Simantov et al., 1978). The most complete characterization of these binding sites in rat atria and ventricles is in a recent study by Krumins et al. (1985). Tritium-labeled diprenorphine binding showed an affinity of about 1 nM. Competition studies do not provide conclusive characterization of the receptor types present, but are suggestive of the presence of delta and kappa binding sites. The mu selective synthetic peptide, DAGO (Tyr-D-Ala-Gly-NMePhe-Gly-ol), produced no inhibition at concentrations of up to 1 μM.

Possible direct actions of opioids on cardiac muscle were evaluated by Saunders and Thornhill (1985). Concentrations of enkephalins up to 100 μM did not affect the tension generated by direct electrical stimulation of rat isolated atrial preparations. Nor did they affect the inotropic effects of norepinephrine or isoproterenol. These results suggest that the opioid binding sites might be located on the autonomic innervation of the heart. Pharmacological evidence provides support for this hypothesis.

4.2. Actions of Opioids on the Vagal Innervation of the Heart

There appear to be considerable differences between species in the effects of opioids on vagal transmission to the heart. Kosterlitz and Taylor (1959) found that intravenous doses of morphine in the range 0.1 to 10 mg/kg reduced the bradycardia produced by stimulation of the vagal nerve in rat and rabbit, whereas in the cat there was a small morphine-induced reduction of the bradycardia. The guinea pig appeared insensitive to this action of morphine; an interesting observation in view of the sensitivity to morphine of cholinergic neurons in the guinea pig myenteric plexus. The response to morphine was most consistent and readily quantified in the rabbit. Resting heart rate was generally not affected by doses of morphine of 0.1 to 1 mg/kg, doses that reduced the bradycardia produced by stimulation of the vagus nerve at frequencies between 2.5 and 40 Hz. Higher morphine doses often also reduced the resting heart rate. The only other opioid tested in this study was nalorphine, which produced a slight reduction in vagal slowing at low doses, but no further slowing at higher doses. The authors were not able to demonstrate consistent antagonism of morphine by nalorphine.

The receptors mediating opioid inhibition of vagal transmission in rabbit heart have been examined in a recent study by Wetzell et al. (1984) in which the effects of morphine and opioid peptides on vagally induced slowing of the isolated rabbit heart perfused by the method of Langedorff were studied. Morphine (IC_{50}, 150 nM), [Met^5]enkephalin (IC_{50}, 25 nM), and DADLE (IC_{50}, 3.2 nM) all reduced the response to vagal stimulation. This effect was antagonized by naloxone, which produced a parallel shift in the opioid dose–response curves. The naloxone K_e against morphine was about 1 nM, against [Met^5]enkephalin, about 30 nM. The delta-selective peptide antagonist ICI 174864 also antagonized the enkephalin (but not morphine) inhibition of vagal transmission, with a K_e of about 30 nM. These results indicate that both mu and delta receptors are able to mediate the inhibition of vagal transmission in rabbit.

The location of these receptors is not yet certain. The opioids did not inhibit the bradycardia induced by acetylcholine administration. In these experiments, the vagus nerve was stimulated preganglionically. It is therefore possible that the receptors are located on preganglionic terminals, and there is autoradiographic evidence supporting the presence of opioid receptors in preganglionic vagal fibers (Young et al., 1980). However, a postganglionic action cannot be excluded. Kennedy and West (1967) studied the effect of opioids on the response of isolated rabbit atria to postganglionic cholinergic stimulation through electrodes located in the sinoatrial node. The initial increase in interbeat interval induced by stimulation was unaffected by hexamethonium, but reduced by atropine and morphine (at about 3 μM). This observation supports a role for mu receptors in inhibiting vagal transmission in the rabbit heart and suggests that at least part of the effect is exerted on the postganglionic cholinergic neurons. The nature and precise location of the opioid receptors inhibiting vagal regulation of heart rate in the rat and cat have not been studied.

4.3. Actions of Opioids on the
Sympathetic Innervation of the Heart

There is accumulating evidence that the sympathetic innervation of the heart can be inhibited by opioids in some species. Kennedy and West (1967) found that sinoatrial node stimulation initially slowed, then increased, the frequency of contraction of isolated rabbit atria. The initial slowing appeared to be cholinergically mediated, since it was inhibited by atropine. The later positive chronotropic effect was inhibited by propranolol, and thus probably mediated by sympathetic adrenergic fibers. The positive inotropic response, unlike the earlier negative inotropic response (*see* section 4.2 above), was insensitive to morphine. In studies with intact perfused rabbit hearts with attached sympathetic nerves, however, it has been shown that ethylketocyclazocine, at concentrations from 0.01 to 1 μM, reduced cardiac acceleration induced by sympathetic nerve stimulation (Starke et al., 1985). This effect was antagonized by naloxone (1 μM). The lack of effectiveness of morphine was confirmed, and [Met[5]]enkephalin and DADLE were also shown to be ineffective. Ethylketocyclazocine had no effect on the increase in heart rate produced by norepinephrine; its action is therefore presumed to be exerted through kappa receptors located on the sympathetic nerve terminals innervating the heart. The ineffectiveness of morphine and the enkephalins suggests that mu and delta receptors are not present.

In guinea pig isolated atria, however, etorphine, DADLE, and [Met[5]]enkephalyl-Arg-Phe inhibited the positive inotropic effect induced by field stimulation (Ledda and Mantelli, 1982; Ledda et al., 1984). The effects of these opioids were antagonized by naloxone (10 μM). Morphine, methadone, and β-endorphin did not produce naloxone reversible effects on heart rate after stimulation. Thus, it appears that guinea pig sympathetic nerves may carry delta opioid receptors. In view of the lack of effects of morphine, methadone, and β-endorphin, it is unlikely that mu or epsilon receptors are present. The possible presence of kappa receptors in this species has not been tested.

4.4. Reflex Regulation of Heart Rate by Opioids

Intravenous administration of morphine and some opioid peptides in rats has been shown to produce a transient bradycardia that is blocked by atropine or vagotomy (Fennessy and Rattray, 1971; Wei et al., 1980). The effect is peripherally mediated, since it has been shown to be antagonized by the quaternary antagonist N-methylnaloxonium (Kiang et al., 1983). Electrophysiological studies have shown that morphine induces increased activity in sensory C-fiber afferents carried in the vagus (Sapru et al., 1981). Thus it seems probable that morphine acts by stimulating sensory afferents to induce a reflex slowing of the heart. Sapru et al. (1981) have suggested that morphine activates pulmonary J receptors. Kiang et al. (1983) showed that a more rapid response to morphine was observed after right atrial than right ventricular injection, and therefore argue that the right atrium is also an important target for morphine.

The sensory fibers activated by morphine appear to be sensitive to mu agonists. Morphine, etorphine, DADLE, and the very mu-selective peptide, PL017 (Tyr-Pro-NMePhe-D-Pro-NH_2) all induce naloxone reversible bradycardias (Kiang and Wei, 1983). [Met^5]- and [Leu^5]enkephalin and dynorphin A (1-13) were substantially less potent (Wei et al., 1980). Subcutaneous administration of subthreshold doses of these peptides, however, appeared to modify the bradycardia response to morphine (Kiang and Wei, 1984). The mechanism of this modulation is not understood. A surprising feature is that although dynorphin A (1-13) and [Leu^5]enkephalin sensitized the rats to morphine, [Met^5]enkephalin induced a desensitization. This dichotomy would not be predicted on the basis of the known receptor selectivities of the two pentapeptide enkephalins. It remains to be established if the proposed modulatory actions of the enkephalins and dynorphin A are mediated through delta or kappa receptors. The site of the proposed modulatory action is also not identified.

4.5. Effects of Opioids on Blood Pressure

It has long been known that opioids produce a fall in blood pressure in mammals (Schmidt and Livingstone, 1933). It has been proposed that, at least in cat, a morphine-induced release of histamine contributes to this effect (Feldberg and Paton, 1951), although the fall in blood pressure cannot be completely reversed by histamine H1 antagonists (Evans et al., 1952). In contrast to morphine, enkephalins produce an increase in blood pressure (Giles and Sander, 1983). Although there are many peripheral sites at which opioids can affect blood pressure, including actions on peripheral blood vessels (*see* section 3.4) and on the heart (*see* sections 4.1, 4.2, and 4.3), studies employing neurotransmitter antagonists and nerve-section suggest that much of the overall effect of opioids on blood pressure can be attributed to central actions that are beyond the scope of this chapter (*see* Giles and Sander, 1983; Holaday, 1983). It has been suggested, however, that ethylketocyclazocine decreases blood pressure in the rabbit through an inhibition of norepinephrine release from peripheral sympathetic nerves (Ensinger et al., 1984).

5. Actions of Opioids on Sensory Nerves

5.1. Endogenous Opioids in Sensory Nerves

There is accumulating evidence that endogenous opioids are present in some sensory nerves. Enkephalins have been found in tooth pulp (Kudo et al., 1983) and in the carotid body (Wharton et al., 1980). The presence of enkephalins and dynorphins in dorsal root ganglia (DRG) of the mouse, rat, and rabbit has been reported (Botticelli et al., 1981; Sweetman et al., 1982). The levels of the peptide were not reduced by rhizotomy, suggesting that the peptide was intrinsic to the DRG and not present in axons originating in the spinal cord (Botticelli et al., 1981). In the spinal cord, there are high concentrations of enkephalins and dynorphins in the substantia gelatinosa (Hunt et al., 1980; Vincent et al., 1982), where collaterals of primary sensory neurons synapse with regulatory interneurons. Thus, endogenous opioids appear to be strategically located for the regulation of transmission from the primary afferent neuron to the central nervous system. Intrathecal administration of opioids of the mu, delta, and kappa types has been shown to reduce the response to various types of noxious stimuli by a local action in the spinal cord (Schmauss and Yaksh, 1984). There remains, however, some doubt as to whether the endogenous opioids of spinal cord act directly on opioid receptors on the terminals of primary sensory neurons (Hunt et al., 1980; Ruda, 1982). The evidence that at least some primary afferent neurons can be regulated by opioids at both their central and peripheral terminals will be discussed below.

5.2. Opioid Receptors on Sensory Neurons

An early autoradiographic study of the binding of intravenously administered [^{3}H]naloxone in the spinal cord of rhesus monkeys in control animals and after section of the dorsal roots suggested that a significant fraction of the opioid binding sites in laminae I–III of the cervical spinal cord were lost 2–4 wk after rhizotomy (Lamotte et al., 1976). It seemed probable that the loss of the binding sites was associated with degeneration of the primary afferent terminals. Direct evidence of opioid binding sites on processes of DRG neurons was provided by the studies of Hiller et al. (1978) on cultures of fetal mouse DRG explants. Binding of [^{3}H]diprenorphine was found to be concentrated in the neuritic outgrowths of the DRG neurons. Fields et al. (1980) demonstrated the binding of both [^{3}H]morphine and [^{3}H]DADLE by homogenates of rat dorsal roots. They concluded that both mu and delta binding sites were therefore present on primary afferent fibers. Since DADLE is known to have high affinity for both mu and delta receptors, further studies are needed to show that the DADLE binding by dorsal roots has the characteristics of delta receptor binding sites. Electrophysiological studies (Werz and Macdonald, 1982; see below) also suggest that the terminals of DRG neurons have delta receptors.

Functional studies support the conclusion that primary afferent neurons can be regulated by opioids. Jessell and Iversen (1977) reported that opioids inhibited the release of substance P from the substantia gelatinosa of the trigeminal nucleus. It is probable that at least part of the released substance P originated from primary afferent terminals, since Mudge et al. (1979) found that enkephalins also inhibited the release of substance P from chick DRG neurons in culture. Yaksh et al. (1980) demonstrated that intrathecal administration of morphine in anesthetized cats and rats inhibited the release of substance P from the spinal cord into the subarachnoid space after sciatic nerve stimulation. Etorphine has been shown to depress synaptic transmission between DRG neurons and spinal cord neurons in explant cultures of mouse DRG and spinal cord (Macdonald and Nelson, 1978). In all these experiments, naloxone reversed the actions of the opioids.

These results suggest that opioids can reduce the output of transmitter from primary afferent neurons, reducing their ability to activate secondary sensory neurons. Electrophysiological studies employing intracellular recording from DRG neurons have provided some indications of the mechanisms underlying this action. Mudge et al. (1979) reported that enkephalin analogs produced a reduction in the duration of the chick DRG action potential and attributed this effect to a reduction in an inward calcium current. They pointed out that this effect might arise either from an increase in outward potassium current or from a direct inhibitory effect on calcium conductance. With the availability of more specific agonists, Werz and Macdonald (1982, 1984) were able to demonstrate that mu-, delta-, and kappa-selective agonists were all capable of reducing the duration of calcium-dependent action potentials in mouse DRG neurons. In neurons inhibited by the mu-selective agonist morphiceptin, the agonist action was readily antagonized by naloxone. In other neurons, the effects of [Leu[5]]enkephalin or dynorphin A often required higher concentrations of naloxone for antagonism to be observed, suggesting a probable action through delta or kappa receptors. Not all neurons were equally sensitive to all types of opioid agonist, suggesting variable ratios of mu, delta, and kappa receptors on different DRG neurons. More neurons responded to dynorphin than to mu or delta agonists. Furthermore, the actions of mu- and delta-selective agonists could be prevented by the intracellular injection of the potassium channel blocker cesium, whereas the dynorphin A response was unaffected by cesium (Werz and Macdonald, 1984). This result suggests that although mu and delta agonists affect the inward flow of calcium indirectly by blocking the opening of potassium channels, dynorphin A and other kappa agonists have a direct inhibitory action on the calcium conductance contributing to the action potential. Cherubini and North (1985) have subsequently demonstrated a similar distinction between the effects of mu and delta agonist on one hand, and kappa agonist on the other, in guinea pig myenteric plexus neurons (*see* section 2 above.). Collectively, these results point to the presence of mu, delta, and kappa receptors on at least some primary sensory neurons. In mouse DRG, more neurons appear to have kappa receptors than mu or delta receptors.

5.3. Peripheral Antinociception by Opioids

Antinociceptive actions of opioids mediated at spinal cord sites are well established (Schmauss and Yaksh, 1984). There is accumulating evidence, however, that the peripheral terminals of primary afferent neurons are also sensitive to opioids. Ferreira and Nakamura (1979) used a modification of the Randall and Sillito test in which pain was produced in a rat paw by the intraplantar injection of prostaglandin E_2 (PGE_2). At various times after injection of the prostaglandin, reaction time in response to increasing pressure applied to the paw was measured. The advantage of this test is that the contralateral paw can act as a control, allowing the location of action of drugs modifying the response to be determined. Ferreira and Nakamura (1979) found that morphine and enkephalins partially prevented the reduction in reaction time (i.e., the hyperalgesia) induced by PGE_2 in the test paw, but had no effect in the contralateral paw unless they were also injected at that site, thus confirming that the analgesic effect of morphine was induced locally. Levorphanol was less potent than morphine, but dextrorphan was completely without effect, demonstrating the stereospecificity of the response (Ferreira, 1981). Naloxone, nalorphine, and pentazocine all produced similar effects to those of morphine in this system, however, thus casting some doubt on the nature of the receptors mediating the antinociceptive effect. The analgesic potency of naloxone was confirmed by Rios and Jacob (1982), using a similar test in which PGE_2 was replaced as the local inflammatory agent by carrageenin. In contrast to the results of Ferreira and Nakamura (1979), Rios and Jacob (1982) also observed that low doses of naloxone partially antagonized the actions of morphine.

The peripheral nature of the antagonism of PGE_2 or carrageenin hyperalgesia has been confirmed by the demonstration that the quaternary analogs of morphine (Smith et al., 1982), naloxone (Rios and Jacob, 1982), and nalorphine (Ferreira et al., 1984) were also active. The interpretation of these results is further complicated by the observation that neither N-methyl naloxone nor N-methyl-nalorphine showed analgesic activity after subcutaneous administration, although N-methyl morphine retained its ability to antagonize the carrageenin hyperalgesia (Smith et al., 1985). It has been shown that very little N-methyl morphine penetrates the brain following subcutaneous administration (Smith et al., 1982). A second analgesic test has provided further evidence of peripheral analgesic actions of opioids. When injected into the peritoneal cavity, morphine and its quaternary analog can inhibit the frequency of abdominal constrictions (or "writhing") induced by the intraperitoneal injection of acetic acid or a stable prostaglandin analog (Bentley et al., 1981; Smith et al., 1982, 1985). Bentley et al. (1981) found that ketocyclazocine was the most potent of the opioids tested. Naloxone and other antagonists were without agonist activity in this test, in contrast to their agonistic activity in reducing PGE_2 hyperalgesia (Smith et al., 1985). These results suggest that opioids can act directly or indirectly on the peripheral terminals of sensory neurons to modulate the response to noxious stimulation, although the nature of the receptors involved is still uncertain.

5.4. Antagonism of Neurogenic Edema

Further evidence for an action of opioids on peripheral sensory neurons has come from studies of their ability to reduce the local edema resulting from increased capillary permeability after sensory nerve stimulation. An experimental procedure based on the increased leakage of Evans blue dye from the circulation into the skin of the foot in anesthetized rat after stimulation of the saphenous nerve (Jancso et al., 1967) has been used to quantify local actions of opioids. Prior treatment of the rats with capsaicin causes a reduction in tissue content of substance P and a much reduced local extravasation of blue dye, suggesting a possible role for substance P as a mediator of this reaction. Morton and Chahl (1980) demonstrated the reduction of neurogenic edema by morphine and antagonism of this effect by naloxone. Because morphine also reduced blood pressure, Morton and Chahl (1980) suggested that the apparent antiinflammatory action of morphine might have resulted from a reduction in local vascular perfusion pressure. Bartho and Szolcsanyi (1981) and Lembeck et al. (1982), however, were able to show that opioids, including a mu-selective enkephalin analog, were able to reduce the neurogenic extravasation of blue dye over a period of time that greatly exceeded the transient fall in blood pressure occurring immediately after administration of the opioids. Lembeck et al. (1982) also showed that the local edema induced by substance P administration was not reduced by opioid treatment. Thus these results suggest that opioids can inhibit the release of local vasoactive substances such as substance P from sensory nerve terminals, which follows antidromic stimulation of the sensory nerves. In these studies, naloxone behaved as a pure antagonist. Among the opioids tested, the activity of morphine and synthetic enkephalin analogs with considerable selectivity for mu receptors indicates that mu receptors are present on the sensory nerve terminals. Kappa receptors are also probably present, however, in view of the high potency of ethylketocyclazocine (Smith and Buchan, 1984) and other kappa-selective agonists, including tifluadom and U50488H (M. J. Rance, personnel communication), in reducing neurogenic extravasation. The activity of delta receptors in this system remains to be demonstrated. All three types of opioid receptor, however, have been shown to be present in the soma of DRG neurons (Werz and Macdonald, 1984). It would therefore not be surprising if they were also present on the peripheral terminals of these neurons. The high potency of ethylketocyclazocine and other kappa agonists may be a consequence of the greater number of DRG neurons shown to responsivity to kappa relative to mu or delta agonists (Werz and Macdonald, 1984) The sensitivity of primary afferent neurons to regulation by locally applied opioids might in the future be exploited to provide selective local pain relief.

6. Opioid Receptors in Pars Nervosa of Pituitary

6.1. Endogenous Opioids in Pars Nervosa

The posterior lobe of pituitary contains high concentrations of opioid peptides derived from each of the opioid peptide genes. High concentrations of β-endorphin-related peptides are present in the pars intermedia, although a large fraction of the β-endorphin peptides are N-acetylated and thus without activity at opioid receptors (Zakarian and Smyth, 1982; Akil et al., 1985). [Leu⁵]enkephalin-like material was reported to be present in the pars nervosa of rat pituitary on the basis of immunocytochemical studies (Rossier et al., 1979). Subsequently, dynorphin and related peptides were isolated from porcine pituitaries and shown to be in very high concentration in pars nervosa (Goldstein and Ghazarossian, 1980). Dynorphins and related peptides have been shown to be cosequestered with vasopressin in the neurosecretory vesicles of the vasopressin (AVP)-containing magnocellular neuron terminals in the pars nervosa (Whitnall et al., 1983). Physiological studies suggest that dynorphin is released together with AVP by stimuli such as dehydration and hemorrhage (Hollt et al., 1981; Cox et al., 1982). In contrast, [Met⁵]enkephalin and other peptides derived from proenkephalin are reported to be concentrated in the oxytocin (OXY)-containing nerve terminals (Martin et al., 1983). The functions of the opioids in pars nervosa are not known. Recent studies, however, have suggested possible roles for the opioids in the regulation of secretion of AVP and OXY.

6.2. Regulation by Opioids of AVP and OXY Secretion

Iversen and coworkers (Iversen et al., 1980) first reported that morphine and other opioids inhibited the electrically stimulated release of AVP from isolated rat pituitary neurointermediate lobes superfused with a physiological saline solution. This inhibition of release was blocked by naloxone. Lutz-Bucher and Koch (1980) showed that morphine inhibited the unstimulated release of AVP and OXY from incubated rat pituitary posterior lobes and also noted that the inhibition was blocked by naloxone. When the pars intermedia was present, naloxone increased peptide secretion in the absence of added opioid, suggesting that β-endorphin or a related peptide released from pars intermedia was producing a tonic inhibition of release of pars nervosa peptides. In subsequent studies of the stimulated release of AVP or OXY, it has often been easier to demonstrate a potentiation of release of AVP or OXY by naloxone treatment than to obtain quantitatively reliable direct inhibitions of AVP or OXY secretion by opioids. Furthermore, Bicknell and Leng (1982; Bicknell et al., 1985a) have found that naloxone increased the electrically stimulated release of OXY, but did not affect the stimulated release of AVP. In contrast, Knepel and Meyer (1983) reported a naloxone-induced potentiation of stimulated release of AVP from rat posterior pituitaries (OXY release was not measured in this study). The reason for these discrepant results is not clear. There are some differences in the electrical stimulation parameters used by the two groups; Bicknell and Leng (1982) used a 13 Hz stimulus for 3 min, whereas Knepel and Meyer (1983) used repeated 10-s trains of 9-Hz stimuli for 5-min periods. It has been suggested that AVP secretion is less well maintained than OXY secretion during sustained electrical stimulation (Bicknell and Leng, 1983). Thus, the different electrical stimulation parameters may in part account for the differences in the observed effects of naloxone.

These studies are complicated by the corelease with AVP or OXY of the endogenous opioids stored in the pars nervosa. The pronounced potentiating effect of naloxone on peptide secretion indicates that the opioid receptors regulating peptide release in the gland are fully or partially saturated with endogenous opioids that have been released prior to or together with AVP and OXY. The sources of the endogenous opioid(s) causing the inhibition of secretion remain to be determined. However, Anhut and Knepel (1982) have demonstrated the presence of dynorphin immunoreactivity in the incubation medium after stimulation of AVP release. Furthermore, Bicknell et al. (1983) have shown that removal of the pars intermedia does not affect the potentiation of electrically stimulated OXY release by naloxone, suggesting that β-endorphin from pars intermedia does not inhibit the stimulated release of OXY (despite its inhibition of the nonstimulated release observed by Lutz-Bucher and Koch, 1980). The delta antagonist,

ICI 174864, had no effect on the stimulated release of OXY, thus suggesting that the receptors mediating the regulation of OXY release are not of the delta type (Bicknell et al., 1985b). Collectively, these studies point to a probable regulation of stimulated OXY and AVP secretion by dynorphin or related peptides.

There are only a few studies of radiolabeled opioid binding by pituitary tissue. Simantov and Snyder (1977) reported the specific binding of several tritium-labeled opioids by membranes prepared from bovine pituitaries. Almost all the specific binding was restricted to the posterior lobe of the pituitary. The small size of rat pars nervosa does not lend itself to conventional radioligand binding studies. Recently, however, Herkenham et al. (1986) have examined rat pituitary opioid binding sites by autoradiography, using tritium ligands selective for mu or delta sites and measured kappa binding with [^{3}H]bremazocine after irreversibly blocking mu and delta binding sites. Their results confirm that specific opioid binding is restricted to the pars nervosa, where virtually all the opioid binding is of the kappa type. These binding sites were reported to be "densely localized to nerve terminals." This observation is in conflict with the report by Lightman et al. (1983) that [^{3}H]etorphine binding in rat pituitary was localized on pituicytes and was not reduced after transection of the pituitary stalk.

In summary, several studies point to a regulation of stimulated OXY and AVP secretion from pars nervosa by endogenous opioids from the pars nervosa. Some evidence suggests that dynorphin or related peptides acting on kappa receptors on the magnocellular nerve terminals may be responsible for this effect. Since dynorphin is contained within the AVP terminals, dynorphin-activated receptors regulating AVP release should be described as autoreceptors. These presumably mediate a feedback inhibition of AVP release. In support of this hypothesis, it has been demonstrated that in intact rats, selective kappa agonists produce a pronounced diuresis associated with a reduction in AVP secretion (Leander, 1983). The site of kappa agonist action in this study was not determined, however. It is possible that kappa agonists also affect AVP secretion by an action in brain. OXY secretion is also regulated by receptors that are not of the delta type (Bicknell et al., 1985b), and therefore might well be kappa in view of the results of Herkenham et al. (1985). Further studies are required, however, to elucidate the detailed mechanisms of opioid regulation of pars nervosa function.

7. Actions of Opioids on Reproductive Tract Tissues

7.1. Endogenous Opioids in Reproductive Tract Tissues

Recent studies have demonstrated the presence of endogenous opioids derived from all three endogenous opioid gene products in tissues of the reproductive tract. β-Endorphin and other peptides derived from POMC have been found in testis (Sharp et al., 1980; Margioris et al., 1983) and ovary (Lim et al., 1983; Shaha et al., 1984). POMC mRNA has also been found in rat testis (Pintar et al., 1984). Proenkephalin mRNA and enkephalin have also been reported to be present in the testes and ovaries of rats, hamsters, and cattle (Kilpatrick et al., 1985). Analysis of extracts of rat testes by radioimmunoassay suggests that dynorphin A is also present (Spampinato and Goldstein, 1983), and prodynorphin mRNA has been found in testis, ovary, and other reproductive tract tissues (Douglass et al., 1987). Endorphins, enkephalins, and dynorphins have also been found in human placenta (Nakai et al., 1978; Rama Sastry et al., 1980; Lemaire et al., 1983).

The functions of reproductive tract endogenous opioids are unknown. A local action on Leydig cell function is possible, since it has been reported that intratesticular injection of naloxone reduced the secretion of testosterone (Gerendai et al., 1984). The local concentration of naloxone may have been as high as 0.1 mM in these studies, however, casting some doubt on the specificity of the naloxone effect. (+)-Naloxone has not been tested.

Some evidence suggests that opioids might be secreted from testis into semen (Sharp and Pekary, 1981; Rama Sastry et al., 1982). Fabri et al. (1985) have reported that human semen inhibits T rosette formation by human lymphocytes. Since the effect was blocked by naloxone, an opioid receptor-mediated mechanism for this action was postulated. Actions of opioids in seminal fluid on blood elements may not play a normal physiological role, although this effect may have some pathological significance. A potentially important site of action of reproductive tract opioids might be the vas deferens, where opioid inhibition of contractions has been unambiguously demonstrated. In addition, opioid receptors have also been found in human placenta.

7.2. Opioid Actions on Vas Deferens

7.2.1. Mouse Vas Deferens

The ability of opioids to inhibit contractions of the vas deferens of the mouse was first reported by Henderson et al. (1972). Using preparations of mouse vas deferens mounted in a physiological saline solution between platinum electrodes, they demonstrated that the contractions of this tissue produced by brief electrical stimuli were inhibited by morphine and that the inhibition was blocked by naloxone. Later studies (Hughes et al., 1975) showed that the inhibition of electrically stimulated contractions was attributable to an inhibition of the release of norepinephrine from the adrenergic nerves innervating this tissue.

The discovery of the enkephalins resulted in the availability of additional opioids chemically unrelated to morphine. When the relative potencies of enkephalins and morphine-like drugs were compared in the isolated mouse vas deferens and guinea pig ileum preparations, significant discrepancies became apparent (Lord et al., 1977). This led to the suggestion that more than one type of opioid receptor was present in each tissue. Since naloxone antagonized normorphine and morphine with a K_e of about 2 nM, but exhibited a K_e of about 20 nM against enkephalins in mouse vas deferens, it was proposed that morphine and related drugs acted on mu-type receptors, whereas enkephalins acted preferentially in this tissue on a different class of receptors, which was named "delta" (Lord et al., 1977). Further evidence for differences in the receptors that mediated the effects of morphine or enkephalins in mouse vas deferens was provided by studies of cross-tolerance. Vas deferens preparations from mice made tolerant to morphine by morphine pellet implantation were less sensitive to inhibition by normorphine than vasa from untreated mice, but there was no difference in their sensitivities to [Leu^5]enkephalin (Cox, 1978). The reverse effect was observed when tolerance was induced by continuous administration (from an implanted reservoir) of a stable peptide with high affinity for delta receptors, DADLE (Schulz et al., 1980). Exposure to this peptide for 6 d produced profound tolerance to enkephalins and other agents acting through delta receptors, but had little effect on the potencies of agonists like normorphine acting through mu receptors. Schulz et al. (1980) also confirmed that sustained exposure to a selective mu agonist (sufentanyl in their experiments) produced selective tolerance to mu agonists, whereas the potencies of delta-selective agonists were almost unchanged. Although the mechanisms by which selective tolerance is produced in this tissue are not yet known, this study provided indirect support for the existence of both mu- and delta-type receptors in mouse vas deferens. Miller and Shaw (1983) have confirmed that mu and delta effects can be discriminated by selective tolerance induction and also noted that a reduction in incubation temperature selectively reduced the maximum inhibition attainable with the mu agonist, normorphine, but had little effect on the maximum inhibition attainable with the delta agonist, DADLE.

Opioids with high affinity for kappa-type receptors also inhibit the electrically stimulated contractions of mouse vas deferens (Lord et al., 1977; Schulz and Wuster, 1981; Cox and Chavkin, 1983). Since naloxone antagonizes both delta and kappa agonist effects with a K_e of 20–30 nM, it was not possible to use sensitivity to naloxone antagonism to determine if the effects of the kappa agonist were mediated through delta or kappa receptors in this tissue. However, vas deferens preparations rendered selectively tolerant to delta agonist effects by chronic administration of DADLE retained their sensitivity for agonists with preferential affinity for kappa receptors (Schulz and Wuster, 1981; Cox and Chavkin, 1983). These results suggest that kappa receptors are also present in mouse vas deferens preparations.

Studies with irreversible opioid antagonists have provided further support for the conclusion that mu, delta, and kappa receptors are all present in mouse vas deferens. Ward et al. (1982) showed that β-FNA initially inhibited the contractions of mouse vas deferens, an effect that was relatively insensitive to antagonism by naloxone (compared to mu receptor-mediated actions), and thus could be mediated by delta or kappa receptors. Since studies in other preparations had demonstrated a kappa agonist effect of β-FNA, Ward et al. (1982) postulated that this reversible effect was the result of kappa receptor activation. This component of β-FNA action was transient. After washing, the electrically stimulated contractions recovered, but now the preparation was selectively insensitive to mu agonists, thus revealing the irreversible occupation of mu receptors by β-FNA. Delta agonists retained their potency (Ward et al., 1982). These results demonstrate the usefulness of β-FNA as a tool for the analysis of mu receptor-mediated effects. Recent studies with higher doses of β-FNA have suggested, however, that this compound may also interact to some extent with delta receptors, resulting in a reduction of delta agonist potency (Hayes et al., 1985).

β-CNA shows only a weak initial agonist effect in mouse vas deferens. Even after repeated washing, β-CNA-treated mouse vas preparations show maintained insensitivity to mu, delta, and kappa agonists, suggesting an irreversible interaction with all three receptor types (Ward et al., 1982; Cox and Chavkin, 1983). The antagonistic effects of increasing doses of β-CNA were not identical for each of these agonists. The dose–response curves for the delta agonist [Leu^5]enkephalin showed a parallel shift to the right, whereas the dose–response curves for the mu agonist normorphine and the kappa agonist dynorphin A(1-13) showed mainly a reduction in maximum response with only a small right-ward shift after β-CNA treatment (Cox and Chavkin, 1986). This result suggests that while there is a large reserve of delta type receptors in mouse vas deferens, there is only a small reserve of mu and kappa receptors. The presence of a large reserve of delta receptors provides an explanation for the high potencies of delta selective agonists in mouse vas deferens since a low fractional occupancy is sufficient to produce maximal inhibition (Cox and Chavkin, 1983).

Schulz and Wuster (1981) have suggested that there may be subtypes, or isoreceptors, of the mu and kappa types in mouse vas deferens. This hypothesis was based on studies of the relative degrees of cross-tolerance exhibited by several receptor-type selective agonists following chronic treatment of the mice with various mu, delta, and kappa agonists. The extent of cross-tolerance between agonists clearly revealed the discrimination between mu, delta, and kappa classes of agonist. Within these sets of agonists, however, the extent of observed cross-tolerance was not identical for all mu- or kappa-selective compounds. Clearly the presence of isoreceptors of the mu and kappa type, with marginally varying configurational requirements for optimal activation by agonists, is a possible explanation of these results. However, the results might also be explained by small but significant differences between the supposed selective mu (or kappa) agonists with regard to their abilities to activate nonpreferred types of opioid receptor. Alternatively, since tolerance development in isolated tissues is associated with a reduction in receptor reserve (Chavkin and Goldstein, 1984), differences in the extent of observed cross-tolerance between different agonists might be related to differences in efficacy (i.e., differences in the fractional occupanies by the various agonists within each class needed to induce an agonist effect; a greater degree of tolerance would be anticipated for agonists with low efficacy). Further studies are needed to confirm that isoreceptors of the mu and kappa type are present in mouse vas deferens.

There are only a few studies of radioligand binding to opioid receptors in mouse vas deferens. Leslie and Kosterlitz (1979) were able to demonstrate the specific binding of [^{3}H][Met^5]enkephalin, [^{3}H]naltrexone, and [^{3}H]dihydromorphine to homogenates of mouse vas deferens at 0°C. Specific binding was not detected at 37°C in this study. Specific binding of [^{3}H]DADLE to homogenates of mouse vas deferens at 25°C has been observed and characterized (Leslie et al., 1980), however. As anticipated, this binding showed a ligand selectivity characteristic of delta-type binding sites. In general, however, the ratio of specific to nonspecific binding is low, limiting the usefulness of this tissue for studies of opioid receptors by radioligand binding.

Electrophysiological studies have confirmed that opioids reduce the electrically stimulated contractions of mouse vas deferens by inhibiting the output of excitatory transmitter. Henderson and North (1976) recorded excitatory junction potentials (ejps) from smooth muscle cells of mouse vas during electrical stimulation, and demonstrated the reduction of ejps amplitude after morphine treatment. A more extensive study showed that normorphine produced a parallel shift of the stimulus–ejps amplitude curve to the right and that naloxone antagonized this effect (Illes and Schulz, 1980). Thus, mu agonists reduced the postsynaptic response to low-intensity stimulation more than the response to higher-intensity stimulation. In contrast, the delta agonist, DADLE, and the very selective kappa agonist, U50488, produced a nonparallel shift in the stimulus–ejps amplitude curve, with greater inhibitions at higher stimulation intensities (Ramme and Illes, 1986). It was concluded that the less readily excited fibers innervating the mouse vas were more sensitive to delta and kappa agonists than mu agonists, although readily excitable fibers were probably equally sensitive to all three classes of agonist. These results suggest that the three classes of opioid receptors found in mouse vas deferens may not all be present on all of the adrenergic fibers innervating the tissue.

7.2.2. Rat, Rabbit, and Hamster Vas Deferens

The isolated rat vas deferens preparation was widely used in the study of adrenergic neurotransmission before Kosterlitz and colleagues (Henderson et al., 1972) demonstrated the inhibitory action of morphine on the mouse vas deferens preparation. Morphine had no inhibitory effect in the rat vas deferens. With the discovery of endogenous opioids, however, additional types of opioid agonist became available for testing. Lemaire et al. (1978) and Wuster et al. (1978) reported that β-endorphin inhibited the electrically stimulated contractions of rat vas deferens. Most other opioids tested were inactive. DADLE and etorphine were capable of producing maximal inhibition of the stimulated contractions, but were less potent than in guinea pig ileum. In view of the relative inactivity of commonly used mu and delta agonists, Wuster et al. (1978) proposed that a different type of opioid receptor, which they designated "epsilon," was present in rat vas deferens. Further studies confirmed that β-endorphin and related compounds were among the most potent compounds in this tissue (Schulz et al., 1979a; Huidobro-Toro et al., 1982). Naloxone antagonized the actions of β-endorphin (Lemaire et al., 1978; Schulz et al., 1979a). The reported K_e values for naloxone against several agonists in this tissue are listed in Table 2. Because of the close similarity of the naloxone dissociation constant against several mu agonists in rat vas to its dissociation constant at mu receptors in guinea pig ileum, it has been argued that the opioid receptors in rat vas deferens are of the mu type (Smith and Rance, 1983). The very weak or absent agonistic action of morphine was explained by the postulate that there are few spare receptors in rat vas deferens. Morphine, it was suggested, does not have adequate efficacy to induce an agonist effect because there is little re-

TABLE 2

Estimates of the Apparent Affinity of Naloxone as an Antagonist in the Isolated Rat Vas Deferens Preparation

Agonist	Estimate of naloxone K_e, nM	Reference
β-Endorphin	27	Lemaire et al., 1978
β-Endorphin	15	Gillan et al., 1981
β-Endorphin	3	Schulz et al., 1979a
DADLE[a]	34	Gillan et al., 1981
Etorphine	3	Schulz et al., 1979a
Normorphine	6	Gillan et al., 1981
DAGO[b]	8	Gillan et al., 1979a
DAGO[b]	3	Smith and Rance, 1983

[a]DADLE, [D-Ala^2-D-Leu^5]enkephalin.
[b]DAGO, Tyr-D-Ala-Gly-N(Me)Phe-Gly-ol.

ceptor reserve in this tissue. This argument requires that morphine behave as an antagonist of more efficacious mu agonists in this tissue, and in fact an antagonist effect of morphine against mu agonists has been observed (Smith and Rance, 1983).

The naloxone K_e values against β-endorphin and DADLE reported by Lemaire et al. (1978) and Gillan et al. (1981) appear to be substantially higher than its K_e values against mu-selective agonists (Table 2). It is possible that β-endorphin and DADLE are acting at delta receptors, but enkephalins generally show very low potency in rat vas, making this unlikely (Schulz et al., 1979a). A novel class of β-endorphin-selective receptors, the "epsilon" receptors of Wuster et al. (1978), may therefore be present. The results of Gillan et al. (1981) and Smith and Rance (1983), however, suggest that mu receptors are also present but that mu receptor-mediated agonist effects are only observed when mu receptors are activated by agonists with high efficacy. The naloxone K_e value against β-endorphin reported by Schulz et al. (1979a) is much lower than those reported by Lemaire et al. (1978) and Gillan et al. (1981), and might indicate that in some rat strains there is a different ratio of mu to epsilon receptors. Ethylketocyclazocine and other related benzomorphans behaved as antagonists in rat vas deferens, displaying greater antagonist potency against mu agonists than against β-endorphin (Gillan et al., 1981). This observation also supports the conclusion that mu agonists and β-endorphin act on different receptors in rat vas deferens. In view of the absence of agonist effects of ethylketocyclazocine, it seems unlikely that kappa receptors are present in significant concentration. The antagonism of mu agonists probably reflects the known affinity of ethyketocyclazocine for mu receptors.

In the isolated rabbit vas deferens, only kappa-selective agonists inhibit the contractile responses induced by electrical stimulation (Oka et al., 1980; Hayes and Kelly, 1985). Naloxone antagonizes this action with a K_e of about 30 nM (Hayes and Kelly, 1985), again suggesting that agonists act through kappa receptors in this tissue. In the hamster, only delta-selective agonists are active (McKnight et al., 1984; Miller and Shaw, 1985; Sheehan et al., 1986), and ICI 174864 is an effective antagonist. These results suggests that only kappa receptors are present in rabbit vas deferens, whereas hamster vas deferens contains only delta receptors. A summary of the opioid receptors contained in vas deferens of different species is presented in Table 3.

TABLE 3
Summary of the Properties of Opioid Receptors Present
in Vas Deferens Preparations

Species	Receptor types present	Evidence
Mouse	Delta	High potency of DSLET, DPDPE; antagonism by naloxone (K_e, approx. 25 nM) and ICI 174864 (K_e, approx. 150 nM); no cross tolerance to mu or kappa agonists (Cotton et al., 1984; Schulz and Wüster, 1981)
	Mu	Agonist action of morphine, sufentanyl; antagonism by naloxone (K_e, approx. 2 nM); no cross tolerance to delta or kappa agonists (Lord et al., 1977; Schulz and Wüster, 1981)
	Kappa	Agonist action of EKC, dynorphin A; antagonism by naloxone (K_e, approx. 20 nM) no cross tolerance to mu and delta agonists (Lord et al., 1977; Schulz and Wüster, 1981; Cox and Chavkin, 1983)
Rat	Mu	Agonist potency of DAGO, normorphine; antagonism by naloxone (K_e, approx. 3–6 nM) (Gillan et al., 1981; Smith and Rance, 1983)
	Epsilon	Agonist potency of β-endorphin, low agonist potency of other opioids; antagonism by naloxone (K_e, 15–30 nM) (Lemaire et al., 1978; Gillan et al., 1981)
Rabbit	Kappa	High agonist potencies of EKC, tifluadom, U50488H; negligible agonist activity of mu and delta agonists; antagonism by naloxone (K_e, approx. 20–30 nM) (Oka et al., 1980; Hayes and Kelly, 1985)
Hamster	Delta	High potency of DADLE, DSLET, DPDPE; low activity of DAGO,

(continued)

TABLE 3 (*continued*)
Summary of the Properties of Opioid Receptors Present
in Vas Deferens Preparations

Species	Receptor types present	Evidence
		U50488H; antagonism by naloxone (K_e, approx. 30 nM) and ICI 174864 (K_e, approx. 30 nM) (McKnight et al., 1984; Miller and Shaw, 1985)

[a]Abbreviations: DADLE, [D-Ala^2-D-Leu^5]enkephalin; DSLET, [D-Ser^2-Leu^5]enkephalyl-Thr; DPDPE, [D-Pen^5-D-Pen^5]enkephalin; EKC, ethylketocyclazocine; U50488H, trans - 3,4 - dichloro - N - methyl - N - 2 - (pyrrolidinyl) - cyclohexyl - benzeneacetamide methansulfonate hydrate; ICI 174864, N,N-diallyl-Tyr-Aib-Aib-Phe-Leu-OH.

7.3. Receptors in Other Reproductive Tract Tissues

Specific binding of [^{3}H]etorphine has been reported in human placenta (Valette et al., 1980). Comparisons of the ability of several opioids to compete for the [^{3}H]etorphine binding sites suggest that the placental binding sites are predominantly of the kappa type (Porthe et al., 1981). Analysis by subcellular fractionation of placental tissues has demonstrated that the opioid binding sites are concentrated on the syncitial brush border membrane (Porthe et al., 1982). The availability of reasonable quantities of placental tissue makes this a very convenient tissue for receptor solubilization studies. Placental opioid binding sites have been solubilized with the zwitterionic detergent, CHAPS, by Ahmed and coworkers (Ahmed et al., 1981; Ahmed, 1983). In general, the solubilized binding material retains the kappa ligand selectivity demonstrated by the membrane-bound receptor, although affinities were all lower after solubilization. The functions of opioid binding sites in placenta are unknown, although a possible facilitatory action on stimulated chorionic gonadotrophin secretion has been suggested (Valette et al., 1983).

Specific binding of [^{3}H]naloxone, [^{3}H]morphine, and [^{3}H]-DADLE has been reported in membranes of the oocytes of the toad *Bufo viridis* (Bakalkin et al., 1984). High- and low-affinity components of binding were observed. These binding sites are not yet well characterized; from a limited range of opioids and opioid peptides, naloxone and bremazocine showed the highest potency in competing against [^{3}H]naloxone binding. Bakalkin et al. (1984) suggest that the high-affinity binding is of the kappa type. Again, the functions of these sites are unknown.

8. Interactions of Opioids with Blood Cells and the Immune System

Early studies of specific opioid binding failed to find evidence of opioid receptors in blood cells (Snyder et al., 1978). More recently, some reports indicating opioid interactions with blood cells have been published. The appropriate classification of the receptors mediating these effects remains uncertain, however. Thus, Yamasaki and Way (1983, 1985) have reported that opioids inhibit a calcium ATPase pump in red cell membranes. They suggest that this is a kappa receptor-mediated effect because of the high potency of some kappa-selective agonists and because naloxone shows an antagonist K_e of 20–30 nM against all the opioids showing activity in this system. The observed relative potencies of agonists are not entirely consistent with their action at kappa receptors. In particular, morphine, levorphanol, dihyromorphine, and β-endorphin are all much more potent than would be predicted from studies of kappa receptors in other tissues if the effect were induced entirely by kappa receptor activation. Thus the possibility that other receptors, or a novel type of receptor, is implicated in this response must be considered. It is noteworthy, however, that in the guinea pig myenteric plexus and elsewhere, kappa receptors have been reported to reduce calcium flux through a calcium channel (Cherubini and North, 1985). Inhibition of calcium transport across cell membranes might be a common feature of these two proposed kappa receptor-mediated events.

There has recently been much interest in the modulation of the function of the immune system by opioids, and a wide range of effects on different components of the system have been reported. Again it has not been possible to demonstrate the role of previously identified types of opioid receptor in these effects, and in some cases the actions of some endogenous opioids involve receptors that are very different from the "classic" opioid receptors that are the subject of this review. The interested reader is referred to two recent short reviews by Chang (1984) and by Teschemacher and Schweigerer (1985), which provide a helpful overview of this rapidly developing field.

9. Summary

There are some common features to the actions of opioids in peripheral tissues. In many different tissues, the effect of the opioids of various types is to reduce the release of neurotransmitter from excitatory or inhibitory neurons. The reduction in transmitter release appears to occur because opioid receptor activation leads, in one way or another, to a reduction in the influx of calcium through voltage-dependent calcium channels. The receptors through which opioids act in the periphery are also similar to the receptors found in the central nervous system. Evidence points to a role for mu, delta, kappa, or epsilon receptors in most of the actions described in this chapter. Although presently available evidence points to considerable similarities between species in the functions employing each type of opioid receptor in the central nervous system, there are very marked differences among species in the sensitivities of various peripheral tissues to different types of opioid. Why is hamster vas deferens inhibited only by opioids with good potency at delta receptors, whereas rabbit vas is only sensitive to kappa agonists? Vasa from other small laboratory animals show different patterns of sensitivity to each type of opioid. Although the vas deferens presents a particularly striking example of species variation in peripheral opioid receptor distribution, similar variations among species are apparent in most other peripheral actions of opioids. How does such diversity arise during evolution and what is its functional significance?

The functions of the endogenous opioid systems are not essential for survival. Chronic treatment with high doses of opioid antagonists does not cause much disturbance in animal behavior, and although adaptive changes in, for example, the density of receptors in particular structures can be discerned, most physiological systems continue to function in apparently normal fashion. This suggests that the endogenous opioids normally serve a modulatory role, fine tuning the regulatory functions exerted by other neurotransmitters and hormones. It may well be that this modulatory role makes agents that mimic the actions of endogenous opioids, that is, opiate drugs, particularly useful as therapeutic agents.

Many of the peripheral actions of opioids are of present or potential therapeutic significance. It has already proved possible to design opioid drugs whose actions are restricted to peripheral tissues since they cannot gain access to the central nervous system. The differential ligand selectivities of the various types of opioid receptor in peripheral tissues make more precise targeting to specific receptors types a feasible goal. If the many peripheral actions of opioids are to be further exploited for drug therapy in humans, however, it will be necessary to determine the distribution and functions of each type of opioid receptor in human peripheral tissues. The marked diversity between lower animal species in the functions of the various types of opioid makes any conclusions based on studies of opioid function in mice, rats, and rabbits of limited significance in predicting potential peripheral targets for opioids in humans.

Acknowledgments

I would like to thank Drs. M. S. Ahmed, R. J. Bicknell, R. Howells, P. Illes, W. Knepel, S. A. Krumins, L. Manara, R. J. Miller, R. A. North, M. J. Rance, R. Schulz, M. B. Tyers, S. Ward, E. L. Way, and E. T. Wei for sending me manuscripts of papers in press, and in some cases allowing me to cite unpublished work. The opinions and assertions expressed herein are the personal views of the author and do not represent the views of the Uniformed Services University or the US Department of Defense.

References

Ahmed, M. S. (1983) Characterization of solubilized opiate receptors from human placenta. *Membrane Biochem.* **5,** 35–47.
Ahmed, M. S., Byrne, W. L., and Klee, W. A. (1981) Solubilization of opiate receptors from human placenta. *Placenta* **3,** 115–121.
Akil, H., Shiomi, H., and Matthews, J. (1985) Induction of the intermediate pituitary by stress: Synthesis and release of a non-opioid form of beta-endorphin. *Science* **227,** 424–426.
Alumets, J., Hakanson, R., Sundler, F., and Chang, K. -J. (1978) Leu-enkephalin-like material in nerves and entero-chromaffin cells in the gut. *Histochemie* **56,** 187–196.
Anhut, H. and Knepel, W. (1982) Release of dynorphin-like immunoreactivity of rat neurohypophysis in comparison to vasopressin after various stimuli in vitro and in vivo. *Neurosci. Lett.* **31,** 159–164.
Awouters, F., Niemegeers, C. J. E., and Janssen, P. A. J. (1983) Pharmacology of antidiarrheal drugs. *Ann. Rev. Pharmacol. Tox.* **23,** 279–301.
Bakalkin, G. Y., Yakovleva, T. V., Korobov, K. P., Bespalova, Zh. D.,

Vinogradov, V. A., and Titov, M. A. (1984) Opiate binding sites and endogenous opioids in oocytes of toad *Bufo viridis. Biokhimya* **49,** 883–888.

Bartho, L. and Szolcsanyi, J. (1981) Opiate agonist inhibit neurogenic plasma extravasation in the rat. *Eur. J. Pharmacol.* **73,** 101–104.

Beckett, A. H. and Casy, A. F. (1954) Synthetic analgesics: Stereochemical considerations. *J. Pharm. Pharmacol.* **6,** 986–999.

Bentley, G. A., Newton, S. H., and Starr, M. J. (1981) Evidence for an action of morphine and the enkephalins on sensory nerve endings in the mouse peritoneum. *Br. J. Pharmacol.* **73,** 325–332.

Bianchi, G., Ferretti, P., Recchia, M., Rochetti, M., Tavani, A., and Manara, L. (1983) Morphine tissue levels and reduction of gastrointestinal transit in rats. *Gastroenterology* **85,** 852–858.

Bicknell, R. J. and Leng, G. (1982) Endogenous opiates regulate oxytocin but not vasopressin secretion from the neurohypophysis. *Nature* **298,** 161–162.

Bicknell, R. J. and Leng, G. (1983) Differential regulation of oxytocin- and vasopressin-secretory nerve terminals. *Prog. Brain. Res.* **60,** 333–341.

Bicknell, R.J., Chapman, C., and Leng, G. (1985a) Effects of opioid agonists and antagonists on oxytocin and vasopressin release in vitro. *Neuroendocrinology* **41,** 142–148.

Bicknell R. J., Chapman, C., and Leng, G. (1985b) Neurohypophysial opioids and oxytocin secretion: Source of inhibitory opioids. *Exp. Brain Res.* **60,** 192–196.

Bicknell, R. J., Ingram, C. D., and Leng, G. (1983) Oxytocin release is inhibited by opiates from the neural lobe, not those from the intermediate lobe. *Neurosci. Lett.* **43,** 227–230.

Binder, H. J., Laurenson, J. P., and Dobbins, J. W. (1984) Role of opiate receptors in regulation of enkephalin stimulation of active sodium and chloride absorption. *Am. J. Physiol.* **247,** G247–G436.

Bitar, K. N. and Makhlouf, G. M. (1982) Specific opiate receptors on isolated mammalian gastric smooth muscle cells. *Nature* **297,** 72–74.

Bitar, K. N. and Makhlouf, G. M. (1985) Selective presence of opiate receptors on intestinal circular muscle cells. *Life Sci.* **37,** 1545–1550.

Black, J. W. and Leff, P. (1983) Operational models of pharmacological agonism. *Proc. Roy. Soc. Lond. (B)* **220,** 141–162.

Blume, A. J., Lichshtein, D., and Boone, A. (1979) Coupling of opiate receptors to adenylate cyclase: Requirement for sodium and GTP. *Proc. Natl. Acad. Sci. USA* **75,** 5626–5630.

Botticelli, L. J., Cox, B. M., and Goldstein, A. (1981) Immunoreactive dynorphin in mammalian spinal cord and dorsal root ganglia. *Proc. Natl. Acad. Sci. USA* **78,** 7783–7786.

Brady, K. T., Balster, R. L., and May, E. L. (1982) Stereoisomers of N-allylnormetazocine: Phencyclidine-like behavioral effects in squirrel monkeys and rats. *Science* **215,** 178–180.

Burks, T. F. (1973) Mediation by 5-hydroxytryptamine of morphine stimulant actions in dog intestine. *J. Pharmacol. Exp. Ther.* **185,** 530–539.

Burks, T. F., Hirning, L. D., Galligan, J. T., and Davis, T. P. (1982) Motility effects of opioid peptides in dog intestine. *Life Sci.* **31,** 2237–2240.

Cairnie, A. B., Kosterlitz, H. W., and Taylor, D. W. (1961) Effect of morphine on some sympathetically innervated effectors. *Br. J. Pharmacol.* **17,** 539–551.

Castanas, E., Giraud, P., Audigier, Y., Drisi, R., Boudouresque, F., Coute-Devolz, B., and Oliver, C. (1984) Adrenal medullary opiate receptors. Pharmacological characterization in bovine adrenal medulla and a human pheochromocytoma. *Mol. Pharmacol.* **25,** 38–45.

Chaminade, M., Foutz, A. S., and Rossier, J. (1984) Co-release of enkephalins and precursors with catecholamines from perfused cat adrenal gland in situ. *J. Physiol.* **353,** 157–169.

Chang, K. -J. (1984) Opioid peptides have actions of the immune system. *Trends Neurosci.* **7,** 234–235.

Chang, K. -J., Miller, R. J., and Cuatrecasas, P. (1978) Interactions of enkephalin with opiate receptors in intact cultured cells. *Mol. Pharmacol.* **14,** 961–970.

Chavkin, C. and Goldstein, A. (1981) Demonstration of a specific dynorphin receptor in guinea pig ileum myenteric plexus. *Nature* **291,** 591–593.

Chavkin, C. and Goldstein, A. (1984) Opioid receptor reserve in normal and morphine-tolerant guinea pig ileum myenteric plexus. *Proc. Natl. Acad. Sci. USA* **81,** 7253–7257.

Chavkin, C., Cox, B. M., and Goldstein, A. (1979) Stereospecific opiate binding in bovine adrenal medulla. *Mol. Pharmacol.* **15,** 751–753.

Cherubini, E. and North R. A. (1985) Mu and kappa opioids inhibit transmitter release by different mechanisms. *Proc. Natl. Acad. Sci. USA* **82,** 1860–1863.

Comb, M., Seeberg, P. H., Adelman, J., Eiden, L., and Herbert, E. (1982) Primary structure of the human Met- and Leu-enkephalin precursor and its mRNA. *Nature* **295,** 663–666.

Corbett, A. D., Sosa, R. P., McKnight, A. T., and Kosterlitz, H. W. (1980) Effects of electrical stimulation on the enkephalins in guinea pig small intestine. *Eur. J. Pharmacol.* **65,** 113–117.

Cotton, R., Giles, M. B., Miller, L., Shaw, J. S., and Timms, T. (1984) ICI 174,864: A highly selective antagonist for the opioid delta receptor. *Eur. J. Pharmacol.* **78,** 385–387.

Coupar, I. M. (1978) Inhibition by morphine of prostaglandin-stimulated fluid secretion in rat jejunum. *Br. J. Pharmacol.* **63,** 57–63.

Cox, B. M. (1978) Multiple Mechanisms in Opiate Tolerance, in *Characteristics and Functions in Opioids* (van Ree, J. and Terenius, L., eds.) Elsevier, Amsterdam.

Cox, B. M., and Baizman, E. R. (1982) Physiological Functions of Endorphins, in *Endorphins; Chemistry, Physiology, Pharmacology, and Clinical Relevance* (Malick, J. B. and Bell, R. M. S., eds.) Dekker, New York.

Cox, B. M. and Chavkin, C. (1983) Comparison of dynorphin-selective kappa receptors in mouse vas deferens and guinea pig ileum. *Mol. Pharmacol.* **23,** 36–43.

Cox, B. M. and Chavkin, C. (1986) Properties of receptors mediating opioid effects: Discrimination of receptor types. Opiate receptor subtypes and brain function. *NIDA Res. Monograph,* **71,** 1–18.

Cox, B. M. and Padhya, R. (1977) Opiate binding and effect in ileum preparations from normal and morphine pretreated guinea pigs. *Br. J. Pharmacol.* **61,** 271–278.

Cox, B. M. and Weinstock, M. (1966) The effect of analgesic drugs on the release of acetylcholine from electrically stimulated guinea pig ileum. *Br. J. Pharmacol.* **21,** 81–92.

Cox, B. M., Baer, A. E., and Goldstein, A. (1982) Dynorphin immunoreactivity in pituitary. *Adv. Biochem. Psychopharmacol.* **33,** 43–50.

Creese, I. and Snyder, S. H. (1975) Receptor binding and pharmacological activity of opiates in the guinea pig intestine. *J. Pharmacol. Exp. Ther.* **194,** 205–219.

Crooks, P. A., Bowdy, B. D., Reinsel, C. L., Iwamoto, E. T., and Gilespie, M. N. (1984) Structure–activity evidence against opiate receptor involvement in Leu[5]-enkephalin induced pulmonary vasoconstriction. *Biochem. Pharmacol.* **35,** 4095–4098.

Currie, M. G., Geller, D. M., Cole, B. R., Boyler, J. G., Yu Sheng, W., Holmberg, S. W., and Needleman, P. (1983) Bioactive cardiac substances: Potent vasorelaxant activity in mammalian atria. *Science* **221,** 71–73.

Davis, T. P., Culling, A. J., Schoemaker, H., and Galligan, J. J. (1983) Beta-endorphin and its metabolites stimulate motility of the dog small intestine. *J. Pharmacol. Exp. Ther.* **227,** 499–507.

Di Giulio, A. M., Yang, H. -Y. T., and Lutold, B., Fratta, W., Hong, J., and Costa, E. (1978) Characterization of enkephalin-like material extracted from sympathetic ganglia. *Neuropharmacology* **17,** 989–992.

Dobbins, J., Racusen, L., and Binder, H. J. (1980) Effect of D-alanine methionine enkephalin amide on ion transport in rabbit ileum. *J. Clin. Invest.* **66,** 19–28.

Donnerer, J., Holzer, R., and Lembeck, F. (1984) Release of dynorphin, somatostatin and substance P from the vascularly perfused small intestine of the guinea pig during peristalsis. *Br. J. Pharmacol.* **83,** 919–925.

Douglass, J., Cox, B. M., Quinn, B., Civelli, O., and Herbert, E. (1987) Expression of the prodynorphin gene in male and female mammalian reproductive tract tissues. *Endocrinology* **120,** 707–713.

Dum, J., Meyer, G., Hollt, V., and Herz, A. (1979) In vivo opiate binding unchanged in tolerant/dependent mice. *Eur. J. Pharmacol.* **58,** 453–460.

Edin, R., Lundberg, J., Terenius, L., Dahlstrom, A., Hokfelt, T., Kewenter, J., and Ahlman, H. (1980) Evidence for vagal enkephalinergic neural control of the feline pylorus and stomach. *Gastroenterology* **78,** 492–497.

Elde, R., Hokfelt, T., Johansson, O., and Terenius, L. (1976) Immunohistochemical studies using antibodies to leucine-enkephalin: initial observations on the nervous system of the rat. *Neuroscience* **1,** 349–351.

Ensinger, H., Hedler, L., Schurr, C., and Starke, K. (1984) Ethylketcyclazocine decreases noradrenaline release and blood pressure in the rabbit at a peripheral opioid receptor. *Naunyn Schmeidebergs Arch. Pharmacol.* **328,** 20–23.

Evans, A. G. J., Nasmyth, P. A., and Stewart, H. C. (1952) The fall of blood pressure caused by morphine in the rat and cat. *Br. J. Pharmacol.* **7,** 542–552.

Fabri, A., Gnessi, L., Perricone, R., de Sanctis, G., Moretti, C., de Carolis,

C., Fontana, L., Isidori, A., and Fraioli, F. (1985) Human semen inhibits T rosette formation through an opiate mediated mechanism. *J. Clin. Endocrinol. Metab.* **60**, 807–809.

Feldberg, W. and Paton, W. D. M. (1951) Release of histamine from skin and muscle of the cat by opium alkaloids and other histamine liberators. *J. Physiol.* **114**, 490–509.

Fennessy, M. R. and Rattray, J. F. (1971) Cardiovascular effects of intravenous morphine in the anesthetized rat. *Eur. J. Pharmacol.* **14**, 1–8.

Ferreira, S. G. (1981) Inflammatory pain, prostaglandin hyperalgesia and the development of peripheral analgesics. *Trends Pharmacol. Sci.* **2**, 183–186.

Ferreira, S. H. and Nakamura, M. (1979) Prostaglandin hyperalgesia: The peripheral analgesic activity of morphine, enkephalins and opioid antagonists. *Prostaglandins* **18**, 191–200.

Ferreira, S. H., Lorenzetti, B. B., and Rae, G. A. (1984) Is methylnalorphinium the prototype of an ideal peripheral analgesic? *Eur. J. Pharmacol.* **99**, 23–29.

Ferretti, P., Bianchi, G., Tavani, A., and Manara, L. (1981) Inhibition of gastrointestinal transit and nociceptive effects of morphine and FK 33-824 in rats are differently prevented by naloxone and by its N-methylquarternary analog. *Res. Commun. Subst. Abuse* **2**, 1–11.

Fields, H. L., Emson, P. C., Leigh, B. K., Gilbert, R. F. T., and Iversen, L. L. (1980) Multiple opiate receptor sites on primary afferent fibers. *Nature* **284**, 351–353.

Fiocchi, R., Bianchi, G., Petrillo, P., Tavani, A., and Manara, L. (1982) Morphine inhibits gastrointestinal transit in the rat primarily by impairing propulsive activity of the small intestine. *Life Sci.* **31**, 2221–2223.

Furchgott, R. F. (1978) Pharmacological characterization of receptors: Its relation to radioligand binding studies. *Fed. Proc.* **37**, 115–120.

Gerendai, I., Shaha, C., Thau, R., and Bardin, C. W. (1984) Do testicular opiates regulate Leydig cell function? *Endocrinology* **115**, 1645–1647.

Giles, T. D. and Sander, G. E. (1983) Mechanism of the cardiovascular response to systemic intravenous administration of leucine enkephalin in the conscious dog. *Peptides* **4**, 171–175.

Gillan, M. C. G., Kosterlitz, H. W., and Magnan, J. (1981) Unexpected antagonism in the rat vas deferens by benzomorphans which are agonists in other pharmacological tests. *Br. J. Pharmacol.* **72**, 13–15.

Gintzler, A. R. and Pasternak, G. (1983) Multiple mu receptors: Evidence for mu_2 sites in the guinea pig ileum. *Neurosci. Lett.* **39**, 51–56.

Gintzler, A. R. and Scalisi, J. A. (1982) Physiological analysis of delta opioid receptors in the guinea pig myenteric plexus. *Life Sci.* **31**, 2363–2366.

Goldstein, A. and Ghazarossian, V. E. (1980) Immunoreactive dynorphin in pituitary and brain. *Proc. Natl. Acad. Sci. USA* **77**, 6207–6210.

Green, A. F. (1959) Comparative effects of analgesics on pain threshold, respiration frequency, and gastrointestinal propulsion. *Br. J. Pharmacol.* **14**, 26–34.

Gubler, U., Seeberg, P., Hoffman, B. J., Gage, L. P., and Udenfriend, S. (1982) Molecular cloning establishes proenkephalin as precursor of enkephalin-containing peptides. *Nature* **295**, 206–208.

Hahn, E. F., Carroll-Buatti, M., and Pasternak, G. W. (1982) Irreversible opiate antagonists: The 14-hydroxydihydromorphinone azines. *J. Neurosci.* **2**, 572–576.

Hanko, J. H. and Hardebo, J. E. (1978) Enkephalin induced dilatation of pial arteries in vitro probably mediated by opiate receptors. *Eur. J. Pharmacol.* **51**, 295–297.

Hayes, A. and Kelly, A. (1985) Profile of activity of kappa receptor agonists in the rabbit vas deferens. *Eur. J. Pharmacol.* **110**, 317–322.

Hayes, A. G., Sheehan, M. J., and Tyers, M. B. (1985) Determination of the receptor selectivity of opioid agonists in the guinea pig ileum and mouse vas deferens using beta-funaltrexamine. *Br. J. Pharmacol.* **86**, 899–904.

Henderson, G. and North, R. A. (1976) Depression by morphine of excitatory junction potentials in the vas deferens of the mouse. *Br. J. Pharmacol.* **57**, 341–346.

Henderson, G., Hughes, J., and Kosterlitz, H. W. (1972) A new example of a morphine-sensitive neuro-effector junction: Adrenergic transmission in the mouse vas deferens. *Br. J. Pharmacol.* **46**, 764–766.

Herkenham, M., Rice, K. C., Jacobsen, A. E., and Rothman, R. B. (1986) Opiate receptors in rat pituitary are confined to the neural lobe and are exclusively kappa. *Brain Res.* **382**, 365–371.

Hervonen, A., Linnoila, I., Pickel, V. M., Helen, P., Pelto-Huikko, M., Alho, H., and Miller, R. J. (1981) Localization of [Met^5]- and [Leu^5]enkephalin-like immunoreactivity in nerve terminals in human paravertebral sympathetic ganglia. *Neuroscience* **6**, 323–330.

Hiller, J. M., Simon, E. J., Crain, S. M., and Peterson, E. R. (1978) Opiate receptors in cultures of fetal mouse dorsal root ganglia (DRG) and spinal cord: Predominance in DRG neurites. *Brain Res.* **145**, 396–400.

Holaday, J. W. (1983) Cardiovascular effects of endogenous opiate systems. *Ann. Rev. Pharmacol. Toxicol.* **23**, 541–594.

Hollt, V., Haarman, I., Seizinger, B. R., and Herz, A. (1981) Levels of dynorphin-(1-13) immunoreactivity in rat neurointermediate pituitaries are concomitantly altered with those of leucine enkephalin and vasopressin in response to various endocrine manipulations. *Neuroendocrinology* **33**, 333–339.

Howells, R. D., Kilpatrick, D. L., Bailey, L. C., Noe, M., and Udenfriend, S. (1985) Pro-enkephalin mRNA in rat heart. *Proc. Natl. Acad. Sci. USA*, in press.

Hughes, J., Kosterlitz, H. W., and Leslie, F. M. (1975) Effects of morphine on adrenergic transmission in the mouse vas deferens. Assessment of agonist and antagonist potencies of narcotic analgesics. *Br. J. Pharmacol.* **53**, 371–381.

Hughes, J., Kosterlitz, H. W., and Smith, T. W. (1977) The distribution of methionine-enkephalin and leucine-enkephalin in the brain and peripheral tissues. *Br. J. Pharmacol.* **61**, 639–647.

Huidobro-Toro, J. P. and Way, E. L. (1981) Contractile effect of morphine and related opioid alkaloids, beta-endorphin, and methionine-enkephalin, on the isolated colon from Long-Evans rats. *Br. J. Pharmacol.* **74**, 681–694.

Huidobro-Toro, J. P., Castanay, E. M., Ling, N., Lee, N. M., Loh, H. H., and Way, E. L. (1982) Studies on the structural prerequisites for the activation of the beta-endorphin receptor on the rat vas deferens. *J. Pharmacol. Exp. Ther.* **222,** 262–269.

Huidobro-Toro, J. P., Yoshimura, K., and Way, E. L. (1982) Application of an irreversible opiate antagonist (beta-FNA) to demonstrate dynorphin selectivity for kappa opioid sites. *Life Sci.* **31,** 2409–2416.

Hunt, S. P., Kelly, J. S., and Emson, P. C. (1980) The electromicroscopic localization of methionine enkephalin within the superficial layers (I and II) of the spinal cord. *Neuroscience* **5,** 1871–1870.

Hutchison, M., Kosterlitz, H. W., Leslie, F. M., and Waterfield, A. A. (1975) Assessment in the guinea pig ileum and mouse vas deferens of benzomorphans which have strong antinociceptive activity but do not substitute for morphine in the dependent monkey. *Br. J. Pharmacol.* **55,** 541–546.

Iijima, I., Minamikawa, J. -I., Jacobsen, A. E., Brassi, A., and Rice, K. E. (1978) Studies in the (+)-morphinan series. 5. Synthesis and biological properties of (+)-naloxone. *J. Med. Chem.* **21,** 398–400.

Illes, P. and Schulz, R. (1980) Inhibition of neuroeffector transmission by morphine in the vas deferens of naive and morphine-treated mice. *Br. J. Pharmacol.* **71,** 195–200.

Illes, P., Pfeiffer, N., Limberger, N., and Starke, K. (1983) Presynaptic opioid receptors in the rabbit ear artery. *Life Sci.* **33** (suppl. 1), 307–310.

Illes, P., Pfeiffer, N., von Kugelen, I., and Starke, K. (1985a) Presynaptic opioid receptor subtypes in the rabbit ear artery. *J. Pharmacol. Exp. Ther.* **232,** 526–533.

Illes, P., Ramme, D., and Starke, K. (1985b) Inhibition of neurotransmitter transmission in the rabbit mesenteric artery by [Met^5]enkephalin. *Eur. J. Pharmacol.* **107,** 397–398.

Iversen, L. L., Iversen, S. D., and Bloom, F. E. (1980) Opiate receptors influence vasopressin release from nerve terminals in rat neurohypophysis. *Nature* **284,** 350–351.

Jaffe, J. H. and Martin, W. R. (1985) Opioid Analgesics and Antagonists, in *The Pharmacological Basis of Therapeutics* Gilman, A. G., Goodman, G. S. Rall, T. W., and Murad, F., (eds.) Macmillan, New York.

Jamieson, J. D. and Palade, G. E. (1964) Specific granules in atrial muscle cells. *J. Cell. Biol.* **23,** 151–172.

Jancso, N., Jancso-Gabor, A., and Szolcsanyi, J. (1967) Direct evidence for neurogenic inflammation and its prevention by denervation and by treatment with capsaicin. *Br. J. Pharmacol.* **31,** 138–151.

Jaquet, Y. F., Klee, W. A., Rice, K. E., Iijima, I., and Minamikawa, J. (1977) Stereospecific and non-stereospecific effects of (+) and (−)-morphine: Evidence for a new class of receptors? *Science* **198,** 842–845.

Jessell, T. M. and Iversen, L. L. (1977) Opiate analgesics inhibit substance P release from rat trigeminal nucleus. *Nature* **268,** 549–551.

Jessen, K. R., Saffrey, M. J., van Noorden, S., Bloom, S. R., Polak, J. M., and Burnstock, G. (1980) Immunohistochemical studies of the enteric nervous system in tissue culture and in situ: Localization of vasoactive intestinal polypeptide (VIP), substance P and enkephalin immunore-active nerves in the guinea pig gut. *Neuroscience* **5**, 1717–1735.

Jonsson, A. – C. (1985) Occurrence of met-enkephalin, met-enkephalin-Arg[6]-Phe[7] and met-enkephalin-Arg[6]-Gly[7]-Leu[8] in gastrin cells of hog antral mucosa. *Cell Tissue Res.* **240**, 361–365.

Kachur, J. F. and Miller, R. J. (1982) Characterization of the opiate receptor in the guinea pig ileal mucosa. *Eur. J. Pharmacol.* **81**, 177–183.

Kachur, J. F., Miller, R. J., and Field, M. (1980) Control of guinea pig intestinal electrolyte secretion by a delta opiate receptor. *Proc. Natl. Acad. Sci. USA* **77**, 2753–2756.

Kennedy, B. L. and West, T. C. (1967) Effect of morphine on electrically induced release of autonomic mediators in the rabbit sinoatrial node. *J. Phamacol. Exp. Ther.* **157**, 149–158.

Kiang, J. G. and Wei, E. T. (1983) Inhibition of an opioid-evoked vagal reflex in rats by naloxone. SMS 201-995, and ICI 154,129. *Reg. Peptides* **6**, 255–262.

Kiang, J. G. and Wei, E. T. (1984) Sensitivity to morphine-evoked bradycardia in rats is modified by dynorphin-(1-13), Leu-, and Met-enkephalin. *J. Pharmacol. Exp. Ther.* **229**, 469–473.

Kiang, J. G., Dewey, W. L., and Wei, E. T. (1983) Tolerance to morphine bradycardia in the rat. *J. Pharmacol. Exp. Ther.* **226**, 187–191.

Kilpatrick, D. L., Howells, R. D., Noe, M., Bailey, C. L., and Udenfriend, S. (1985) Expression of pre-proenkephalin mRNA and its peptide products in mammalian testis and ovary. *Proc. Natl. Acad. Sci. USA* **82**, 7467–7469.

Klee, W. A. and Streaty, R. A. (1974) Narcotic receptor sites in morphine dependent rats. *Nature* **248**, 61–63.

Knepel, W. and Meyer, D. F. (1983) The effect of naloxone on vasopressin release from rat neurohypophysis incubated in vitro. *J. Physiol.* **341**, 515–516.

Knoll, J. (1976) Neuronal peptide (enkephalin) receptors in the ear artery of the rabbit. *Eur. J. Pharmacol.* **39**, 403–407.

Konishi, S., Tsunoo, A., and Otsuka, M. (1979) Enkephalins pre-synaptically inhibit cholinergic transmission in sympathetic ganglia. *Nature*, **282**, 515–516.

Konishi, S., Tsunoo, A., and Otsuka, M. (1981) Enkephalin as a transmitter for presynaptic inhibition in sympathetic ganglia. *Nature* **294**, 80–82.

Kosterlitz, H. W. and Robinson, J. A. (1958) The inhibitory action of morphine on the contraction of the longitudinal muscle coat of the isolated guinea pig ileum. *Br. J. Pharmacol.* **13**, 296–303.

Kosterlitz, H. W. and Taylor, D. W. (1959) The effect of morphine on vagal inhibition of the heart. *Br. J. Pharmacol.* **14**, 209–214.

Kosterlitz, H. W. and Watt, A. (1968) Kinetic parameters of narcotic agonists and antagonists, with particular reference to N-allylnoroxymorphone (naloxone). *Br. J. Pharmacol.* **33**, 266–276.

Kromer, W., Hollt, V., Schmidt, H., and Herz, A. (1981) Release of immunreactive dynorphin from the isolated guinea pig small intestine is reducued during peristaltic activity. *Neurosci. Lett.* **25**, 53–56.

Krumins, S. A., Faden, A. I., and Feuerstein, G. (1985) Opiate binding in rat hearts: Modulation of binding after hemorrhagic shock. *Biochem. Biophys. Res. Commun.* **127**, 120–128.

Kudo, T., Chang, H. -L., Maeda, S., Makamae, J., and Inoki, R. (1983) Changes of the Met-enkephalin-like peptide content induced by noxious stimuli in the rat incisor pulp. *Life Sci.* **33**, (suppl. I), 677–680.

Kumakara, K., Karoum, F., Guidotti, A., and Costa, E. (1980) Modulation of nicotinic receptors by opiate receptor agonists in cultured adrenal chromaffin cells. *Nature* **283**, 489–492.

Kurose, H., Katada, T., Amano, T., and Ui, M. (1983) Specific uncoupling by islet-activating protein, pertussis toxin, of negative signal transduction via alpha-adrenergic, cholinergic and opiate receptors in neuroblastoma × glioma hybrid cells. *J. Biol. Chem.* **258**, 4870–4875.

Lamotte, C., Pert, C. B., and Snyder, S. H. (1976) Opiate receptor binding in primate spinal cord: Distribution and changes after dorsal root section. *Brain Res.* **112**, 407–412.

Lang, R. E., Hermann, K., Dietz, R., Gaida, W., Ganten, D., Kraft, K., and Unger, T. (1983) Evidence for the presence of enkephalins in the rat. *Life Sci.* **32**, 399–406.

Law, P. Y., Hom, D. S., and Loh, H. H. (1983) Opiate regulation of adenosine 3', 5'-cyclic monophosphate level in neuroblastoma × glioma NG 108-15 hybrid cells. Relationship between receptor occupancy and effect. *Mol. Pharmacol.* **23**, 26–35.

Leander, J. (1983) A kappa opioid effect: Increased urination in the rat. *J. Pharmacol. Exp. Ther.* **224**, 89–94.

Ledda, F. and Mantelli, L. (1982) Possible pre-synaptic inhibitory effect of etorphine on sympathetic nerve terminals of guinea pig heart. *Eur. J. Pharmacol.* **85**, 247–250.

Ledda, F., Mantelli, M., Corti, V., and Fantozzi, R. (1984) Inhibition of the cardiac response to sympathetic nerve stimulation by opioid peptides and its potentiation by morphine and methadone. *Eur. J. Pharmacol.* **102**, 443–450.

Lemaire, S., Livett, B., Tseng, R., Mercier, R., and Lemaire, I. (1981) Studies on the inhibitory action of opiate compounds in isolated bovine adrenal chromaffin cells. *J. Neurochem.* **36**, 886–892.

Lemaire, S., Magnan, J., and Regoli, D. (1978) Rat vas deferens: A specific bioassay for endogenous opioid peptides. *Br. J. Pharmacol.* **64**, 327–329.

Lemaire, S., Valette, A., Chouinard, L., Depuis, N., Day, R., Porthe, G., and Cros, J. (1983) Purification and identification of multiple forms of dynorphin in human placenta. *Neuropeptides* **3**, 181–191.

Lembeck, F., Donnerer, J., and Bartho, L. (1982) Inhibition of neurogenic vasodilatation and plasma extravasation by substance P antagonists, somatostatin, and [D-Met^2,Pro^5]enkephalin amide. *Eur. J. Pharmacol.* **85**, 171–176.

Leslie, F. M. and Kosterlitz, H. W. (1979) Comparison of the binding of [^{3}H]methionine-enkephalin, [^{3}H]naloxone, and [^{3}H]dihydromorphine in the mouse vas deferens and the myenteric plexus and brain of the guinea pig. *Eur. J. Pharmacol.* **56**, 379–383.

Leslie, F. M., Chavkin, C., and Cox, B. M. (1980) Opioid binding properties of brain and peripheral tissues: Evidence for heterogeneity in opioid ligand binding sites. *J. Pharmacol. Exp. Ther.* **214**, 395–402.

Lewis, R. V., Stern, A. S., Kimura, S., Rossier, J., Stein, S., and Udenfriend, S. (1980) An about 50,000-dalton protein in adrenal medulla; a common precursor of [Met]- and [Leu]-enkephalin. *Science* **208**, 1459–1461.

Lightman, S. L., Ninkovic, M., Hunt, S. P., and Iversen, L. L. (1983) Evidence for opiate receptors on pituicytes. *Nature* **305**, 235–237.

Lim, A. T., Lolait, S., Barlow, J. W., Wai Sum, O., Zois, I., Toh, B. H., and Funder, J. W. (1983) Immunoreactive beta-endorphin in sheep ovary. *Nature* **303**, 709–711.

Linnoila, R. I., DiAugustine, R. P., Miller, R. J., Chang, K. -J., and Cuatrecasas, P. (1978) An immunohistochemical and radioimmunological study of the distribution of [Met]- and [Leu]-enkephalin in the gastrointestinal tract. *Neuroscience* **3**, 1187–1196.

Lopez-Ruiz, M. P., Arilla, E., Gomez-Pan, A., and Prieto, J. C. (1985) Interaction of leu-enkephalin with isolated enterocytes from guinea pig: Binding to specific receptors and stimulation of cAMP accumulation. *Biochem. Biophys. Res. Commun.* **126**, 404–411.

Lord, J. A. H., Waterfield, A. A., Hughes, J., and Kosterlitz, H. W. (1977) Endogenous opioid peptides: Multiple agonists and receptors. *Nature* **267**, 495–499.

Lujan, M., Lopez, E., Ramirez, R., Aguilar, H., Martinez-Olmedo, M. A., and Garcia-Sainz, J. A. (1984) Pertussis toxin blocks the action of morphine, norepinephrine and clonidine on isolated guinea pig ileum. *Eur. J. Pharmacol.* **100**, 377–380.

Lutz-Bucher, B. and Koch, B. (1980) Evidence for a direct inhibitory effect of morphine on the secretion of posterior pituitary hormones. *Eur. J. Pharmacol.* **66**, 375–378.

Lux, B. and Schulz, R. (1985) Opioid dependence prevents the action of pertussis toxin in the guinea pig myenteric plexus. *Naunyn Schmeidelbergs Arch. Pharmacol.* **330**, 184–186.

Macdonald, R. L. and Nelson, P. G. (1978) Specific-opiate-induced depression of transmitter release from dorsal root ganglion cells in culture. *Science* **199**, 1449–1451.

Manara, L. and Bianchetti, A. (1985) The central and peripheral influences of opioids on gastrointestinal propulsion. *Ann. Rev. Pharmacol. Toxicol.* **25**, 249–273.

Margioris, A. N., Liotta, A. S., Vaudry, H., Bardin, C. W., and Krieger, D. T. (1983) Characterization of immunoreactive pro-opiomelanocortin-related peptides in rat testes. *Endocrinology* **113**, 663–671.

Martin, R., Geis, R., Holl, R., Schafer, M., and Voight, K. H. (1983) Coexistence of unrelated peptides on oxytocin and vasopressin terminals of rat neurohypophyses: Immunoreactive methionine-enkephalin, leucine-enkephalin, and chylocystokin-like substances. *Neuroscience* **8**, 213–227.

Martin, W. R., Eades, C. G., Thompson, J. A., Huppler, R. E., and Gilbert, P. E. (1976) The effects of morphine- and nalorphine-like drugs in the non-dependent and morphine-dependent chronic spinal dog. *J. Pharmacol. Exp. Ther.* **197**, 517–532.

McKay, J. S., Linaker, B. D., and Turnberg, L. A. (1981) Influence of opiates on ion transport across rabbit ileal mucosa. *Gastroenterology* **80**, 279–284.

McKnight, A. T., Corbett, A. D., Marcoli, M., and Kosterlitz, H. W. (1984) Hamster vas deferens contains delta-opioid receptors. *Neuropeptides* **5**, 97–100.

Mihara, S. and North, R. A. (1986) Opioids increase potassium conductance in submucous neurons of guinea pig caecum by activating delta receptors. *Br. J. Pharmacol.*, **88**, 315–322.

Miller, L. and Shaw, J. S. (1983) Multiple opiate receptors in mouse vas deferens. *Eur. J. Pharmacol.* **90**, 257–261.

Miller, L. and Shaw, J. S. (1985) Characterization of the delta opioid receptor on the hamster vas deferens. *Neuropeptides* **6**, 531–536.

Miller, R. J., Brown, D. R., Chang, E. B., and Friel, D. D. (1985) The Pharmacological Modification of Secretory Responses, in *Microbial Toxins and Diarrheal Disease*. Ciba Foundation Symposium 112, Pittman, London.

Morita, K. and North, R. A. (1982) Opiate activation of potassium conductance in myenteric neurons; inhibition by calcium ion. *Brain Res.* **242**, 145–150.

Morton, C. R. and Chahl, L. A. (1980) Pharmacology of the neurogenic edema response to electrical stimulation of the saphenous nerve in the rat. *Naunyn Schmeidebergs Arch. Pharmacol.* **314**, 271–276.

Mudge, A. W., Leeman, S. E., and Fischbach, G. D. (1979) Enkephalin inhibits release of substance P from sensory neurons in culture and decreases action potential duration. *Proc. Natl. Acad. Sci. USA* **76**, 526–530.

Nakai, Y., Nakao, K., Oka, S., and Imura, H. (1978) Presence of immunoreactive beta-endorphin in human placenta. *Life Sci.* **23**, 2013–2018.

Nijkamp, F. P., and van Ree, J. M. (1980) Effects of endorphins on different parts of the gastrointestinal tract of rat and guinea pig in vitro. *Br. J. Pharmacol.* **68**, 599–606.

Noda, M., Furutani, Y., Takahashi, H., Toyosato, M., Horose, T., Inayama, S., Nakanishi, S., and Numa, S. (1982) Cloning and sequence analysis of cDNA for bovine adrenal preproenkephalin. *Nature* **295**: 202–206.

Oka, T. (1980) Enkephalin receptor in the rabbit ileum. *Br. J. Pharmacol.* **68**, 193–195.

Oka, T., Negishi, K., Suda, M., Matsumiva, T., Inazu, T., and Ueki, M. (1980) Rabbit vas deferens: A specific bioassay for opioid kappa-agonists. *Eur. J. Pharmacol.* **73**, 235–236.

Paton, W. D. M. (1957) The action of morphine and related substances on contraction and on acetylcholine output of coaxially stimulated guinea pig ileum. *Br. J. Pharmacol.* **12**, 119–127.

Pfaffinger, P. J., Martin, J. M., Hunter, D. D., Nathanson, N. M., and Hille, B. (1985) GTP-binding proteins couple cardiac muscarinic receptors to a potassium channel. *Nature* **317**, 536–540.

Pintar, G. E., Schachter, B. S., Herman, A. B., Durgerian, S., and Krieger, D. T. (1984) Characterization and localization of pro-opiomelanocortin messenger RNA in the adult rat testis. *Science* **225**, 632–634.

Polak, J. M., Sullivan, S. N., Bloom, S. R., Fater, P., and Pearse, A. G. E. (1977) Enkephalin-like immunoreactivity in the human gastrointestinal tract. *Lancet* **i**, 972–974.

Porreca, F. and Burks, T. F. (1983) Affinity of normorphine for its pharmacologic receptor in the naive and morphine-tolerant guinea pig isolated ileum. *J. Pharmacol. Exp. Ther.* **225**, 688–693.

Porthe, G., Valette, A., and Cros, J. (1981) Kappa opiate binding sites in human placenta. *Biochem. Biophys. Res. Commun.* **101**, 1–6.

Porthe, G., Valette, A., Moisand, A., Tafani, M., and Cros, J. (1982) Localization of human placental opiate binding sites on the syncitial brush border membrane. *Life Sci.* **31**, 2647–2645.

Portoghese, P. S., Larson, D. L., Jiang, J. B., Caruso, T. P., and Takemori, A. E. (1979) Synthesis and pharmacologic characterization of an alkylating analogue (chlornaltrexamine) of naltrexone with ultra long-lasting narcotic antagonist properties. *J. Med. Chem.* **22**, 168–173.

Powell, D. W. (1981) Muscle or mucosa: The site of action of antidiarrheal opiates? *Gastroenterology* **80**, 406–408.

Puig, M. M., Gascon, P., Craviso, G. L., and Musacchio, J. M. (1977) Endogenous opiate receptor ligand: Electrically induced release in the guinea pig ileum. *Science* **195**, 419–420.

Rama Sastry, B. V., Janson, V. E., Owens, L. K., and Tayeb, O. S. (1982) Enkephalin and substance P-like immunoreactivities of mammallian sperm and accessory sex glands. *Biochem. Pharmacol.* **31**, 3519–3522.

Rama Sastry, B. V., Tayeb, O. S., Barnwell, S. L., Janson, V. E., and Owens, L. K. (1980) Occurrence of methionine-enkephalin in human placental villus. *Biochem. Pharmacol.* **29**, 475–478.

Ramme, D. and Illes, P. (1986) Differential effect of stimulation strength in mouse vas deferens on inhibition of neuroeffector transmission by receptor type selective opioids. *Naunyn Schmeidebergs Arch. Pharmacol.* **332**, 57–61.

Rattan, S. and Goyal, R. K. (1983) Identification and localization of opioid receptors in the opussum lower esophageal sphincter. *J. Pharmacol.* **224**, 391–397.

Rezvani, A. and Way, E. L. (1984) Dynrophin-(1-13) restores the potency of morphine on the tolerant guinea pig ileum. *Eur. J. Pharmacol.* **102**, 475–479.

Rios, L. and Jacob, J. J. C. (1982) Inhibition of inflammatory pain by naloxone and its N-methyl quaternary analogue. *Life Sci.* **31**, 1209–1212.

Ronai, A. Z., Harsing, L. G., Bersetai, I. P., Bajusz, S., and Vizi, E. S. (1982) [Met⁵]enkephalin-Arg-Phe acts on vascular opiate receptors. *Eur. J. Pharmacol.* **79**, 337–338.

Rossier, J., Battenberg, E., Pittman, Q., Bayon, A., Koda, L., Miller, R., Guillemin, R., and Bloom, F. (1979) Hypothalamic enkephalin neurons may regulate the neurohypophysis. *Nature* **277**, 653–655.

Ruckebusch, Y., Bardon, T., and Pairet, M. (1984) Opioid control of the ruminant stomach motility: Functional importance of mu, kappa, and delta receptors. *Life Sci.* **35**, 1731–1738.

Ruda, M. A. (1982) Opiates and pain pathways: Demonstration of enkephalin synapses on dorsal horn projection neurons. *Science* **215**, 1523–1525.

Saiani, S. and Guidotti, A. (1982) Opiate receptor mediated inhibition of catecholamine release in primary cultures of bovine adrenal chromaffin cells. *J. Neurochem.* **39**, 1669–1676.

Sapru, H. N., Willette, R. N., and Krieger, A. J. (1981) Stimulation of pulmonary J receptors by an enkephalin analog. *J. Pharmacol. Exp. Ther.* **217,** 228–234.

Saunders, W. S. and Thornhill, J. A. (1985) No inotropic action of enkephalin or enkephalin derivatives on electrically stimulated atria isolated from lean and obese rats. *Br. J. Pharmacol.* **85,** 513–522.

Sawynok, J. and Jhamandas, K. (1979) Interactions of methylxanthines, nonxanthine phosphodiesterase inhibitors, and calcium with morphine in the guinea pig myenteric plexus. *Can. J. Physiol. Pharmacol.* **57,** 853–859.

Schaumann, O., Giovanni, M., and Jochum, K. (1952) Morphinahnlich wirkende Analgeticka und Darmmotorik. I. Spasmolyse und Peristaltik. *Naunyn Schmeidebergs Arch. Exp. Path. Pharmacol.* **215,** 460–463.

Schick, R. and Schusdziarra, V. (1985) Physiological, pathophysiological and pharmacological aspects of exogenous and endogenous opiates. *Clin. Physiol. Biochem.* **3,** 43–60.

Schild, H. O. (1949) pA_x and competitive drug antagonism, *Br. J. Pharmacol.* **4,** 277–280.

Schmauss, C. and Yaksh, T. (1984) In vivo studies on spinal opiate receptor systems mediating antinociception. II. Pharmacological profiles suggesting a differential association of mu, delta, and kappa receptors with visceral chemical and cutaneous thermal stimuli in the rat. *J. Pharmacol. Exp. Ther.* **228,** 1–12.

Schmidt, C. F. and Livingston, A. E. (1933) The action of morphine on the mammalian circulation. *J. Pharmacol. Exp. Ther.* **47,** 411–441.

Schultzberg, M., Hokfelt, T., Nilsson, G., Terenius, L., Rehfeld, J. F., Brown, M., Elde, R., Goldstein, M., and Said, S. (1980) Distribution of peptide and catecholamine-containing neurons in the gastrointestinal tract of rat and guinea pig. Immunohistochemical studies with antisera to substance P, vasoactive intestinal polypeptide, enkephalins, somatostatin, gastrin, cholecystokinin, neurotensin, and dopamine hydroxylase. *Neuroscience* **5,** 689–744.

Schultzberg, M., Hokfelt, T., Terenius, L., Elfvin, L. -G., Lundberg, I. M., Brandt, J., Elde, R. P., and Goldstein, M. (1979) Enkephalin immunoreactive nerve fibers and cell bodies in sympathetic ganglia of the guinea pig and rat. *Neuroscience* **4,** 249–270.

Schultzberg, M., Lundberg, J. M., Hokfelt, T., Terenius, L., Brandt, T., Elde, R., and Goldstein, M. (1978) Enkephalin-like immunoreactivity in gland cells and nerve terminals in sympathetic ganglia and adrenal medulla. *Neuroscience* **3,** 1169–1180.

Schulz, R., Faase, E., Wuster, M., and Herz, A. (1979a) Selective receptors for beta-endorphin on the rat vas deferens. *Life Sci.* **24,** 843–850.

Schulz, R. and Wuster, M. (1981) Are there subtypes (isoreceptors) of multiple opiate receptors in the mouse vas deferens? *Eur. J. Pharmacol.* **76,** 61–66.

Schulz, R., Wuster, M., and Herz, A. (1979b) Centrally and peripherally mediated inhibition of intestinal motility by opioids. *Naunyn Schmeidebergs Arch. Pharmacol.* **308,** 255–260.

Schulz, R., Wuster, M., Kreuss, H., and Herz, A. (1980) Lack of cross-tolerance on multiple opiate receptors in the mouse vas deferens. *Mol. Pharmacol.* **18,** 395–401.

Schulz, R., Wuster, M., Rubini, P., and Herz, A. (1981) Functional opiate receptors in the guinea pig ileum. Their differentiation by means of selective tolerance development. *J. Pharmacol. Exp. Ther.* **219,** 547–550.

Shaha, C., Margioris, A., Liotta, A. S., Krieger, D. T. and Bardin, C. W. (1984) Demonstration of immunoreactive beta-endorphin and gamma-melanocyte stimulating hormone-related peptides in the ovaries of neonatal, cyclic and pregnant mice. *Endocrinology* **115,** 378–384.

Sharp, B. and Pekary, A. E. (1981) Beta-endorphin-(61-91) and other beta-endorphin immunoreactive peptides in human semen. *J. Clin. Endocrinol. Metab.* **52,** 586–588.

Sharp, B., Pekary, A. E., Meyer, N. V. and Hershman, J. M. (1980) Beta-endorphin in male rat reproductive organs. *Biochem. Biophys. Res. Commun.* **95,** 618–623.

Shaw, J. S. (1979) Characterization of opiate receptors in the isolated rat rectum. *Br. J. Pharmacol.* **67,** 428–429P.

Shaw, J. S., Miller, M., Turnbull, M. J., Gormley, J. J., and Morley, J. S. (1982) Selective antagonists at the opiate delta-receptor. *Life Sci.* **31,** 1259–1269.

Sheehan, M. J., Hayes, A. G., and Tyers, M. B. (1986) Pharmacology of opioid receptors in the hamster vas deferens. *Eur. J. Pharmacol.* **130,** 57–64.

Simantov, R. and Snyder, S. H. (1977) Opiate receptor binding in the pituitary gland. *Brain Res.* **124,** 178–184.

Simantov, R., Childers, S. R., and Snyder, S. H. (1978) [^{3}H]Opiate binding: Anomalous properties in kidney and liver membranes. *Mol. Pharmacol.* **14,** 69–76.

Smith, C. F. C. and Rance, M. J. (1983) Opiate receptors in the rat vas deferens. *Life Sci.* **33,** (suppl. 1), 327–330.

Smith, T. W. and Buchan, P. (1984) Peripheral opioid receptors located on the rat saphenous nerve. *Neuropeptides* **5,** 217–220.

Smith, T. W., Buchan, P., Parsons D. N., and Wilkinson, S. (1982) Peripheral antinociceptive effects of N-methyl morphine. *Life Sci.* **31,** 1205–1208.

Smith, T. W., Follenfant, R. L., and Ferreira, S. H. (1985) Antinociceptive models displaying peripheral opioid activity. *Int. J. Tiss. Reac.* **7,** 61–67.

Snyder, S. H., Pasternak, G. W., and Pert, C. B. (1978) Opiate Receptor Mechanisms, in *Handbook of Psychopharmacology* vol. 5 (Iversen, L. L. Iversen, S. D., and Snyder, S. H., eds.) Plenum, New York.

Spampinato, S. and Goldstein, A. (1983) Immunoreactive dynorphin in rat tissues and plasma. *Neuropeptides* **3,** 193–212.

Starke, K., Schoffel, E., and Illes, P. (1985) The sympathetic axons innervating the sinus node of the rabbit possess presynaptic opioid kappa- but not mu- or delta- receptors. *Naunyn Schmeidebergs Arch. Pharmacol.* **329,** 206–209.

Sun, F. and Zhang, A. (1985) Dynorphin receptor in the blood vessel. *Neuropeptides* **5,** 595–598.

Sweetman, P. M., Neale, J. H., Barker, J. L., and Goldstein, A. (1982) Localization of immunoreactive dynorphin in neuronal cultures from spinal cord and dorsal root ganglia. *Proc. Natl. Acad. Sci. USA* **79**, 6742–6746.

Tachibana, S., Araki, K., Ohya, S., and Yoshida, S. (1982) Isolation and structure of dynorphin, an opioid peptide, from porcine duodenum. *Nature* **295**, 339–340.

Tavani, A., Bianchi, G., and Manara, L. (1979) Morphine no longer blocks gastrointestinal transit but retains antinociceptive action in diallylnormorphine-pretreated rats. *Eur. J. Pharmacol.* **59**, 151–154.

Terenius, L. (1973) Stereospecific uptake of narcotic analgesics by a subcellular fraction of the guinea pig ileum. *Ups. J. Med. Sci.* **78**, 150–152.

Teschemacher, H. and Schweigerer, L. (1985) Opioid peptides: Do they have immunological significance? *Trends Pharmacol. Sci.* **6**, 368–370.

Trendelenburg, P. (1917) Physiologische und pharmakologische Versusche uber die Dunndarmperistaltik. *Naunyn Schmeidebergs Arch. Exp. Path. Pharmakol.* **81**, 55–129.

Trendelenburg, U. (1957) The action of morphine on the superior cervical ganglion and on the nictitating membrane of the cat. *Br. J. Pharmacol.* **12**, 79–85.

Tucker, J. F. (1984) Effect of pertussis toxin on normorphine-dependence and on acute inhibitory effects of normorphine and clonidine in guinea pig isolated ileum. *Br. J. Pharmacol.* **83**, 326–328.

Uddman, R., Hakanson, R., Sundler, F., and Walles, B. (1980) Peptidergic (enkephalin) innervation of the mammalian esophagus. *Gastroenterology* **78**, 732–737.

Valette, A., Reine, J. M., Pontonnier, G., and Cros, J. (1980) Specific binding for opiate like drugs in the placenta. *Biochem. Pharmacol.* **29**, 2657–2661.

Valette, A., Tafani, M., Porthe, G., Pontonnier, G., and Cros, J. (1983) Placental kappa binding site: Interaction with dynorphin and its possible implication in hCG secretion. *Life Sci.* **33**, (suppl. I), 523–526.

Van Neuten, J. M., Janssen, P. A. J., and Fontaine, J. (1976) Unexpected reversal effects of naloxone on the guinea pig ileum. *Life Sci.* **18**, 803–810.

Vaughan Williams, E. M. (1954) The mode of action of drugs upon intestinal motility. *Pharmacol. Rev.* **6**, 159–190.

Vinayek, R., Brown, D. R., and Miller, R. J. (1983) Inhibition of the antisecretory effect of [D-Ala[2], D-Leu[5]]enkephalin in the guinea pig ileum by a selective delta opioid antagonist. *Eur. J. Pharmacol.* **94**, 159–161.

Vincent, S. R., Dalsgaard, C. -J., Schultzberg, M., Hokfelt, T., Christensson, I., and Terenius, L. (1984) Dynorphin-immunoreactive neurons in the autonomic nervous system. *Neuroscience* **11**, 973–987.

Vincent, S. R., Hokfelt, T., Christensson, I., and Terenius, L. (1982) Dynorphin immunoreactive neurons in the central nervous system of the rat. *Neurosci. Lett.* **33**, 185–190.

Viveros, O. H., Diliberto, E. J., Hazum, E., and Chang, K. -J. (1979) Opiate like materials in the adrenal medulla: Evidence for storage and secretion with catecholamines. *Mol. Pharmacol.* **16**, 1101–1108.

von Kugelen, I., Illes, P., Wolf, D., and Starke, K. (1985) Presynaptic inhibitory delta- and kappa-receptors in a branch of the rabbit ileocolic artery. *Eur. J. Pharmacol.* **118,** 97–105.

Ward, S. J., Portoghese, P. S., and Takemori, A. E. (1982) Pharmacological profiles of beta-funaltrexamine (beta-FNA) and beta-chlornaltrexamine (beta-CNA) on the mouse vas deferens preparation. *Eur. J. Pharmacol.* **80,** 377–384.

Watson, S. J., Akil, H., Ghazarossian, V. E., and Goldstein, A. (1981) Dynorphin immunocytochemical localization in brain and peripheral nervous system: Preliminary studies. *Proc. Natl. Acad. Sci. USA* **78,** 1260–1263.

Wei, E. T., Lee, A., and Chang, J. -K. (1980) Cardiovascular effects of peptides related to the enkephalins and beta-casomorphin. *Life Sci.* **26,** 1517–1522.

Weihe, E., McKnight, A. T., Corbett, A. D., and Kosterlitz, H. W. (1985) Proenkephalin and prodynorphin-derived opioid peptides in guinea pig heart. *Neuropeptides* **5,** 453–456.

Werz, M. A. and Macdonald, R. L. (1982) Heterogeneous sensitivity of cultured dorsal root ganglion neurons to opioid peptides selective for mu- and delta-opiate receptors. *Nature* **299,** 730–733.

Werz, M. A. and Macdonald, R. L. (1984) Dynorphin reduces calcium-dependent action potential duration by decreasing voltage dependent calcium conductance. *Neurosci. Lett.* **46,** 185–190.

Wetzell, R., Illes, P., and Starke, K. (1984) Inhibition via opioid mu- and delta-receptors of vagal transmission in rabbit isolated heart. *Naunyn Schmeidebergs Arch. Pharmacol.* **328,** 186–190.

Wharton, J., Polak, J. M., Pearse, A. G. E., McGregor, G. P., Bryant, M. G., Bloom, S. R., Emson, P. C., Bisgard, G. E., and Will, J. E. (1980) Enkephalin-, VIP- and substance P-like immunoreactivity in the carotid body. *Nature* **284,** 269–271.

Whitnall, M. H., Gainer, H., Cox, B. M., and Molineaux, C. J. (1983) Dynorphin A(1-8) is contained within vasopressin neurosecretory vesicles in rat pituitary. *Science* **222,** 1137–1139.

Wuster, M., Schulz, R., and Herz, A. (1978) Specificity of opioids towards the mu, delta, and epsilon opiate receptors. *Neurosci. Lett.* **15,** 193–198.

Yaksh, T., Jessell, T. M., Gamse, R., Mudge, S. W., and Leeman, S. E. (1980) Intrathecal morphine inhibits substance P release from mammalian spinal cord in vivo. *Nature* **286,** 155–157.

Yamasaki, Y. and Way, E. L. (1983) Possible inhibition of Ca^{++} pump of rat erythrocyte ghosts by opioid kappa agonists. *Life Sci.* **33,** (suppl. I), 723–726.

Yamasaki, Y. and Way, E. L. (1985) Inhibition of calcium ATPase of rat erythrocyte membranes by kappa-opioid agonists. *Neuropeptides* **5,** 359–362.

Young, W. S., Walmsley, J. K., Zarbin, M. A., and Kuhar, M. J. (1980) Opioid receptors undergo axonal flow. *Science* **210,** 76–78.

Zakarian, S. and Smyth, D. G. (1982) Beta-endorphin is processed differently in specific regions of rat pituitary and brain. *Nature* **296,** 250–252.

Zukin, R. S. and Gintzlerr, A. R. (1980) Guanyl nucleotide interaction with opiate receptors in guinea pig brain and ileum. *Brain Res.* **186,** 486–491.

SECTION 6
REGULATION OF
OPIOID RECEPTORS

Chapter 12

Regulation of Opioid Receptors

Steven G. Blanchard and Kwen-Jen Chang

1. Introduction

Two processes by which the response of cells to hormones and transmitters is modulated are (1) regulation of the number of cellular receptors or (2) regulation of their sensitivity to applied ligand. The opioid receptors have been found to exhibit both types of modulation. In some systems, chronic treatment with opioid ligands results in alterations in the number of cell surface receptors; receptor numbers are decreased on treatment with agonists and increased on antagonist treatment. Additionally, both ligand affinity and receptor coupling to effector systems can be modulated by agents such as cations and guanyl nucleotides.

2. Modulation of Receptor–Ligand Interactions

Although the effects of cations and guanyl nucleotides have been examined in large part on membrane preparations in vitro, these studies have an important bearing on the understanding of opioid actions on intact preparations for two reasons. First, the "sodium shift" is a useful predictor of the agonist or antagonist properties of a particular ligand. That is, the affinity of opioid agonists, but not antagonists, is greatly reduced in the presence of sodium and GTP. Second, it has become increasingly clear that the effects of guanyl nucleotides on opioid binding are mediated through the interaction of the receptor with the inhibitory guanyl nucleotide binding protein N_i or G_i [or related protein(s)]. This protein is believed to be responsible for the coupling of opioid receptor occupation to inhibition of adenylate cyclase activity. In addition, recent evidence from other receptor systems suggests that the N proteins may also be involved in the coupling of receptors to other effector systems. The following sections will briefly review the phenomena of guanyl nucleotide and cation regulation of opioid receptors, and then will attempt to explain the relationship of these effects to the coupling protein N_i.

2.1. Effects of Cations on Opioid Binding

Early studies of opioid receptor binding showed that addition of sodium to binding assays results in a decrease of affinity for agonists, but not antagonists (Pert and Snyder, 1974; Simon and Groth, 1975). This decrease of affinity appears to be caused by an increase in the rate of ligand dissociation in the presence of sodium (Blume, 1978). Recently, however, careful kinetic studies using membranes from NG108-15 cells have shown that the effect of sodium is more complicated. Law et al. (1985a) found that the apparent decrease in affinity caused by sodium could be better described in terms of a shift in the relative populations of different affinity states. Because Na^+ is required for inhibition of adenylate cyclase (Blume et al., 1979), these authors attributed the appearance of a very-high-affinity state in the presence of sodium and ligand to the formation of a complex between receptor and N_i. The nature of the site responsible for the effects of sodium remains unclear, however, since neither the existence of a separate sodium binding component nor of a sodium binding site on the receptor or on N_i has been demonstrated. It should be noted that multiple affinity states for agonists have also been observed with intact cells (Costa et al., 1985).

The effects of Na^+ can be reversed by divalent cations such as Mn^{2+} or Mg^{2+} (Pasternak et al., 1975). Additionally, both Na^+ and Mg^{2+} are necessary for opioid stimulation of GTP hydrolysis (Koski and Klee, 1981) and inhibition of cyclase (Blume et al., 1979). Recent evidence on coupling of the opioid receptor with N_i has suggested that the hydrolysis of GTP mediated by opioids is caused by the intrinsic GTPase activity of N_i (see below).

2.2. Regulation of Opioid Binding
by Guanyl Nucleotides

Guanosine triphosphate (GTP) decreases the affinity of ligand binding to opioid receptor by increasing the rate of ligand dissociation (Blume, 1978; Childers and Snyder, 1980; Blume et al., 1979). GTP potentiates the effects of sodium on agonist binding (Childers and Snyder, 1980) and is necessary for the inhibition of adenylate cyclase activity by opioids (Blume et al., 1979). Both μ- and δ-receptors are sensitive to GTP, although effects on the μ-type receptor (rat brain membranes) are more pronounced than are those on the δ-receptor from neuroblastoma cell lines (Chang et al., 1981). Guanyl nucleotides and sodium also inhibit agonist binding to κ-receptors in membranes from guinea pig cerebellum (Frances et al., 1985). Furthermore, the effects of guanyl nucleotides depend on the particular incubation conditions used. That is, inclusion of guanyl nucleotides during the binding assay results in decreased ligand binding, whereas pretreatment of membranes with GTP or GDP followed by removal of excess nucleotide results in a magnesium-dependent increase in ligand binding (Chang et al., 1983). All of the above effects of guanyl nucleotides and cations have been postulated to be mediated through an inhibitory guanyl nucleotide binding protein N_i, analogous to the stimulatory nucleotide binding protein N_s responsible for coupling between adenylate cyclase and receptors that stimulate this enzyme. Recently, two lines of evidence have served to support this hypothesis. First, the N_i protein has been purified and characterized by several laboratories (Bokoch et al., 1984; Codina et al., 1984). Second, the ability of pertussis toxin (IAP, islet activating protein) to inactivate N_i by ADP ribosylation of its α-subunit (Katada and Ui, 1982; Bokoch et al., 1983; Hildebrandt et al., 1983; Codina et al., 1983, 1984) has provided a useful tool in defining the coupling of this protein with opioid receptors (as well as many other receptor systems).

2.3. Relationship of Opioid Binding to N_i

Sharma et al. (1975) first reported inhibition of adenylate cyclase by morphine and noted that the activity of this enzyme returned to its basal level on prolonged treatment. Subsequently, removal of morphine results in an increase of cyclase activity above the basal level. These phenomena are also observed for other opioids and opioid peptides (Lampert et al., 1976; Klee and Nirenberg,

1976). The return of cyclase activity to its basal level and the "overshoot" phenomenon on opioid removal have been suggested to be biochemical correlates for opioid tolerance and withdrawal, respectively (Sharma et al., 1975). Thus, examination of the mechanism of opioid-mediated inhibition of adenylate cyclase has been an important aspect of the study of opioid action.

It is now known that the inhibition of adenylate cyclase by receptors such as the opioid, α_1-adrenergic, and muscarinic cholinergic receptor is mediated through N_i, one of a family of nucleotide binding proteins (for reviews, see Gilman, 1984a,b). This family is composed of transducin (involved in signal transduction in the visual system), the stimulatory and inhibitory coupling proteins of adenylate cyclase, N_s and N_i, and N_o. N_o copurifies with N_i in brain and some other tissues (Sternweis and Robishaw, 1984; Neer et al., 1984; Malbon et al., 1985), but its function is unknown. These proteins are heterotrimeric, consisting of an α-subunit that differs for each member of the family (M_r = 39,000–45,000), and β- and γ-subunits of M_r 35,000 and $\sim$ 10,000, respectively. The β- and γ-subunits appear to be identical in the various complexes. Study and purification of these proteins have been possible in large part because of the availability of bacterial toxins that catalyze transfer of an ADP-ribose moiety from NAD to the α-subunits of the N proteins. This results in perturbation of the activity and coupling of the complex, and also gives a means of identifying these proteins in complex systems by use of radiolabeled NAD. Cholera toxin specifically labels N_s (Cassel and Pfeuffer, 1978; Gill and Meren, 1978; Northrup et al., 1980), whereas IAP specifically labels N_i and N_o (Katada and Ui, 1982; Bokoch et al., 1983; Sternweis and Robishaw, 1984). Transducin has specific ADP-ribosylation sites for both toxins (Abood et al., 1982; Manning et al., 1984). Several lines of evidence have shown that the cation and nucleotide effects on opioid binding mentioned in the above discussion are mediated through receptor coupling to N_i.

Treatment of NG108-15 cells with pertussis toxin resulted in a loss of opioid-mediated inhibition of adenylate cyclase (Kurose et al., 1983; Costa et al., 1983). Such treatment did not cause a change in the number of binding sites assayed by opioid antagonists. The binding of agonists, however, was greatly decreased because of a decreased affinity, and guanyl nucleotides no longer had an effect on agonist binding (Costa et al., 1983; Kurose et al., 1983; Hsia et al., 1984). Similar effects have been reported for other inhibitory receptor systems (Cote et al., 1984; Kurose et al., 1983). In addition, the effect of guanyl nucleotides on ligand binding to purified muscarinic cholinergic receptors is lost. Reconstitution of purified receptor with N_i resulted in an increased agonist affinity and return of guanyl nucleotide sensitivity (Florio and Sternweis, 1985). Further evidence for coupling of N_i to opioid receptors comes from studies of opioid-stimulated GTPase activity (Koski and Klee, 1981). Pertussis toxin inhibits enkephalin-stimulated GTPase (Burns et al., 1983), and purified N_i exhibits high-affinity GTPase activity (Sunyer et al., 1984; Milligan and Klee, 1985). Reconstitution of N_i with purified muscarinic cholinergic receptor, another inhibitory system, results in restoration of ligand-sensitive GTPase activity (Haga et al., 1985).

The above results suggest, therefore, that the observed effects of guanyl nucleotides and cations on opioid binding result from changes in the coupling of receptor with the guanyl nucleotide-binding protein N_i. The ultimate demonstration of this interaction will come from reconstitution studies using N_i and purified receptor preparations. Because of recent progress in this area (*see* chapter by Simon and Hiller, in this volume), these experiments may be expected in the near future.

3. Ligand-Induced Down-Regulation

In addition to regulation of affinity or coupling as described above, many receptor systems also undergo ligand-induced changes in receptor numbers. Incubation of cells with polypeptide ligands causes an internalization of receptor–ligand complex with a corresponding decrease of surface receptor numbers, but no change in affinity (for reviews, *see* Brown et al., 1983; Hazum et al., 1981; King and Cuatrecasas, 1981; Pastan and Willingham, 1983). In contrast, chronic in vivo administration of morphine followed by subsequent in vitro measurements of opioid binding showed no changes in either numbers or affinity of opioid receptors (Pert et al., 1973; Klee and Streaty, 1974; Hollt et al., 1975).

3.1. Opioid Peptides and Neuroblastoma Cells

Direct receptor binding studies (Chang et al., 1978) and experiments using a rhodamine-labeled enkephalin analog (Hazum et al., 1979a,b, 1980) suggested that there was no down-regulation or internalization of ligand–receptor complexes in the mouse neuroblastoma cell line N4TG1, which contains a homogeneous population of δ- (enkephalin) receptors (Chang and Cuatrecasas, 1979). Because these results were obtained under suboptimal conditions for down-regulation of other receptors [i.e., low temperatures (24°C) and nonadherent cells (Zidovetski et al., 1981)], they were reinvestigated under more appropriate experimental conditions. Incubation of monolayers of neuroblastoma cells with [D-Ala^2-D-Leu^5]enkephalin at 37°C resulted in a rapid ($t_{1/2} \approx 30$ min) decrease in number of enkephalin binding sites with no change in affinity (Chang et al., 1982). This reduction in receptor numbers was specific for the peptides tested and was antagonized both by opioid antagonists and by alkaloid agonists such as morphine. Opioid receptors in these cells are also down-regulated by nonpeptide agonists such as etorphine (Gwynn and Costa, 1982). Similar results have been reported for the hybrid cell line NG108-15 (Law et al., 1982; Simantov et al., 1982). Although the mechanistic reasons underlying the ligand selectivity of down-regulation are not clear, Law et al. (1983a) have noted a relationship between intrinsic activity and ability to cause down-regulation. Thus morphine, which is only a partial agonist with respect to adenylate cyclase inhibition in NG108-15 cells (Law et al., 1983b), does not cause down-regulation in any of the systems tested. Additionally, it should be noted that opioid receptor down-regulation is homologous. That is, down-regulation of opioid receptors was not accompanied by loss of either alpha-2 adrenergic or muscarinic receptors, two other inhibitory systems present on the hybrid cells (Law et al., 1983a).

3.2. Mechanism of Down-Regulation

In both the neuroblastoma and neuroblastoma-glioma cells lines, down-regulation is dependent on dose, temperature, and time of incubation (Chang et al., 1982; Law et al., 1983a). These characteristics are all consistent with a mechanism involving internalization of receptor–ligand complexes. Furthermore, down-regulation is blocked by the inhibitors of metabolic energy production, sodium azide, and 2,4-dinitrophenol (Blanchard et al., 1982, 1983). In the N4TG1 line, [^{3}H][D-Ala^2-D-Leu^5]enkephalin is taken up by a receptor-mediated process with time, dose, and temperature dependencies similar to those for down-regulation (Blanchard et al., 1983). Under these conditions, ligand is accumulated in the cells in apparent excess over receptor number, suggesting receptor recycling (Blanchard et al., 1983). In contrast, Law et al. (1984) found accumulation of [^{3}H]DADLE in NG108-15 cells only in the presence of the inhibitor of lysosomal processing, chloroquine. This accumulation was accompanied by the appearance of a population of ligand in the lysosomal compartment as measured by centrifugation of cellular homogenates on Percoll gradients. This difference in results between the two cell lines probably reflects a difference in the direction of intercellular shuttling of receptors through the recycling versus degradative lysosomal pathways. At this point, the biochemical "traffic signs" responsible for directing the internalized opioid receptor are unknown. Furthermore, we do not know if one pathway is preferentially utilized over the other in normal (i.e., nontumor) tissues. The route of receptor internalization has not been investigated; however, the finding of ligand-induced clustering of opioid receptors as assayed by fluorescent ligands (Hazum et al., 1979a,b, 1980; Blanchard et al., 1984), together with the fact that a fluorescent enkephalin analog can cause down-regulation (Blanchard et al., 1984), suggest that coated pits may be involved. The recent observation of the presence of opioid binding sites in coated vesicles purified from bovine brain (Bennett et al., 1985) gives support to this hypothesis.

3.3. Down-Regulation in Other Tissues

Although the amount of material available is too limited to allow mechanistic studies, down-regulation has been observed in normal tissues such as hippocampal slices (Dingledine et al., 1983) and an aggregated fetal brain cell preparation (Lenoir et al., 1983). In both cases, morphine did not cause down-regulation, in agreement with earlier results on chronic morphine administration (Pert et al., 1973; Klee and Streaty, 1974; Hollt et al., 1975; Simon and Hiller, 1978). It should be noted that both of these heterogenous preparations would be expected to contain μ- (morphine) type receptors. Thus the lack of effect of morphine cannot be attributed to an absence of receptors for this opioid. In the hippocampal system, this constancy of μ-receptors was directly demonstrated using binding of a μ-selective ligand (Dingledine et al., 1983). The lack of effect on μ-receptors was not caused by the use of an alkaloid (morphine), since the μ-selective peptide, morphiceptin, was also ineffective at inducing down-regulation. In light of these findings, it is tempting to conclude that ligand-induced down-regulation is a property of only δ-receptors. However, electroconvulsive shock has been shown to cause down-regulation of both δ- and μ-receptors in specific areas of rat brain (Nakata et al., 1985). Although the mechanism of this down-regulation is not known, it is reasonable to assume that it is mediated through endogenous opioids released by the electroconvulsive shock.

3.4. Possible Significance of Down-Regulation

The present state of knowledge does not allow us to make many statements on the significance of opioid down-regulation. We can, however, point out some processes in which down-regulation is not involved. First, the lack of down-regulation by morphine suggests that it is not involved in the mechanisms of morphine tolerance and dependence. Second, down-regulation is not required for inhibition of adenylate cyclase since some compounds (e.g., morphine) are partial agonists with respect to cyclase inhibition, but antagonists of down-regulation (Law et al., 1983a). It should be noted, however, that inhibition of adenylate cyclase and desensitization of this response precede down-regulation in a temporal sense (Law et al., 1983a) and may be required, but not sufficient, for subsequent down-regulation. Finally, internalization of receptor does not appear to be coupled to internalization of N_i (Law et al., 1985b). This could result in long-term changes in the activity of N_i or effector systems coupled to it. Again, however, data are not yet available on these questions.

4. Receptor Up-Regulation

In contrast to the effects of agonists, acute administration of antagonist had no effect on receptor numbers in the neuroblastoma and neuroblastoma-glioma cell lines (Chang et al., 1982; Law et al., 1983a). Chronic administration of antagonists to rodents, however, results in an increase in opioid binding (Hitzemann et al., 1974; Zukin et al., 1982; Lahti and Collins, 1978; Schulz et al., 1979). The receptors induced by up-regulation seem to be functional, since animals treated chronically with antagonist exhibit an increased sensitivity to morphine (Schulz et al., 1979; Tang and Collins, 1978). In addition, agonists showed an increased sensitivity to guanyl nucleotides in treated animals (Zukin et al., 1982). In contrast to the studies with adult brain, naloxone treatment of rats aged 1–21 d, followed by assay on day 22, showed an increased number of receptors, but no increase in morphine sensitivity (Bardo et al., 1982).

The functional nature of up-regulated receptors is also suggested by the regional specificity of the new binding sites. Thus binding studies to membranes from specific brain regions showed the largest increases in mesolimbic and frontal cortex areas, whereas there was very little increase in the periaqueductal gray and dorsal hippocampus (Zukin et al., 1982). These studies have recently been extended by use of brain-slice autoradiography at the light-microscopy level (Tempel et al., 1984). At this level, very large increases were seen in the substantia nigra compacta, ventromedial hypothalamus, and ventral tegmental area. It should also be noted that increased receptor numbers in a specific brain region (amygdala) have been noted on 6-hydroxydopamine lesion of substantia nigra (Gardner et al., 1980). This suggests that up-regulation may not be caused by receptor occupation with antagonist, but by lack of normal receptor inputs (i.e., by lack of agonist occupation). Finally, the process of up-regulation may not be specific for a particular type of receptor since Zukin et al. (1982) found increased binding for both a μ-ligand (dihydromorphine) and a δ-ligand (DADLE). Further work will be required on this point, however, since the selectivity of these ligands for their respective receptor types is not extremely great.

Although the studies detailed above suggest that the up-regulated receptors are functional, the subcellular distribution of up-regulated receptors reveals a more complicated picture. Roth et al. (1981) have shown that brain opioid receptors can be resolved into two subcellular populations, a plasma membrane fraction and one enriched in endoplasmic reticulum and Golgi. Analysis of up-regulated receptors showed that the receptor numbers increased in the microsomal fraction to a greater extent than in the plasma membrane fraction (Moudy et al., 1985). Thus, most of the receptor increase occurs in internalized receptors not available for ligand binding and not on the plasma membrane. In agreement with earlier results (Tempel et al., 1983), cycloheximide did not block this up-regulation (Moudy et al., 1985). These studies then suggest that up-regulation is not simply the result of transfer of internal receptors to the plasma membrane. At this time, significance of the increased number of internal receptors is unclear.

References

Abood, M. E., Hurley, J. B., Pappone, M.-C., Bourne, H. R., and Stryer, L. (1982) Functional homology between signal-coupling proteins: Cholera toxin inactivates the GTPase activity of transducin. *J. Biol. Chem.* **257,** 10540–10543.

Bardo, M. T., Bhatnagar, R. K., and Gebhart, G. F. (1982) Differential effects of chronic morphine and naloxone on opiate receptors, monoamines, and morphine-induced behaviors in preweanling rats. *Dev. Brain Res.* **4,** 139–147.

Bennett, D. B., Spain, J. W., Laskowski, M. B., Roth, B. L., and Coscia, C. J. (1985) Stereospecific opiate-binding sites occur in coated vesicles. *J. Neurosci.* **5,** 3010–3015.

Blanchard, S. G., Chang, K.-J., and Cuatrecasas, P. (1982) Studies on the mechanism of enkephalin receptor down regulation. *Life Sci.* **31,** 1311–1314.

Blanchard, S. G., Chang, K.-J., and Cuatrecasas, P. (1983) Characterization of the association of tritiated enkephalin with neuroblastoma cells under conditions optimal for receptor down regulation. *J. Biol. Chem.* **258,** 1092–1097.

Blanchard, S. G., Chang, K.-J., and Cuatrecasas, P. (1984) Visualization of enkephalin receptors by image-intensified fluorescence microscopy. *Meth. Enzymol.* **103,** 219–227.

Blume, A. J. (1978) Interaction of ligands with the opiate receptors of brain membranes: Regulation by ions and nucleotides. *Proc. Natl. Acad. Sci. USA* **75,** 1713–1717.

Blume, A. J., Lichtshtein, D., and Boone, G. (1979) Coupling of opiate receptors to adenylate cyclase: Requirement for Na$^+$ and GTP. *Proc. Natl. Acad. Sci. USA* **76,** 5626–5630.

Bokoch, G. M., Katada, T., Northup, J. K., Hewlett, E. L., and Gilman, A. G. (1983) Identification of the predominant substrate for ADP-ribosylation by islet activating protein. *J. Biol. Chem.* **258,** 2072–2075.

Bokoch, G. M., Katada, T., Northup, J. K., Ui, M., and Gilman, A. G. (1984) Purification and properties of the inhibitory guanine nucleotide-binding regulatory component of adenylate cyclase. *J. Biol. Chem.* **259,** 3560–3567.

Brown, M. S., Anderson, R. G. W., and Goldstein, J. L. (1983) Recyling receptors: The round-trip itinerary of migrant membrane proteins. *Cell* **32,** 663–667.

Burns, D. L., Hewlett, E. L., Moss, J., and Vaughan, M. (1983) Pertussis toxin inhibits enkephalin stimulation of GTPase of NG108–15 cells. *J. Biol. Chem.* **258,** 1435–1438.

Cassel, D. and Pfeuffer, T. (1978) Mechanism of cholera toxin action: Covalent modification of the guanyl nucleotide-binding protein of the adenylate cyclase system. *Proc. Natl. Acad. Sci. USA* **75,** 2669–2673.

Chang, K.-J. and Cuatrecasas, P. (1979) Multiple opiate receptors: Enkephalins and morphine bind to receptors of different specificity. *J. Biol. Chem.* **254,** 2610–2618.

Chang, K.-J., Miller, R. J., and Cuatrecasas, P. (1978) Interaction of enkephalin with opiate receptors in intact cultured cells. *Mol. Pharmacol.* **14,** 961–970.

Chang, K.-J., Hazum, E., Killian, A., and Cuatrecasas, P. (1981) Interactions of ligands with morphine and enkephalin receptors are differentially affected by guanine nucleotide. *Mol. Pharmacol.* **20,** 1–7.

Chang, K.-J., Eckel, R. W., and Blanchard, S. G. (1982) Opioid peptides induce reduction of enkephalin receptors in cultured neuroblastoma cells. *Nature* **296,** 446–448.

Chang, K.-J., Blanchard, S. G., and Cuatrecasas, P. (1983) Unmasking of magnesium-dependent high-affinity binding sites for [D-Ala^2, D-Leu^5]enkephalin after pretreatment of brain membranes with guanine nucleotides. *Proc. Natl. Acad. Sci. USA* **80,** 940–944.

Childers, S. R. and Snyder, S. H. (1980) Differential regulation by guanine nucleotides of opiate agonist and antagonist receptor interactions. *J. Neurochem.* **34,** 583–593.

Codina, J., Hildebrandt, J., Iyengar, R., Birnbaumer, L., Sekura, R. D., and Manclark, C. R. (1983) Pertussis toxin substrate, the putative N_i component of adenylyl cyclases, is an $\alpha\beta$ heterodimer regulated by guanine nucleotide and magnesium. *Proc. Natl. Acad. Sci. USA* **80,** 4276–4280.

Codina, J., Hildebrandt, J. D., Birnbaumer, L., and Sekura, R. D. (1984) Effects of guanine nucleotides and Mg on human erythrocyte N and N_s, the regulatory components of adenylyl cyclase. *J. Biol. Chem.* **259,** 11408–11418.

Costa, T., Aktories, K., Schultz, G., and Wuster, M. (1983) Pertussis toxin decreases opiate receptor binding and adenylate inhibition in a neuroblastoma × glioma hybrid cell line. *Life Sci.* **33** (suppl. 1), 219–222.

Costa, T., Wuster, M., Gramsch, C., and Herz, A. (1985) Multiple states of opioid receptors may modulate adenylate cyclase in intact neuroblastoma × glioma hybrid cells. *Mol. Pharmacol.* **28,** 146–154.

Cote, T. E., Frey, E. A., and Sekura, R. D. (1984) Altered activity of the inhibitory guanyl nucleotide-binding component (N_i) induced by pertussis toxin: Uncoupling of N_i from receptor with continued coupling of N_i to the catalytic unit. *J. Biol. Chem.* **259,** 8693–8698.

Dingledine, R., Valentino, R. J., Bostock, E., King, M. E., and Chang, K.-J. (1983) Down-regulation of δ but not μ opioid receptors in the hippocampal slice associated with loss of physiological response. *Life Sci.* **33** (suppl. 1), 333–336.

Florio, V. A. and Sternweis, P. C. (1985) Reconstitution of resolved muscarinic cholinergic receptors with purified GTP-binding proteins. *J. Biol. Chem.* **260,** 3477–3483.

Frances, B., Moisand, C., and Meunier, J.-C. (1985) Na$^+$ ions and Gpp(NH)p selectively inhibit agonist interactions at μ- and κ-opioid receptor sites in rabbit and guinea-pig cerebellum membranes. *Eur. J. Pharmacol.* **117,** 223–232.

Gardner, E. L., Zukin, R. S., and Makman, M. H. (1980) Modulation of opiate receptor binding in striatum and amygdala by selective mesencephalic lesions. *Brain Res.* **194,** 232–239.

Gilman, A. G. (1984a) Guanine nucleotide-binding regulatory proteins and dual control of adenylate cyclase. *J. Clin. Invest.* **73,** 1–4.

Gilman, A. G. (1984b) G proteins and dual control of adenylate cyclase. *Cell* **36**, 577–579.

Gill, D. M. and Meren, R. (1978) ADP-ribosylation of membrane proteins catalyzed by cholera toxin: Basis of the activation of adenylate cyclase. *Proc. Natl. Acad. Sci. USA* **75**, 3050–3054.

Gwynn, G. J. and Costa, E. (1982) Opioids regulate cGMP formation in cloned neuroblastoma cells. *Proc. Natl. Acad. Sci. USA* **79**, 690–694.

Haga, K., Haga, T., Ichiyama, A., Katada, T., Kurose, H., and Ui, M. (1985) Functional reconstitution of purified muscarinic receptors and inhibitory guanine nucleotide regulatory protein. *Nature* **316**, 731–733.

Hazum, E., Chang, K.-J., and Cuatrecasas, P. (1979a) Opiate (enkephalin) receptors of neuroblastoma cells: Occurrence in clusters on the cell surface. *Science* **206**, 1077–1079.

Hazum, E., Chang, K.-J., and Cuatrecasas, P. (1979b) Role of disulphide and sulphydryl groups in clustering of enkephalin receptors in neuroblastoma cells. *Nature* **282**, 626–628.

Hazum, E., Chang, K.-J., and Cuatrecasas, P. (1980) Cluster formation of opiate (enkephalin) receptors in neuroblastoma cells: Differences between agonists and antagonists and possible relationships to biological functions. *Proc. Natl. Acad. Sci. USA* **77**, 3038–3041.

Hazum, E., Chang, K.-J., and Cuatrecasas, P. (1981) Receptor redistribution induced by hormones and neurotransmitters: Possible relationships to biological functions. *Neuropeptides* **1**, 217–230.

Hildebrandt, J. D., Sekura, R. D., Codina, J., Iyengar, R., Manclark, C. R., and Birnbaumer, L. (1983) Stimulation and inhibition of adenylyl cyclases mediated by distinct regulatory proteins. *Nature* **302**, 706–709.

Hitzemann, R. J., Hitzemann, B. A., and Loh, H. H. (1974) Binding of ^{3}H-naloxone in the mouse brain: Effect of ions and tolerance development. *Life Sci.* **14**, 2393–2404.

Hollt, V., Dum, J., Blasig, J., Schubert, P., and Herz, A. (1975) Comparison of *in vivo* and *in vitro* parameters of opiate receptor binding in naive and tolerant/dependent rodents. *Life Sci.* **16**, 1823–1828.

Hsia, J. A., Moss, J., Hewlett, E. L., and Vaughan, M. (1984) ADP-ribosylation of adenylate cyclase by pertussis toxin: Effects on inhibitory agonist binding. *J. Biol. Chem.* **259**, 1086–1090.

Katada, T. and Ui, M. (1982) ADP ribosylation of the specific membrane protein of C6 cells by islet-activating protein associated with modification of adenylate cyclase activity. *J. Biol. Chem.* **257**, 7210–7216.

King, A. C. and Cuatrecasas, P. (1981) Peptide hormone-induced receptor mobility, aggregation and internalization. *N. Eng. J. Med.* **305**, 77–88.

Klee, W. A. and Nirenberg, M. (1976) Mode of action of endogenous opiate peptides. *Nature* **263**, 609–612.

Klee, W. A. and Streaty, R. A. (1974) Narcotic receptor sites in morphine-dependent rats. *Nature* **248**, 61–63.

Koski, G. and Klee, W. A. (1981) Opiates inhibit adenylate cyclase by stimulating GTP hydrolysis. *Proc. Natl. Acad. Sci. USA* **78**, 4185–4189.

Kurose, H., Katada, T., Amano, T., and Ui, M. (1983) Specific uncoupling by islet-activating protein, pertussis toxin, of negative signal transduction via α-adrenergic, cholinergic, and opiate receptors in neuroblastoma × glioma hybrid cells. *J. Biol. Chem.* **258**, 4870–4875.

Lahti, R. A. and Collins, R. J. (1978) Chronic naloxone results in prolonged increases in opiate binding sites in brain. *Eur. J. Pharmacol.* **51**, 185–186.

Lampert, A., Nirenberg, M., and Klee, W. A. (1976) Tolerance and dependence evoked by an endogenous opiate peptide. *Proc. Natl. Acad. Sci. USA* **73**, 3165–3167.

Law, P.-Y., Hom, D. S., and Loh, H. H. (1982) Loss of opiate receptor activity in neuroblastoma × glioma NG108-15 hybrid cells after chronic opiate treatment: A multiple-step process. *Mol. Pharmacol.* **22**, 1–4.

Law, P.-Y., Hom, D. S., and Loh, H. H. (1983a) Opiate receptor downregulation and desensitization in neuroblastoma × glioma NG108-15 hybrid cells are two separate cellular adaptation processes. *Mol. Pharmacol.* **24**, 413–424.

Law, P.-Y., Hom, D. S., and Loh, H. H. (1983b) Opiate regulation of adenosine 3':5'-cyclic monphosphate level in neuroblastoma × glioma NG108-15 hybrid cells: Relationship between receptor occupancy and effect. *Mol. Pharmacol.* **23**, 26–35.

Law, P.-Y., Hom, D. S., and Loh, H. H. (1984) Down-regulation of opiate receptor in neuroblastoma × glioma NG108-15 cells: Chloroquine promotes accumulation of tritiated enkephalin in the lysosomes. *J. Biol. Chem.* **259**, 4096–4104.

Law, P.-Y., Hom, D. S., and Loh, H. H. (1985a) Multiple affinity states of opiate receptor in neuroblastoma × glioma NG108-15 hybrid cells: Opiate agonist association rate is a function of receptor occupancy. *J. Biol. Chem.* **260**, 3561–3569.

Law, P.-Y., Lovie, A. K., and Loh, H. H. (1985b) Effect of pertussis toxin treatment on the down-regulation of opiate receptors in neuroblastoma × glioma NG108-15 hybrid cells. *J. Biol. Chem.* **260**, 14818–14823.

Lenoir, D., Barg, J., and Simantov, R. (1983) Down-regulation of opiate receptors in serum-free cultures of aggregating fetal brain cells. *Life Sci.* **33** (suppl. 1), 337–340.

Malbon, C. C., Mangano, T. J., and Watkins, D. C. (1985) Heart contains two substrates (M_r = 40,000 and 41,000) for pertussis toxin-catalyzed ADP-ribosylation that co-purify with N_s. *Biochem. Biophys. Res. Comm.* **128**, 809–815.

Manning, D. R., Fraser, B. A., Kahn, R. A., and Gilman, A. G. (1984) ADP-ribosylation of transducin by islet-activating protein: Identification of asparagine as the site of ADP-ribosylation. *J. Biol. Chem.* **259**, 749–756.

Milligan, G. and Klee, W. A. (1985) The inhibitory guanine nucleotide-binding protein (N_i) purified from bovine brain is a high affinity GTPase. *J. Biol. Chem.* **260**, 2057–2063.

Moudy, A. M., Spain, J. W., and Coscia, C. J. (1985) Differential up-regulation of microsomal and synaptic membrane μ-receptors. *Biochem. Biophys. Res. Comm.* **132**, 735–741.

Nakata, Y., Chang, K.-J., Mitchell, C. L., and Hong, J. S. (1985) Repeated electroconvulsive shock down regulates the opioid receptors in rat brain. *Brain Res.* **346**, 160–163.

Neer, E. J., Lok, J. M., and Wolf, L. G. (1984) Purification and properties of the inhibitory guanine nucleotide regulatory unit of brain adenylate cyclase. *J. Biol. Chem.* **259,** 14222–14229.

Northup, J. K., Sternweis, P. C., Smigel, M. D., Schleifer, L. S., Ross, E. M., and Gilman, A. G. (1980) Purification of the regulatory component of adenylate cyclase. *Proc. Natl. Acad. Sci. USA* **77,** 6516–6520.

Pastan, I. and Willingham, M. C. (1983) Receptor-mediated endocytosis: Coated pits, receptosomes and the golgi. *TIBS* **8,** 250–254.

Pasternak, G. W., Snowman, A. M., and Snyder, S. H. (1975) Selective enhancement of [³H]opiate agonist binding by divalent cations. *Mol. Pharmacol.* **11,** 735–744.

Pert, C. B. and Snyder, S. H. (1974) Opiate receptor binding of agonists and antagonists affected differentially by sodium. *Mol. Pharmacol.* **10,** 868–879.

Pert, C. B., Pasternak, G. W., and Snyder, S. H. (1973) Opiate agonists and antagonists discriminated by receptor binding in brain. *Science* **182,** 1359–1361.

Roth, B. L., Laskowski, M. B., and Coscia, C. J. (1981) Evidence for distinct subcellular sites of opiate receptors: Demonstration of opiate receptors in smooth microsomal fractions isolated from rat brain. *J. Biol. Chem.* **256,** 10117–10123.

Schulz, R., Wuster, M., and Herz, A. (1979) Supersensitivity to opioids following chronic blockade of endorphin activity by naloxone. *Naunyn Schmiedebergs Arch. Pharmacol.* **306,** 93–96.

Sharma, S. K., Klee, W. A., and Nirenberg, M. (1975) Dual regulation of adenylate cyclase accounts for narcotic dependence and tolerance. *Proc. Natl. Acad. Sci. USA* **72,** 3092–3096.

Simantov, R., Levy, R., and Baram, D. (1982) Down regulation of enkephalin (δ) receptors: Demonstration in membrane bound and solubilized receptors. *Biochim. Biophys. Acta.* **721,** 478–484.

Simon, E. J. and Groth, J. (1975) Kinetics of opiate inactivation by sulfhydryl reagents: Evidence for a conformational change in the presence of sodium ions. *Proc. Natl. Acad. Sci. USA* **72,** 2404–2407.

Simon, E. J. and Hiller, J. M. (1978) *In vitro* studies on opiate receptors and their ligands. *Fed. Proc.* **37,** 141–146.

Sternweis, P. C. and Robishaw, J. D. (1984) Isolation of two proteins with high affinity for guanine nucleotides from membranes of bovine brain. *J. Biol. Chem.* **259,** 13806–13813.

Sunyer, T., Codina, J., and Birnbaumer, L. (1984) GTP hydrolysis by pure N_i, the inhibitory regulatory component of adenylyl cyclases. *J. Biol. Chem.* **259,** 15447–15451.

Tang, A. H. and Collins, R. J. (1978) Enhanced analgesic effects of morphine after chronic administration of naloxone in the rat. *Eur. J. Pharmacol.* **47,** 473–474.

Tempel, A., Crain, S., Simon, E. J., and Zukin, R. S. (1983) Opiate receptor upregulation in explants of spinal cord-dorsal root ganglia. *Soc. Neurosci. Abst.* **9,** 327.

Tempel, A., Gardner, E. L., and Zukin, R. S. (1984) Visualization of opiate receptor upregulation by light microscopic autoradiography. *Proc. Natl. Acad. Sci. USA* **81,** 3893–3897.

Zidovetski, R., Yarden, Y., Schlessinger, J., and Jovin, T. M. (1981) Rotational diffusion of epidermal growth factor complexed to cell surface receptors reflects rapid microaggregation and endocytosis of occupied receptors. *Proc. Natl. Acad. Sci. USA* **78,** 6981–6985.

Zukin, R. S., Sugarman, J. R., Fitz-Syage, M. L., Gardner, E. L., Zukin, S. R., and Gintzler, A. R. (1982) Naltrexone-induced opiate receptor supersensitivity. *Brain Res.* **245,** 285–292.

Chapter 13

Role of Opioid Receptors in Narcotic Tolerance/ Dependence

Andrew P. Smith, Ping-Yee Law, and Horace H. Loh

1. Introduction

The signal feature of opioid drugs is their ability to induce tolerance and dependence when given chronically to humans or experimental animals. Tolerance may be defined as a state in which the dose of drug required to achieve a given effect is larger than normal. Dependence is a state in which regular doses of the drug are required to prevent withdrawal symptoms.

Opioid dependence or addiction is, of course, one of the major health problems of our time, and a hindrance to the effective use of opioids as clinical analgesics. It is also, however, a phenomenon with some similarities to memory: The brain, as a result of repeated exposure to an agent, alters its response to that agent. Thus it may be a useful model of long-term, adaptive changes in the nervous system. The recent discovery that the brain contains endogenous opioids with neurotransmitter-like properties (Zieglgansberger et al., 1976; Henderson et al., 1978; Rossier and Bloom, 1979) reinforces the belief that the kinds of processes that result in opioid tolerance/dependence are not unique to these

441

substances, but probably occur in some form throughout the central nervous system.

Opiate addiction has been known for over 2000 yr, but only in the last dozen, beginning with the discovery of opioid receptors in the brain (Pert and Snyder, 1973; Terenius, 1973; Simon et al., 1973), has it been possible to attempt to elucidate the molecular processes involved. Increasing evidence suggests that changes in opioid receptors, as well as in certain other functional macromolecules with which they are closely associated, are involved in tolerance and dependence. In this chapter, we will review the most important of these studies, then attempt to reconstruct some of the molecular processes involved in tolerance/dependence in their light.

Much of the work to be discussed has been carried out not with whole animals, but with isolated cell or tissue preparations, in which molecular and cellular processes can be analyzed more readily and in which factors such as drug accessibility to receptors can be controlled. Because such systems do not exhibit analgesia, they obviously cannot provide a complete understanding of the actions of opioids in whole animals. At the very least, however, studies with these model systems have provided us with testable hypotheses about the molecular basis of tolerance and dependence in whole animals.

2. Chronic Opioid Effects in Clonal Neuroblastoma–Glioma Cell Lines

The simplest system currently known for studying both acute and chronic effects of opioids is the neuroblastoma–glioma hybrid cell culture, particularly the NG108-15 cell line. About 10 yr ago, Sharma et al. (1975a) showed that opioid agonists administered to these cells inhibited both basal and prostaglandin E_1 (PGE_1)-stimulated adenylate cyclase. This inhibition was dose-dependent and naloxone-antagonizable, and the inhibitory potencies of a series of opioid agonists correlated well with their binding affinities to these cells, as well as with their in vivo pharmacological potencies.

Subsequently, this group found that chronic opioid agonist treatment resulted in a gradual loss of opioid inhibition of adenylate cyclase, with cyclic AMP levels returning to normal (Sharma et al., 1975b). Furthermore, withdrawal of agonist at this time resulted in an increased adenylate cyclase activity, above that of control level. These effects are at least superficially analogous to opiate tolerance and dependence, respectively, suggesting that NG108-15 cells would constitute a useful model system in which to study these phenomena.

In seeking to understand the molecular processes underlying the chronic effects of opioids in NG cells, researchers have been aided greatly by previous studies of the receptors for other ligands, particularly β-adrenergic agonists and glucagon. In many clonal cell lines, as well as in erythrocytes and certain isolated primary cell preparations, acute administration of these ligands stimulates adenylate cyclase, whereas chronic treatment results in a progressive loss of this stimulatory effect. The acute effect is mediated by a GTP-binding subunit (G_s or N_s), which couples the receptor to the catalytic subunit of adenylate cyclase (Rodbell, 1980). The chronic effect, on the other hand, appears to involve at least two steps (Su et al., 1980; Lefkowitz et al., 1980). In the first step, called *desensitization* in this chapter, the receptor becomes uncoupled from the GTP-binding subunit, with an accompanying reduction of affinity for agonist binding. In the second step, *down-regulation*, the receptors are removed from the cell surface, passing into the cell interior where they may be degraded or later recycled to the surface. This step, then, results in a loss of receptor binding sites, or a reduction in B_{max}.

Studies of opioid action in NG108-15 cells, carried out in our own as well as other laboratories, have indicated that these ligands act through generally similar mechanisms. Opioid agonist inhibition of adenylate cyclase is now recognized to be mediated through a GTP-binding subunit called N_i (G_i). Thus opioid receptor-mediated inhibition of cyclase is not seen if GTP is replaced by its non-hydrolyzable analog Gpp(NH)p, and the potencies of various opioids to inhibit cyclase are closely correlated with their stimulation of GTP hydrolysis (Koski and Klee, 1981; Koski et al. 1982). The chronic effects of opioids in NG cells likewise appear to take place through a multistep process, involving desensitization and down-regulation as well as an increased adenylate cyclase observed upon withdrawal (Law et al., 1984b). Below, we will consider each of these processes in more detail.

Before we do, however, one other study that was essential to the understanding of chronic opioid effects in this system should be mentioned. It is now well recognized that the brain contains multiple types of opioid receptors that are selective for mu (morphine-like), delta (enkephalin-like), and kappa (ethylketocyclazocine-like) opioid agonists (Lord et al., 1977; Iwamoto and Martin, 1981; Wood, 1982). NG cells, in contrast, contain only delta-type receptors (Chang and Cuatrecasas, 1979; Chang, 1984). Although mu and kappa, as well as delta, agonists can inhibit adenylate cyclase in this system, only the latter (and the alkaloids etorphine and keto-cyclazocine) act as full agonists. This was demonstrated in a study comparing the ratios of K_d (binding affinity) to K_i (inhibition of cyclase) for a series of opioids (Law et al., 1983a). Delta agonists (and etorphine) had ratios ranging from 4 to 5–10 or more, whereas other opioid agonists had ratios of 2.5 or less.

Further studies, which will be discussed below, demonstrated that delta agonists also differed from most alkaloids with respect to their chronic effects in this system. Specifically, whereas full agonists could induce both desensitization and down-regulation, partial agonists could induce only the former step. This finding was thus not only critical to establishing that both of these steps can occur in NG108-15 cells, but that the two processes are distinct.

2.1. Desensitization

Law et al. (1982, 1983b) first demonstrated that chronic opioid effects on NG108-15 cells, using nonsaturating concentrations of a full agonist, could be dissociated into two processes, a relatively rapid desensitization, occurring within 2 h, and a slower down-regulation, apparent after 24 h. Desensitization was initially defined as simply a loss of agonist inhibition of adenylate cyclase, whereas down-regulation was measured as a reduction in binding of the antagonist diprenorphine. However, subsequent studies showed that desensitization to opioid agonists, as had earlier been reported with catecholamines (Su et al., 1980), involved a reduction of agonist affinity and an uncoupling of receptor from adenylate cyclase.

In detailed studies of the process, Law et al. (1985b) reported that opioid receptors on NG108-15 cells could exist in multiple affinity states, depending on conditions. Control membranes, incubated in the presence of 10 mM Mg^{2+}, exhibited a single high affinity site for D-Ala^2-D-Leu^5-enkephalin (DADLE), with a K_d of about 2 nM. Addition to the incubation mixture of guanyl nucleotide and 100 mM Na$^+$, which are known to be essential to coupling, converted the receptor to multiple affinity states, the highest of which had a K_d for DADLE of about 0.4 nM. When a similar analysis was carried out on membranes prepared from NG cells that had been de-sensitized by incubation with 100 nM DADLE for 3 h, the multiple sites still existed in the presence of Na^+ and guanyl nucleotide, but the percentage of receptors in the highest affinity state was significantly reduced.

On the basis of these results, the authors postulated the follow-ing scheme. In the absence of Na^+ and guanyl nucleotide, opioid re-ceptor and N_i are uncoupled, and a single population of opioid bind-ing sites is observed. Upon addition of these coupling promoters, the coupled receptor–N_i complex is formed, resulting in the appear-ance of a new, higher affinity site. This coupled form is in equilib-rium with the uncoupled form of the receptor—hence the existence of multiple binding sites—but since the coupled form has a higher affinity for opioid agonists, the latter bind preferentially to it and shift the equilibrium further in the direction of coupling. Finally, upon prolonged treatment with opioid agonist, GTP is hydrolyzed to GDP, and the equilibrium is shifted back toward the uncoupled form—hence the decrease in high affinity binding sites.

Still to be elucidated is how chronic agonist treatment promotes this uncoupling of receptor from N_i. Since desensitization in this sys-tem is homologous—that is, the sensitivity to nonopioid agonists, which also mediate their effects through N_i, is unchanged (Law et al., 1983b)—presumably the change must occur in the receptor, rather than in N_i. Desensitization of other receptors, such as the β-adrenergic receptor (Sibley et al., 1985), is thought to involve phosphorylation, but experiments in our laboratory suggest that this is not the mechanism for opioid desensitization. Indeed, using a cell-free system, we have found that opioid desensitization is promoted by incubation of NG108-15 cell membranes in the presence of the nonhydrolyzable ATP analog App(NH)p, suggesting that dephos-phorylation may be involved (Louie et al., 1986).

2.2. Down-Regulation

Down-regulation is defined as a loss of receptor number, mani-fested as a decrease in B_{max} of ligand binding, upon chronic treat-ment. It has been described for several receptor systems, includ-ing those for catecholamines (Lefkowitz et al., 1980) and peptide hormones (Brown et al., 1983), and was reported for opioids by both our laboratory (Law et al., 1983b) and by Chang et al. (1982). Although we found this process to be relatively slow, Chang et al. (1982) reported down-regulation of opioid receptors within 2 h.

This may be a result of the different cell lines used by the two groups, as well as the saturating concentration of agonist used by the Chang group.

Studies with peptide hormone receptors have revealed that down-regulation occurs by a well-defined process, involving (1) clustering of the receptors in special areas on the cell surface known as coated pits; (2) their endocytotic movement into the cell; and (3) degradation of recycling back to the outer surface of the membrane (Goldstein et al., 1979; Brown et al., 1983). Studies with opioids have confirmed that at least some of these steps also occur with down-regulation of opioid receptors. Hazum et al. (1979) first reported clustering of enkephalin receptors on the surface of their N4TG1 cell line, a process that can occur independently of down-regulation. Evidence of internalization was obtained in experiments showing that down-regulation was energy dependent and accompanied by accumulation of radioactive agonist in N4TG1 cells (Blanchard et al., 1983).

Law et al. (1984a), in contrast, were initially unable to observe an accumulation of agonist in cells during down-regulation of opioid receptors in NG108-15 cells. Subsequent experiments, however, in which the lysosomotropic agent chloroquine was added to the cultures, revealed a time-dependent translocation of ligand from plasma cell membrane to a lysosome-enriched fraction, manifested in a shift in density of the fraction with which the ligand was associated. From these results it was concluded that the ligand–receptor complex was transported into lysosomes, where under normal conditions it was degraded, releasing free ligand to be extruded by the cells.

As pointed out above, evidence indicates that changes in the opioid receptor, rather than in N_i, underlie desensitization. The same appears to be true with regard to down-regulation. Inactivation of N_i by pertussis toxin, which prevents receptor coupling with this component (Murayama and Ui, 1983), resulted in no detectable effect on down-regulation or internalization (Law et al., 1985c). Furthermore, using the ADP-ribosylation that is catalyzed by the toxin as a marker for N_i, it was established that there was no internalization of this component. Thus is appears that the receptor–agonist complex internalizes by itself.

Further studies by this group attempted to define the role of protein synthesis and modification in down-regulation (Law et al., 1985a). Earlier studies by other groups had shown that down-regulation of muscarinic receptors could be potentiated by protein synthesis inhibitors such as cycloheximide (Klein et al., 1979), whereas the levels of insulin receptors were affected by glycosylation inhibitors such as tunicamycin (Rosen et al., 1979). Since the cell surface concentration of receptors presumably represents a dynamic equilibrium between synthesis and degradation, this is the result one would expect if chronic opioid treatment affected one or both of these processes. Treatment of NG108-15 cells with either agent, however, though it resulted in a time- and inhibitor concentration-dependent decrease in opioid binding, had no effect on agonist inhibition of adenylate cyclase, nor on the rate or magnitude of down-regulation. Thus it appears that in opioid down-regulation, neither synthesis nor degradation of receptors is a rate-limiting step, but rather some intervening process is. For example, one could postulate that down-regulation alters the rate at which internalized receptors are recycled.

Perhaps the most important lesson from these studies, however, is that they reemphasize the point that down-regulation is not an entirely novel process. Like desensitization, it simply represents a normal process that has been slightly altered. Individual receptors are constantly being internalized. Chronic treatment, apparently by inactivating the receptor is one way, simply alters the balance between this internalization process and the replacement of receptors, so that there is a net observable decrease in the cell surface population of receptors.

2.3. Increase of Adenylate Cyclase Activity

The studies discussed in the previous two sections have firmly established that the changes in sensitivity to opioids that occur during chronic treatment of NG108-15 cells with these ligands reflect changes in receptors, or in receptor–effector coupling, and not simply a compensatory increase in adenylate cyclase, as had originally been believed (Sharma et al., 1977). This conclusion is also supported by studies of another cell line, N18TG2, chronic opioid treatment of which reduces opioid sensitivity without any increase in adenylate cyclase activity (Law et al., 1982). The fact remains, however, that such an increase does occur in NG108-15 cells and must therefore be considered part of the adaptive response of these cells.

Early studies by Nirenberg's group had indicated that this increase resulted from a change in the activity of adenylate cyclase, rather than in the number of enzyme molecules (Sharma et al., 1977). This conclusion was based on the fact that the cyclase activity of membranes from control and chronically treated cells did not differ when assayed in the presence of agents that directly stimulate the enzyme, such as NaF. Subsequent studies by Wilkening and Nirenberg (1980) suggested that certain lipids might be necessary, since culturing cells in delipidated serum reduced the magnitude of increase. In support of this, we found that treatment of cells with phospholipase C, which hydrolyzes the polar head groups of lipids, reduced the cyclase increase, whereas treatment with phospholipase A_2, which removes acyl chains, did not (Griffin et al., 1986). We also found, however, that culturing the cells in a chemically defined serum-free medium had no effect on the adenylate cyclase increase (Griffin et al., 1985a). This led us to conclude that the role of lipid head groups in this process was an indirect one.

One possible role of these lipids could be to bind calcium. Earlier studies in our laboratory (Chapman and Way, 1980) and by other groups (Ross and Cardenas, 1979) had established that opioid binding and calcium binding are closely related and may regulate each other. Opioids can also inhibit in a dose-dependent, naloxone-antagonizable manner the NG108-15 plasma membrane levels of the calcium-binding protein calmodulin (Baram and Simantov, 1983); this protein has been implicated in a wide range of cellular processes (Cheung, 1981), including the stimulation of adenylate cyclase (Brostrom et al., 1978). We found that the increase of cyclase activity could be reduced or eliminated by calcium antagonists such as EGTA and La^{3+} (Law et al., 1984b). By mixing fractions from such altered cells with those of normal cells, we were able to localize a fraction in the cytosol necessary for the increase. Gel filtration of this fraction resolved it into two components, one consisting of adenosine and the other a larger molecular weight species with the properties of calmodulin (Griffin et al., 1983; Law et al., 1984b). Since both of these substances can stimulate cyclase, they might conceivably be involved in the process by which the activity of this enzyme is increased.

Any complete model of the opioid-induced increase in adenylate cyclase activity, however, will have to account for an apparently paradoxical observation: In cells chronically treated with opioid agonist, the ability of the latter to inhibit cyclase is eventually lost completely (Law et al., 1983b). This latter observation seems to indicate that opioid receptors are completely uncoupled from N_i; if this were true, however, then how could opioid antagonism result in an increase in cyclase activity? In other words, although the inability of opioids to inhibit adenylate cyclase in chronically treated cells indicates that receptors have lost the ability to regulate enzyme, the naloxone-induced increase in activity indicates that they have retained some form of regulation.

A possible solution to this problem was suggested, again, by studies of catecholaminergic receptors. Manning and Gilman (1983) showed that both N_i and N_s, upon activation by stimulatory or inhibitory receptors, respectively, dissociate into several sub-units; one of these (alpha$_s$ or alpha$_i$) is responsible for mediating the stimulation or inhibition, whereas at least one of the others (beta) appears to be common to the two GTP-binding proteins. This led Gilman (1984) to propose that the enzyme is normally under dual regulation by these two proteins. Each N-protein, in addition to having a direct effect on the enzyme through its alpha-subunit, can have an indirect effect on it through its beta-subunit; the latter effect is mediated by the combining of beta with the alpha-subunit of the other N-species, which prevents its activation.

Accordingly, Griffin et al. (1985b) proposed a model in which opioids initially inhibit adenylate cyclase both directly and indirectly. During chronic agonist treatment, it was suggested, opioids lose the ability to couple to N_i and inhibit the enzyme directly; however, they retain the ability to inhibit the enzyme indirectly, through blocking N_s. Because of this latter effect, opioids are still effectively regulating cyclase activity, and thus naloxone antagonism results in an increase in this activity. However, since they are only preventing a tonic stimulation of the enzyme, their acute administration does not inhibit the enzyme.

To test this model, Griffin et al. (1985b) treated cells with pertussis toxin, which is known to inactivate N_i (Murayama and Ui, 1983). Consistent with their hypothesis, this resulted in an increase in adenylate cyclase activity that was quite similar to that observed in cells chronically treated with opioid agonist. Furthermore, this increase (or that induced simply by chronic opioid treatment) could be prevented by chronic treatments with stimulatory ligands such as adenosine, which desensitize, or uncouple, receptor–mediated stimulation of cyclase. This supports the hypothesis that activation of N_s is required for the adenylate cyclase increase. This latter finding is also consistent with the earlier observation of increased adenosine levels in these cells (see above), which might mediate stimulation of the cyclase.

This scheme does have some problems, however. For example, it is not clear how, if opioids lose the ability to activate N_i, they can nevertheless continue to block activation of N_s, since both processes are supposed to depend on dissociation of N_i into subunits. It appears that one must postulate that the opioid receptor interacts with alpha$_i$, even after the latter's dissociation from N_i, and that this interaction is altered in chronically treated cells, because of an alteration in the receptor.

2.4. Summary and Conclusions

Opioid regulation of adenylate cyclase in NG108-15 cells has proved to be the most accessible system for studying the biochemical mechanisms underlying chronic opiate effects. Even in this relatively simple system, however, the changes in sensitivity to opioids that accompany their long-term administration are clearly complex, involving several distinct steps. Each of these steps is in fact quite complex in itself, and is not yet completely understood.

Adaptive systems such as this presumably evolved because they were able to protect cells from over-stimulation in the continuous presence of a ligand. Thus opiate desensitization and down-regulation prevent the cell from completely shutting down adenylate cyclase over extended periods of time. At the same time, however, such adaptation has costs of its own, for it forces the cell to undergo certain metabolic changes that may be energetically expensive, both to initiate and to reverse.

In this light, a multiple-step process clearly has advantages, since it enables the cell to temper its response to an agent. For example, desensitization, the first step in the response to chronic opioid observed by Law et al. (1983b), involves uncoupling of the receptor from cyclase; this is a relatively easy step to reverse, for it involves simply a shift in an equilibrium. If contact with opiate is more prolonged, on the other hand, the cell experiences an actual decrease in receptor number. This is a more difficult process to reverse, since it requires acceleration of certain processes within the cell, and since it takes some time to replenish the missing receptors. In some cases, such as treatment with opiate alkaloids, adenylate cyclase may be up-regulated without down-regulation of receptors, thus increasing its activity in still another way.

To the extent that analogies with whole animals are valid, desensitization and down-regulation, both of which reduce the sensitivity of the cells to agonist, are equivalent to tolerance, whereas the increase in adenylate cyclase observed upon challenge with naloxone is a form of dependence. Thus the studies discussed above suggest that tolerance and dependence, classically considered to be different manifestations of a single phenomenon, may to some extent be dissociable. As noted above, opioid desensitization is homologous—that is, it does not affect the cell's response to other classes of ligands—so the change responsible for it presumably must occur in the receptors themselves; down-regulation, of course, also involves changes at the receptor level. The increase in adenylate cyclase, in contrast, seems to require processes subsequent to receptor binding, such as, perhaps, changes in adenosine or calmodulin levels. Evidence that a similar dissociation of tolerance and dependence may also be the case in more complex isolated tissue systems, as well as in whole animals, has recently been reported, and will be discussed in following sections of this article.

However, it is clear that the analogies between chronic phenomena in cultured cells and in whole animals have serious limitations. In the first place, opioid regulation of adenylate cyclase in brain has been firmly established only in the striata (Law et al., 1981; Cooper et al., 1982), where opioids do not have analgesic effects. Furthermore, in all cases it has been the delta-type receptor that has been linked to cyclase; however, increasing evidence indicates that opioid analgesia, at least supraspinally, is mediated exclusively through mu-type receptors (Ward and Takemori, 1983; Chaillet et al., 1983, 1984).

On the other hand, a recent study in our laboratory found that N_i is present in many brain regions besides the striatum (Abood et al., 1985). Thus it is conceivable that mu receptors are linked to cyclase in these other regions, but that this association is not observed in binding assays because of the absence of some critical cofactor (Lambert and Childers, 1984). Alternatively, since GTP is known to regulate binding to mu as well as delta receptors (Blume, 1978), N_i, or some other GTP-binding protein (Sternweis and Robishaw, 1984), may mediate analgesia through its interactions with molecules other than adenylate cyclase. Of particular interest in this regard are ion channels. Several studies have shown that opioids may activate potassium or calcium channels (Mudge et al., 1979; Williams et al., 1982; North and Williams, 1983), which presumably underlies their ability to alter the firing rates of some brain neurons (Zieglgansberger et al., 1976). Other evidence suggests that calcium gating may be mediated by GTP-binding proteins (Gomperts, 1983). Thus studies of opiate receptor coupling to N_i in NG108-15 cells could be relevant to mechanisms of opiate action in these neurons.

A potentially more serious problem that arises in attempting to use NG cell data to understand opiate action in the brain is that whole animal phenomena such as analgesia are mediated by multicellular networks, which to some extent have properties that transcend those of their individual members. This means that even if the responses of individual brain neurons to opiates were identical to that of NG cells, their collective response might be quite different. Recent evidence that tolerance might be based on such a collective response was reported by Williams and North (1983). They found that acute administration of opiates to either whole animals or to slices of the locus ceruleus (LC) induced a hyperpolarization in the LC neurons. In animals chronically treated with morphine, a high degree of tolerance to this response was seen, but the tolerance was much lower in cells of isolated LC. Apparently, connections of these cells with other neurons are vital to the full development of tolerance.

3. Chronic Opioid Effects in Isolated Tissue Systems

As model systems with which to study the acute and chronic effects of opioids, isolated tissue systems offer a level of analysis between that of cultured cells, on the one hand, and whole animals, on the other. Unlike cultured cells, they retain nervous transmission and a physiological response, so that studies can proceed beyond simply the elucidation of receptor mechanisms and ask how these mechanisms are transduced into physiological phenomena. Yet they are still considerably simpler than the whole brain, and so lend themselves better to dissection of cellular and intercellular processes affected by opioids. A further advantage over whole animals is that the concentration of opioids and other molecules (such as ions) that are in contact with receptors can be rigorously controlled.

In this section we will discuss primarily work carried out with the guinea pig ileum (GPI) and mouse vas deferens (MVD), since these are the best-characterized isolated tissue systems with regard to opioid effects, and particularly with regard to chronic effects. However, some mention will also be made of studies of central nervous system tissue preparations, since these have recently commanded more attention among opioid pharmacologists and may ultimately provide deeper insights into tolerance and dependence.

3.1. Guinea Pig Ileum and Mouse Vas Deferens

Both the GPI and MVD are smooth muscle preparations that undergo a series of contractions upon electrical stimulation. Opioid agonists inhibit these contractions in a dose-dependent, naloxone-reversible fashion, and with some important exceptions, there is a good correlation between their potency in these systems and their ability to induce analgesia (Lord et al., 1977). Furthermore, upon chronic treatment with opioid agonist in vivo or in vitro, these preparations develop tolerance to and, at least in the case of the GPI, dependence on opiates (Goldstein and Schulz, 1973; Hammond et al., 1976; Schulz et al., 1980).

Unfortunately, studies of the GPI and MVD have not yet established the second messenger(s) responsible for opioid effects, although some evidence implicates adenylate cyclase (see below). This has hindered attempts to understand tolerance and dependence in these systems by preventing the kind of detailed studies of receptor–effector relationships that have been possible in NG cells. However, researchers have gained important insights into these chronic phenomena by taking advantage of receptor multiplicity in these systems. Unlike NG cells, which contain a single opioid receptor type, these isolated tissue systems contain several; the GPI has mu and kappa receptors, whereas the MVD, though it has predominantly delta receptors, also has mu and kappa types. This has made it possible to examine the questions of cross-tolerance and cross-dependence; that is, to determine whether chronic activation of one receptor type results in tolerance and dependence only with respect to ligands that interact with that receptor type, or to opioids specific for other types as well. From these studies, as we will discuss below, inferences can be made about the site of tolerance and dependence in these systems.

3.1.1. Cross-Tolerance

Herz and colleagues (Schulz et al., 1980; Schulz and Herz, 1984) investigated the question of cross tolerance between multiple opioid receptors in the MVD. Tolerance to the selective agonists sufentanil (mu), DADLE (delta), or EKC (kappa) was induced in mice by means of implanted osmotic minipumps. The vasa were then removed from the tolerant animals and set up in an organ bath in the presence of the same concentration of agonist present in the serum of the tolerant animal (to prevent withdrawal), and their response to a range of acute doses of various agonists was determined.

Under these conditions a high degree of selectivity in the development of tolerance was observed. Thus in vasa from mice infused with DADLE (5 μg,/h for 6d), the IC_{50} value for this ligand increased about 800-fold, from 0.4 nM to 300 nM; the IC_{50} values for other delta ligands, such as Met- and Leu-enkephalin, experienced similar large increases. In contrast, the IC_{50} for sufentanil increased only about fivefold, and that for EKC less than twofold. Analogous results were obtained with vasa from animals made tolerant to sufentanil or EKC; tolerance to mu or kappa agonists, respectively, was far greater than that to other types of opioids.

These results are so clear-cut that the conclusion of selective tolerance appears unassailable; yet there is one odd feature of them that has emerged as a result of subsequent research. Although the ligands that Herz and colleagues used in their studies were the most selective then available for particular opioid receptor types, it is now well recognized that all of them have appreciable affinity for more than one receptor type. This is particularly true of EKC, which binds to mu and delta receptors almost as well as it does to kappa receptors, and DADLE, which has fairly high affinity for mu as well as delta receptors (Pfeiffer and Herz, 1981; Zukin and Zukin, 1981; Landahl et al., 1985). The concentrations of these agonists, and probably of sufentanil as well, that were present chronically in vivo and in vitro should have been high enough to activate more than one receptor. Why, then, was such a high degree of selectivity observed? One possibility is that tolerance development in this system is not linear. In this study, the IC_{50} values for various specific agonists were not determined at different levels of tolerance, but only at one level. Thus it is conceivable that the ratios of tolerance obtained do not accurately reflect the relative amounts of receptor occupancy. This possibility could easily be tested, of course, by determining IC_{50} values after larger or more prolonged infusions of the ligand used to produce tolerance.

Another possible explanation is based on evidence that mu and delta receptors are allosterically linked (Lee and Smith, 1980; Rothman and Westfall, 1982), such that occupation of one receptor may alter the affinity of ligands for the other. Under these conditions, chronic treatment of a ligand selective for one receptor type might be expected to reduce the amount of ligand specific for another type of receptor that is necessary to inhibit contractions. As a result, its change in IC_{50} value, and apparent degree of tolerance, would be underestimated.

Although the degree of selectivity observed in these studies may be puzzling, it seems clear that the concept of selectivity itself is valid. This conclusion, which was also supported by studies of the GPI (Wuster et al., 1981) and of whole animal analgesia (Schulz et al., 1981; Von voightlander and Lewis, 1982; see below), challenges the classical notion that cross-tolerance exists among all opioids, an idea that was formulated long before any opioid receptors, let alone multiple receptors, had been identified. In retrospect, it appears that the reason this rule seemed to be valid is that the opioids tested all acted through a common receptor type, mu (Chaillet et al., 1983, 1984; see below).

Perhaps the most important implication of these findings, however, is for our understanding of tolerance. In the GPI and MVD different opioid receptor types trigger a common physiological response—inhibition of electrically induced contractions; thus it follows that the processes resulting in tolerance must occur somewhere before this step in the chain of events beginning with receptor activation. Although it is conceivable that each receptor type mediates inhibition of contractions through a different second messenger system, it seems more likely that all work through a common process, such as an ion channel (see below). Thus these findings of selective tolerance lend support to the conclusion that tolerance occurs at the receptor level, as it appears to in NG108-15 cells. However, there is no direct evidence for this conclusion yet. Rubini et al. (1982) measured opioid binding in MVD following chronic treatment with agonist, and found no changes in number or affinity of receptors. These results are somewhat suspect, however, in that binding could only be measured in the absence of agonist, under which conditions the tissue is withdrawn. Furthermore, as we shall discuss later, a model of tolerance development based on changes in opioid receptors can be formulated that specifically predicts that these changes would not be found when binding to isolated tissue is analyzed.

3.1.2. Cross-Dependence

The Herz group has also attempted to investigate the question of cross dependence in the GPI (Schulz et al., 1982; Schulz and

Herz, 1984). Dependence in this system is measured by determining the intensity of contractions that occur upon withdrawal of opioid agonist from a chronically treated preparation, in the absence of any electrical stimulation. In their studies, Herz and collaborators used naloxone to precipitate withdrawal. Since this antagonist is not very selective for different receptor types, however, they compared its effect on receptors occupied by different specific agonists. The approach was to prepare ilea from animals treated chronically with a selective agonist (mu or kappa), as in the tolerance experiments, remove the agonist by washing, then incubate for 30 min in the presence of that or another agonist type. Naloxone challenge was then used to elicit withdrawal contractions. These were found to be of similar intensity regardless of whether the agonist used in vitro was the same type or a different type from that used in vivo.

This study establishes that dependence occurs to either mu or kappa agonist in this system, but it is not certain that it proves, as the Herz group has claimed, that cross dependence exists between these two types of receptors. The problem is not simply that the degree of specificity of the ligands used is such that they may activate both receptors simultaneously, a problem Schulz et al. (1982) attempted to eliminate by first selectively blocking one set of receptors with a covalent ligand. The problem is that by washing the ilea after removal from the dependent animal, much of the initial dependence is eliminated (this reduction of dependence was in fact monitored in some studies by demonstrating the inability of naloxone to precipitate withdrawal contractions after washing). Thus one could argue that the dependence revealed by naloxone challenge after 30 min incubation with agonist was in fact largely caused by this in vitro exposure. (Or, if one wishes to argue that the washing did not eliminate most of the original dependence, then one must assume that it did not eliminate most of any dependence because of activation of other receptors.) In fact, Schulz et al. (1980) have demonstrated that a very high tolerance to DADLE in vitro develops within 3 h.

3.1.3. Relationship of Tolerance to Dependence

Studies of the GPI and MVD have not only provided insight into the relationships of different opioid receptor types in tolerance and dependence, but may be used to examine the relationship of these two adaptive phenomena to each other. A classical tenet of opiate pharmacology has been that tolerance and dependence represent a unitary phenomenon; that is, that they are simply different manifestations of a single underlying process. Several observations made in these isolated tissue systems, however, seem to challenge this notion. These are: (1) the existence of cross dependence, but not cross tolerance in the GPI; (2) the existence of tolerance, but not dependence, in MVD chronically treated with opioids (Gillan et al., 1979); and (3) a lack of correlation between the appearance of tolerance and that of dependence in GPI (Schulz et al., 1982). On this basis, it has been argued that tolerance and dependence are separate phenomena in these isolated tissue systems (Schulz and Herz, 1984; Wuster et al., 1985).

A closer look at each of these points, however, suggests that this conclusion, though suggestive, is not yet compelling. The first line of evidence has already been discussed in the preceding section, where it was pointed out that the evidence for cross-dependence in the GPI is not conclusive. It was also pointed out that tolerance for different types of opioid ligands is probably not as selective as the data imply, because of the limited selectivity of the ligands employed. Taking these points together, one might reasonably conclude that a partial cross-tolerance as well as a partial cross dependence occurred under the conditions of these experiments. With respect to the second line of evidence, lack of dependence in tolerant MVD, this point is still a little controversial. Herz' group has argued strongly for this case, yet their own data cast some doubt on it (Schulz et al., 1980). Vasa prepared from DADLE- and sufentanil-tolerant mice did in fact show a significant increase in twitch tension upon naloxone challenge in some cases, but not in others. Furthermore, electrophysiological studies of tolerant MVD have revealed changes that might reflect dependence (North and Vitek, 1979). On the other hand, these studies do offer some support for the thesis that tolerance and dependence are distinct processes, in that any dependence that does develop in this system is not observed as clearly and reproducibly as tolerance.

The third line of evidence comes from studies by the Herz group in which both tolerance and dependence were determined in GPI of animals exposed to various chronic dosages of morphine (Schulz and Herz, 1984). These investigators reported that the two phenomena did not develop in parallel. In fact, a significant degree of dependence was observed before any tolerance was seen. At higher doses of chronic agonist, dependence leveled off, whereas tolerance continued to increase.

The results of this last study seem, at first glance, paradoxical. A little thought about what tolerance and dependence mean shows that it is impossible for the latter to occur in the absence of the former. Dependence is defined as a state in which drug is required to prevent withdrawal symptoms; but if an animal or tissue system requires drug to maintain its normal state, it follows that it is also tolerant to that level of drug. If it requires drug, then it must be tolerant to the drug. To explain this, Schulz and Herz (1984) suggested that there might be two chronic processes in this system, one involving tolerance and dependence, and the other involving tolerance only. The first process could involve a parallel development of tolerance and dependence, with the relationship between the two such that dependence is much larger and more easily detected, even though both processes occur simultaneously. Subsequently, tolerance would continue to increase without any change in dependence levels. This proposed sequence of events is consistent with the definitions of tolerance and dependence, although of course it remains hypothetical.

In conclusion, there is significant evidence that tolerance and dependence are distinct phenomena in these isolated tissue systems, although it is not yet compelling. This conclusion is consistent with the findings in NG cells, discussed above, and likewise, suggests that tolerance in this system may take place at the receptor level, although dependence occurs at some subsequent process.

3.1.4. Relationship of Opioid and Nonopioid Dependence

Electrically induced contractions in the GPI can be inhibited not only by opioids, but by two other classes of agonists: adrenergic ligands such as clonidine and purines such as adenosine. Furthermore, chronic treatment of ilea in vivo or in vitro with these agonists leads to dependence, as it does with opioids. Thus the GPI can be used to ask whether cross dependence exists between opioid and nonopioid ligands.

Collier and Tucker (1984) examined this question by preparing ilea dependent on each type of agonist, then testing the effects of an antagonist specific for a particular receptor type. The antagonists used were naloxone for the opioid receptor, yohimbine for the adrenergic receptor, and 8-phenyltheophylline for the purine receptor. These studies found that withdrawal could be precipitated only by an antagonist specific for the dependence-producing agent. This result is not unexpected, for it simply confirms the notion that each type of ligand acts at a specific receptor. It was also found, however, that withdrawal could be prevented by an agonist of any of these three classes. This suggests that the dependence induced by these agonists is mediated through a common process "downstream" from the receptor.

The nature of this common process is still unknown. Collier and Tucker (1984) reported that pertussis toxin, a specific inhibitor of N_i, reduced withdrawal, which suggests involvement of adenylate cyclase. Lux and Schulz (1985) repeated this finding, and showed that the toxin had no effect on withdrawal if given after dependence had developed. Pertussis toxin had no effect on the acute response to opioid in this system, however, which it should have had if opioid receptors are coupled to adenylate cyclase in the manner found in NG108-15 cells and in striatum. In fact, it should be recalled that Griffin et al. (1985b) found that in NG108-15 cells, pertussis toxin actually induced a withdrawal-like increase in adenylate cyclase when given by itself. The failure to observe an increase in cyclase in cells treated with both toxin and chronic agonist was because of the fact that cyclase levels had already reached those found in cells withdrawing from agonist alone. So it appears that the processes underlying both acute and chronic effects of opioids in the GPI are significantly different from those in NG cells. However, in light of the fact that the GPI is a more complex, multicellular system, it is too soon to compare it directly with NG cells in this regard.

Collier's work is nonetheless significant in that it establishes that the process responsible for dependence takes place subsequent to receptor activation. This is consistent with the situation in NG cells, and adds further support to the idea that tolerance and dependence may be distinct phenomena. Although the question of cross tolerance of opioid and nonopioid ligands has not been addressed in this system, one would predict, in light of the apparently selective tolerance of different opioid receptor types in this system (see above), that it would not be found.

3.2. Central Nervous System Tissue

Although the GPI and MVD have proved to be useful model systems in which to study the acute and chronic actions of opioids, the fact that they are peripheral nervous system preparations may limit their relevance to analgesia and other central effects of opioids. For this reason, investigators have recently begun to study opioid action in cultures of central nervous system tissue. In whole animals, opioids given acutely have well-defined effects on the activity of many types of central neurons, usually inhibitory, but sometimes excitatory (Zieglgansberger et al., 1975; Nicoll et al., 1977). Moreover, tolerance- and dependence-like phenomena can often be observed. Thus these effects are frequently reduced in animals treated chronically with morphine (Satoh et al., 1975, 1976), whereas they may be reversed by naloxone under the same conditions (Frederickson et al., 1975; Fry et al., 1980).

Application of this same approach to in vitro preparations has revealed, in most respects, similarities in the responses to opioids. French and Zieglgansberger (1982) reported that both normorphine and methionine-enkephalin potentiated field potentials of pyramidal neurons in hippocampal slices, as previously had been shown in vivo. Slices from morphine-tolerant animals showed tolerance to normorphine, but not to Met-enkephalin, suggesting a lack of cross tolerance between mu and delta agonists. Andrade et al. (1983) showed that tolerance could develop to the decrease in spontaneous activity induced by acute morphine in neurons of locus ceruleus slices. In contrast to the results of in vivo experiments, however, they did not observe withdrawal-like increases in firing upon addition of naloxone. Thus they concluded that tolerance and dependence could be dissociated, with the latter perhaps depending on inputs from brain regions outside the LC. As pointed out earlier, a study by Williams and North (1983), in which the ability of opioids to open K^+ channels was studied, concluded that external circuits were required for tolerance. This thus constitutes further evidence that the kind of single-cell tolerance/dependence phenomena observed in NG108-15 cells may not be directly relevant to changes in the brain.

In order to see whether receptor changes could underlie these chronic effects of opioids, Dingledine et al. (1983) recently analyzed binding to mu and delta sites in hippocampal slices. Incubation of slices for 4 h with DADLE resulted in a decrease of delta receptors, but not mu receptors. Incubation with the mu agonists morphine or morphiceptin had no effect on either mu or delta receptors, although physiological tolerance to morphiceptin was observed. Dingledine et al. (1983) concluded that desensitization could account for tolerance to delta agonists in this preparation, but not tolerance to mu agonists.

Another tissue culture preparation that has been useful for studying the acute and chronic effects of opioids is the spinal cord

(Crain, 1984). In explants of spinal cord cross-sections, dorsal root ganglia stimuli evoke slow wave responses over the dorsal horn. These responses are inhibited by morphine and various opioid peptides (Crain et al., 1978) and antagonized by calcium as well as by naloxone (Crain et al., 1982a). These results are consistent with the ability of morphine to inhibit noxious stimuli when injected into the substantia gelatinosa of the cord of whole animals (Duggan et al., 1977), and also with studies that show high levels of opioid receptors in the dorsal region (Lamotte et al., 1976). In fact, the spinal cord is the best isolated tissue preparation currently available that possesses receptors known to mediate analgesia in vivo.

Tolerance to the effects of opioids could be observed after 2 d of culture in the presence of 1 μM morphine, and there appeared to be cross tolerance between different classes of agonist (Crain, 1984). This finding thus differs from that observed in GPI and MVD, as discussed above as well as from what has been reported in the spinal cord in vivo (Tung and Yaksh, 1982); Yaksh, 1983). There was also cross-tolerance to the effects of serotonin, though not to other depressants of cord responses (Crain et al., 1982b). Although no clear-cut sign of dependence could be elicited, the investigators did report an increase in slow wave amplitude in tolerant cultures. Electrophysiological studies of this preparation indicate that opioids may act by blocking a Ca^{2+}-dependent action potential in DRG neurons (Crain, 1984). This conclusion is also supported by the observation that Ca^{2+} inhibits the acute response to opioids, as does 4-aminopyridine, which enhances Ca^{2+} efflux indirectly by depressing K^+ conductance (Illes and Thesleff, 1978). Opioids do not, however, have these acute effects on action potentials in adult DRG neurons (Williams and Zieglgansberger, 1981). Thus the relevance of this system to our understanding of spinal analgesia is still open to debate.

3.3. Summary and Conclusions

Most, though not all, of the studies of isolated tissue systems discussed above are consistent with two important conclusions derived from the studies of NG108-15 cells: (1) tolerance is mediated at, or near, the receptor level, with selective tolerance exhibited by different opioid receptor types; and (2) dependence is distinct from tolerance, and is mediated at some step subsequent to receptor activation. Unlike the case with NG cells, however, the acute effects of opioids do not appear to be mediated by inhibition of adenylate cyclase in any of these isolated tissue systems, though GTP-binding proteins may very well be involved.

As with NG cells, studies of these isolated tissue systems may be criticized on the grounds that they are not directly relevant to analgesia. This is obviously true with respect to the GPI and MVD, but it is probably also so for central neurons. The brain regions that have been best studied in vitro, such as the hippocampus and locus ceruleus, are not known to be part of the classic pain pathway, whereas the spinal cord changes that have been observed, as noted above, were found only in fetal tissue. Furthermore, as emphasized earlier, some evidence indicates that tolerance and dependence may depend in some cases on extensive nervous connections that are not present in these isolated systems. Nevertheless, it seems highly likely that the general processes described in these systems, such as the effects of opioids on ion channels, are very similar to those underlying analgesia, because these processes have been observed in so many different kinds of cells. Thus these isolated tissue preparations, particularly those from the central nervous system, should be extremely useful in future research.

4. Chronic Opioid Effects in Whole Animals

Compared to the isolated cell and tissue systems discussed in the preceding sections, study of the processes underlying tolerance and dependence in whole animals is extremely difficult. To begin with, the brain contains a vast assortment of different types of cells, only a small portion of which are involved in analgesia. Thus any biochemical changes accompanying tolerance and dependence are likely to be obscured unless small, discrete portions of the brain are analyzed. As discussed above, however, some evidence suggests that tolerance and dependence may depend on extensive pathways in large areas of the brain. In fact, it has been recognized for many years that several other neurotransmitter systems are involved in mediating both the acute and chronic effects of opioids in whole animals (Iwamoto and Way, 1979; Domino, 1979; Brase, 1979). Thus the study of discrete portions of the brain may also be misleading.

A further problem is that, even within a discrete region of the brain, the biochemical situation is likely to be considerably more complex than that in most of the isolated systems discussed in the preceding sections. Opioid interaction with receptors is subject to numerous controls, such as modulation by various endogenous opioids (Vaught and Takemori, 1979; Lee and Smith, 1984) and nonopioids (Faris et al., 1983; Contreras and Takemori, 1984; Yang et al., 1985a,b), as well as interaction with various effector systems (Clouet and Yonehara, 1984). Our ignorance in this area can hardly be overstated. At this time, we do not even know the identity of the endogenous ligand that morphine and other analgesic alkaloids presumably mimic, let alone the endogenous substances that may modulate this interaction under physiological conditions. We also do not know the biochemical effector system or systems that are involved in the initial steps leading to analgesia.

A final problem, which has been fully appreciated only in recent years, is that there are several levels of the CNS at which analgesia can be mediated. It is now believed that pain regulation occurs at three main centers: the dorsal horn of the spinal cord, the rostral-ventral medulla, and the periaqueductal gray in the brain (Basbaum and Fields, 1984). Although the mu receptor seems to mediate analgesia exclusively in the brain (Chaillet et al., 1983, 1984; Ward and Takemori, 1983), mu, delta, and possibly kappa receptors mediate it in the spinal cord (Yaksh, 1983). Moreover, the processes mediated by these systems are to some extent not independent, but synergistic. If a given dose of morphine is administered chronically to an animal both intracerebroventricularly (icv) and intrathecally (ith), the degree of tolerance that develops is greater than the sum of tolerances obtained from administration through either route alone (Yeung and Rudy, 1980). One consequence of this is that it is very difficult to interpret studies of cross-tolerance and cross-dependence using different selective opioids, as was done for the GPI and MVD (see preceding section). In fact, some studies of this kind have indicated selective tolerance to mu, delta, and kappa agonists (Schulz et al., 1981; Von voightlander and Lewis, 1982), which support the conclusion that tolerance may occur at the receptor level. Since these agonists may have different effects in the whole animal, however, it is not possible to conclude from such studies that tolerance occurs at the receptor level; if the effector systems are different, tolerance could occur at this level. Furthermore, since these studies administered opioid systemically, both spinal as well as supraspinal systems would have been affected, so it is obviously not possible to conclude anything about tolerance processes at either site alone.

Despite these complexities in the whole animal, however, studies of opioid receptors during chronic treatment with opioids can at least suggest possible processes involved, especially when the results are consistent with those obtained in simpler systems. In this section, we shall consider some of this work.

4.1. Down-Regulation of Opioid Receptors in the Brain

Soon after the identification of opioid receptors in the brain, many laboratories attempted to demonstrate changes in the affinity or number of these receptors in tolerant-dependent animals. The results of these studies, however, were disappointing. In almost all cases, investigators observed either no changes or changes that did not correlate well, in magnitude or time course, with tolerance development (Klee and Streaty, 1974; Hitzemann et al., 1974; Hollt et al., 1975; Harris and Kazmierowski, 1975; Pert and Snyder, 1976; Creese and Sibley, 1981).

Most of these studies, however, examined opioid binding in whole brain, and because opioid receptor heterogeneity was not appreciated at this time, binding to specific receptor types was not analyzed. Thus it could be argued that changes in binding to specific receptor types in discrete brain regions would have been missed. In fact, as discussed earlier, a study of receptor changes following chronic in vitro opioid treatment of hippocampal slices found decreases in delta, but not mu, receptors (Dingledine et al., 1983).

Recently, our laboratory considered another possible factor that might be important to the development of desensitization or down-regulation of opioid receptors in brain. In our earlier studies of NG108-15 cells (see section 2, above), we had shown that morphine did not induce down-regulation, apparently because it was only a partial agonist in this delta-receptor system. We reasoned that a similar situation might exist in certain parts of the brain, particularly in light of the fact that we had shown opioid regulation of adenylate cyclase in the striate, similar to that earlier demonstrated in NG cells (Law et al., 1981). Accordingly, we prepared rats tolerant to etorphine, which is a full agonist in NG cells (Tao et al., 1984). Under these conditions, we observed a time-dependent decrease in [^{3}H]diprenorphine binding in all three brain regions examined: cortex, midbrain, and striate. This decrease was caused by a decrease in receptor number, rather than affinity, and was accompanied by a twofold increase in the IC_{50}

for etorphine inhibition of striatal adenylate cyclase. Analysis of specific receptor types revealed that mu receptor binding was decreased in all three brain regions examined, whereas delta binding was significantly decreased only in the midbrain. In agreement with others, however (see above), no changes in receptor number or affinity accompanied chronic morphine treatment.

These results establish that the levels of both mu and delta opioid receptors in the brain can be regulated by certain agonists. The receptor number reached minimum levels, however, within 3 d of chronic treatment, although tolerance continued to develop for at least 7 d. This observation, together with the fact that no changes were observed to accompany the chronic administration of morphine, call into question the relevance of these findings to morphine tolerance. Possibly, such down-regulation could be the basis of tolerance to other, nonanalgetic effects of certain opioids.

Before completely ruling out the possibility of opioid receptor changes in morphine-tolerant animals, however, one other potentially complicating factor should be considered. When brain tissue is removed from a tolerant animal, in preparation for the opioid binding assay, any changes in receptors that might have developed in vivo could conceivably be reversed as a result of withdrawal of the chronic opioid. Some support for this idea is provided by a study by Davis et al. (1979), who found that when binding was assayed in unwashed brain stem slices of chronic animals before homogenization, a reduction in binding occurred in tolerant animals. The presence of opioid of course interferes with the binding assay, so very careful controls must be carried out to demonstrate that a real change in opioid receptors has in fact occurred. This kind of study, however, is one that deserves to be pursued further, applying it particularly to regions such as the periaqueductal gray.

4.2. Up-Regulation of Opioid Receptors in the Brain

In contrast to down-regulation, opioid receptor up-regulation in brain is well established (Hitzemann et al., 1974; Pert and Snyder, 1976; Tang and Collins, 1978; Schulz et al., 1979; Zukin et al., 1982, 1984). As with up-regulation that has been reported in other receptor systems (Creese et al., 1977), this appears to be an adaptive response to treatments that block opioid agonist activity, for it is induced by both lesions of certain brain pathways (Gardner et al., 1980; Young et al., 1982; Simantov and Amir, 1983) and, most commonly, by chronic administration of antagonist (Zukin et al., 1982).

In a detailed characterization of the phenomenon, Zukin et al., (1984) found an increase of nearly 100% in ^{3}H-etorphine binding in rats chronically treated with the opiate antagonist naltrexone, this maximum being reached after 8 d. The increase was caused entirely by a change in receptor number, with no change in affinity. It was parallelled by an increase in sensitivity of the animals to morphine, suggesting functional significance of the up-regulation. There was also an increased sensitivity of opiate binding to guanine nucleotides, suggesting an increase in receptor coupling to adenylate cyclase or to some other functional molecule. Autoradiographic studies indicated an uneven distribution of up-regulation, with ventromedial hypothalamus, ventral tegmental area, substantia nigra compacta, and amygdala showing the most increase in etorphine binding; there were also increases in Met-enkephalin in some areas. And most significantly, the up-regulation was observed with both mu and delta receptors, but not with kappa receptors (Tempel et al., 1985). Zukin and colleagues have also demonstrated up-regulation in the isolated spinal cord–dorsal root ganglion preparation, where the underlying processes can be examined under more controlled conditions (Tempel et al., 1983). The time course of this phenomenon in the presence of 10 μM naloxone (50% up-regulation in 5 d) was similar to that observed in spinal cord in vivo. The up-regulation was not blocked by cycloheximide, leading these investigators to conclude that up-regulation results from unmasking of previously inactive receptors, rather than from synthesis of new ones.

Very recently, Holaday et al. (1985) have reported up-regulation of opioid receptors in the brain following chronic agonist (morphine) treatment. The up-regulation was region and delta-receptor specific, and could also be induced by repeated electroconvulsive shock treatments, which the authors found produced many of the effects of opioids. Furthermore, there was cross-tolerance between the effects of the two treatments.

In theory, agonist-induced up-regulation of opioid receptors could account for tolerance, although such a model has major difficulties explaining certain data (see below). The major significance of these (antagonist- as well as agonist-induced) up-regulation studies, however, is that they suggest that opioid receptors in brain are in a state of dynamic flux, which can be altered by receptor occupation. Since opioid agonists are present in the brain, treatment with antagonists presumably inhibits agonist binding to opioid receptors. If this results in up-regulation of the receptors, the presence of agonist can be seen as a down-regulating factor. These studies thus support those of Dingledine et al. (1983) and Tao and Law (1984), suggesting that although opioid receptor down-regulation may not be involved in opioid tolerance, it nevertheless plays an important role in brain function.

5. Toward a Theory of Opioid Tolerance/ Dependence

From the studies discussed above, it is clear that our understanding of the molecular processes underlying tolerance and dependence is for the most part still quite rudimentary. In NG108-15 cells, which constitute the simplest system to analyze, the picture is now fairly clear, although many important details, such as the processes responsible for receptor–N_i uncoupling and for the increase in adenylate cyclase activity, remain to be filled in. But in isolated tissue systems, not to mention whole animals, the field is wide open: we still do not have compelling evidence for the existence of any process that could account for the effects of chronic opioids in these systems.

In this state of affairs, an attempt to propose a specific model of tolerance/dependence would be premature. Nevertheless, we believe that a general discussion of the kinds of models that might be proposed is a useful way to conclude this article, for it puts into perspective the data that have been obtained so far, as well as clarifies the directions that future research needs to take. Conventionally, theories of opioid tolerance/dependence have been grouped into two major classes, receptor models and homeostatic models (though in fact all theories of tolerance must invoke some kind of homeostatic process) (Goldstein, 1974). Several years ago, we suggested a third kind of theory, combining aspects of the first two, which we called the combined model (Smith and Loh, 1981). Below, we will briefly describe each model and its strengths and weaknesses (summarized in Table 1). For the sake of abbreviating a discussion that has in some part been presented before, we will confine it largely to the issue of tolerance.

TABLE 1
Models of Tolerance/Dependence

	Strong Points	Weak points
Receptor models	Account for lack of cross-tolerance between different types of opioid agonists Receptor changes observed in simple systems and in brain under certain conditions	No receptor changes of the required size and direction observed in brains of tolerant animals
Desensitization (affinity decrease)		Very large increases in tolerance difficult to explain
Down-regulation (population decrease)		Tolerance becomes infinite (i.e., point reached at which no amount of drug can achieve effect seen in naive system)
Up-regulation (population increase)		Receptor increase required is very high
		Up-regulation observed to date has been accompanied by increased sensitivity to morphine
Homeostatic models	Consistent with lack of receptor changes observed during tolerance	Tolerance cannot increase indefinitely
Combined models	Tolerance can increase continuously and indefinitely Can account for lack of observed changes in receptors during tolerance	No evidence of tolerance-associated increase in postulated endogenous opioid antagonist

5.1. Receptor Models

Receptor models, best exemplified by those proposed by the Goldsteins over 20 yr ago (Goldstein and Goldstein, 1961, 1968), postulate that tolerance results from changes in either the number or the affinity of opioid receptors. For example, if the number of receptors were reduced during chronic opioid administration, or if their affinity for opioid were reduced, then a greater amount of the opioid would be necessary to achieve the same effect. Tolerance could also conceivably result from an increase or up-regulation of opioid receptors, and, in fact, this was proposed in the Goldstein's original model. This could occur, for example, if the acute effect of opioids were to block some process normally mediated by unoccupied receptors. In this case, up-regulation would result in more unoccupied receptors, so that a higher dose of opioid would be necessary to reduce the number to the original level. Although it would be difficult to envision this process occurring with a receptor that exerted its effect through coupling to another molecule, such as adenylate cyclase, this scheme would work quite well if the opioid receptor were an enzyme.

Although receptor models can account for tolerance in an elegantly simple manner, they encounter major difficulties in explaining certain data. One problem, which was discussed in the previous section, is the lack of reproducible changes in opioid receptor number or affinity associated with tolerance. The exceptions to this, such as the work by Dingledine et al. (1983) and by Tao and Law (1984), have generally been observed under conditions that are not relevant to morphine-induced analgesia, though they may be relevant to other opioid effects. The inability of investigators to detect significant changes in opioid receptors during tolerance could be explained by the reversal of these changes during tissue isolation. Most receptor models, however, also have difficulty in explaining other data. For example, if we assume that there is a one-to-one relationship between receptor occupation and effect, the down-regulation model predicts a definite limit to tolerance development. When receptor number falls to below 50% of the original level, it will no longer be possible, no matter how high the dose is raised, to achieve an effect observed with an ED_{50} dose in the naive animal. Even worse, calculations show that under these conditions very little tolerance would be observed until down-regulation closely approached this level, at which point the degree of tolerance would rise sharply (Table 2). In other words, most of the tolerance increases observed in animals

TABLE 2
Degree of Tolerance as a Function of Receptor Number
in Down-Regulation Model

Number of receptors, arb. units	Required fractional occupancy	Degree of tolerance, relative ED_{50}
1.0	0.50	1.0
0.9	0.55	1.25
0.8	0.625	1.67
0.7	0.714	2.5
0.6	0.833	5.0
0.55	0.909	10.0
0.54	0.926	12.5
0.53	0.943	16.7
0.52	0.962	25.0
0.51	0.980	50.0

would have to result from very small decreases in receptor number, taking place at levels between 60 and 50% of the original number.

Of course the assumption that there is a one-to-one relationship between receptor occupation and effect may not be correct; however, it is not clear that any other assumption makes this model more attractive. For example, if spare receptors exist, so that only a tiny fraction of receptors must be occupied to have an effect, then extensive down-regulation would occur with little effect on tolerance at all. And as in the case with no spare receptors, the ED_{50} would rise sharply as a function of down-regulation as the number of remaining receptors approached the number needing to be occupied to produce the pharmacological effect.

In the case of tolerance mediated by receptor up-regulation, any original level of acute effect could theoretically be attained by a sufficiently high dose. In this case, however, there is a problem raised by the amount of increase in receptor number that would be necessary to account for tolerance. This model predicts that, for tolerance more than a fewfold, the degree of tolerance will increase at the same rate as the increase in receptor number (Table 3); that is, for every two-fold increase in tolerance, there must be a two-fold increase in receptor number. Since tolerance in animals and humans can raise the ED_{50} of opioids as much as 100- or even 1000-fold (Goldstein, 1974), this model of tolerance clearly requires enormous increases in receptor number.

In addition to this argument against the up-regulation model, there is another, provided by the very studies that have demon-

TABLE 3
Degree of Tolerance as a Function of Receptor Number
in Up-Regulation Model

Number of receptors, arb. units	Required fractional occupancy	Degree of tolerance, relative ED_{50}
1.0	0.5	1.0
2.0	0.75	3.0
3.0	0.83	5.0
5.0	0.9	9.0
10	0.95	19
20	0.975	39
50	0.99	99
100	0.995	199

strated up-regulation of opioid receptors in the brain (Zukin et al., 1984). This work has shown that the naloxone-induced increase in receptor number is accompanied by an increase, not a decrease, in morphine sensitivity. This result thus strongly suggests that, even if chronic opioid agonist treatment could induce receptor up-regulation (Holaday et al., 1985), this up-regulation could not be the basis of tolerance to the agonist.

Finally, there are tolerance models based on a decrease in affinity of the receptor for opioids, or desensitization. These appear to be the most plausible kind of receptor model, in that they can in theory account for very high levels of tolerance. Another point in their favor is that it is much easier to envision changes in receptor affinity, as opposed to changes in receptor number, being reversed during isolation of tissue from brain, which would explain why such changes are not observed in tolerant animals. Desensitization models do have some trouble explaining one aspect of tolerance, however. It is a commonplace observation that tolerance develops more or less continuously, as demonstrated by a linear or smooth curve plot of ED_{50} vs. time. It is highly unlikely, however, that a single binding site could change in such a way as to manifest a continuously decreasing affinity for ligand. Continuity might be explained by the development of a second binding state of much lower affinity, as in fact has been reported to occur during desensitization of NG108-15 cells (Law et al., 1985b). In this case, continuous changes in the *apparent* affinity for agonist could be manifested by a continuous change in the proportions of the two binding sites. However, to explain the large ED_{50} increases that can occur during tolerance, it would be necessary to postulate that this second site has a much lower affinity

TABLE 4
Degree of Tolerance as a Function of Proportions
of Two Receptors in Desensitization Model[a]

Fraction of receptors in high affinity state	Degree of tolerance, relative ED_{50}
1.0	1.0
0.9	1.25
0.8	1.65
0.7	2.5
0.6	5.0
0.5	30
0.4	200
0.3	400
0.2	600
0.1	800

[a]The model assumes a high-affinity site of K_d 1 nM, which gradually converts to a low-affinity site of K_d 1 μM during tolerance development.

than the first, say a K_d of at least 1 μM. Under these conditions, tolerance would develop much as in the down-regulation model, with a very slow increase as the high-affinity receptor initially converted to the low-affinity form, followed by a very steep rise as the latter form became more predominant (Table 4).

In summary, of the theories that account for opioid tolerance in terms of changes in opioid receptors, those based on desensitization appear to be the most attractive, although it is not yet clear that they can account for very high levels of tolerance development. It should also be emphasized that a more satisfactory theory could be formulated by combining or modifying these simple receptor models. For example, a model based on both down-regulation and desensitization might explain tolerance better than either of these latter models alone. Another factor that could make any of these models fit reality much better is the presence of multiple nervous pathways contributing to various aspects of tolerance, as one could imagine that different pathways might be activated at different concentrations of chronic opioid.

5.2. Homeostatic Models

Homeostatic models of tolerance explain this phenomenon by postulating the existence of a process subsequent to, or "downstream" from, the receptor, which opposes the process mediating analgesia. The original proposal by Sharma et al. (1977) that "tolerance" (decreased sensitivity to opioid-mediated adenylate cyclase inhibition) in NG cells results from a compensating increase in adenylate cyclase activity is an example of a homeostatic model of tolerance. For whole animal tolerance, examples of homeostatic models are theories that postulate that chronic opioid treatment results in increased levels of a nonopioid peptide that antagonizes analgesia (Yang et al., 1985a,b).

Homeostatic models are of course consistent with the substantial body of data that indicates changes in opioid receptors do not occur during tolerance. Like receptor models, however, they fail to provide an adequate explanation for certain characteristic features of tolerance. In this case, the problem is the almost limitless degree of tolerance that animals can develop under certain conditions. It is well known that tolerance to opioids can reach levels as high as 100-fold or even 1000-fold, based on the change in ED_{50} value for morphine (Goldstein, 1974). Furthermore, after a given level of tolerance has been developed and maintained, a further increase is possible by further increasing the dose (Williams and Oberst, 1946; Martin and Fraser, 1961). What this shows is that tolerance can continue to develop after doses have been reached that are sufficient to saturate all the opioid receptors present in the naive animal. Since any homeostatic process must be initiated by binding to these receptors, however, this is inconsistent with any theory of tolerance that does not postulate some kind of change in these receptors. If there is no change, then as soon as the receptors are saturated, the homeostatic process, whatever it is, should reach its peak. There could of course be some time lag, because of protein synthesis or some other relatively slow process. Kinetics of both the development and decline of tolerance demonstrate that this lag is at most a few days, however, and thus cannot account for changes that can develop over months. The fact that a tolerance plateau can be reached by maintaining a constant, chronic dose schedule also shows that the lag time is relatively short (Martin and Fraser, 1961).

Since this is a point that many investigators in opioid research seem not to appreciate, it is worth explaining in a little more detail, with the help of a specific example. As mentioned above, a popular current theory of opioid tolerance is that it is mediated by an increase in levels of an endogenous nonopioid (Yang et al., 1985a,b). Since these peptides are thought not to bind to opioid receptors, their antagonism of analgesia probably takes place at a step subsequent to receptor activation. For the sake of simplicity, we could assume that the peptide closes ion channels that opioids open (Williams and North, 1983). Administration of opioid agonist, then, initially results in opening of ion channels, which in turn produces analgesia. In the continued presence of opioid, however, levels of the nonopioid peptide gradually rise, resulting in reclosing of the channels. Consequently, a higher dose of opioid agonist is required to reopen the channels. This leads to a still higher level of the inhibiting nonopioid, and so forth.

The problem with this model of tolerance lies in the fact that the levels of nonopioid can only be raised by increased activation of opioid receptors. This is true regardless of how many steps intervene between this activation and the increase. If it were not true—if, for example, levels of the nonopioid could rise indefinitely in the presence of a saturating concentration of opioid— then it would not be possible to observe a plateau in tolerance development when a given dose is maintained. Therefore, as soon as these receptors are saturated—and this will effectively occur at a dose of opioid of about ten times the ED_{50} level in the naive animal—the nonopioid levels reach a plateau, and no further development of tolerance is possible.

As with receptor models it might be possible to rescue this simple homeostatic model by making it more complex. For example, if more than one nonopioid inhibitor were involved, and levels of these nonopioids were controlled by separate (but always opioid receptor-mediated) processes, then the range of possible tolerance development could be significantly increased. Nonopioid peptides could also play a role in tolerance development if they were able to interact directly or indirectly with the opioid receptor, as some recent evidence suggests may be the case (Zhu and Raffa, 1986). In this case, however, tolerance is no longer being mediated by a purely homeostatic process, but rather by a combined process which we shall now discuss.

5.3. Combined Models

Because of the problems both receptor and homeostatic models have in fully explaining opioid tolerance, we proposed several years ago a different kind of model that combines features of both (Smith and Loh, 1981). In this model, chronic opioid treatment results in the synthesis of a molecule that combines reversibly with the opioid receptor, preventing its binding agonist. Consequently, a higher concentration of the latter is required to achieve a given degree of binding and of pharmacological effect. Because this model incorporates features of both the traditional kinds of models, it can explain all the data that they were designed to explain. At the same time, however, it avoids the difficulties inherent in the traditional models. For example, this model is like receptor models in that it postulates changes in opioid receptors during tolerance. Thus unlike homeostatic models, it has no difficulty accounting for the very high levels of tolerance that animals can develop. The combined model differs from receptor models, however, in that these changes are not physical or *intrinsic* to the receptor, but *extrinsic*, arising from competition of agonist with another molecule. Thus this model is consistent with the lack of receptor changes that have been observed in most studies of tolerant animals, since it is necessary only to assume that the process of isolating brain membranes would remove any inhibitory factors. Furthermore, this model accounts much better than receptor models for the continuity of tolerance development and the high levels that it can attain. Both of these conditions can be satisfied by a continuous synthesis of the inhibitory molecule.

When we first presented this model of tolerance, we proposed that the inhibitory molecule was a protein subunit similar to one of the subunits of the opioid receptor; by displacing the latter subunit, it would prevent agonist binding (Smith and Loh, 1981). Subsequent work, however, has brought to the fore a much more obvious candidate and a much simpler and more plausible process: competition by an endogenous opioid peptide. Endogenous opioids are of course present in regions of the brain that have opioid receptors (Kuhar and Uhl, 1979; Rossier and Bloom, 1979), and thus any process that increased either their levels or their accessibility to these receptors could easily account for tolerance. Their action could either be competitive, directly competing with agonist for the binding site like a classical antagonist, or noncompetitive, interacting with another site on the receptor to alter the affinity of the latter for agonist.

Recent work has made it clear that there are several endogenous opioids in the brain that can antagonize morphine-induced analgesia, and that therefore could be considered candidates for playing a role in tolerance development. These include met-enkephalin (Vaught and Takemori, 1979), dynorphin (Friedman et al., 1981; Tulunay, et al., 1981), and several β-endorphin fragments (Hammonds et al., 1984). Of these, the β-endorphin fragments may be of particular interest, since they are derived from a molecule with agonist activity, making possible a simple process of regulating agonist/antagonist ratio. To date, however, changes in the brain content of these or other endogenous opioids have not been observed to occur during tolerance, although changes in the messenger RNA for the β-endorphin precursor proopiomelanocortin have been reported (Morchetti et al., 1985).

There are also several nonopioid peptides in the brain that modulate opioid analgesia, though it is not yet clear that any of them satisfy the requirement of binding to opioid receptors. These include adrenocorticotropic hormone (Smock and Fields, 1981), melanocyte inhibitory factor (Kastin et al., 1979), cholecystokinin (Faris et al., 1983), and α-melanocorticotropin (Contreras and Takemori, 1984). Perhaps the leading candidates, however, are several peptides possessing the Phe-Met-Arg-Phe-NH$_2$ (FMRF-NH$_2$) terminus. In addition to inhibiting morphine-induced analgesia (Yang et al., 1985a), they appear to be concentrated in brain and spinal cord regions associated with analgesia (Majane and Yang, 1986), and antibodies to them inhibit tolerance development (Yang et al., 1985b). Also encouraging is recent evidence that FMRF-NH$_2$ can bind to low-affinity opioid receptors (Zhu and Raffa, 1986).

In conclusion, although there is currently no direct evidence to support any particular theory of opioid tolerance/dependence, certain kinds of theories are better able to account for this phenomenon than others. These include theories that postulate changes in opioid receptor affinity (desensitization) and those that envision the increased action of an endogenous opioid antagonist. And although it is unlikely that any one of these simple models can account entirely for such a complex phenomenon, as it is manifested in the whole animal, it appears that receptor changes play a key role in the process, changes that are gradually becoming open to direct testing.

References

Abood, M. E., Law, P. Y., and Loh, H. H. (1985) Pertussis toxin treatment modifies opiate action in the rat brain striatum. *Biochem. Biophys. Res. Comm.* **127,** 477–483.

Andrade, R., Vandermaelen, C., and Aghajanian, G. (1983) Morphine tolerance and dependence in the locus coeruleus: single cell studies in brain slices. *Eur. J. Pharmacol.* **91,** 161–169.

Baram, D. and Simantov, R. (1983) Enkephalins and opiate agonists control calmodulin distribution in neuroblastoma-glioma cells. *J. Neurochem.* **40,** 55–63.

Basbaum, A. I. and Fields, H. L. (1984) Endogenous pain control systems:

Brainstem spinal pathways and endorphin circuitry. *Ann. Rev. Neurosci.* **7**, 309–338.

Blanchard, S. G., Chang, K.-J., and Cuatrecasas, P. (1983) Characterization of the association of tritiated enkephalin with neuroblastoma cells under conditions optimal for receptor down-regulation. *J. Biol. Chem.* **258**, 1092–1097.

Blume, A. J. (1978) Interaction of ligands with the opiate receptors of brain membranes: Regulation by ions and nucleotides. *Proc. Natl. Acad. Sci. USA* **75**, 1713–1717.

Brase, D. E. (1979) Roles of serotonin and gamma-aminobutyric acid in opioid effect. *Adv. Biochem. Psychopharmacol.* **20**, 409–428.

Brostrom, M. A., Brostrom, C. O., Breckenridge, B. M., and Wolff, D. L. (1978) Calcium-dependent regulation of brain adenylate cyclase. *Adv. Cyclic Nucleotide Res.* **9**, 85–99.

Brown, M. S., Anderson, R. G. W., and Goldstein, J. L. (1983) Recycling receptors: The round-trip itinerary of migrant membrane proteins. *Cell* **32**, 663–667.

Chaillet, P., Coulaud, A., Fournie-Zaluski, M. C., Gacel, G., Roques, B. P., and Costentin, J. (1983) Pain control by endogenous enkephalins is mediated by mu opioid receptors. *Life Sci.* **33**, (Suppl. I), 685–688.

Chaillet, P., Coulaud, A., Zajac, J.-M., Fournie-Zaluski, M. C., Costentin, J., and Roques, B. P. (1984) The mu rather than the delta subtype of opioid receptors appears to be involved in enkephalin-induced analgesia. *Eur. J. Pharmacol.* **101**, 83–90.

Chang, K.-J. (1984) Opioid receptors: Multiplicity and sequelae of ligand-receptor interactions, in *The Receptors* vol. I, Academic, New York.

Chang, K.-J. and Cuatrecasas, P. (1979) Multiple opiate receptors: Enkephalins and morphine bind to receptors of different specificity. *J. Biol. Chem.* **254**, 2610–2618.

Chang, K. J., Eckel, R. W., and Blanchard, S. G. (1982) Opioid peptides induce reduction of enkephalin receptors in cultured neuroblastoma cells. *Nature* **296**, 446–448.

Chapman, D. B. and Way, E. L. (1980) Metal ion interactions with opiates. *Ann. Rev. Pharmacol. Toxicol.* **20**, 553–579.

Cheung, W. Y. (1981) Discovery and recognition of calmodulin: A personal account. *J. Cyclic Nucleotide Res.* **7**, 71–84.

Clouet, D. H. and Yonehara, N. (1984) Biochemical Reactions Between Opiate Receptor Binding and Inhibition of Neurotransmission, in *Mechanisms of Tolerance and Dependence* (C.W. Sharp, ed.) NIDA Research Monograph 54, US Government Printing Office, Washington DC.

Collier, H. O. J. and Tucker, J. F. (1984) Sites and Mechanisms of Dependence in the Myenteric Plexus of the Guinea Pig Ileum, in *Mechanisms of Tolerance and Dependence* (C. W. Sharp, ed.) NIDA Research Monograph 54, US Government Printing Office, Washington, DC, pp. 81–94.

Contreras, P. C. and Takemori, A. E. (1984) Antagonism of morphine-induced analgesia, tolerance and dependence by alpha-melanocyte-stimulating hormone. *J. Pharmacol. Exp. Ther.* **229**, 21–26.

Cooper, D. M. F., Londos, C., Gill, D. L., and Rodbell, M. (1982) Opiate receptor-mediated inhibition of adenylate cyclase in rat striatal plasma membranes. *J. Neurochem.* **38**, 1164–1167.

Crain, S. M. (1984) Spinal cord tissue culture models for analyses of opioid analgesia, tolerance and plasticity. In *Mechanisms of Tolerance and Dependence* (Sharp, C. W., ed.) NIDA Research Monograph 54, US Government Printing Office, Washington, DC, pp. 260–292.

Crain, S. M., Crain, B., Peterson, E. R., and Simon, E. J. (1978) Selective depression by opioid peptides of sensory-evoked dorsal horn network responses in organized spinal cord cultures. *Brain Res.* **157,** 196–201.

Crain, S. M., Crain, B., Peterson, E. R., Hiller, J. M., and Simon, E. J. (1982a) Exposure to 4-aminopyridine prevents depressant effects of opiates on sensory-evoked dorsal horn network responses in spinal cord cultures. *Life Sci.* **31,** 235–240.

Crain, S. M., Crain, B., and Peterson, E. R. (1982b) Development of cross-tolerance to 5-hydroxytryptamine in organotypic cultures of mouse spinal cord-ganglia during chronic exposure to morphine. *Life Sci.* **51,** 241–247.

Creese, I. and Sibley, D. R. (1981) Receptor adaptations to centrally acting drugs. *Ann. Rev. Pharmacol. Toxicol.* **21,** 357–391.

Creese, I., Burt, D., and Snyder, S. (1977) Dopamine receptor binding enhancement accompanies lesion-induced behavioral super-sensitivity *Science* **197,** 596–598.

Davis, N. E., Akera, T., and Brody, T. M. (1979) Reduction of opiate binding to brainstem slices associated with the development of tolerance to morphine in rats. *J. Pharmacol. Exp. Ther.* **211,** 112–119.

Dingledine, R., Valentino, R. J., Bostock, E., King, M. E., and Chang, K.-J. (1983) Down-regulation of delta but not mu opioid receptors in the hippocampal slice associated with loss of physiological response. *Life Sci.* **33** (suppl. I), 333–336.

Domino, E. F. (1979) Opiate interactions with cholinergic neurons. *Adv. Biochem. Psychopharmacol.* **20,** 339–355.

Duggan, A. W., Hall, J. G., and Headley, P. M. (1977) Suppression of transmission of nociceptive impulses by morphine: Selective effects of morphine administered in the region of the substantia gelatinosa. *Br. J. Pharmacol.* **61,** 65–76.

Faris, P. L., Komisaruk, B. R., Watkins, L. R., and Mayer, D. L. (1983) Evidence for the neuropeptide cholecystokinin as an antagonist of opiate analgesia. *Science* **219,** 310–312.

Frederickson, R. C. D., Norris, F. H., and Hewes, C. R. (1975) Effects of naloxone and acetylcholine on medial thalamic and cortical units in naive and morphine-dependent rats. *Life Sci.* **17,** 81–82.

French, E. and Zieglgansberger, W. (1982) The excitatory response of *in vitro* hippocampal pyramidal cells to normorphine and methionine-enkephalin may be mediated by different receptor populations. *Exp. Brain Res.* **48,** 238–244.

Friedman, H. J., Jen, M. F., Chang, J. K., Lee, N. M., and Loh, H. H. (1981) Dynorphin: A possible modulatory peptide on morphine or beta-endorphin analgesia in mouse. *Eur. J. Pharmacol.* **69,** 351–360.

Fry, J. P., Herz, A., and Zieglgansberger, W. (1980) A demonstration of naloxone-precipitated withdrawal on single neurons in the morphine-tolerant/dependent rat brain. *Br. J. Pharmacol.* **68,** 585–592.

Gardner, E. L., Zukin, R. S., and Makman, M. (1980) Modulation of opiate receptor binding in striatum and amygdala by selective mesencephalic lesions. *Brain Res.* **194,** 233–239.

Gillan, M. G. C., Kosterlitz, H. W., Robson, L. E., and Waterfield, A. A. (1979) The inhibitory effects of presynaptic alpha-adrenoceptor agonists on contractions of guinea pig ileum and mouse vas deferens in the morphine-dependent and withdrawn states produced *in vitro. Br. J. Pharmacol.* **66,** 601–608.

Gilman, A. G. (1984) Guanine nucleotide-binding regulatory proteins and dual control of adenylate cyclase. *J. Clin. Invest.* **73,** 1–4.

Goldstein, A. (1974) Drug tolerance and physical dependence, in *Principles of Drug Action* (A. Goldstein, L. Aronow, and S. M. Kalman, eds.) Harper & Row, New York.

Goldstein, D. B. and Goldstein, A. (1961) Possible role of enzyme inhibition and repression in drug tolerance and addiction. *Biochem. Pharmacol.* **8,** 48.

Goldstein, A. and Goldstein, D. B. (1968) Enzyme expansion theory of drug tolerance and physical dependence. *Res. Publ. Assoc. Ment. Dis.* **46,** 265–267.

Goldstein, A. and Schulz, R. (1973) Morphine tolerant longitudinal muscle strip from guinea pig ileum. *Br. J.Pharmacol.* **48,** 655–666.

Goldstein, J. L., Anderson, R. G. W., and Brown, M. S. (1979) Coated pits, coated vesicles and receptor-mediated endocytosis. *Nature* **279,** 679–685.

Gomperts, B. D. (1983) Involvement of guanine nucleotide binding proteins in the gating of calcium by receptors. *Nature* **306,** 64.

Griffin, M. T., Law, P. Y., and Loh, H. H. (1983) Modulation of adenylate cyclase activity by a cytosolic factor following chronic opiate exposure in neuroblastoma × glioma NG108-15 hybrid cells. *Life Sci.* **33,** 365–369.

Griffin, M. T., Law, P. Y., and Loh, H. H. (1985a) Neuroblastoma × glioma hybrid cells cultured in a serum-free chemically defined medium: Effects on acute and chronic opiate regulation of adenylate cyclase activity. *Brain Res.* **360,** 370–373.

Griffin, M. T., Law, P.-Y., and Loh, H. H. (1985b) Involvement of both inhibitory and stimulatory guanine nucleotide binding proteins in the expression of chronic opiate regulation of adenylate cyclase activity in NG108-15 cells. *J. Neurochem.* **45,** 1585–1589.

Griffin, M. T., Law, P. Y., and Loh, H. H. (1986) Effects of phospholipases on chronic opiate action in neuroblastoma × glioma NG108-15 hybrid cells. *J. Neurochem.* **47,** 1098–1105.

Hammond, M. D., Schneider, C., and Collier, H. O. J. (1976) Induction of Opiate Tolerance in Guinea Pig Ileum and Its Modification by Drugs. in *Opiates and Endogenous Opioid Peptides* (H. W. Kosterlitz, ed.) Amsterdam, Elsevier/North Holland.

Hammonds, R. G., Nicolas, P., Jr., and Li, C. H. (1984) Beta-endorphin-(1-27) is an antagonist of beta-endorphin analgesia. *Proc. Natl. Acad. Sci, USA* **81,** 1389–1390.

Harris, J. and Kazmierowski, D. T. (1975) Morphine Tolerance and Naloxone Receptor Binding. *Life Sci.* **16,** 1831–1836.

Hazum, E., Chang, K.-J., and Cuatrecasas, P. (1979) Opiate (enkephalin) receptors of neuroblastoma cells: Occurrence in clusters on the cell surface. *Science* **206**, 1077–1079.

Henderson, G., Hughes, J., and Kosterlitz, H. W. (1978) *In vitro* release of Leu- and Met-enkephalin from the corpus striatum. *Nature* **271**, 677–679.

Hitzemann, R. J., Hitzemann, B. A., and Loh, H. H. (1974) Binding of [^{3}H] naloxone in the mouse brain: Effect of ions and tolerance development. *Life Sci.* **14**, 2393–2404.

Holaday, J. W., Rothman, R. B., Danks, J. A., Hitzemann, R. J., and Tortella, F. C. (1985) Repeated electroconvulsive shock and chronic morphine: Upregulation of opioid receptors. *Abstr. Ann. Meet. Am. Coll. of Neuropsychopharmacol.* 74.

Hollt, V., Dum, J., Blasig, J., Schubert, P., and Herz, A. (1975) Comparison of *in vivo* and *in vitro* parameters of opiate receptor binding in naive and tolerant/dependent rats. *Life Sci.* **16**, 1823–1828.

Illes, P. and Thesleff, S. (1978) 4-Aminopyridine and evoked transmitter release from motor nerve endings. *Br. J. Pharmacol.* **64**, 623–629.

Iwamoto, E. T. and Martin, W. R. (1981) Multiple opioid receptors. *Medicinal Res. Rev.* **1**, 411–440.

Iwamato, E. T. and Way, E. L. (1979) Opiate actions and catecholamines. *Adv. Biochem. Psychopharmacol.* **20**, 357–407.

Kastin, A. J., Olson, R. D., Ehrensing, R. H., Beizas, M. C., Schally, A. V., and Coy, D. H. (1979) MIF's differential actions as an opiate antagonist. *Phamacol. Biochem. Behav.* **11**, 721–723.

Klee, W. A. and Streaty, R. A. (1974) Narcotic receptor sites in morphine-dependent rats. *Nature* **248**, 61–63.

Klein, W. L., Nathanson, N. M., and Nirenberg, M. (1979) Muscarinic acetylcholine receptor regulated by accelerated rate of receptor loss. *Biochem. Biophys. Res. Comm.* **90**, 506–512.

Koski, G. and Klee, W. A. (1981) Opiates inhibit adenylate cyclase by stimulating GTP hydrolysis. *Proc. Natl. Acad. Sci. USA* **78**, 4185–4189.

Koski, G., Streaty, R.A., and Klee, W. A. (1982) Modulation of sodium-sensitive GTPase by partial opiate agonist: An explanation for the dual requirement for Na$^+$ and GTP in inhibitory regulation of adenylate cyclase. *J. Biol. Chem.* **257**, 14035–14040.

Kuhar, M. J. and Uhl, G. R. (1979) Histochemical localization of opiate receptors and the enkephalins. *Adv. Biochem. Psychopharmacol.* **20**, 53–68.

Lambert, S. M. and Childers, S. R. (1984) Modification of guanine nucleotide-regulatory components in brain membranes. I. Changes in guanosine 5'-triphosphate regulation of opiate receptor binding sites. *J. Neurosci.* **4**, 2755–2763.

Lamotte, C., Pert, C. B., and Snyder, S. H. (1976) Opiate receptor binding in primate spinal cord: Distribution and changes after dorsal root section. *Brain Res.* **112**, 407–412.

Landahl, H. D., Garzon, J., and Lee, N. M. (1985) Mathematical modeling of opiate binding to mouse brain membrane. *Bull. Math. Biol.* **47**, 503–512.

Law, P. Y., Wu, J., Koehler, J. E., and Loh, H. H. (1981) Demonstration and characterization of opiate inhibition of the striatal adenylate cyclase. *J. Neurochem.* **36**, 1834–1846.

Law, P. Y., Koehler, J. E., and Loh, H. H. (1982) Comparison of opiate inhibition of adenylate cyclase activity in neuroblastoma N18TG2 and neuroblastoma × glioma NG108-15 hybrid cell lines. *Mol. Pharmacol.* **21**, 483–491.

Law, P. Y., Hom, D.S., and Loh, H. H. (1983a) Opiate regulation of adenosine 3'5'-cyclic monophosphate level in neuroblastoma × glioma NG108-15 hybrid cells. *Mol. Pharmacol.* **23**, 26–35.

Law, P. Y., Hom, D. S., and Loh, H. H. (1983b) Opiate receptor down-regulation and desensitization in neuroblastoma × glioma NG108-15 hybrid cells are two separate cellular adaption processes. *Mol. Pharmacol.* **25**, 413–424.

Law, P. Y., Hom, D.S., and Loh, H. H. (1984a) Down-regulation of opiate receptor in neuroblastoma × glioma NG108-15 hybrid cells: Chloroquine promotes accumulation of tritiated enkephalin in the lysosomes. *J. Biol. Chem.* **259**, 4096–4104.

Law, P. Y., Griffin, M. T., and Loh, H. H. (1984b) Mechanisms of multiple cellular adaptation processes in clonal cell lines during chronic opiate treatment, in *Mechanisms of Tolerance and Dependence* (Sharp, C. W., ed.) NIDA Research Monograph 54, US Government Printing Office, Washington, DC, pp. 119–135.

Law, P. Y., Ungar, H. G., Hom, D. S., and Law, P. Y. (1985a) Effect of cycloheximide and tunicamycin on opiate receptor activities in neuroblastoma × glioma NG108-15 hybrid cells. *Biochem. Pharmacol.* **34**, 9–17.

Law, P. Y., Hom, D. S., and Loh, H. H. (1985b) Multiple affinity states of opiate receptor in neuroblastoma × glioma NG108-15 hybrid cells. *J. Biol. Chem.* **260**, 3561–3569.

Law, P. Y., Louie, A. K., and Loh, H. H. (1985c) Effect of pertussis toxin treatment on down-regulation of opiate receptors in neuroblastoma × glioma NG108-15 hybrid cells. *J. Biol. Chem.* **260**, 14818–14823.

Lee, N. M. and Smith, A. P. (1980) A protein-lipid model of the opiate receptor. *Life Sci.* **26**, 459–464.

Lee, N. M. and Smith, A. P. (1984) Possible regulatory function of dynorphin and its clinical implications. *Trends Pharmacol. Sci.* **5**, 108–110.

Lefkowitz, R. J., Wessels, M. R., and Stadel, J. M. (1980) Hormones, receptors and cyclic AMP; their roles in target cell refractoriness. *Curr. Top. Cell. Regul.* **17**, 205–230.

Lord, J. A. H., Waterfield, A. A., Hughes, J., and Kosterlitz, H. W. (1977) Endogenous opioid peptides: Multiple agonists and receptors. *Nature* **267**, 495–499.

Louie, A. K., Law, P. Y., and Loh, H. H. (1986) Cell free desensitization of opiate inhibition of adenylate cyclase in neuroblastoma × glioma NG108-15 hybrid cell membranes. *J. Neurochem.* **47**, 733–737.

Lux, B. and Schulz, R. (1985) Opioid dependence prevents the action of pertussis toxin in the guinea pig myenteric plexus. *Naunyn Schmiedebergs Arch. Pharmacol.* **330**, 184–186.

Majane, E. A. and Yang, H.-Y. T. (1986) Distribution and characterization of two non-opioid peptides with morphine modulating activity in the brain. *Fed. Proc.* **45**, 1052.

Manning, D. R. and Gilman, A. G. (1983) The regulatory components of adenylate cyclase and transducin: A family of structurally homologous guanine nucleotide-binding proteins. *J. Biol. Chem.* **258**, 7059–7063.

Martin, W. R. and Fraser, H. F. (1961) A comparative study of physiological and subjective effects of heroin and morphine administered intravenously in postaddicts. *J. Pharmacol. Exp. Ther.* **133**, 388–399.

Morchetti, I., Giorgi, O., Schwartz, J. P., and Costa, E. (1985) Regulation of hypothalamic proopiomelanocortin system by morphine treatment. *Trans. Soc. Neurochem.* **16**, 253.

Mudge, A. W., Leeman, S. E., and Fischbach, G. D. (1979) Enkephalin inhibits release of substance P from sensory neurons in culture and decreases action potential duration. *Proc. Natl. Acad. Sci. USA* **76**, 526–530.

Murayama, T. and Ui, M. (1983) Loss of the inhibitory function of the guanine nucleotide regulatory components of adenylate cyclase due to its ADP ribosylation by islet-activating protein pertussis toxin in adipocyte membranes. *J. Biol. Chem.* **258**, 3319–3326.

Nicoll, R. A., Siggins, G. R., Ling, N., Bloom, F., and Guillemin, R. (1977) Neuronal actions of endorphins and enkephalins among brain regions: A comparative microiontophoretic study. *Proc. Natl. Acad. Sci. USA* **74**, 2584–2588.

North, R. A. and Vitek, L. (1979) The effect of chronic morphine treatment on excitatory junction potentials in the mouse vas deferens. *Br. J. Pharmacol.* **68**, 399–406.

North, R. and Williams, J. T. (1983) Opiate activation of potassium conductance inhibitory calcium action potentials in rat locus coeruleus neurons. *Br. J. Pharmacol.* **80**, 225–228.

Pert, C. B. and Snyder, S. H. (1973) Opiate receptor: Its demonstration in nervous tissue. *Science* **179**, 1011–1014.

Pert, C. B. and Snyder, S. H. (1976) Opiate receptor binding enhancement by opiate administration *in vivo. Biochem. Pharmacol.* **25**, 847–853.

Pfeiffer, A. and Herz, A. (1981) Demonstration and distribution of an opiate binding site in rat brain with high affinity for ethylketocyclazocine and SKF 10047. *Biochem. Biophys. Res. Comm.* **101**, 38–44.

Rodbell, M. (1980) The role of hormone receptors and GTP regulatory proteins in membrane transduction. *Nature* **284**, 17–22.

Rosen, O. M., Chia, G. H., Fung, C., and Rubin, C. S. (1979) Tunicamycin-mediated depletion of insulin receptors in 3T3-L1 adipocytes. *J. Cell Physiol.* **99**, 37–42.

Ross, D. H. and Cardenas, H. L. (1979) Nerve cell calcium as a messenger for opiate and endorphin actions. *Adv. Biochem. Psychopharmacol.* **20**, 301–336.

Rossier, J. and Bloom, F. (1979) Central neuropharmacology of endorphins. *Adv. Biochem. Psychopharmacol.* **20**, 165–185.

Rothman, R. B. and Westfall, T. C. (1982) Allosteric coupling between morphine and enkephalin receptors *in vitro. Mol. Pharmacol.* **21**, 548–557.

Rubini, P., Schulz, R., Wuster, M., and Herz, A. (1982) Opiate receptor binding studies in the mouse vas deferens exhibiting tolerance without dependence. *Naunyn Schmiedebergs Arch. Pharmacol.* **319**, 142–146.

Satoh, M., Zieglgansberger, W., and Herz, A. (1975) Interaction between morphine and putative excitatory neurotransmitters in cortical neurons in naive and tolerant rats. *Life Sci.* **17**, 75–80.

Satoh, M., Zieglgansberger, W., and Herz, A. (1976) Actions of opiates upon single unit activity in the cortex of naive and tolerant rats. *Brain Res.* **115**, 99–110.

Schulz, R. and Herz, A. (1984) Opioid Tolerance and Dependence in Light of the Multiplicity of Opioid Receptors. In *Mechanisms of Tolerance and Dependence* (Sharp, C. W., ed.) NIDA Research Monograph 54, U.S. Government Printing Office, Washington, DC., pp. 70–80.

Schulz, R., Wuster, M., and Herz, A. (1979) Supersensitivity to opioids following chronic blockade of endorphin activity by nalaxone. *Naunyn Schmiedebergs Arch. Pharmacol.* **306**, 93–96.

Schulz, R., Wuster, M., Krenss, H., and Herz, A. (1980) Lack of cross-tolerance on multiple opiate receptors in the mouse vas deferens. *Mol. Pharmacol.* **18**, 395–401.

Schulz, R., Wuster, M., and Herz, A. (1981) Differentiation of opiate receptors in the brain by the selective development of tolerance. *Pharmacol. Biochem. Behav.* **14**, 75–79.

Schulz, R., Seidl, E., Wuster, M., and Herz, A. (1982) Opioid dependence and cross-dependence in the isolated guinea pig ileum. *Eur. J. Pharmacol.* **84**, 33–40.

Sharma, S., Nirenberg, M., and Klee, W. (1975a) Morphine receptors are regulators of adenylate cylcase activity. *Proc. Natl. Acad. Sci. USA* **72**, 590–594.

Sharma, S. K., Klee, W. A., and Nirenberg, M. (1975b) Dual regulation of adenylate cyclase accounts for narcotic dependence and tolerance. *Proc. Natl. Acad. Sci. USA* **72**, 3092–3096.

Sharma, S. K., Klee, W. A., and Nirenberg, M. (1977) Opiate-Dependent modulation of adenylate cyclase. *Proc. Natl. Acad. Sci. USA* **74**, 3365–3369.

Sibley, D. R., Strasser, R. H., Caron, M. G., and Lefkowitz, R. J. (1985) Homologous desensitization of adenylate cyclase is associated with phosphorylation of the beta-adrenergic receptor. *J. Biol. Chem.* **260**, 3883–3886.

Simon, E. J., Hiller, J. M., and Edelman, J. (1973) Stereospecific binding of the potent narcotic analgesic [³H] etorphine to rat brain homogenate. *Proc. Natl. Acad. Sci. USA* **70**, 1947–1949.

Simantov, R. and Amir, S. (1983) Regulation of opiate receptors in mouse brain: Arcuate nuclear lesion induces receptor up-regulation and supersensitivity to opiates. *Brain Res.* **262**, 168–171.

Smith, A. P. and Loh, H. H. (1981) The Opiate Receptor, in *Hormonal Proteins and Peptides* vol. 10 (C. H. Li, ed.) Academic, New York.

Smock, T. and Fields, H. L. (1981) ACTH (1-24) antagonizes opiate induced analgesia in the rat. *Brain Res.* **212**, 202–206.

Sternweis, P. C. and Robishaw, J. D. (1984) Isolation of two proteins with high affinity for guanine nucleotides from membranes of bovine brain. *J. Biol. Chem.* **259,** 13806–13813.

Su, Y. F., Harden, T. K., and Perkins, J. P. (1980) Cathecholamine-specific desensitization of adenylate cyclase: Evidence for a multi-step process. *J. Biol. Chem.* **255,** 7410–7419.

Tang, A. and Collins, R. (1978) Enhanced analgesic effects of morphine after chronic administration of naloxone in the rat. *Eur. J. Pharmacol.* **47,** 473–474.

Tao, P. L. and Law, P. Y. (1984) Down-regulation of opiate receptor in rat brain after chronic etorphine treatment. *Proc. West. Pharmacol. Soc.* **127,** 557–560.

Tempel, A., Crain, S. M., Simon, E. J., and Zukin, R. S. (1983) Opiate receptor upregulation in explants of spinal cord-dorsal root ganglia. *Soc. Neurosci. Abst.* **9,** 327.

Tempel, A., Gardner, E. L., and Zukin, R. S. (1985) Neurochemical and functional correlates of naltrexone-induced opiate receptor upregulation. *J. Pharmacol. Exp. Ther.* **232,** 439–444.

Terenius, L. (1973) Stereospecific interaction between narcotic analgesics and synaptic plasma membrane fraction of rat cerebral cortex. *Act Pharmacol. Toxicol.* **32,** 317–320.

Tulunay, F. C., Jen, M. F., Chang, J. K., Loh, H. H., and Lee, N. M. (1981) Possible regulatory role of dynorphin on morphine- and endorphin-dependent analgesia. *J. Pharmacol. Exp. Ther.* **219,** 296–298.

Tung, A. S. and Yaksh, T. L. (1982) In vivo evidence for multiple opiate receptors mediating analgesia in the rat spinal cord. *Brain Res.* **247,** 75–83.

Vaught, J. L. and Takemori, A. E. (1979) Differential effects of leucine and methionine enkephalin on morphine-induced analgesia, acute tolerance and dependence. *J. Pharmacol. Exp. Ther.* **208,** 86–90.

Von Voightlander, P. F. and Lewis, R. A. (1982) U50,488, a selective kappa opioid agonist: Comparison to other reported kappa agonists. *Prog. Neuropsychopharmacol. Biol. Psychiatry* **6,** 467–470.

Ward, S. J. and Takemori, A. E. (1983) Relative involvement of mu, kappa, and delta receptor mechanisms in opiate-mediated antinociception. I. Mu and delta receptor profiles in the primate. *J. Pharmacol. Exp. Ther.* **224,** 525–530.

Wilkening, D. and Nirenberg, M. (1980) Lipid requirement for long-lived morphine-dependent activations of adenylate cyclase of neuroblastoma × glioma hybrid cells. *J. Neurochem.* **34,** 321–326.

Williams, E. G. and Oberst, F. W. (1946) A cycle of morphine addiction, biological and psychological studies. I. Biological studies. *Public Health Rep.* **61,** 1–20.

Williams, J. and North, R. A. (1983) tolerance to opiates in locus coeruleus actions? *Abst. Int. Narc. Res. Conf.* **16,** 49.

Williams, J. T. and Zieglgansberger, W. (1981) Neurons in the frontal cortex of the rat carry multiple opiate receptors. *Brain Res.* **226,** 304–308.

Williams, J. T., Egan, T. M., and North, D. (1982) Enkephalin opens potassium channel on mammalian central neurons. *Nature* **229,** 74–77.

Wood, P. L. (1982) Multiple opiate receptors: Support for unique mu, delta, and kappa sites. *Neuropharmacology* **21,** 487–497.

Wuster, M., Rubini, P., and Schulz, R. (1981) The preference of putative pro-enkephalins for different types of opiate receptors. *Life Sci.* **29,** 1219–1227.

Wuster, M., Schulz, R., and Herz, A. (1985) Opioid tolerance and dependence: Re-evaluating the unitary hypothesis. *Trends Pharmacol. Sci.* **6,** 64–67.

Yaksh, T. L. (1983) *In vivo* studies on spinal opiate receptor systems mediating antinociception. I. Mu and delta receptor profiles in the primate. *J. Pharmacol. Exp. Ther.* **226,** 303–316.

Yang, H.-Y., Tang, J., and Costa, E. (1985a) Role of endogenous non-opioid peptides which may modulate opiate analgesia. *Abstr. Ann. Meet. Coll. Neurophsycopharm.* 105.

Yang, H.-Y. T., Fratta, W., Majane, E. A., and Costa, E. (1985b) Isolation, sequencing, synthesis and pharmacological characterization of two brain neuropeptides that modulate the action of morphine. *Proc. Natl. Acad. Sci. USA* **82,** 7757–7761.

Yeung, J. C. and Rudy, T. A. (1980) Sites of antinociceptive action of systemically injected morphine: Involvement of supraspinal loci as revealed by intracerebroventricular injection of naloxone. *J. Pharmacol. Exp. Ther.* **215,** 626–632.

Young, E., Olney, J., and Akil, H. (1982) Increase in delta, but not mu receptors in MSG-treated rats. *Life Sci.* **31,** 1343–1346.

Zieglgansberger, W., Satoh, M., and Bayerl, J. (1975) Actions of microelectrophoretically applied opiates on cortical and spinal neurons. *Naunyn Schmiedebergs Arch. Exp. Path. Pharmacol.* **287** (suppl.), RR16.

Zieglgansberger, W., Fry, J. P., Herz, A., Moroder, L., and Wunsch, E. (1976) Enkephalin-induced inhibition of cortical neurons and the lack of this effect in morphine tolerant/dependent rats. *Brain Res.* **115,** 160–164.

Zhu, X. Z. and Raffa, R. B. (1986) FMRFamide: Low affinity inhibition of opioid binding to rabbit brain membranes. *Fed. Proc.* **45,** 797.

Zukin, R. S. and Zukin, S. R. (1981) Demonstration of [^{3}H] cyclazocine binding to multiple opiate receptor sites. *Mol. Pharmacol.* **20,** 246–254.

Zukin, R. S., Sugarman, J. R., Fitz-Syage, M. L., Gardner, E. L., Zukin, S. R., and Gintzler, A. R. (1982) Naltrexone-induced opiate receptor supersensitivity. *Brain Res.* **245,** 285–292.

Zukin, R. S., Tempel, A., and Gardner, E. L. (1984) Opiate Receptor Upregulation and Functional Supersensitivity, in *Mechanisms of Tolerance and Dependence* (Sharp, C. W., ed.) NIDA Research Monograph 54, U.S. Government Printing Office, Washington, DC, pp. 146–161.

SECTION 7
FUTURE
VISTAS

Chapter 14

Opiate and Opioid Peptide Receptors:
The Past, the Present, and the Future

Gavril W. Pasternak

1. The Classical Era

The study of opiate action is one of the oldest areas of pharmacological research. Although many scientists consider 1973 the breakthrough year, with the description of opiate binding sites in brain, this discovery was only one in a long progression of studies. Classical approaches provided essential insights into opiate action and, in most cases, molecular studies merely confirmed prior hypotheses.

Much of opiate pharmacology is based upon the availability of antagonists. Unlike other areas of neuropharmacology, no natural antagonists are available. The synthesis at the turn of the century of N-allylnorcodeine, the first opiate antagonist (Von Braun, 1916; Pohl, 1915), provided a major milestone in opiate research. The subsequent synthesis of nalorphine (N-allylnormorphine; McCawley et al., 1941) opened many avenues of opiate research and was soon followed by naloxone, the first pure antagonist (Blumberg et al., 1961). Studies of morphine/nalorphine combinations by Houde and Wallenstein (1956) and Lasagne and Beecher (1954) led Martin to propose the existence of two classes of opiate receptors: Receptor Dualism (Martin, 1967), which was followed by his proposal of three opiate receptor subtypes: mu, kappa, and sigma opiate receptors (Martin et al., 1976). Confirmation of these subtypes using binding approaches took over 5 more years. In addition to attesting to the abilities of the investigators, these studies emphasize the importance of classical pharmacological approaches.

One of the major advantages of working in the opiate system has been the availability of assays of opiate action. The development of antinociceptive assays (Woolfe and MacDonald, 1944; D'Amour and Smith, 1941; Haffner, 1929) provided rapid and accurate assessments of analgesic activity. The muscle contraction assays, such as the guinea pig ileum contraction assay (Paton, 1955, 1957; Gyang and Kosterlitz, 1966; Kosterlitz and Robinson, 1955), however, have played an exceptionally important role in opiate pharmacology. These systems require very little compound and eliminate most of the pharmacokinetic variability among compounds, enabling a more accurate assessment of receptor affinity. Even today, these bioasays play an integral role in assessing opiate and opioid peptide action.

Behavioral approaches have also proven important in understanding opiate systems. Beecher (1946), in his classic study, compared the analgesic requirements of wounded soldiers to civilian patients undergoing elective surgery and found that far fewer soldiers needed pain relief. Clearly, situational factors can alter pain perception. Twenty years later, Reynolds (1969) reported that electrical stimulation of specific brain regions can elicit a profound analgesia. The subsequent discovery that this stimulation-produced analgesia (SPA) can be reversed by the selective opiate antagonist naloxone implied that SPA worked by activating an endogenous opiate system within the brain (Akil et al., 1976).

Thus, classical approaches provided the foundation for our understanding of multiple opioid receptors and the presence within the brain of endogenous opioid systems capable of modulating pain perception. These classical studies still provide the framework upon which opiate and opioid peptide research is based today and open important avenues of research that can be best studied in conjunction with molecular approaches.

2. The Molecular Era

The initial demonstrations of opiate binding sites in 1973 (Pert and Snyder, 1973; Simon et al., 1973; Terenius, 1973) opened the field of molecular opioid pharmacology. Overcoming the technical problems faced by earlier groups in attempting to demonstrate biochemically opiate receptors enabled basic studies not possible previously. The initial surge of papers revealed the association of opiate receptors with neurons in general and synaptic regions in particular. In addition to their presence in brain regions known to be important in pain modulation, the high density of binding sites in a wide range of other areas provided the first glimmer of how important opioid systems were in general to neuropharmacology.

Many of these early studies are difficult to interpret today since they did not address the issue of multiple receptor subtypes. Several observations remain important, however. The ability of sodium ions to selectively inhibit the binding of agonists (Pert et al., 1973; Simon et al., 1975) was first demonstrated with opiate receptors and soon followed by guanine nucleotide sensitivity (Blume, 1978a,b; Childers and Snyder, 1979, 1980), both closely associated with the coupling of receptors with guanine nucleotide-binding proteins (N proteins). The subsequent differentiation of agonist from antagonist binding by divalent cations, enzymes, and reagents (Pasternak et al., 1975a,b; Pasternak and Snyder, 1975b; Wilson et al., 1975) also provided important evidence for differing agonist and antagonist receptor conformations.

Clearly, one of the most important breakthroughs in binding was the identification of distinct morphine (mu) and enkephalin (delta) receptors (Lord et al., 1977; Chang and Cuatrecasas, 1979; Chang et al., 1979). The differentiation of mu and delta sites provided the first unequivocal biochemical evidence for multiple receptor subtypes. Again, it is interesting to note that classical bioassay approaches implied the presence of these different subtypes prior to the binding studies.

The proposal of multiple mu receptors (Pasternak and Snyder, 1975a; Wolozin and Pasternak, 1981; Pasternak and Wood, 1986) is also an important advance for a number of reasons. First, this subtype (mu_1) appears to be responsible for supraspinal opioid analgesia, among other actions. Second, it is a very unique idea and may illustrate a more general concept in neuropharmacology. Despite the strong evidence supporting this proposal, more information is needed before it can be considered proven.

3. The Future

The future of opiate research is bright. Important, new discoveries are coming at an ever-increasing pace. Several important issues have now emerged that it is hoped can be addressed in coming years.

3.1. Receptor Heterogeneity

Although most investigators now accept the existence of multiple subtypes of opiate and opioid peptide receptors, the relationship of one subtype to another remains unknown. Both mu and delta receptors appear to interact with N proteins, as evident from their sensitivity to sodium ions and GTP. The degree of homology between them remains a basic question. Indeed, we do not even know if they represent different gene products or whether differentiation between mu and delta sites results from posttranslational processing.

The issue of multiple mu receptors also leaves many issues unresolved. Based upon the available information, this proposal best explains both the binding and in vivo data. The concept of receptor convergence needs special attention in future studies. Do these sites possess a distinct gene product? Are they related to the morphine-selective mu_2 and enkephalin-preferring delta receptors? Again, these are fundamental questions that need to be addressed.

Obviously, to answer these questions, the genes for these receptor subtypes must be cloned and compared. Much progress has been made in the purification of mu and delta receptors, and a number of laboratories will probably clone them in the very near future. Of course, the primary sequence of the receptor is just the start in understanding its structure.

3.2. Receptor Function

The molecular events following opiate and opioid peptide binding remain unclear. The sensitivity of binding to sodium ions and GTP suggests that mu and delta receptors are coupled to N proteins, but we know little about their second messengers. Evidence has suggested an association of delta receptors with cyclase inhibition. Although this effect is highly reproducible, recent studies comparing inactivation of binding sites with cylcase effects raise some questions regarding this correlation. Mu receptors clearly do not influence cyclase action in a wide variety of systems studies to date, and kappa receptors do not even show the binding sensitivities that suggest interactions with N proteins. Attempts by several laboratories to examine opiate modulation of phosphotitdylinositol turnover have also been unsuccessful. Thus, the second messengers associated with opioid action remain, for the most part, completely unknown. This area remains one of the most important to address.

3.3. Tolerance and Dependence

Tolerance and dependence play a major role in opiate pharmacology. These two factors greatly interfere with the clinical utility of the drugs and influence their abuse. Again, we are faced with a monumental question, a large amount of data, and much work to do. We still do not understand the basic mechanisms involved with either effect. Much information is now emerging regarding both up and down regulation of opioid receptors. It is hoped that this area will see much progress in future years.

3.4. Clinical Perspectives

A major end point of all studies of opiate and opioid peptide action is the development of new compounds with clinical utility. To date, opiates have been used primarily as analgesics and antidiarrheals. The importance of opioid mechanisms in a wide range of neuropharmacological actions, however, suggests that these agents may have a much wider use, including treating obesity and cardiovascular and septic shock. In addition to their potential expanded clinical role, the identification of multiple receptors offers the potential of more selective compounds capable of producing desired actions with fewer side effects.

References

Akil, H., Mayer, D. L., and Liebeskind, J. C. (1976) Antagonism of stimulation-produced analgesia by naloxone, a narcotic antagonist. *Science* **191**, 961–962.

Beecher, H. K. (1946) Pain in men wounded in battle. *Ann Surg.* **123,** 96–105.

Blumberg, H., Dayton, H. B., George, M., and Rapaport, D. N. (1961) N-Allylnoroxymorphone: A potent narcotic antagonist. *Fed. Proc.* **20,** 311.

Blume, A. J. (1978a) Opiate binding to membrane preparations of neuroblastoma-glioma hybrid cells NG108-15: Effects of ions and nucleotides. *Life Sci.* **22,** 1843–1852.

Blume, A. J. (1978b) Interactions of ligands with opiate receptors of brain membranes: Regulation by ions and nucleotides. *Proc. Natl. Acad. Sci. USA* **75,** 1713–1717.

Chang, K.-J. and Cuatrecasas, P. (1979) Multiple opiate receptors: Enkephalins and morphine bind to receptors of different specificity. *J. Biol. Chem.* **254,** 2610–2618.

Chang, K.-J., Cooper, B. R., Hazum, E., and Cuatrecasas, P. (1979) Multiple opiate receptors: Different regional distribution in the brain and differential binding of opiates and opioid peptides. *Mol. Pharmacol.* **16,** 91–104.

Childers, S. R. and Snyder, S. H. (1979) Guanine nucleotides differentiate agonist and antagonist interactions with opiate receptors. *Life Sci.* **32,** 759–762.

Childers, S. R. and Snyder, S. H. (1980) Differential regulation by guanine nucleotides of opiate agonist and antagonist interactions. *J. Neurochem.* **34,** 683–593.

D'Amour, F. E. and Smith, D. L. (1941) A method for determining loss of pain sensation. *J. Pharmacol. Exp. Ther.* **72,** 74–79.

Gyang, E. A. and Kosterlitz, H. W. (1966) Agonist and antagonist actions of morphine-like drugs on the guinea pig isolated ileum. *Br. J. Pharmacol. Chemother.* **27,** 514–527.

Haffner, F. (1929) Experimentille Prufung schmerzstillenden. *Mittel. Dtsch. Med. Wochenschr.* **55,** 731–733.

Houde, R. W. and Wallenstein, S. L. (1956) Clinical studies of morphine-nalorphine combinations. *Fed. Proc.* **15,** 440–441.

Kosterlitz, H. W. and Robinson, J. A. (1955) Mechanism of the contraction of the longitudinal muscle of the isolated guinea pig isolated ileum, caused by raising the pressure in the lumen. *J. Physiol.* **129,** 18p–19p.

Lasagne, L. and Beecher, H. K. (1954) The analgesic effectiveness of nalorphine and nalorphine-morphine combinations in man. *J. Pharmacol. Exp. Ther.* **112,** 356–363.

Lord, J. H., Waterfield, A. A., Hughes, J., and Kosterlitz, H. W. (1977) Endogenous opioid peptides: Multiple agonists and receptors. *Nature* **267,** 495–499.

Martin, W. R., Eades, C. G., Thompson, J. A., Huppler, R. E., and Gilbert, P. E. (1976) The effects of morphine- and nalorphine-like drugs in the nondependent and morphine dependent chronic spinal dog. *J. Pharmacol. Exp. Ther.* **197,** 517–532.

Martin, W. R. (1967) Opioid antagonists. *Pharmacol. Rev.* **19,** 463–521.

McCawley, W. L., Hart, E. R., and Marsh, D. F. (1941) The preparation of N-allylnormorphine. *J. Am. Chem. Soc.* **62,** 314.

Pasternak, G. W. and Snyder, S. H. (1975a) Opiate receptor binding: Enzymatic treatments discriminate between agonist and antagonist interactions. *Mol. Pharmacol.* **11**, 478–484.

Pasternak, G. W., Snyder, S. H. (1975b): Identification of novel high affinity opiate receptor binding in rat brain. *Nature* **253**, 563–565.

Pasternak, G. W., and Wood, P. L. (1986) Multiple mu opiate receptors. *Life Sci.* **38**, 1889–1898.

Pasternak, G. W., Snowman, A., and Snyder, S. H. (1975a) Selective enhancement of ^{3}H-opiate agonist binding by divalent cations. *Mol. Pharmacol.* **11**, 735–744.

Pasternak, G. W., Wilson, H. A., and Snyder, S. H. (1975b) Differential effects of protein-modifying reagents on receptor binding of opiate agonists and antagonists. *Mol. Pharmacol.* **11**, 340–351.

Paton, W. D. M. (1955) The response of the guinea pig ileum to electrical stimulation. *J. Physiol.* **127**, 40p–41p.

Paton, W. D. M. (1957) The action of morphine and related substances on contraction and on acetylcholine output of coaxially stimulated guinea pig ileum. *Br. J. Pharmacol.* **12**, 119–127.

Pert, C. B., and Snyder, S. H. (1973) Opiate receptor: Demonstration in nervous tissue. *Science* **179**, 1011–1014.

Pert, C. B., Pasternak, G. W., and Snyder, S. H. (1973) Opiate agonists and antagonists discriminated by receptor binding in brain. *Science* **182**, 1359–1361.

Pohl, J. (1915) Uber das N-allylnorcodein, einen antagonisten des morphins. *Z. Exp. Pathol. Ther.* **17**, 370–382.

Reynolds, D. V. (1969) Surgery in the rat during electrical analgesic induced by focal brain stimulation. *Science* **164**, 444–445.

Simon, E. J., Hiller, J. M., and Edelman, I. (1973) Stereospecific binding of the potent narcotic analgesic ^{3}H-etorphine to rat brain homogenates. *Proc. Natl. Acad. Sci. USA* **70**, 1947–1949.

Simon, E. J., Hiller, J. M., Groth, J., and Edelman, I. (1975) Further properties of stereospecific opiate binding sites in rat brain: On the nature of the sodium effect. *J. Pharmacol. Exp. Ther.* **192**, 531–537.

Terenius, L. (1973) Characteristics of the "receptor" for narcotic analgesics in synaptic plasma membrane fractions from rat brain. *Acta Pharmacol. Toxicol.* **33**, 377–384.

Von Braun, J. (1916) Untersuchengen uber morphium-alkaloid. III. *Mitteilung. Ber. Deut. Chem. Ges.* **49**, 977–989.

Wolozin, B. L. and Pasternak, G. W. (1981) Classification of multiple morphine and enkephalin binding sites in the central nervous system. *Proc. Natl. Acad. Sci. USA* **78**, 6181–6185.

Woolfe, D. and MacDonald, A. D. (1944) The evaluation of the analgesic action of pethidine hydrochloride (Demerol). *J. Pharmacol. Exp. Ther.* **80**, 300–307.

Wilson, H. A., Pasternak, G. W., and Snyder, S. H. (1975) Differentiation of opiate agonist and antagonist receptor binding by protein—modifying reagents. *Nature* **253**, 448–450.

Index

A

Acetylcholine, 279, 330
Adenylate cyclase, 246,
    250–256, 291, 442, 447
Adrenal gland, 25, 32, 35, 379
Adrenocorticotropin hormone
    (ACTH), 24, 26, 317
Affinity labeling, 173–182
α-Neoendorphin, 43
Amidorphin, 37
Analgesia, 48, 50, 54, 55, 390
    delta, 308
    kappa, 310
    mu_1 receptors and, 309
    spinal, 54
    stimulation-produced, 490
    supraspinal, 308
Antidiarrheal mechanisms,
    375
Autoradiography, 199, 201
    epsilon receptor
        distribution, 215
    kappa receptor distribution,
        120, 211
    mu_1 and mu_2 receptor
        distribution, 207, 208
    mu vs delta receptor
        distributions, 100, 206
    strain differences, 208

B

β-Chlornaltrexamine, 105, 116,
    174
β-Endorphin, analgesia, 52
    receptors, 51, 218
    synthesis, 24, 31
β-Funaltrexamine, 105, 277
Benzomorphan, 116
Bremazocine, 112

C

Calcium, 260
Calmodulin, 260
Cardiovascular system
    opioids and, 383–388
Catalepsy, 314
Cholera toxin, 235
Cyclase, see Adenylate cyclase

D

Dependence, 3, 6, 112, 441
    cross, 455
Detergents, 127, 166, 168
Dopamine, 332–337
Dorsal horn of spinal cord,
    282
Dynorphin 25, 41–43, 55, 57,
    115, 131, 220, 221

E

Enkephalin
  analgesia, 52
  analogs, 24, 53
  synthesis, 34
Enkephalinase, 46, 49

F

Feeding, 316

G

G-proteins, 232, 239, 292, 427,
  491
Gastrointestinal motility,
  361–372
Gastrointestinal secretion, 373
Growth hormone, 326
GTPase, 256–258
Guanine nucleotides, 223, 240,
  427

H

Heart, 383
Hippocampus, 284–291

I

Immunology, 405

L

Leutinizing hormone, 329
Locus coeruleus, 280

M

Metorphamide, 40
Morphine
  endogenous, 26

N

Nalorphine, 4
Naloxazone, 89, 105, 111, 120,
  277
Naloxonazine, 89, 105, 111,
  176
NMDA receptor, 154

O

Opioid receptors, 75
  biochemical characterization
    and demonstration, 76,
    78
  delta, 17, 99, 115
  development, 128, 129, 202
  epsilon, 119, 121
  kappa, 17, 120
  mu, 17, 99, 491
  mu_1, 89, 107–112, 325
  mu_2, 107
  pharmacological correlations
    of, 82
  regional distribution, 79, 80,
    119, 120, 149
  sigma, 116, 143
  solubilization and
    purification, 167,
    182–187
  upregulation and
    downregulation,
    429–433, 443–445,
    464–466
Oxytocin, 393

P

Pertusis toxin, 449
Phencyclidine, 117, 145
Phosphoinositide, 236
Phospholipase A, 86, 124
Phospholipid, 77

Phosphorylation, 259
Potassium conductance, 278, 279, 281
Prolactin, 323
Proopiomelanocorticotropin (POMC), 26–30, 218, 220

R

Receptor binding assays
  techniques and theory of, 11, 97
Respiratory depression, 12, 112, 312–314

S

Schild plots, 276
Serotonin, 337, 338
Sodium, 83, 124, 239, 243, 425
Sympathetic nervous system, 377

T

Thyroid stimulating hormone, 321
Tolerance, 6, 441, 463
  cross, 453
Transducin, 235
Trypsin, 77

U

U50488, 115

V

Vas Deferens
  mouse, 397
  rat and rabbit, 400
Vasopressin, 393

W

Wheat germ agglutinin, 124, 170